ROUTLEDGE HANDBOOK OF CRITICAL OBESITY STUDIES

The *Routledge Handbook of Critical Obesity Studies* is an authoritative and challenging guide to the breadth and depth of critical thinking and theory on obesity. Rather than focusing on obesity as a public health crisis to be solved, this reference work offers divergent and radical strategies alongside biomedical and positivist discourses.

Comprised of thirty nine original chapters from internationally recognised academics, as well as emerging scholars, the Handbook engages students, academics, researchers and practitioners in contemporary critical scholarship on obesity; encourages engagement of social science and related disciplines in critical thinking and theorising on obesity; enhances critical theoretical and methodological work in the area, highlighting potential gaps as well as strengths; relates critical scholarship to new and evolving areas of obesity-related practices, policies and research.

This multidisciplinary and international collection is designed for a broad audience of academics, researchers, students and practitioners within the social and health sciences, including sociology, obesity science, public health, medicine, sports studies, fat studies, psychology, nutrition science, education and disability studies.

Michael Gard is Associate Professor of Sport, Health and Physical Education in the School of Human Movement and Nutrition Sciences at the University of Queensland, Australia.

Darren Powell is a Senior Lecturer in the Faculty of Education and Social Work, University of Auckland, New Zealand.

José Tenorio is an Associate Lecturer at the School of Human Movement and Nutrition Sciences, University of Queensland, Australia.

ROUTLEDGE HANDBOOK OF CRITICAL OBESITY STUDIES

Edited by
Michael Gard, Darren Powell
and José Tenorio

Routledge
Taylor & Francis Group
LONDON AND NEW YORK

First published 2022
by Routledge
2 Park Square, Milton Park, Abingdon, Oxon OX14 4RN

and by Routledge
605 Third Avenue, New York, NY 10158

Routledge is an imprint of the Taylor & Francis Group, an informa business

British Library Cataloguing-in-Publication Data
A catalogue record for this book is available from the British Library

Library of Congress Cataloging-in-Publication Data
Names: Gard, Michael, 1965– editor. | Powell, Darren (Educator) editor. | Tenorio, José, editor.
Title: Routledge handbook of critical obesity studies / edited by Michael Gard, Darren Powell, and José Tenorio.
Description: Milton Park, Abingdon, Oxon; New York, NY: Routledge, 2022. | Includes bibliographical references and index.
Identifiers: LCCN 2021032280 (print) | LCCN 2021032281 (ebook) | ISBN

ISBN: 978-0-367-36244-7 (hbk)
ISBN: 978-1-032-16219-5 (pbk)
ISBN: 978-0-429-34482-4 (ebk)

DOI: 10.4324/9780429344824

Typeset in Bembo
by codeMantra

The Open Access version of chapter 3 was funded by Spritzer Family Trust.
The Open Access version of chapter 19 was funded by University of Auckland.

From Michael Gard
To Beverley and Ralph Gard, thank you for giving me everything, including Yamba!
To Eimear Enright and Fiadh Gard, thank you for giving me a home,
and apologies for my snoring.

From Darren Powell
For Harvey, Matilda and Maddy.

From José Tenorio
Para las incansables guerreras que han entregado sus vidas para
hacer brillar la de otros.

CONTENTS

Contents

FIGURES

TABLES

CONTRIBUTORS

Eva Barlösius is Professor of Sociology with a focus on food studies, social inequality and science studies at the Leibniz Universität Hannover. She founded the Leibniz Center for Science and Society (LCSS) and is the speaker of the Forum Wissenschaftsreflexion. For several years, she has been working on obesity, the sociology of food and the sociological conception of infrastructures and public services.

Denise Bernuzzi de Sant'Anna is Full Professor of History at the Pontifícia Universidade Católica de São Paulo (PUC-SP) and Researcher at the National Council for Scientific and Technological Development of Brazil (CNPq).

Lisette Burrows is a Professor in Community Health at Te Huataki Waiora, University of Waikato. Her research explores the place and meaning of physical culture and health in young people's lives. She is currently working on a project that explores the intersection of school-based health messages with family life.

Patricia Cain's research is informed by both qualitative and quantitative methodology, with a focus on critical health psychology, specifically weight stigma and stigma intervention research. Patricia's research has developed and validated the Fat Attitudes Assessment Toolkit.

Graeme Ditchburn is a Chartered Organisational Psychologist and Supervisor, registered and endorsed in Australia and the United Kingdom. My research interests focus on performance and well-being at work and the design of valid and reliable measures for employees and organisations.

Ngaire Donaghue's research investigates questions concerning gender, body image and obesity from the perspective of critical-feminist psychology. I work with a large and active group of research students, and our work explores how social understandings of concepts such as gender and body image shape and constrain the kinds of identities that are developed by men and women of different shapes and sizes.

Dorothea Dumuid is a Research Fellow at the University of South Australia, who has pioneered the use of compositional data analysis in time-use studies. She develops novel analytical models that explore how to get the balance right, not only for one aspect of health such as obesity but also for overall health and well-being.

Jenny Ellison is the Curator of Sport and Leisure at the Canadian Museum of History. As curator, Dr. Ellison's work has included exhibitions, events, scholarly and popular articles on women's sport, hockey, Rick Hansen and public history.

Katherine M. Flegal had a long career as a senior scientist in the United States at the National Center for Health Statistics of the Centers for Disease Control and Prevention, largely working with the National Health and Nutrition Examination Survey program. She currently has an unpaid appointment in the Prevention Research Center at Stanford University. She has published over 180 peer-reviewed articles and book chapters.

Isabel Fletcher is a Senior Research Fellow in Science, Technology and Innovation Studies at the University of Edinburgh. Isabel is a qualitative social scientist whose research is based in science and technology studies, and also incorporates approaches from sociology and food policy. She has research interests in policy approaches to food, nutrition and eating and the ways in which interdisciplinary research is used to address complex social problems.

Simone Fullagar is Chair of the Sport and Gender Equity research hub at Griffith University. As an interdisciplinary sociologist, Simone works with feminist new materialist theories and (post)qualitative methods to pursue change across sport, health and physical cultures. She is a co-editor of the new Routledge book series *Postqualitative, New Materialist and Critical Posthumanist Research*.

Michael Gard is an Associate Professor of Sport, Health and Physical Education in the School of Human Movement and Nutrition Sciences at the University of Queensland. He teaches, researches and writes about how the human body is and has been used, experienced, educated and governed.

Mabel Gracia-Arnaiz is a Professor in the Department of Anthropology, Philosophy and Social Work at the Universitat Rovira i Virgil in Tarragona, Spain. Her research line is at the intersection of food anthropology and medical anthropology. Her works focus on the analysis of food security and the medicalization of food and body practices.

Susan Greenhalgh is John King and Wilma Cannon Fairbank Research Professor of Chinese Society in the Anthropology Department at Harvard University. Her work focuses on the corporate management of the global obesity epidemic through the US production and global circulation of a distorted corporate science of obesity and its solution.

Julie Guthman is a Professor of social sciences at the University of California, Santa Cruz. Her research has broadly been about how neoliberal-inflected capitalism shapes the conditions of possibility for food system transformation. She has also studied the influence of California's agrarian past on contemporary efforts to reduce pesticide use.

Travis Hay is a historian of Canadian settler colonialism who was born and raised in Thunder Bay, Ontario. He is currently a Postdoctoral Fellow in the Indigenous Learning Department at Lakehead University and is working collaboratively with First Nations and Inuit communities to write histories of service gaps in the Canadian north.

Fetaui Iosefo is the youngest daughter of Fuimaono Luse Vui Siope and Sua Muamai Vui Siope. Her parents migrated from Samoa to Aotearoa in the late 1950s. Fetaui has taught in South Auckland for over 20 years and is a PhD Candidate and a Teaching Fellow in the University of Auckland.

Anna Kirkland is Arthur F. Thurnau Professor of Women's and Gender Studies at the University of Michigan, USA.

Nicole Land is an Assistant Professor in the School of Early Childhood Studies at Ryerson University. Thinking with early childhood educators and children, and within a commitment to craft and nourish post-developmental pedagogies, Nicole's work is curious about the inherited and inventive relations we might create with fats, muscles and movement.

Cyrille Laporte is Associate Professor at the University of Toulouse Jean Jaurès (France). He conducts research on sociology of food, focusing on the changes of food systems organisation and their impact on eating patterns and practices.

Deana Leahy is an Associate Professor of Health Education in the Faculty of Education at Monash University, Melbourne, Australia. Her interdisciplinary research interrogates the politics and practices of health education with a focus on food pedagogies.

Jessica Lee is a Senior Lecturer in the School of Medicine at Griffith University. Her research is informed by critical approaches to health knowledge and practice. She has specific interests in the uptake of knowledge from a critical perspective in health policy.

Jo Lindsay is Professor of Sociology in the School of Social Sciences at Monash University. Jo specialises in research on families, consumption and environmental sociology. She is currently researching household innovation and the transition to the low waste city and food and healthy eating in families and communities.

JaneMaree Maher is Professor in the Centre for Women's Studies and Gender Research, Sociology and Associate Dean Academic Development, Faculty of Arts, Monash University. Her research addresses women's paid and unpaid work, family structures and gendered violences.

Niamh Ni Shuilleabhain is currently working as a lecturer in culture, media and sport at the University of Bath. Her research has focused on exploring critical and creative approaches to addressing youth health. Her PhD research was a collaboration with a UK national charity for eating disorders, and aimed to develop alternative approaches to health education that are more responsive to body dissatisfaction.

Moss E. Norman is an Assistant Professor in the School of Kinesiology at the University of British Columbia. He uses a socio-cultural approach to the study of the intersection between physical culture, youth and gender. Recently, his research has focused on the relationship between Indigenous masculinity and physical culture, with a focus on the place-specific context of Fisher River Cree Nation (Manitoba).

Tim Olds is an Australian Professor of behavioural epidemiology, with a particular interest in how people use their time and how that affects their health. He led the 2007 National Children's Nutrition and Physical Activity Survey and was Australian lead of the 12-nation ISCOLE study and the 49-nation Active Healthy Kids network. His recent work focuses on the concept of the 24-hour day and trade-offs that people make in time use.

Tania Orellana is an art historian, geographer and flower therapist. Her research explores the configuration of corporeality in medical discourses and its socialization and representation in different historical moments and social contexts. She teaches courses at the intersections of art, science, technology, health and beauty stereotypes at the University of Chile.

Bonnie Pang is curious about human subjectivities as they relate to the psycho-socio-material-discursive conditions in health and physical cultures, including their leisure, sport, physical education and health. She ponders over Chineseness, reflexivity, identity and race, embodiment and affect, and diversity and inclusion.

George Parker is Lecturer in Health Service Delivery – Pūkenga Ratoa Hauora in the School of Health at Victoria University of Wellington, Aotearoa New Zealand. A registered midwife, George researches at the intersection of sexual and reproductive health, fatness, health equity and social justice.

Cat Pausé is a Fat Studies scholar at Massey University in New Zealand. Her research is focused on the effects of fat stigma on health and well-being of fat individuals and how fat activists resist the fatpocalypse. She has called for a new fat ethics, acknowledging the role science has played in the oppression of fat people and ensuring that research around fatness centres fat epistemology.

LeAnne Petherick is an Assistant Professor in the Department of Curriculum and Pedagogy in the Faculty of Education at the University of British Columbia. LeAnne's research program draws on a feminist post-structural lens to examine curriculum policy and pedagogy, planned and lived, in health and physical education.

Jennifer Poudrier is a Metis sociologist and community-based researcher in the Department of Sociology at the University of Saskatchewan. Her innovative research has deployed 'photovoice' as a way of examining Indigenous conceptions of body image and health body weight in First Nations communities.

Jean Pierre Poulain is Professor in sociology and anthropology at the University of Toulouse Jean Jaurès (France). He conducts research on sociology of food, focusing on the changes of eating patterns, their links with health and food crises in the frame of CERTOP (Research Center on Work, Organizations and Policies), a unit of CNRS (French National Center for Scientific Research) and University of Toulouse.

Darren Powell, formerly a primary school teacher, is a Senior Lecturer of Health Education in the Faculty of Education and Social Work, University of Auckland. Darren's research focuses on the intersections of public education and public health, with a particular interest in how corporations and charities are re-inventing themselves as part of the solution to the 'childhood obesity epidemic'.

Richard Pringle is Professor of Sport Sociology and Health and Physical Education at Monash University, Melbourne, where he is currently the Associate Dean of Graduate Research. He is a critical qualitative researcher who examines diverse socio-cultural and pedagogical issues associated with sport, exercise, health, sexualities, bodies and genders.

Valeria Radrigán is a cultural studies researcher. Her works address the relationships of the body with technology, science, society and contemporary art. Currently, she is conducting research in digital sexuality and transhumanism, financed by the National Fund for Scientific and Technological Development of Chile (ANID-FONDECYT Chile).

Emma Rich is Chair of the Physical Culture, Sport and Health research group at the University of Bath. Working across sociology and critical pedagogies, her works advance theoretical frameworks to understand how people learn about health and their bodies and the impact on their identities, health practices and physical activity.

Abigail C. Saguy is UCLA Professor of Sociology, with a courtesy appointment in the Department of Gender Studies. Saguy is currently studying – with Juliet A. Williams and with support from the National Science Foundation – how lawyers, activists and journalists invoke the principle of gender neutrality to advance (or oppose) gender equality.

Hillel Schwartz is a cultural historian, poet and translator. His current research on the changing concepts and experience of "emergency" since the 18th century led to a 2014 Berlin Prize in Cultural History at the American Academy in Berlin.

Gyorgy Scrinis is Associate Professor of Food Politics and Policy in the School of Agriculture and Food, Faculty of Veterinary and Agricultural Sciences at the University of Melbourne. His research has examined the politics, policy and philosophy of food and nutrition, with a focus on nutrition science, dietary advice, functional foods, food labelling, animal welfare regulations, the role of transnational corporations, alternative proteins and new technologies of production.

Aimee B. Simpson has a sociology PhD from the University of Auckland. She is interested in sociology of medicine, the body and issues relating to health. Currently, she is working on an analysis of obesity discourses and their effects on understandings of fatness, health and identity using a fat studies lens.

Peter N. Stearns is University Professor of History at George Mason University. His book, *Fat History: Bodies and Beauty in the Modern West*, was published (2nd ed.) in 2002. More recent work deals with fat shaming and the tensions between dignity claims and health standards.

Sian Supski is a freelance researcher and project manager specialising in cultural sociology. She is an Adjunct Research Fellow in Sociology, College of Arts, Social Sciences and Commerce, La Trobe University, Melbourne, Australia.

Claire Tanner is a Senior Lecturer in Sociology and Gender Studies in the Faculty of Arts at Monash University, Melbourne, Australia. Her work sits at the intersection of the sociology of gender, health and science and tackles socio-ethical questions around science innovation, gender inequity, obesity and exploitative commercial health industries.

José Tenorio is an Associate Lecturer in the School of Human Movement and Nutrition Sciences at the University of Queensland. His research and teaching interests sit at the intersection of food studies, education and public health.

Karen Throsby is an Associate Professor in Gender Studies in the School of Sociology and Social Policy at the University of Leeds (UK), where she is also Director of the Centre for Interdisciplinary Gender Studies (CIGS). Her research focuses on the intersections of gender, technology, bodies and health.

Signild Vallgårda is a historian and Professor of Health Policy Analysis at the Department of Public Health, University of Copenhagen. Her recent research focuses on obesity policies and policies on reducing social inequalities in health.

Melissa Wake is an Australasian paediatrician whose "population pediatrics" research spans common childhood conditions and antecedents of diseases of ageing. Her work triangulates multiple methodologies (trials, registries, health services research and screening, cohorts and open science longitudinal data resources).

Megan Warin is a Professor and social anthropologist at the University of Adelaide. Her research focuses on the gendered dynamics of disordered eating, structural disadvantage and obesity, public health interventions, and the politics of gender and race in the fields of developmental origins of health and disease and epigenetics in the context of nutritional (and other) exposures.

T. M. Wilkinson is Professor of Politics and International Relations at the University of Auckland. He is a political theorist who has worked on applied ethics for years.

Benjamin Williams is a Lecturer in the School of Education and Professional Studies at Griffith University. His research addresses the topics of evidence, experts and expertise as they concern policy and practice in health and physical education. This research is informed by sociological approaches to health, bodies, physical activity, science and technology.

Jan Wright is an Emeritus Professor in the Faculty of Arts Social Sciences and Humanities at the University of Wollongong, Australia. Her research draws on feminist and post-structuralist theory to critically engage issues associated with the relationship between embodiment, culture and health.

PART A

Introduction

1

THE WORLDS OF CRITICAL OBESITY STUDIES

Darren Powell, José Tenorio and Michael Gard

In 2018, when we first started to develop the idea for this edited volume, we were cognisant that the term 'critical obesity studies' was problematic. This was mostly due to the fact that we did not really know – or certainly could not easily define – what 'critical obesity studies' means or not. As we wrote in our proposal to the publisher, we did not necessarily see even our own work as 'critical obesity studies', but understood that our work – and others – contributed to this 'field', for want of a better word. Alongside the interesting problem with the word 'critical', we wanted to provide a breadth and depth of critical thinking and critical theory on 'obesity', a book that did not adhere to one critical orientation (e.g., poststructuralism) or that focused on a single issue or topic (e.g., education, fat studies or public health). Ultimately, we wanted to present a range of critical issues, theories and perspectives, and we wrote in our proposal to the publishers:

> The volume is about ideas that are 'critical' of diverse obesity issues, discourses, policies, practices, and research. However, unlike other books on obesity, we are not pushing for one particular agenda, ideology, theory or method; not conservative, liberal, progressive, queer, feminist, posthumanist or any other perspectives. We argue that there are diverse ideas about what makes obesity research 'critical'.

Based on these ideas, we invited many international scholars to contribute to this volume, people we believed would offer diverse perspectives, including those who would challenge, even contradict, what is currently understood as being 'critical' obesity research, as well as authors whose work we did not always agree with. Then we waited.

A month or two passed with a steady stream of positive and negative responses, before we received a couple of interesting messages. The messages were from colleagues who had noticed online conversations between fat studies scholars and fat activists, some of whom were perturbed, even angered, by our proposed book. There were comments such as 'nobody had heard of us', that we are not fat, that we are men and that we are 'not critical'. As one commentator said: 'If you're using the word "obesity", then you're not critical at all'. Since then, we have wrestled with the term 'critical obesity studies' over time, and we now offer the following reflections about what this 'field' actually means to us and, potentially, to the authors and readers of this text.

DOI: 10.4324/9780429344824-2

What do we mean by the words 'critical' and 'obesity'?

In a paradoxical way, some of the scholars, who were attracted by the opportunities that a space of scholarship and debate like critical obesity studies offered, had concerns about being excluded from other academic venues if they decided to list their names next to scholars who use inverted commas around 'obesity'. Therefore, we were many times urged to clarify, what does critical mean. At a basic level, to be critical is to assess claims of knowledge in terms of their validity, or at a broader level, to critique policies, practices, institutions, inequalities and injustices, including taken-for-granted assumptions and specific socio-cultural contexts (Hammersely, 2000).

As editors with diverse backgrounds, politics and perspectives on life, we do not share a completely aligned standpoint on what critical, in a broad sense, actually means. In theoretical terms, some of us are predominantly influenced by the stream of critical thinking shaped by postmodernism. Contradictorily, the Frankfurt School, decolonial theories and poststructuralism were fundamental in the development of a critical perspective for others. Combined with our own life experiences, however, our ways of understanding and engaging with critical scholarship have been in constant change. Today, we cannot subscribe, neither individually nor collectively, to a particular critical tradition. Without trying to propose a bounded definition, we would say that, for us, critical means the art of systematically questioning everything, the duty of being receptive to ideas that trouble our own thinking and the will to embrace change.

In this way, 'critical obesity studies' does not merely provide a critique or criticism of the validity of scientific knowledge or act in opposition to it, but seeks to understand how social, cultural and political contexts (among others) work to produce (or at least attempt to produce) particular ways of thinking, knowing, acting and being. It can also be critical in the sense of seeking to understand how relations of power work, which may include criticism of oppression and exploitation, and the struggle of social and political changes. To this end, the critical can be radical and transformative.

As we reflect on some of our own research, we understand the 'critical' to involve a number of interconnected elements. For instance, a key aspect of critical obesity studies is to make dominant obesity discourses visible; challenge 'regimes of truth' (Foucault, 2003); examine the effects of discourses (and discursive practices); provide challenges to these discourses by pointing out tensions and contradictions; disentangle the complex assemblage of ideologies, moralities, technologies, organisations, subjectivities and practices; reveal unequal and unjust power relations; and imagine the potential for resistance, counter-politics and change.

The use of the word obesity without quotation marks or scare quotes (i.e. 'obesity') is also important for some, but not all, critical obesity studies researchers. We understand the ways in which the term obesity can be highly problematic, and has been used and abused to concomitantly normalise and value thin bodies, and demonise and oppress fat people (e.g., Cameron & Russell, 2016; Cooper, 2010; Rothblum & Solovay, 2009). We also recognise the power of the 'f-word' (Wann, 1998) as a means to reclaim fatness, to resist the stigmatisation and pathologisation of fat people. We do not contest the importance of the power of language. What we do challenge, however, is the assumption that anyone who uses the term obesity cannot be critical. And although we are well aware that using obesity may maintain dominant obesity discourses and the effects of such discourses, we argue that obesity is still a useful rhetorical device for the critical project – for critical obesity studies. For us, anyway, we cannot provide an effective challenge to wealthy institutions, dominant discourses, 'dangerous' practices or unequal power relations without using the word that makes all of this possible: obesity.

Furthermore, using the 'O-word' can be an effective strategy to provide a form of counter-politics (Youdell, 2011) to dominant biomedical discourses and potentially harmful practices. For instance, in our own research, we show how corporations and other organisations exploit notions of 'childhood obesity' and a 'childhood obesity epidemic' to teach children about healthy lifestyles, shape public policy and ultimately profit (see Gard, 2011; Powell, 2020; Tenorio, 2021). These organisations employ 'obesity' as a particularly useful rhetoric device, trading off public and political fears about 'obesity' (such as children living shorter lives than their parents, the threat to economies and national security) to meet their own interests and needs. Therefore, there is a dire need to interrogate and illuminate how *obesity* is used (as well as misused and abused) in ways that benefit certain players (e.g., multinational food and drink corporations, academics and government agencies), often at the expense of marginalised groups in society. In other words, there is a need to be *critical*. In our view, to be critical about obesity is not just an attempt to critique, but to develop a greater understanding of socio-cultural and political contexts, to demonstrate how power 'works' and to ultimately address issues of social injustice and inequity.

What does we mean by the word 'studies'?

The inclusion of the word *studies* in the title of this volume is somewhat ambitious. It has been enriched by the contributions of scholars who, through various analytical lenses and from diverse geographical and cultural locations, have challenged taken-for-granted ideas about obesity. But this volume falls short in capturing the diversity of research which, broadly speaking, has critically interrogated the construction of body weight as a public health 'problem'. In the context of this volume, therefore, the word *studies* does not have to be understood as an already bounded field of inquiry. Rather, it can be seen as a collection of ideas seeking to grow into space of scholarship, inviting the reader to think about obesity and the study of obesity differently.

This task is not an entirely novel one. From the late 2000s, a series of edited collections have made visible the work of scholars from different disciplines who are challenging mainstream obesity ideas (not limited by, but some examples to consult are Ellison, McPhail & Mitchinson, 2016; McCullough & Hardin, 2013; Rothblum & Solovay, 2009; Wright & Harwood, 2009). These edited books benefit from multiple authors taking different, usually in some form or other 'critical', approaches to issues such as health and medicine, social inequality, education, social construction of fatness, feminism, weight stigma and fat activism. However, the contributors to the aforementioned collections largely hail from and do research at universities in often English-speaking countries, which provides only a partial outlook of the critical obesity research that has taken place in diverse contexts.

Our volume includes what we believe is a wider breadth and depth of international scholarship that employs critical, multi-disciplinary approaches to researching obesity. In an attempt to partially fill this geographical gap affecting the production of knowledge, our volume includes contributions from Brazilian, Danish, German, Samoan, French, Chilean, Spanish and Mexican authors who have critically researched obesity from their own contexts. This, we believe, has the potential of enhancing the global critical conversations about obesity.

Naturally, this geographical diversity implied challenges for us as editors. The hegemony of the English language in academia sometimes works as a barrier to ideas that are generated in other languages. While for most of our contributors speaking and writing English is common practice, for some others this is a task that requires time, effort and money. Most of our non-English speaking contributors incurred in translating or proofreading expenses to bring their chapter to best possible quality. They also patiently addressed the many editorial comments and requests. We were attracted by the diverse uses of language to refer to obesity and the meanings they convey. We especially thank the non-English authors who contributed to this volume.

We invited contributors from non-English speaking countries to use key words within their chapters in their own language and, if applicable, to discuss how the meaning of these words contrasted with the English word 'obesity'. In Chapter 27, for example, Fetaui Iosefo exposes how the obesity discourse works among Samoans as a 'derogatory reminder' that they are 'being exposed as a people who have failed in their health'. Unlike the violence that obesity exerts in classifying Samoan bodies as 'ill' within Western standards for health, Samoan words '*puta*' (fat) and '*lapoa*' (large) are used in 'context of endearment or with humour', not with the aim of stigmatising. In Chapter 22, Eva Barlösious discusses how they used a flyer entitled '*Dicke Freunde*' ('Fat Friends' or 'Best Friends') to recruit participants. The German word for '*dicke*' can mean both 'close' or 'best', when used for people who enjoy being together and 'fat' for bodily descriptions. Barlösius designed this world play for the flyer to 'ensure that mainly fat young people would feel addressed by, and that the flyer would convey, a positive meaning of fat, namely "best friends"'. From a historical perspective, Denisse Bernuzzi de Sant'Anna shows in Chapter 5 that in Brazil the pathologisation of body weight by using the word obesity became possible only after the emergence of scientific paradigms, political changes and economic reforms in the 1970s. In the predominantly rural and hungry Brazil of the 1920s, in exchange, large bodies were appreciated as 'spectacular "phenomena"' because they looked like an '*armazém*' [warehouse] with the 'capacity to store food for times of shortage'. The words *dicke*, *puta* and *lapoa*, and the socially constructed idea that '*corpos armazém*' [warehouse bodies] were to be celebrated, show us how bodies are appreciated differently across cultures and periods of time, and that body weight does not need to be exclusively spoken about in negative terms. This is also a reminder that language is always evolving and that obesity as a discourse that pathologises body weight is a relatively recent construction.

The inclusion of non-English authors and their words in this handbook is, in itself, a reminder of the power, ambivalence and uses of language, which might help to challenge words that, like obesity, convey a reductionist meaning and stigmatise people. Our effort to include critical perspectives on obesity beyond the usual geographical places of discussion, however, is limited. Although we worked hard, we were not successful in recruiting to this volume scholars researching obesity critically in, for example, South-East Asia, Middle-East, Africa and Eastern Europe. Language also was a natural barrier. Our knowledge beyond English, Spanish, Portuguese and French languages is limited or completely lacking. Thus, although our handbook is expanding the reach of the obesity debate to other areas, more work is to be done to gain insights into how other cultures conceive and debate the idea that large bodies can be a sign of bad health.

Conscious of these limitations, then, the word *studies* in our title needs to be understood as a diversity of ideas, plurality of approaches and competing perspectives that, in different geographical spaces, challenge what is sometimes taken as univocal truths about obesity. The list of contributors to this volume is another expression of its diversity. In disciplinary terms, this collection brings together anthropologists, historians, sociologists, epidemiologists, as well as scholars working in the fields of education, science and technology studies and others whom refuse to be 'labelled'. The theories and methodologies that these authors employ to question, in one or another way, obesity are as diverse as their backgrounds and research interests are.

Under the idea of critical obesity *studies*, we are bringing together diverse forms of scholarships that would be hard to be found together in other already bounded disciplines. Contributors to this volume develop their arguments drawing from poststructuralism, social constructivism, neo-Marxism, posthumanism or from none of these. For us, it is not about theory *per se*, but about how the dialogue between works underpinned by different theories can expand the critical understanding of obesity and its proposed solutions.

However, we anticipated that our decision to use the word *obesity*, rather than 'weight' or 'fat', has the potential to trouble scholars doing critical work, including authors in this collection (see above our discussion of the word 'obesity' in this chapter). More than once, we were asked to clarify why we had, as one contributor put it, 'embraced' obesity in naming our chosen area of scholarship. The word obesity, understood as biomedical concept that is used to categorise people's health based on their body weight, can be offensive for some people. The word fat therefore has been the preference of some scholars who critically interrogate, among other issues, the affects that the obesity language has on people's, particularly women and poor people, lives.

However, using this language is our strategy to invite diverse voices to speak about obesity and to reach audiences that would be inaccessible otherwise. Naming this space of scholarship and debate critical obesity *studies* afforded us a broader integration of perspectives to challenge the making and workings of the obesity word. We also wanted to read others work, but without adopting one single interpretation of, or position towards, obesity and without pursuing a unified set of beliefs or politics. While, as we discussed above, languages are crucial for us, we are not prioritising a particular one. Contributors to this volume freely use obesity, fat or 'obesity', in inverted commas. For us, it is not so important which language is used, but rather how it is used to challenge taken-for-granted ideas.

The reasons why we deliberately decided to use obesity might not satisfy many readers (see Gard's second chapter in this volume, Chapter 12), but let us be clear: we are aiming to form neither a movement nor a jealously guarded field of knowledge; we simply want to share the possibilities that this space of scholarship and debate offers to people who want to think differently about obesity. In short, for the three of us, *obesity* works as an umbrella under which many different perspectives, methods, theories and politics can be brought together to interrogate the construction of body weight as a marker of illness, immorality and its multiple effects on people's lives. This, we believe, has enriched this theoretically, methodologically, politically and geographically diverse collection of *critical obesity studies* to expand the obesity debate.

A summary of this volume

The editing of this volume was performed by people who have biases, including their genders, socio-economic classes, races, busy schedules and lives to lead. Perhaps, the connection between the editors is the 'hunger' for knowledge, although, having said this, the editors of this volume do not claim any special quality. The 'hunger' is everywhere. But, to begin with, our previous work in school physical and health education disciplines and our desire for critical thinking about obesity partly explain the emergence of this volume. Having decided to take on this major task, which would partly take at least three years out our lives, we wanted to include, for example, older and newer authors who have interesting perspectives on obesity. We also wanted to sketch out where the 'field', as it were, has been and where it is going. Our idea was also to include contributions from feminism, fat people, science, public health, sport, education and many others.

We also want to emphasise that name of this volume is not, by extension, 'fat studies'. Of course, there are many authors from fat studies whom, although would not agree with us on many issues, we still have a positive and academic relationships with them (see further discussion by Gard, Chapter 12). For example, we have included chapters written by Cat Pausé (Chapter 8), Aimee Simpson (Chapter 20), George Parker (Chapter 23) and Abigail Saguy (Chapter 28). These researchers, as others, have produced standard reading material for anyone who wants to think critically about fat or obesity. But, although we do not see the academic knowledge as 'field' to be 'claimed' and 'argued over', we think that critical obesity studies are, in some ways, larger than fat studies. In this particular situation, the emphasis, at least for us, is on the word 'critical'. For example, some of the authors draw from cultures which they think about obesity differently, including José Tenorio (Chapter 15), Bonnie Pang (Chapter 16), Eva Barlösius (Chapter 22) and Fetaui Iosefo (Chapter 27). Some authors look at the evidence and come up with different, and even radical, conclusions, including Isabel Fletcher (Chapter 6), Michael Gard (Chapter 7), Karen Throsby (Chapter 13), Darren Powell (Chapter 19) and Patricia Cain, Ngaire Donaghue, and Graeme Ditchburn (Chapter 38). It might come from their cultural situations, including Nicole Land (Chapter 11) and Jean-Pierre Poulain and Cyrille Laporte (Chapter 18), or it comes from the more individual perspectives, including Hillel Schwartz (Chapter 2), Michael Gard (Chapter 12) and Anne Kirkland (Chapter 37). Some authors have different perspectives on, for example, weight 'management' practices, but it comes from critical perspective, including Susan Greenhalgh (Chapter 14) and Jenny Ellison (Chapter 26). We might agree or disagree with them, but we want to know their outlook on, say, weight, fatness, fitness, health and mental health. We might be wrong about all this, so we are never becoming comfortable with our views. We want to read fat studies scholarship, but we also want to read historical (Peter Stearns, Chapter 4), theoretical (Richard Pringle, Chapter 9; Simone Fullagar, Emma Rich, and Niamh Ni Shuilleabhaina, Chapter 10), ethics (Martin Wilkinson, Chapter 36), social science (Julie Guthman, Chapter 14; Lisette Burrows, Chapter 24), cultural (Denise Bernuzzi de Sant'Anna, Chapter 5) or science voices (Katherine Flegal, Chapter 3; Tim Olds, Dorothea Dumuid, and Melissa Wake, Chapter 25; Gyorgy Scrinis, Chapter 39).

We have also included some printed and electronic media studies, for example, Valeria Radrigán and Tania Orellana (Chapter 29), Travis Hay and Jennifer Poudrier (Chapter 30) and Jessica Lee and Benjamin Williams (Chapter 31). And, of course, slightly closer to our home discipline, we have educators who have taken this area of obesity scholarship seriously for many years (Deana Leahy, Jan Wright, Jo Lindsay, Claire Tanner, JaneMaree Maher and Sian Supski, Chapter 17; LeAnne Petherick and Moss Norman, Chapter 35).

With respect to the section titles of this volume, we found it extremely difficult to categorise each chapter. There will be commentary introductory notes for each sections and for each individual chapter. We also worked tirelessly to produce section titles that might make some sense to a reader. For example, we stayed fairly 'conservative' with titles such as 'History' (Section B), 'Theory' (Section C) and 'Future directions' (Section H). In some cases, we asked authors to address particular historical issues (e.g., Peter Stearns, Chapter 4), areas of theory (e.g., Pringle, Chapter 9; Fullager *et al.*, Chapter 10). But there were other issues in play, including the reviews of our original proposal to the publishers and more 'creative' reading by us for some chapters (e.g., SantaAnna, Chapter 5; Cain, *et al.*, Chapter 38; Scrinis, Chapter 39).

We then had to make further decisions and, after much 'negotiation', we arrived at four section titles: Food (Section D), Bodies (Section E), Media (Section F) and Policies (Section

G). Again, some chapters were basically straightforward. For example, we chose Tenorio (Chapter 15) and Pang (Chapter 16) to be the basis of the 'Food' section. We also used Saguy's chapter (Chapter 28) to build a section called 'Media' section.

But, having said all this, most, or even all, chapters are really about 'bodies', talk either formally or informally. So, we had no trouble finding eight chapters to create 'Bodies' as a section. But the problem became more serious, especially for some authors and potentially all readers, why not stop at eight chapters for Bodies? With apologies in advance to each authors who might be slightly or extremely worried about our section title (!), we would humbly register that we just had to make these decisions and those decisions, either by ourselves or by the reader, can be argued forcibly for good reasons. In other words, each chapter can be read in multiple ways; each chapter can be interpreted in terms of its historical, theoretical, physical, ethical, artistic, political and cultural (or other fields of activity) importance which one could choose. Each chapter, then, embodies a world on its own.

To sum up our arguments for this chapter, 'critical obesity studies' should be an area of debate where, within limits, rules do not apply. Whatever reasons that people might have against these terms, authors should be free to use *their* language and technical terms without being accused of being 'not critical'. We understand the complexity of this area of knowledge, and in language, there are contexts, politics, history and bodies. Whatever our starting position begins from, one's position does not rule out any perspectives. We want to think with our own mind rather than use somebody else's mind or language. We want to use our mind, and therefore, our minds will take us where it wants to go. There are many disadvantages here, but, at least for the editors of this volume, ideas are very important, perhaps because or in spite of one's position. There are many voices and arguments about 'fat' and 'overweight' and 'obesity'. We, as readers or authors or as a person, want to think carefully and want to hear them but with our own ears.

References

Cameron, E. & Russell, C. (Eds.) (2016). *The fat pedagogy reader: Challenging weight-based oppression through critical education*. New York: Peter Lang.

Cooper, C. (2010). Fat studies: Mapping the field. *Sociology Compass*, 4(12), 1020–1034. doi:10.1111/j.1751-9020.2010.00336.x

Ellison, J., McPhail, D. & Mitchinson, W. (Eds.) (2016). *Obesity in Canada: Critical perspectives*. Toronto, ON: University of Toronto Press:

Foucault, M. (2003). Truth and power. In P. Rabinow & N. Rose (Eds.), *The essential Foucault: Selections from essential works of Foucault 1954–1984* (pp. 300–318). London: The New Press.

Gard, M. (2011). *The end of the obesity epidemic*. Oxon: Routledge.

Hammersley, M. (2000). *Critical or uncritical, is that the Question? On researchers as public intellectuals engaged in social criticism*. Paper presented at the British Educational Research Association Annual Conference, Cardiff University.

McCullough, M.B. & Hardin, J.A. (Eds.) (2013). *Reconstructing obesity: The meaning of measures and the measure of meanings* (Vol. 2). New York: Berghahn Books.

Powell, D. (2020). *Schools, corporations, and the war on childhood obesity: How corporate philanthropy shapes public health and education*. London: Routledge.

Rothblum, E. D. & Solovay, S. (Eds.) (2009). *The fat studies reader*. New York: New York University Press.

Tenorio, J. (2021). Cooking 'healthy lifestyles' as a *dispositif*: Obesity policies, school food politics and corporations in neoliberal Mexico. PhD Thesis. University of Queensland.

Wann, M. (1998). *Fat!So? Because you don't have to apologize for your size!* Berkeley, CA: Ten Speed Press.

Wright, J. & Harwood, V. (Eds.) (2009). *Biopolitics and the 'obesity epidemic': Governing bodies*. London: Routledge.

Youdell, D. (2011). *School trouble: Identity, power and politics in Education*. New York: Routledge.

PART B

History

We have opened this volume with a section called 'history.' Obviously, this can be seen as a quite conservative choice to begin this volume, and there were many forceful editorial arguments for and against this inclusion. Having read them carefully, we could see different emergent approaches to reading and, therefore, grouping these chapters. One possible direction for was to use 'standard' language section titles which an alert reader will see in later sections in this volume. For example, we have used 'standard' language like 'bodies' and 'food' as section titles. But obvious questions appeared. Having received chapters which often would be classified as 'history,' what other approaches are there to categorizing these chapters? Should we move away from a having 'history' section and 'farm' these chapters out to other sections. In other words, should we have a disciplinary title like 'history' or move toward section titles which, in some cases, shift the labor slightly to the reader?

Our decision, ultimately, was that we should keep a singular section for history flavored chapters, understanding that this decision may court accusations of intellectual conservatism. We think that history as a discipline and, particularly in the context of the chapters in this volume, represents a special case. The reader might read these chapters differently, and certainly, we are not presenting a textbook with a series of chapters connecting a narrative or ideas. These six chapters take different approaches to history and reflect different philosophical positions, of which we will not be the umpires. As we have already suggested, those debates between authors and disciplines, in this section and the volume in general, are part of the business of being a critical obesity reader and researcher. Their different approaches notwithstanding, an educated reader will garner from this section the deep historical and connected reasons why obesity has long been the subject of critical research.

Take Hillel Schwartz's chapter. He has definitely *not* written a standard history chapter. Rather, it is series of 'dictionary' meanings of technical terms and slang words although the historical reasons are for the reader to encode. Of course, for an interested reader, some ideas are fairly obvious. But, like a dictionary which uses terms in alphabetical order, sometimes, the meanings are somewhat buried, waiting to be found, discussed, and argued over. There are no sub-headings to direct the reader's attention. Rather, this chapter offers the reader various suggesting routes through many cultures and 'obesity' literatures.

The second chapter comes from Katherine M. Flegal, a widely cited author who has worked in the United States and in disciplines as varied as nutrition, anthropology, and

DOI: 10.4324/9780429344824-3

public health. But, within this chapter, she is writing about an historical and essential issue for the reader to consider: how body size became a disease? This chapter also connects her work that crosses the disciplinary boundaries and gives a reader a possible historical starting point for a very modern 'crisis.'

Peter N. Stearns gives us another way to understanding what is going with obesity today. His chapter focuses on the period between the late 19th century and the early decades of the 20th century. He tries to describe the interweaving of fashion, medical, and moral culture that emerged in the United States.

In the following chapter, we are presented with a quite radical departure from previous chapters. Denise Bernuzzi de Sant'Anna writes about Brazil and long and deep historical battles between 'liberties and pathologies.' In some senses, this chapter is contrasting and connecting piece from, say, Stearns' chapter. North America and Latin America are always closely related. But, as Sant'Anna amply demonstrates, this chapter presents new stories about race, gender, social class, and the way different Brazilians see, for example, popular culture and public health policies.

In the next chapter, Isabel Fletcher presents historical findings from her medical and research history. But as good history always performs many roles, the focus on modern obesity is partly a historical question. For example, the changes in the way 'we' live have to be interpreted, and therefore, critical questions have to be raised and, therefore, answered. Further, the way in which epidemiology research studies have their own 'culture' or, rather, 'cultures' and its relationships with broader society. This chapter encapsulates the connections between many often misunderstood areas of life.

The final chapter, written by Michael Gard, hones on the emergence of 'obesity epidemic' at the beginning of the 21st century. Following the previous chapters in this section, in many ways, Gard writes about the exaggerations and mistakes in the obesity science literature. But Gard also wants to describe the likeness between the obesity science literature and the print and electronic media. We are often told that the differences between the science and its reporting in the media are very numerous and varied, but the subject of this chapter is the reverse; Gard wants to argue that the obesity 'viruses' either the science or the media; sometimes, it is quite hard to tell the difference. This chapter comes mostly from the second chapter of the book called 'The End of Obesity Epidemic' (Gard, 2011, published by Routledge).

2

A CRITICAL OBESIDARIUM (IN ENGLISH)

Hillel Schwartz

adipose. Adjective (1684), noun (1814), with associated word-cluster (adipal, adipescent, adipocere, adipocyte, adiposity) posing fat as a surplus, excess, dross, or zombie. Surplus: *adipocyte* cells specialize in the storage of fat in the form of triglycerides. Excess: "It is commendable in the author [of *Cursory Remarks on Corpulence*], considering the adipose nature of his pursuit, that he did not extend it to more obesity of bulk," from a review in the *Universal Magazine* 213 (March 1810). Dross: "He grew thinner and thinner, but was delighted with his emaciation, since all adipose tissue, he informed me, was perfectly useless, except for purposes of warmth," from E. F. Benson, *Windsor Magazine* (March 1911). Zombie: *adipocere*, that greyish or yellowish-white waxy substance that forms on dead bodies during decomposition.[1] Since the 1600s, anglophone writers and speakers have often framed fat in sumptuary terms, at once insubstantial and overmuch, a contradiction intrinsic to the rhetoric surrounding obesity.

baby fat. (1899), fat that should be outgrown unless in calves raised for veal. Infants should be neither lean nor hungry, but shifting norms, independent of nutritional status, establish the age at which a child is no longer an infant—and fat, as a residual of healthy birth or nursing, no longer a welcome sign. Indeed, since the late 20th century, "baby fat" has had to contend with the ascendancy of BMI (*q.v.*), lung-power, reaction times, and concentrations of proteins and trace minerals in the blood as a primary tally of "thriving." Although obstetricians have liberally expanded the normal range of *in utero* weights for a fetus, the popular disposition to identify "pudgy" newborns as "overweight" threatens to reduce even further the period during which parents may expect to delight in baby fat.

Blob, The. B–film of 1958, starring Steve McQueen in his first leading role, with theme music by Burt Bacharach, "Beware the Blob." As a globule of viscid substance, "blob" appeared in 1725 and then lay in wait for 233 years under cover of Impressionist paint and Australian slang for "someone of no account." Even as it begins to absorb the unassuming residents of a small Pennsylvania town, no one actually calls it "the Blob." A nameless monster ("Indescribable... Indestructible! Nothing Can Stop It!") oblivious to all weapons ("It Eats You Alive!), the Blob was as red as cherry Jello™ and Communism™ and equally amorphous at the height of the Cold War. The horror it invoked was less of an alien life-form than of unstoppable expansion and unremitting hunger. Wherefore, the next year, 1959, Mead Johnson and Company launched a national advertising campaign for a product

DOI: 10.4324/9780429344824-4

usually restricted to medical journals. Metrecal™ was itself, in taste, texture, and genus, a blob. "Not exactly a drug product, not exactly a food product," it was a thick amorphous shake—a meal "replacement" that made you feel too full to overeat. Metrecal sales grew after weekly spots were inserted into "The Valiant Years," a television series about a portly Winston Churchill. "We hold our freedom by extending it, and by deserving it every day," said the soft-spoken overvoice for Mead Johnson. By 1961, Metrecal was surpassing $100 million in sales, and *The Blob* was gaining cult status.[2]

BMI. (1940, "index of bodily mass," 1969–1972 for the abbreviation of Body-Mass Index.)

One of the several formulae relating weight to height, used to define comparative "fatness" as well as cardiovascular risk (*q.v.*). The original formula, weight in kilograms divided by the square of height in meters, was known as the Quetelet Index, after Adolphe Quetelet, a Belgian statistician (1796–1874) who contrived the formula in order to fit data on the weights of Dutch newborns, children, and adults to what we call a "normal" (Gaussian, or Bell) curve. This act of violence he performed in 1832 in pursuit of demographic averages that would, he believed, lay bare the laws of development physiological, intellectual, and social. Seven score years later, relying upon weight and height samples from the United States, England, Finland, Italy, Japan, and South African Bantu, researchers led by Ancel Keys of the University of Minnesota School of Public Health confirmed the utility of what they termed the Body Mass Index. Although their base population was entirely male, versions of the BMI have since been applied globally, across genders and cultures, in programs to reduce malnutrition, heart disease, and adult-onset diabetes. And although neither the statistical correlations nor the epidemiological data withstand scrutiny, BMI remains vital to fitness chains, clinical nutritionists, scale manufacturers, pharmaceutical giants, and retailers of fat-burning supplements. Aside from economic interests, the 50-year success of the BMI may be attributed to desires to obviate ethical and scientific concerns about surveys of obesity based on body shape or mere poundage. Finally, the BMI prevails because it invokes a something—mass—which seems as indisputable and ineluctable as it is, for most people, imponderable.[3]

Carbohydrate-Insulin Model (CIM). (2013, formally.) A model proposed by David S. Ludwig and Cara B. Ebbelling, designed to remedy the lack of a "satisfactory explanation for the obesity epidemic, beyond the difficulty many people have maintaining self-control in the modern environment." Since self-control is a perennial thorn and so-called addictive behaviors have been manifest for millennia, neither accounts for the increase of 25–30 lbs. in average adult weight in the US and Western Europe over the past half-century. Whether or not one regards the new poundage as proof of "obesity," let alone of an epidemic, and whether these averages accommodate class issues of poverty or the uncertainty of secure work, an historical explanation for the ostensible increase in poundage is worth hearing out. CIM attends to hormonal responses provoked by changes in dietary quality during the last 50 years, such that our calories ("metabolic fuels") tend to be deposited in fat tissue rather than circulated through the bloodstream, leaving the body hungry and entreating overeating. Foods with a high "glycemic index" (1981)—carbohydrates that digest quickly and stimulate insulin secretion—are the culprit, for insulin exerts anabolic control of the body's energy exchange system. Insulin prompts glucose uptake into tissues, suppresses the release of fatty acids from adipose tissue, and promotes fat deposition, leading to weight gain. The more refined grains, potato products, and added sugars that we consume, the higher our glycemic load and the greater the amount of circulating insulin. And it is exactly these foods whose consumption has markedly increased since the 1960s. Worse, the prevailing low-calorie, low-fat diets may "exacerbate the underlying metabolic problem by further restricting energy available in the blood—triggering the starvation response comprised of rising hunger, falling metabolic rate, and elevated stress hormone levels." Critics find that CIM neglects neuroendocrine and genetic components of obesity and the powerful role of plasma triglycerides while overplaying its hand concerning free fatty acids and ignoring the fact that "diets varying widely in glycemic index and load do not reliably result in differences in hunger." Still, the CIM deserves credit for enabling a full-on critique of the homeostatics of late Capitalism, whose carbohydrate menu for the 21st-century precariat (shantytown proletariats, rootless peasantries, a gig-economy cognetariat) may be challenged in the light of other drastic changes affecting individual and collective energy balance: declining hours of full-body physical exercise; declining hours of REM sleep; mounting levels of anxiety; mounting levels of pollution in the air, ground, and water; stresses of urbanization; the prohibitive cost of protein, whole grains, and fresh vegetables vis-à-vis sugars and processed foods, especially for those with no time for food preparation while working three jobs. It is not sloth that conduces toward fat, however deposed.[4]

corpulence, corpulent. Noun and adjective (by 1398 as "solid, dense, gross"; by 1440 as "large or bulky of body"), and etymologically neutral in the Latin, rooted as it is in "the nature of a physical or material body." I am most interested here in what the Philadelphia gynecologist George Henry Napheys had to say about corpulence in his *Prevention and Cure of Disease* (1871): "The dryness of the air is not favourable to corpulence in our country." What was he thinking? A man well ahead of his time, publishing sensible sexual counsel for women (*The Physical Life of Woman*, 1869) and men (*Transmission of Life*, 1871), Napheys died young, in 1876, at the age of 34, but not before penning 20 explicit pages on how to gain or lose weight. In his *Laws of Health in Relation to the Human Form* (1870), he discouraged weight-loss dieters from drinking much of anything, for a goodly proportion of the putative fat and poundage in a body consisted in fact of water that could be sweated out with exercise or eliminated through personal drought. It followed that a dry climate promoted thinner bodies, which was why he expected that the majority of his readers would desire to add to their weight. Perhaps, the United States was on the whole dryer in 1870 than it is now, and perhaps, we would be wise to consider climatic correlations to average weights or BMI (*q.v.*) of diverse populations. However, more to the point is the question of how best to frame alarms about obesity *and* about devastating thinness or malnutrition (see **kwashiorkor**) in the context of climate change, global food waste, and loss of habitat. Wrote Napheys:

> the precise medium between corpulence and leanness is hard to attain and harder to keep....and when such a condition of body goes on to the extent of obesity on one hand, or emaciation on the other, what charms can survive the heavy change?

What charms indeed?[5]

diet. Noun and verb, a portmanteau word combining "to die" with the past tenses of "eat," and understood sometimes as "dying to eat," sometimes as "dying while eating," and sometimes as "not having et, died." Alright, this is the sort of etymology that Ambrose Bierce would suggest, but it captures the cultural–historical ambiguity of diet as a strategy for weight loss, weight gain ("bulking up"), optimal performance (sports, stock-trading), healthy ageing, reduction of nausea (during chemotherapy or at sea), reduction of morning sickness or migraines, political protest, and adolescent defiance. And there can be fatal consequences far beyond cases of anorexia/bulimia or overdosing on dietary supplements. According to a study in the Global Burden of Disease series, poor diet (high in sodium, low in whole grains, fruits, nuts, vegetables, seafood) was a direct risk factor in 19% of deaths worldwide in 2017, poor child and maternal malnutrition in 6% of deaths. Since other risk factors are diet-related (high blood glucose, high LDL cholesterol, use of tobacco and alcohol to cope with hunger, loss of vitality or stamina, food insecurity), and since together these factors play a significant role in figures for morbidity as well as mortality, diet is no mean advance agent for the acute care, hospital, and mortuary industries.[6] If we have surprisingly little evidence pointing to higher mortality as a result of the weight cycling (*q.v.* yo-yo) inherent in weight-loss practices,[7] we have even less data about the burden of morbidity incident to a history of dieting for weight-loss, for body-sculpting, or for disease prevention or mitigation (e.g., colon cancer, arthritis, and severe cramps). We do have suspicions in social theory and accusations in critical media that putting the onus of dietary remediation on the individual is a corporate sleight of hand, diverting attention from the additives and food processing industries and their advertising campaigns for high-profit, low-nutritional-value goodies. Instead of blaming consumers for "risky behavior" (*q.v.* risk) when faced with mounds of sweet, fatty, salty, or "empty calorie" foods, much remains to be done by food activists (see **slow food**) to reinstall **diet** as a legislative body.

dopamine. (1951). The handier name for 3-hydroxytyramine given by Sir Henry Dale, who had studied its pharmacology back in 1910, when first synthesized. The name stems from its position as the metabolic intermediate, formed from L-dopa, in the biosynthesis of norepinephrine and adrenaline. In 1957, Arvid Carlsson showed that dopamine was a neurotransmitter ever-present in the basal ganglia of the brain and not just a precursor of norepinephrine. The functions of the basal ganglia have been slow to show themselves, but once dopamine was identified by Paul Greengard with the neuroendocrinal reward system, psychiatrists and pharmaceutical labs took notice (Intropin, Dopastat, methylphenidate and neuroleptic drugs, L-dopa). In 2010, Johnson and Kenny inspired biochemists and ad agencies to pursue the "hedonic mechanisms" common to drug addiction and overeating when they proved that giving rats access to a Western-style diet promotes compulsive food-seeking and eating by downregulating dopamine receptors.[8] See next entry.

eating contests. (Well before 1900, although the *OED* is fixated on turn-of-the-century pigeon-eating contests in Europe and the United States). Eating a single pie at speed, rather than many over a set time, was the ambition of contestants at county fairs during the 1800s, but pastry- and meat-eating contests are certain to be traced back at least as far as medieval Carnival, perhaps with pies of 4-and-20 blackbirds. Attitudes toward such contests have fluctuated, with a particularly grim aspect in the Jim Crow South as whites rounded up blacks for eating contests that made racist coinage of what Vivian Nun Halloran calls the "gustatory abject." These days, eating contests are not won by the fattest (or darkest) but by the fastest eaters, who do not mean to enjoy what they eat but to entertain as magicians entertain, by making things disappear before our eyes. It makes sense, then, that the first modern eating contests with commercial sponsors were held at that mecca of sad magic, Coney Island. A spurious date of 1916 for the original contest was intended to establish it as an American Independence Day tradition, but dedicated speed-eating at Coney Island began no earlier than 1972 at Nathan's Hot Dogs stand. In 2018, before a worldwide ESPN audience, Joey Chestnut downed 74 dogs in 10 minutes; Miki Sudo swallowed 37 to win on the women's side, as sanctioned by Major League Eating. MLE is an arm of IFOCE, the International Federation of Competitive Eating (founded 1997), which ranks professional competitors and arranges a circuit of contests, such as the Glutton Bowl (2002) and the Tour de Gorge.[9]

fat, colors of. White fat (as butter, 1686). White fat cells store energy in the form of lipids (*q.v.*). In visuals produced by anti-fat campaigners, white fat looks to be a sickly yellow.[10] **Brown fat** (<German *braunes Fettgewebe*, J. A. Hammar, 1895). Brown fat is a type

of adipose tissue, highly cellular and vascular, found initially in hibernating mammals and the newborns of many species. It is thermogenic, capable of generating heat through lipid oxidation to help the body adapt to cold weather; in other words, it can burn calories, a property that has spurred researchers to look to increase the proportion of brown fat in those with a predisposition toward diabetes or obesity. **Beige fat**, described in 2012, is found interspersed among strata of white fat, and unlike brown fat, it burns both lipids and glucose. A beige adipocyte newly identified in 2018 has such a "sweet tooth" that under the thermal stress of chronic cold it burns glucose (sugar) in preference to lipids. After studies in 2014 revealed that subcutaneous white fat can be "browned" via immune signaling pathways activated by eosinophils, which stain pink, Lee and Tontonoz wrote that "**Pink [Fat] is the New Brown.**"[11] This rush to color is exemplary of a double-fisted cultural drive to bestow upon fat an unheralded activity and agency.[12] One fist shapes fat into a mercenary or terrorist; the other fist may eventually free the "fat," "overweight," and "obese" from stereotypes of passivity, lethargy, and drabness.

Fat, location of. Fat has been jumping around of late, trying to get our attention. Should we pay more heed to hip fat or belly fat? Do the risks of heart attack rise with a greater waist-to-hip ratio or with droopier abdominal fat? Are love handles the grab-bars for adult-onset diabetes? What pattern of body fat distribution should most alarm postmenopausal women? What topography of fat is most prophetic of disaster for men in their 60s?[13] If weight-loss sieges and fat-melting compounds have miserable records over the long run,[14] they have failed most miserably at targeted fat removal. Wherefore, the geographers and engineers of fat must be plastic surgeons.

glutton, gluttony. (1200, from Old French.) One of the seven deadly sins, riding side by side with Idleness in Spenser's *The Faerie Queene* (1590, I, iv. sig D3). At its most punishing extreme, gluttony is all-consuming: "He lives only to digest, and, while the organs of gluttony perform their office, he has not a wish beyond."[15] Yet, John Garrow, writing in the *British Medical Journal* in 1996, took up the cudgel in defense of gluttony as the least offensive of the mortal sins, for it bespeaks resistance to satiation, which may translate into a noble refusal to compromise and a drive whose unslaked ambitions can be admirable when in defense of the downtrodden and divorced from sloth. Nor is gluttony to be blamed for the accumulation of fat, which piles up more often through near-unconscious if incessant snacking than through a well-considered if intransigent feasting.[16] From this prospect, gluttony is the intellectual's (the book-lover's, the philosopher's) sin; what's more, the brain is the most gluttonous of organs, demanding up to 20% of the body's energy haul in order to fuel the electrical impulses through which neurons communicate and to maintain cell health, AKA cerebral "housekeeping."[17]

heaviness. (Since 1000.) Another word laying contradictory historical claims: from one direction, "serious, deep, profound, intense"; from a second, "that which weighs or presses sorely on the feelings;" from a third, "Of persons: oppressive; troublesome; angry; violent" from a fourth, "Causing or occasioning sorrow; distressing, grievous, saddening; sorrowful." That's heavy-duty, man, and it would take some heavy industry (1888), if not some heavy metal (1964), to parse it all and still leave room for heavy petting (1960). The same split is found in theater and cinema, where the "heavy" may be handed a part sober or tragic (1814), tyrannical (1828), or villainous (1885). In any case, neither comedy nor drama, even in the West, demands an obese heavy; melodramas often had thin actors playing the part. The Dance of Death was led by a skeleton.

image, body. AKA body schema. (1934, Paul Schilder). The subjective picture or mental image which a person has of his or her body—its contours, its weak and strong points, its missing or ill-fitting pieces, its invisible strengths or glaring faults. Obsession with body image may be narcissistic or an aspect of Stockholm Syndrome in which hostages come to sympathize with their captors (*viz.*, the fashion industry, mainstream cinema, and the designers of exercise machines).

jumbo. *See* **mumbo-jumbo.**

kwashiorkor. (1933, from the Gold Coast language of Ga, *kwa ni oshi korkor*, "pretend not to mind the second one," referring to what happens to a baby when the next in the family is born and it, the weanling, no longer has access to its mother's milk.[18]) A condition of severe malnutrition, chiefly affecting children under the age of five, and characterized by pitting edema, loss of pigmentation, diarrhea, apathy, and stunted growth. Neglected, it can be fatal. If the symptoms are obvious, the etiology is contested. Once thought to be caused by protein poverty as a result of monoculture diets (maize, rice milk), hence easily remedied through high-protein, high-profit supplements produced and promoted by agri-business for distribution by UN agencies and NGOs, subsequent research has suspected micronutrient deficiencies, microbial gut infections, or insufficient calories. Recent studies of kwashiorkor, acknowledging a spectrum of diseases under the rubric of PEM (Protein-Energy Malnutrition), have returned to the hypothesis of very low levels of all essential amino acids and also of choline, a nutrient requisite for lipid synthesis.[19] The roots of widespread malnutrition, however, whether kwashiorkor, marasmus, or zinc or vitamin A deficiency (together afflicting perhaps a third of children worldwide), have more to do with the political economy of famine, postcolonial labor and settlement policies, and the ongoing exploitation of women. Just as the distended bellies of starving children appear as visual oxymorons that deserve a cultural analysis well beyond amino acids, so does the low "nutritional status" of populations long-resident in some of the most fertile areas of the planet.[20] Why the scare quotes? Because the phrase itself may be used to induce preternatural emergencies.

lipids. (1925, W. R. Bloor,[21] deciding against "lipins," "lipides," "lipoids.") Any of the group of fats and fat-like compounds that occur in living organisms as their most concentrated source of energy, "yielding per gram over twice as many calories as do carbohydrates and proteins."[22] So much for the association of fat with lethargy and sloth.

mumbo-jumbo. (1738, as an English transliteration of Mandingo *maamajomboo* or *mama-gyo-mbo,* meaning, "magician who makes the troubled spirits of ancestors go away.")[23] Consider the compound-complexity that has given rise to a lexical vortex of divinity and idols, ritual song and doubletalk, confidence game, and supersizing (cf. **XL, XXL**). So the giant **jumbo** of big clumsy people (1823) and captive elephants (1882), of great movable drilling platforms (1908) and passenger jets (1966), of enormous California peaches (1897) and daunting burgers (1959), had to be cut away from the mumble-**mumbo** of the sorcerer-dancer who looked twice as large in mask and costume as any other Mandingo along the Gambia's banks… Cut away for good reason: for centuries, the Mandingo perplexed the English with their syncretic embrace of Islam, their lazy casual approach to farming, their regime of slaves, and above all the employment of magicians by husbands to keep their women in line—"a dreadful Bugbear to the Women, call'd Mumbo-Jumbo, which is what keeps the women in awe"—because Mandingo women were noisier, more headstrong, and more powerful than those of neighboring Wolofs or Jolas. The historical baggage of **jumbo** resurfaces in the hype of size and in the gendered binaries of proud **jumbo** for things masculine, laughable **jumbo** for appurtenances female, and **mumbo-jumbo** for talk that must be squelched.[24]

noise, fat and. Aren't fat people noisier because more awkward (moving in shambles), more gluttonous (chomping with open mouths), and louder (with the vocal power of a barrel organ or diva)? And when the proudly fat become vociferous in claiming rights to clothing that fits, chairs that hold, safety belts that wrap around, isn't this the noise of yet another self-defining group that wants to have it both ways: sociolegal acceptance of manifest difference and ability, yet expensive accommodation to their disability? Isn't fat itself the proprioceptive equivalent of data noise, inherently interfering with access to information and truth? Thin people are quiet, clear-sighted, moderate, mobile, and adaptable to a just-in-time world. Right?[25]

Obecity. (2006, Simon Marvin and Will Medd[26]). A neologism for the flow of fats through the clogged arteries (sewers) and hearts (pumping stations) of sprawling megalopoli. The cardiovascular analogy is explicit, but the difficulties of "breaking down" and disposing of the waste of residents and their pets, restaurants and their grease, cars and their oil, industries and their effluents are far more troubling. Why are we displacing our frustration with waste disposal and pollution onto the bodies of those corralled into an "epidemic" of obesity, when all of us are facing most immediately the scandal of obecity?

phat. (1963, slang, esp. hip-hop, among African Americans.) In Old English, fat connoted "the richest or best part of anything," as in "the fat of the land," but the *OED* insists that this connotation is obsolete. Perhaps, it simply has another orthography. His (surely male) informants were surely ribbin' an jivin' Hal Foster when they told him that "phat" was an acronym for "pussy, hips, ass, and tits," or "pretty hole at all time,"[27] given that the word was current a decade earlier with reference to cool music, and had such precursors as Fats Waller, of stride and swing, and Fats Domino, of boogie-woogie and, in 1949, the first rock-and-roll record to sell a million copies, "The Fat Man." Myself, I would move phat into the realm of what Malinowski in 1936 called "phatic communion," a type of speech whose principal aim is creating or maintaining social bonds,[28] the kind of chit-chat that becomes improv and scat in jazz, or the rhythmic rhyming repeats replete in hip-hop. Phat, then, as both grease and glue, reversing the negative spin on fat, so, a form of turntabling.

quarter-pounder. (1847, the weight of a fish; by 1972, a proprietary McDonald's burger.) Does a Quarter Pounder® weigh a quarter pound? Yes, and no. Until 2017, its raw ground beef patty weighed 4 oz.; that patty has since been beefed up to 4.25 oz.[29] But due to the fat that drips out during cooking, the patty's weight at first bite is 2.8 to 3 oz. McDonald's website furnishes nutritional values for a Quarter Pounder® with slivered onions, ketchup, and mustard on a toasted sesame seed bun: 430 calories, 20 g fat (8 g saturated fat, 1 g transfat, 75 mg cholesterol), 37 g total carbs, 26 g protein, 700 mg sodium, 2 g dietary fiber, 9 g sugars, 150 IU Vitamin A, 2 mg Vitamin C, 30 mg calcium, and 4.5 mg iron. Most of these values are accompanied by a parenthetical percentage of recommended Daily Value based on a 2000 calorie diet—for example, cholesterol: 75 mg (24% DV). With medium fries and a sweet drink, the calories double, as do milligrams of total fat. Anyone seeking a dissertation topic need look no further, for the questions raised by this capsule c.v. of a meal are manifold: How and when did the West arrive at such nutritional categories? How and why have the categories changed? When did it become essential to know about transfat or dietary fiber? How do the values compare to minimum adequate nutrition for net-fishermen, for women selling bibles door-to-door, and for farmworkers picking vegetables? To what degree have the demands for reasonable military rations influenced nutritional standards, and how have new tactics, weaponry, or women in the ranks affected these standards? For whose benefit are nutritional numbers provided? Dieters? Doctors? The homeless? Homemakers? Dozens more questions lurk. If there is research that begins to address each individually, no scholar has put the answers together into one big unhappy meal. *See also* **jumbo**.

risk. (Dating the word itself would demand another dissertation by someone who has mastered Arabic [*rizq, rezq*, "fortune, luck, destiny, chance, portion divinely allotted to each man"], postclassical Latin [*resicum, risicum,* "danger, hazard"] from? classical Latin [*resecum,* "cutting," implying sharpness or jaggedness], and medieval French [*risque,* "danger or inconvenience, predictable or otherwise," 1578 as a feminine noun, 1633 as a masculine noun; 1690 as a legal term], but my mouth waters at the Middle Persian *rozik,* "daily provision" (*see* quarter-pounder)). Since proof of direct causal links between sheer poundage and increased mortality are hard to come by, life insurance companies and the public health community refocused their concerns about obesity from weight to fat [*see* BMI]. For half a century, fat bodies have been constrained and contoured by risk, that is, by calculations of the higher chances of heart attack, stroke, liver disease, diabetes, and kidney failure.[30] These calculations may be exemplary of a "risk society" and late Capitalism's provocations of anxiety;[31] they are also an outcome of the love–hate relationships between family medicine and merchandising and between surgery and the aesthetics industries (sanitation, cosmetics, ergonomics). Although our biome is now at existential risk, with global warming, extreme weather, and loss of habitat challenging every species except perhaps extremophiles, risk is currently used to divide us, body from body.

slow food. (Before 1974.) Food prepared in a customary or thoughtful manner, as opposed to "fast food," whether instant, ready-to-eat, drive-in, or stand-up. Since 1986, slow food has also been the slogan and moniker of an environmental, social justice, and fair trade movement, stemming from initiatives in Northern Italy to preserve local culinary traditions and agricultural diversity, further promoted since 1989 by Slow Food International, a non-profit.[32] Partisans direct attention to the mistreatment of farmworkers, the ravages of industrialized farming, and such unsustainable ironies as the estimate by Patrick Holden that it takes ten calories of fossil fuel energy to produce, in general, each calorie of edible food.[33] From this perspective, what is obese in the most terrible of senses (i.e., ponderous, bloated, unresponsive, and potentially fatal) are systems of food production that rely on very-low-wage labor, tankers of biocides, subsidies for the least environmentally or nutritionally sound crops, and the underbudgeting of safety inspectors and regulators. Slow eating does assist digestion and reduce constipation, but as a movement, slow food must speed up and sharpen its teeth.

Thinner. (1984.) A novel by Stephen King, the last he published under the pseudonym Richard Bachman. Like many successful thrillers, the plot pushes a commonplace toward its extreme, in this case, dieting (*q.v.*). An arrogant, obnoxious man who cannot seem to lose his bulk or curb his appetite gets off without so much as a reprimand after having run over a Gypsy woman. Leaving the courtroom, where he has colluded with the judge, he is met by the dead woman's father, who utters a single word: "Thinner." This is a curse in the form of a *pharmakon,* a gift and a poison: the gift, a dieting regime that works; the poison, a regime that will not quit, driving him toward incorporeality, AKA death.[34] However much the antagonistic protagonist may gorge, his appetite is no match for the curse, where all calories are literally "empty" calories. The novel was supposedly inspired by King's own life: when he rose to 236 pounds, his physician commanded him to lose weight. He did, and while he kept the weight off, he began to mull over the tyranny of such a command. Oddly, the curse was reversed for the book itself, which has gained pages over the years, from an initial 282 pages to 318 in the Signet edition of 1995, 340 pages in the Hodder edition of 2007, and 423 pages in the Pocket Books edition of 2016. Even more oddly, critics tore into the book, dismissing it as an inflated short story. Janis Eidus wrote, "*Thinner,* for all its padding, can be seen for what it is—a pretty thin book." Don Herron reduced it to "a great short gimmick story lost in novel-length packaging." In art as in bariatrics, it seems that there must be a thin man inside every fat man.[35]

underweight. *See* **kwashiorkor;** *Thinner*.

voluminous. (1611, from the Latin *volume*, coil, wreath, roll of parchment or papyrus.) The word began innocently enough: "The manifold turnings and windings of the way like a company of voluminous Meanders." Then came connotations of length, of "writing so much as to fill volumes," a copiousness which by 1664 could be extended to intimidating beasts ("The larger and more voluminous sort of Animals, as Bulls, Bears, Tygers, &c."). It veered toward the human body circa 1680 ("His Legs are stuck in his great voluminous Britches"), whence voluminous skirts, volumizing shampoo, and mascara. What's peculiar in this genealogy is how the word eluded the gravitational pull of the black hole of obesity. Did its infancy among scrolls, imperial or sacred, confer immunity?

WALL-E (2008.) An animated sci-fi satire produced by Pixar Studios, directed by Andrew Stanton, story by Andrew Stanton and Peter Docter. In the barrens of the 29th century, we find WALL-E, a trash compactor robot, cleaning up the garbage left after humanity evacuated an unredeemable Earth in 2110 at the prompting of Buy-N-Large megacorp. Remnant humans are now voluminous adipose blobs with scant limbs and no jobs, couch potato captives of the *Axiom* starliner that doubles as a mall and a giant survival bubble. But Wall-E is hard at work, gleaning what can be saved from a lost civilization of mass consumerism and criminal neglect. Every so often, the *Axiom* automatically sends a probe back to look for signs of life on the dead home planet. This time, probe EVE happens on a small green plant that Wall-E has recently discovered and coaxed toward health inside his corrugated shed. This is big news, but the bigger news is that WALL-E has fallen in love with EVE. When she confiscates his plant as evidence of Earth's incipient renewal, WALL-E pursues her across the galaxy, back to the *Axiom*, where things get complicated—secret directives, holo-detectors, rabble-rousing robots, garbage chutes, all that stuff. The film was "an instant blockbuster," grossing half a billion dollars and winning Golden Globe, Hugo, and Academy Awards. In 2016, film critics worldwide placed *WALL-E* 29th among 100 films considered the best yet of the new century.[36] Just thought you'd want to know.

XL. (1950, extra large, a garment size.) Caitlin Moran: "A world where a size 12 is 'XL'— is another piece of what strident feminists can technically dismiss as 'total bullshit'."[37] She's wrong: protests against sizing practices are hardly strident or finicky. *See* XXL.

XXL. (1952, extra extra large, a label now assigned to figures merely stocky.) Shaming ordinary bodies by forcing upon them totems of anonymous monstrosity is a variant of Disaster Capitalism, which profits from devastation and disempowerment.[38] But there has been push back toward more comfortable clothing for larger people, in more styles, and an occasional public embrace of "outsize" silhouettes. The map may not be the territory, but it has always been grounds for action, often for war. *See also* zero zero (00).

yo-yo diet. (1915, from one of the Philippine languages, describing an indigenous toy; before 1976, describing cycles of weight loss and weight gain.) A yo-yo demonstrates the laws of momentum through which a body can be made to fall under its own weight and rise again. Figuratively and figurally, yo-yos are icons of resurrection, crucial to imaginations that propel perpetual dieting and recursive plastic surgery.

zero zero (00), size. (Before 2000.) Traditionally, the size that would fit a 23-inch waist; recently, the size apt to an eight-year-old,[39] though sewn into lines of expensive women's wear as asymptote to the fantasies of the fashion industry and here and there a tight-lacing fetishist. The premise of **00** is the inverse of the premise of *Thinner* (q.v.): the end of thinness is not incorporeality and a wasting death but universatility[40] and the photogenic immortality of the person who can fit (i.e., vanish) into anything.

Notes

1 Unless otherwise noted, I draw dates for word usage and all exemplary quotations from the online edition of the Oxford English Dictionary (Oxford University Press, 2000-), 3rd edition (March 2004), accessed August through December 2018. Most dating for the earliest use of any word that is neither a conscious neologism nor a newly patented technology must be considered decades late.

2 Hillel Schwartz, *Never Satisfied: A Cultural History of Diets, Fantasies and Fat* (Free Press, 1986) 252–253.

3 Garabed Eknoyan, "Adolphe Quetelet (1796–1894)—The Average Man and Indices of Obesity," *Nephrology Dialysis Transplantation* 23 (2008) 47–51, doi:10.1093/ndt/gfm517; Ancel Keys et al., "Indices of Relative Weight and Obesity," *Journal of Chronic Diseases* 25 (1972) 329–343, reprinted in *International Journal of Epidemiology* 43, 3 (2014) 655–755, doi: 10.1093/ije/dyu058; Jenn Anderson, "Whose Voice Counts? A Critical Examination of Discourses Surrounding the Body Mass Index," *Fat Studies* 1, 2 (2012) 195–207, doi: 10.1080/21604851.2012.656500; Keith Devlin, "Top 10 Reasons Why THE BMI Is Bogus," *National Public Radio* (4 July 2009) Weekend Edition Saturday, accessed 27 December 2018 at https://www.npr.org/templates/story/story.php?storyId=106268439.

4 David S. Ludwig and Cara B. Ebbeling, "The Carbohydrate-Insulin Model of Obesity: Beyond 'Calories In, Calories Out,'" *JAMA Internal Medicine* (2 July 2018) E1–E6, doi:10.1001/jamainternmed.2018.2933, with rebuttal by Kevin D. Hall, Stephan J. Guyenet, and Rudolph L. Leibel, "The Carbohydrate-Insulin Model of Obesity Is Difficult to Reconcile with Current Evidence," E1–E2.

5 George Henry Napheys, Prevention and Cure of Disease: A Practical Treatise on the Nursing and Home Treatment of the Sick (W. J. Holland, 1871) iii. I. 615; idem, The Laws of Health in Relation to the Human Form (W. J, Holland, 1870) quote on p. 37.

6 Nicola Davis, "Poor diet a factor in one-fifth of global deaths in 2017 study," *The Guardian* (8 November 2018), reporting on the Global Burden of Disease study, at www.theguardian.com/society/2018/nov/08/poor-diet-a-factor-in-one-fifth-of-global-deaths-in-2017-study.

7 Victoria L. Stevens, et al. "Weight Cycling and Mortality in a Large Prospective US Study," *American Journal of Epidemiology* 175, 8 (15 April 2012) 785–792, doi.org/10.1093/aje/kwr378; Caitlin Mason et al., "History of Weight Cycling Does Not Impede Future Weight Loss or Metabolic Improvements in Postmenopausal Women," *Metabolism* 62, 1 (January 2013) 127–136, doi.org/10.1016/j.metabol.2012.06.012.

8 O. Hornykiewicz, "Brain Dopamine: A Historical Perspective," in *Dopamine in the CNS*, ed. G. Di Chiara (Springer, 2002) 1–5; Arvid Carlsson, "Thirty Years of Dopamine Research," *Advances in Neurology* 60 (1993) 1–10; S. D. Iversen and L. L. Iversen, "Dopamine: 50 Years in Perspective," *Trends in Neuroscience* 30, 5 (May 2007) 188–193, doi: 10.1016/j.tins.2007.03.002; Paul M. Johnson and Paul J. Kenny, "Dopamine D2 Receptors in Addiction-Like Reward Dysfunction and Compulsive Eating in Obese Rats," *Nature Neuroscience* 13 (2010) 635–641, doi: 10.1038/nn.2519.

9 Jason Fagone, *Horsemen of the Esophagus: Competitive Eating and the Big Fat American Dream* (Crown/Archetype, 2006) 17–21; Itai Vardi, "Feeding Race: Eating Contests, the Black Body, and the Social Production of Group Boundaries through Amusement in Turn of the Twentieth Century America," *Food, Culture & Society* 13, 3 (2010) 371–396; Vivian Nun Halloran, "Biting Reality: Extreme Eating and the Fascination with the Gustatory Abject," *Iowa Journal of Cultural Studies* 4, article 5 (2004) 24–42, https://ir.uiowa.edu/cgi/viewcontent.cgi?article=1047&context=ijcs; Wikipedia entries for "competitive eating," "Major League Eating," and Nathan's Hot Dog Eating Contest: https://en.wikipedia.org/wiki/Competitive_eating; https://en.wikipedia.org/wiki/Nathan%27s_Hot_Dog_Eating_Contest; www.majorleagueeating.com/contests.php.

10 Christopher E. Forth, "On Fat and Fattening: Agency, Materiality, and Animality in the History of Corpulence," *Body Politics: Zeitschrift für Körpergeschichte* 3, 5 (2015) 51–74, at 53–54.

11 Paul Cohen and Bruce M. Spiegelman, "Brown and Beige Fat: Molecular Parts of a Thermogenic Machine," *Diabetes* (7 June 2015), doi: 10.2337/db15-0318; J. Wu et al., "Beige Adipocytes Are a Distinct Type of Thermogenic Fat Cell in Mouse and Human," *Cell* 150 (2012) 366–376; Wenfei Sun and Christian Wolfrum, "Fat Cells with a Sweet Tooth," *Nature* (19 December 2018) News & Views, doi: 10.1038/d41586-018-07739-6, summarizing Yong Chen et al., "Thermal Stress Induces Glycolytic Beige Fat Formation via a Myogenic State," *Nature* (19 December 2018), doi.org/10.1038/s41586-018-0801-z; Stephen D. Lee and Peter Tontonoz, "Eosinophils in Fat: Pink

Is the New Brown," *Cell* 157, 6 (5 June 2014) 1249–1250, doi.org/10.1016/j.cell.2014.05.025, summarizing Rajesh R. Rao et al., "Meteorin-Like Is a Hormone That Regulates Immune-Adipose Interactions to Increase Beige Fat Thermogenesis," *Cell* 157 (5 June 2014) 1279–1291, doi: 10.1016/j.cell.2014.03.065

12 Cf. Nina Mackert, "Writing the History of Fat Agency," *Body Politics: Zeitschrift für Körpergeschichte* 3, 5 (2015) 13–24.

13 Luca A. Lotta, et al., "Association of Genetic Variants Related to Gluteofemoral vs Abdominal Fat Distribution With Type 2 Diabetes, Coronary Disease, and Cardiovascular Risk Factors," *JAMA* 320, 24 (2018) 2553–2563, doi: 10.1001/jama.2018.19329.

14 On the political economics of weight-loss-dieting failures, see esp. Anna Mollow and Robert McRuer, "Fattening Austerity," *Body Politics: Zeitschrift für Körpergeschichte* 3, 5 (2015) 25–50.

15 Sidney Smith, *The Works: Including his Contributions to the Edinburgh Review* (Longman, Brown, Green, Longmans, and Roberts, 1859) I, 39, from an essay of 1803.

16 John Garrow, "Gluttony," *British Medical Journal* 313, 7072 (21 December 1996) 1595. http://www.bmj.com/archive/

17 Nikhil Swaminathan, "Why Does the Brain Need So Much Power?" *Scientific American* (29 April 2008), summarizing Fei Du et al., "Tightly Coupled Brain Activity and Cerebral ATP Metabolic Rate," *Proceedings of the National Academy of Sciences USA* 105, 17 (29 April 2008) 6409–6414, doi.org/10.1073/pnas.0710766105.

18 Cicely D. Williams, "Kwashiorkor: A Nutritional Disease of Children Associated with a Maize Diet," *Lancet* (1 November 1935) 1151–1152, reprinted in the *Bulletin of the World Health Organization* 81, 12 (December 2003) 912–913; Geert Tom Heikens and Mark Manary, "75 Years of Kwashiorkor if [*sic*: in] Africa," *Malawi Medical Journal* 21, 3 (September 2009) 96–100.

19 Donald S. McLaren, "The Great Protein Fiasco," *Lancet* 304, 7872 (13 July 1974) 93–96, doi.org/10.1016/S0140-6736(74)91649-3; idem, "The Great Protein Fiasco Revisited," *Nutrition* 16, 5 (June 2000) 464–465, doi.org/10.1016/S0899-9007(00)00234-3; Alan A. Jackson, "Severe Undernutrition in Jamaica. Kwashiorkor and Marasmus: The Disease of the Weanling," *Acta Paediatrica Scandinavica* (Supplement) 323 (1986) 43–51, doi: 10.1111/j.1651-2227.1986.tb10349.x; Richard D. Semba et al., "Child Stunting Is Associated with Low Circulating Essential Amino Acids," *EBioMedicine* 6 (April 2016) 246–252, doi.org/10.1016/j.ebiom.2016.02.030.

20 Cf. John Nott, "Malnutrition in a Modernising Economy: The Changing Aetiology and Epidemiology of Malnutrition in an African Kingdom, Buganda, c. 1940–73," *Medical History* 60, 2 (April 2016) 229–249, doi: 10.1017/mdh.2016.5.

21 W. R. Bloor, "Biochemistry of the Fats," *Chemical Reviews* 2 (1925) 243–300, at 243–244, doi: 10.1021/cr60006a003.

22 Abraham White et al., *Principles of Biochemistry* (McGraw-Hill, 1954) 453.

23 Ishmael Reed, Mumbo-Jumbo (Macmillan, 1972) end of prologue, citing the then-current edition of the American Heritage Dictionary of the English Language, but see Johnnella E. Butler, "*Mumbo Jumbo*, Theory, and the Aesthetics of Wholeness," in *Aesthetics in a Multicultural Age*, eds. Emory Elliot, Louis F. Caton, and Jeffrey Rhyne (Oxford University Press, 2002) 175–192, note 5.

24 In addition to the OED entries under "jumbo" and "mumbo-jumbo," I am using Paul Nugent, "Putting the History Back into Ethnicity: Enslavement, Religion and Cultural Brokerage on the Construction of Mandinka/Jola and Ewe/Agotime Identities in West Africa c.1650–1930," *Comparative Studies in Society and History* 50, 4 (2008) 920–48, doi: 10.1017/S001041750800039X; John G. Wood, *The Uncivilized Races of Men in All Countries of the World* (J.B. Burr, 1875) I, 607–608.

25 Hillel Schwartz, "Fat and Noise," *Dimensions* 12 (June/July 1996) 18–19, accessible at www.academia.edu/7824736/Fat_and_Noise_one_of_a_series_of_23_bi-monthly_columns_published_1993-2001_on_issues_related_to_cultural_notions_of_the_body

26 Simon Marvin and Will Medd, "Metabolisms of Obecity: Flows of Fat through Bodies, Cities, and Sewers," *Environment and Planning A* 38, 2 (2006) 313–324, doi/10.1068/a37272.

27 Hal Foster, *Ribbin' Jivin' and Playin' the Dozens: The Persistent Dilemma in Our Schools*, 2nd ed. (Ballinger, 1990 [1974]) 63, 78 note 75.

28 Gunter Senft, "Phatic communion," in *Handbook of Pragmatics*, eds. Jef Verschueren, Jan-Ola Östman, and Jan Blommaert (John Benjamins, 1995) 1–10, quoting from Malinowski's "The Problem of Meaning in Primitive Languages," in *The Meaning of Meaning*, eds. C. K. Ogden and I. A. Richards (Kegan Paul, 1936 [1923]), Supplement I, 296–336.

29 Joe Satran, "McDonald's Quarter Pounders Will Soon Weigh More Than A Quarter Pound," *Huffington Post* (6 December 2017), accessed 27 December 2018 at www.huffpost.com/entry/mcdonalds-quarter-pounder_n_7691010.

30 A comprehensive endnote here would list thousands of citations. Instead, see simply the National Institute of Diabetes and Digestive and Kidney Diseases, "Health Risks of Being Overweight," conflating weight and fat and meant to scare you out of your wits, accessed 31 December 2018 at www.niddk.nih.gov/health-information/weight-management/health-risks-overweight.

31 Again, a vast literature. Start perhaps with Barbara Adam, Ulrich Beck, and Joost van Loon, eds., *The Risk Society and Beyond: Critical Issues for Social Theory* (Sage, 2000) and, most aptly, Michael Gard and Jan Wright, "Managing Uncertainty: Obesity Discourses and Physical Education in a Risk Society," *Studies in Philosophy and Education* 20 (2001) 535–549.

32 Koen van Bommel and André Spicer, "Hail the Snail: Hegemonic Struggles in the Slow Food Movement," *Organization Studies* 32, 12 (2011) 1717–1744, doi: 10.1177/0170840611425722.

33 Eric Schlosser, "Slow Food for Thought," *The Nation* (22 September 2008), accessed 30 December 2018 at https://www.thenation.com/article/slow-food-thought/.

34 Jacques Derrida, "Plato's Pharmacy (1968)" in *Disseminations*, trans. Barbara Johnson (Continuum, 1981) 67–186. Derrida was a thin man, and like the cinematic Thin Man of the Thirties, a self-parodic detective. If only more critical inquiry were made of thinness in men and women beyond such works as Sharlene J. Hesse-Biber's Am I Thin Enough Yet? The Cult of Thinness and the Commercialization of Identity (Oxford University, 1996). Where are the journals devoted to Thin Studies? Slim Investigations?

35 "*Thinner* (novel)," Wikipedia, https://en.wikipedia.org/wiki/Thinner_(novel), last edited–and accessed--31 Dec 2018; Don Herron, "Stephen King: The Good, the Bad, and the Academic (1982)," in *Stephen King*, ed. Harold Bloom (Infobase, 2006), 39 for gimmick and 22 for Eidus quote.

36 All this from my repeated viewings of the film and from the Wikipedia entry, accessed 31 December 2018 at https://en.wikipedia.org/wiki/WALL-E.

37 Caitlin Moran, *How to Be a Woman* (Ebury, 2011; Harper, 2012) 111.

38 Naomi Klein, *The Shock Doctrine: The Rise of Disaster Capitalism* (Metropolitan/Henry Holt, 2007).

39 Starsinthetwilight, "Size 0," Urban Dictionary (19 February 2009), accessed 31 December 2019 at www.urbandictionary.com/define.php?term=Size%200

40 My portmanteau word, and I stand by it.

3

HOW BODY SIZE BECAME A DISEASE

A history of the body mass index and its rise to clinical importance

Katherine M. Flegal

Introduction

Taller people tend to weigh more than shorter people. But how does weight vary with height? The body mass index (BMI, calculated as weight (W) divided by height (H) squared) is one way to express weight adjusted for height. It is widely used, with the advantages of being technically uncomplicated, non-invasive, easy to measure and calculate. Where did it come from? How did it become the definition of a disease?

Quetelet and the relation of weight to height

The 19th-century Belgian statistician Adolphe Quetelet (1796–1874), originally trained as an astronomer, had wide-ranging interests in social and physical characteristics of human populations, addressing topics such as natality, mortality, crime, education and more. Stigler (1986) provides an extensive account of Quetelet's contributions; see also Eknoyan (2008) and Weigley (2000). A pioneer in statistical data gathering and statistical thinking, Quetelet wanted to discover the mathematical laws governing social as well as physical phenomena. A minor aspect of his work was the investigation of development of body measurements from birth through adulthood, and among these was the relation of weight to height in adults. In a brief footnote in his 1835 book "Sur l'homme," Quetelet observed that, for adults, weight varied as the square of height (Quetelet, 1835, Vol. 2, p. 54).

He derived this from empirical observations, not from theoretical considerations. Quetelet recognized that "if man increased equally in all his dimensions, his weight at different ages would be as the cube of his height. Now this is not what we really observe" (Quetelet, 1835, Vol. 2, p 52). He took the 12 tallest and the 12 shortest men within a data set and found their average heights and also their average weight/height values. He observed that the ratio of mean height of the shortest men to the tallest men was in the proportion of 5 to 6. He observed that the ratio of mean weight/height of the shortest men to the tallest men was also in the proportion of 5 to 6. As long as these two proportions are the same as each other, then, as Quetelet's footnote points out, it can be shown that weight increases as the square of stature.[1] He repeated these observations for women, with the same finding. Quetelet was interested in the properties of what he called the "l'homme moyen" (the average or typical individual)

DOI: 10.4324/9780429344824-5

23

and did not attempt to investigate departures of weight from what was expected based on stature. Quetelet did not propose an index. However, because of his observations, the ratio of weight divided by height squared (W/H^2) later became known as Quetelet's index.

Other early empirical investigations agreed with Quetelet's findings that weight varied as the square of height. In 1869, Benjamin Gould, the actuary for the US military, published extensive data on newly demobilized Civil War soldiers (Gould, 1869). Beyond investigations of topics ranging from ages at enlistment, place of birth and extending even to topics such as hair and eye colours, Gould also addressed anthropometry (body measurements), not only weight and height but also many other physical dimensions. As had Quetelet before him, Gould observed empirically that weight did not vary as the cube of height but rather as the square. According to Gould, "... we are irresistibly led to the singular and interesting discovery that the mean weights, vary strictly as the squares of the statures. ... The fact here elicited was observed by Quetelet" (Gould, 1869, p. 409).

Quetelet's index – just one of many

Quetelet's index was just one of a number of different indicators used for descriptive and research purposes in the 19th and early 20th centuries to express weight adjusted for height. Such indicators were simply ways to standardize weight for height, so that descriptions and comparisons of weight could be made across individuals of different heights. As noted by Gray and Mayall (1920) and by Billewicz, Kemsley, and Thomson (1962), the nomenclature attached to these indicators is not always consistent, and it would require a good deal of historical research to establish their origins.

The Broca index, *weight (kg) = height (cm) −100*, is said to have been developed around 1871 (Laurent et al., 2020; Rössner, 2007) by the French neuroscientist Paul Pierre Broca (1824–1880), although its origins are obscure (Gray & Mayall, 1920). In 1898, the Italian doctor Ridolfo Livi (1856–1920) argued that because weight is a measure of volume, the correct index would be the cube root of weight, divided by height, which he called the "indice ponderal" or ponderal index (Livi, 1898). Swiss physician Fritz Rohrer (1888–1926) developed the Rohrer index, weight divided by height cubed, that also used the cube rather than the square (Rohrer, 1908, 1921). In a later version, William H. Sheldon (1898–1977), the influential creator of the concept of somatotypes (Vertinsky, 2002, 2007), used an inverted form of the index, which he also called ponderal index.

In a very large sample of US military conscripts, however, Davenport observed, "Were short people and tall people of the same shape, then it would be true that their weight would be expected to vary with the cube of any one dimension. But this assumption is not true" (Davenport, 1920, p. 470). He summarized his findings by saying, "for young adult males the best index of build is apparently obtained by dividing weight by the square of stature" (Davenport, 1920, p. 475).

In these discussions, weight for height indicators was viewed as a method of standardizing weight for height for descriptive purposes. For instance, Livi (1898) felt that his index could be used to examine how weight varied by factors such as sex, age, race or environmental conditions after adjusting for differences in height.

Life insurance and the beginnings of "ideal weight" standards

On a different track, weight for height tables began to be developed and then to be used as an indicator of risk for life insurance purposes. Czerniawski (2007) provides a detailed analysis of the development of such tables between the 1830s (when Quetelet published what is perhaps the first example of a weight for height table) and 1943, when the Metropolitan Life Insurance company presented tables of "ideal weights" by height for men and women. Beginning as descriptive, such tables were transformed to a tool used for actuarial purposes by life insurance companies and then to recommendations for the general population going from "average" to "ideal" weights. Shephard (1907) presented a table compiled in 1897 of the average heights and weights by age of men who had been accepted for life insurance, stating that weights of 20 percent above or below those average weights indicated a poor actuarial risk. In 1908, Symonds (1908), discussing the same table, asserted that someone who was 20 percent or more above the standard weight for age should be considered overweight. Since the 1897 standard weights increased with age, the weight considered overweight on this basis also increased with age. Later, Armstrong, Dublin, Wheatley, and Marks (1951), discussing the 1943 Metropolitan Life tables, recommended a fixed set of standards based on the ideal weight for ages 25–30, with 10 percent over that weight considered overweight and 20 percent over ideal weight being pathological overweight or obesity.

Throughout the 1960s and 1970s, the 1959 Metropolitan Life tables (Metropolitan Life Insurance Company (MLIC), 1959) played a dominant role in identifying what were called "desirable" weights (Weigley, 1984). Seltzer (1965) commented on the severity and often unrealistic requirements of the desirable weights in these tables. A discussion and critique of some of the shortcomings of the 1959 version of the Metropolitan Life tables and the later 1983 version (MLIC, 1983) was presented at the 1985 NIH Conference on the Health Implications of Obesity (Harrison, 1985). Knapp critiqued both the concept of "ideal weight" and the construction of the Metropolitan Life tables, calling the methods by which the tables were constructed "almost unfathomable" (Knapp, 1983, p. 507). Jarrett (1986) quoted Knapp but added that he questioned the "almost." Andres, Elahi, Tobin, Muller, and Brant (1985) reanalyzed the data on which the 1983 Metropolitan Life tables were based and concluded that weight standards should be adjusted for age and should be higher for older adults, a finding that was the subject of some controversy (Willett, Stampfer, Manson, & Vanitallie, 1991).

Weight–height indices and fatness

Early attempts to use weight and height to create an indicator of adiposity (body fatness) were limited by the methods of measuring adiposity then available before the advent of methods such as dual-energy x-ray absorptiometry (DXA) and magnetic resonance imaging. One method involved weighing a person underwater and then following the principles set out by Archimedes to determine body density (Forbes, 1999). Although this method, called hydrodensitometry or hydrostatic weighing, provided accurate estimates of body density, converting body density to a measure of fatness required assumptions about body composition that might not be accurate at the individual level. Another method was to use callipers to measure the thickness of subcutaneous fat levels at different body sites (skinfold measurements). With these, one approach was to characterize adiposity simply by the sum of the skinfold measurements; another approach was to use prediction equations (e.g., Wilmore and Behnke 1969) to generate estimates of body fat from skinfold measurements. Because of the difficulties in obtaining measures of adiposity, much of the discussion in the 1960s and 1970s about weight–height indices was based on theoretical considerations or on comparisons of different indicators against population distributions of weight for height, not on comparisons with measures of adiposity. These discussions typically evaluated different values for the power of height in power-type indices of the general form W/H^p, generally including W/H, W/H^2 and some index using a power of 3, such as H/W$^{1/3}$.

An early attempt to address the issue of indices of adiposity (Billewicz et al., 1962) had adiposity data from densitometry only for 81 men and women from Taiwan and 98 American infantrymen in training, not enough for a detailed analysis. Therefore, Billewicz et al. (1962) primarily compared various functions of weight and height to the distribution of weight for height in several other population samples, making the assumption that, in a normal unselected population, the distribution of body weight at each level of height would reflect, in a general way, the distribution of adiposity. This is really the same problem of describing how weight varies with height that Quetelet had already addressed without making any assumptions about adiposity. Billewicz et al. (1962) concluded that, of the weight–height indices, Quetelet's index was the best approximation to adiposity but that a better approximation to adiposity would be to use the ratio of weight to standard weight from a life insurance table of standard weights for height.

As had Billewicz et al., Khosla and Lowe (1967) also evaluated weight–height indices in the absence of any measures of adiposity, simply by comparing them to the distributions of weight for height and inferring their relationship to adiposity from this comparison. They felt that Quetelet's index was the best and used it to compare groups within an industrial population that differed in height. This comparison demonstrated that the senior staff weighed more than the wage-earners because they were taller and thus not necessarily because they were more obese.

Other discussions similarly evaluated weight–height indices as indicators of adiposity despite not using any actual measures of adiposity. Evans and Prior (1969) extended Khosla and Lowe's approach to Rarotongans and Pukapukans, two Polynesian populations in the Cook Islands. They concluded that weight/height^2 was satisfactory as a method of adjusting weight for height within genetically homogeneous groups but that it should be interpreted with caution to compare different racial groups. Similar conclusions were reached by Lee, Kolonel, and Hinds (1981) who compared weight for height among five different ethnic groups in Hawai'i – Caucasians, Chinese, Filipinos, native Hawaiians, and Japanese – and felt that the relation of BMI to height differed across groups, therefore preferring the approach suggested by Benn (1971) of calculating a specific power of height for a given population to minimize correlations with height for an index.

Florey compared three different power-type indices but firmly rejected the idea that an index of weight and height could serve as a measure of adiposity: "One must conclude that the indices are at most weight corrected for height, and should not be used as indices of adiposity or physique in the belief that they are valid measures of these qualities" (Florey, 1970, p. 102). Florey felt that the appropriate nomenclature would be an "index of corrected weight" to remove any idea that these were indices of fatness and concluded that all three indices were poor measures of adiposity.

Quetelet's index gets a new name and a lukewarm recommendation

In 1972, American physiologist Ancel Keys studied four indicators of weight for height (three weight–height indices and the percent of standard weight-for-height) and their correlation with body fat, as assessed by skinfold measurements in a healthy all-male sample from five countries, including Japanese farmers and fishermen, Bantu workers in South Africa, university students and executives from Minnesota, railroad workers in Italy and the US, and samples of rural populations in Finland and Italy (Keys, Fidanza, Karvonen, Kimura, & Taylor,

1972). Of these indicators, he felt that the best was W/H^2, which he renamed the "body mass index" (BMI) and suggested as an approximate indicator of fatness for research purposes. But Keys' recommendation was lukewarm: "the body mass index, W/H^2, proves to be, if not fully satisfactory, at least as good as any other relative weight index as an indicator of relative obesity" (Keys, et al., p. 339). Keys rejected the idea of using BMI to label people as over-weight and characterized such value judgments as "scientifically indefensible" (1972, p. 341).

BMI categories began to be used as labels

Bray (1978) recommended a cut point for overweight at a BMI of 25 and for obesity at a BMI of 30. These values were loosely based on an adaptation of the 1959 Metropolitan Life tables from the "Obesity in Perspective" conference held in 1973 at the Fogarty Center (Bray, 1975). The value of 25 approximately corresponded to the top of the range of acceptable or recommended range of weights for height and the value of 30–120 percent of the top of the range. Garrow (1981) suggested that obesity be classified as follows: Grade 0, BMI 20–24.9; Grade I, BMI 25–29.9; Grade II, BMI 30–40; and Grade III, BMI > 40. He went on to say that "the choice of 25, 30 and 40 as boundaries between grades 0, I, II and III is arbitrary and can be justified only on grounds of convenience" (Garrow, 1981, p. 3). These arbitrary cut points at 5-unit or 10-unit intervals ending in 0 or 5 are more likely to represent a form of digit preference than to correspond to any specific biological reality. These recommendations were intermittently used but not considered definitive.

BMI continued to be just one among numerous possible indicators of weight for height. The *Obesity in America* conference held in 1977 at the Fogarty Center recommended the use of an adaptation of the 1959 Metropolitan Life insurance tables to evaluate relative weight for clinical purposes and suggested that investigators should in addition consider using the BMI (Bray, 1979). A 1982 workshop on body weight, health, and longevity sponsored by the Nutrition Coordinating Committee of the National Institutes of Health (NIH) and the Centers for Disease Control (CDC) recommended that, in order to establish age-related desirable weights, data on weight and height should be analysed and presented separately by sex, age, and duration of follow-up, with age divided by decades (Simopoulos & Van Itallie, 1984). The committee also recommended that data on weight and height be additionally expressed as the BMI with a median, range, and standard deviation presented for each age and gender group.

Explicit definitions of overweight in terms of BMI were created in 1985 and began to be used for US government publications and research studies. In 1985, as part of its series of consensus conferences on a wide variety of topics, NIH convened a short conference on the health effects of obesity (*Health Implications*, 1985). As part of this effort, the panel investigated several methods to express weight adjusted for height, such as weight–height tables, and suggested that physicians consider the use of BMI as an additional factor in evaluating patients. The panel described BMI as a simple measurement that minimized the effect of height and would be useful for descriptive or evaluative purposes. This recommendation, along with Keys' observations, contributed to the gradual adoption of BMI over the next decade as a standard international measure of weight for height for adults. A practical factor at the time that limited the use of BMI was the difficulty in calculating such an index before the advent of pocket calculators; thus, the panel recommended that nomograms be used to facilitate calculations of body mass index.

The 1985 conference recommended a definition of overweight as a BMI equal to or greater than 27.8 for men or 27.3 for women. To arrive at this definition, the panel combined information from life insurance tables with national survey data on measured weight and height. These BMI cutoffs represented the sex-specific 85th percentile of the BMI distribution for persons aged 20–29 years in the second National Health and Nutrition Examination Survey (NHANES II). The rationale for selecting this age group as the reference population was that young adults are relatively lean, and the increase in body weight that usually occurs with age is due almost entirely to fat accumulation. The panel also noted that these values corresponded approximately to a weight 20 percent above the midpoint of the sex-specific median weight range across all heights for a medium frame in the 1983 Metropolitan Life weight-for-height tables (MLIC, 1983). These definitions were adopted within the US government and widely used within the US, but not elsewhere.

There was still no real consensus over what categories to use (Kuczmarski & Flegal, 2000). The overweight criteria based on the BMI cutoffs of ≥27.8 for men and ≥27.3 for women were used to report the prevalence of overweight among US adults in every annual edition of the government publication "Health United States" beginning in 1985 and continuing through 1998. The quinquennial US Dietary Guidelines, beginning in 1980, conformed pretty closely to a BMI of 25 as the dividing line to define overweight (Flegal, Troiano, & Ballard-Barbash, 2001). Yet, different BMI levels were suggested in the report "Diet and Health: Implications for Reducing Chronic Disease Risk" (National Research Council, 1989), which suggested a "desirable BMI" of 20–25 for those 25–34 years old, increasing with age to a desirable BMI of 24–29 for those over 65.

Weight loss treatments become a medical issue

Weight loss was not always seen as a salient medical issue (Maddox, Anderson, & Bogdonoff, 1966; Maddox & Liederman, 1969; Puhl & Brownell, 2001). For tax purposes, the IRS did not allow costs of weight loss as a medical deduction until 2002. Health insurance did not cover weight loss treatments (Gibbs, 1995). Research showed that, in more than half of doctor visits, weight and height were not even measured (Graham, 2012). A timeline review (Kyle, Dhurandhar, & Allison, 2016) shows the changes that took place over time to further the concept of obesity first as a medical issue and then as a disease.

Weight-loss drugs had a checkered history (Colman, 2005). It was difficult to define clinical efficacy, and there were concerns about possible side effects. Fenfluramine had been approved in 1973, but only for short-term use. Renewed interest in weight-loss drugs increased in the 1990s with the advent of several new drugs. The drug combination fenfluramine/phentermine, known as fen-phen, was an anti-obesity treatment that utilized two anorectics (Weintraub, 1992a, 1992b). In addition to popularizing off-label use of these two drugs, the fen-phen studies began a transition from short-term to long-term drug treatment of obesity. The first drug to garner Food and Drug Administration (FDA) approval in the US for the long-term treatment of obesity was dexfenfluramine, an isomer of fenfluramine. In 1996, dexfenfluramine (marketed as Redux) was approved for longer term use. The use of these medicines exploded, with approximately 14 million prescriptions written for fenfluramine or dexfenfluramine from 1995 until they were withdrawn for safety reasons in 1997 (Yanovski, 2005). Although these medicines were intended for weight loss, 25 percent or more of users were not overweight (Blanck, Khan, & Serdula, 2004; Khan, Serdula, Bowman, & Williamson, 2001). Other medications appeared. Sibutramine, a norepinephrine and serotonin reuptake inhibitor, marketed in the US as Meridia, was approved by the FDA in 1997 but withdrawn in 2010 for safety reasons. Orlistat, marketed by Roche as Xenical, was approved by the FDA in 1999. Xenical was described as a potential blockbuster by an industry analyst who predicted that the market could be between $5 billion and $10 billion (Sharpe, 1999). Sales, however, proved disappointing.

The limited medical concern for obesity was seen as a barrier for wider acceptance of the use of weight-loss medications. According to a Reuters report (Bruton, 2000) entitled "Quest for blockbuster obesity drug vexes firms," companies believed that, for drugs like Xenical and Meridia to reach their potential, the possibility of a pharmaceutical treatment for obesity had to be more widely accepted. Many consumers still saw obesity more as a cosmetic concern than as a health issue. The Reuters report quoted Terence Hurley, a Roche spokesman, as saying "Part of our challenge moving forward with Xenical is to "medicalize" weight management to physicians."

WHO and NIH use BMI to define "obesity"

An important step towards international standardization occurred in 1993. A World Health Organization (WHO) expert committee met in Geneva for a week and produced a lengthy report on the uses of anthropometry (body measurements) to assess health and nutritional conditions including malnutrition, stunting, thinness, and overweight for all segments of the population – from newborn infants to older adults ("Physical Status", 1995). For adults, the panel used BMI to define three grades of overweight. They selected the tidy cut points of 25, 30, and 40, describing the method used to establish cut-off points as largely arbitrary and noting that Grade 2 overweight (BMI 30–40) was relatively common in industrialized countries. The panel noted that, "in essence, it has been based upon visual inspection of the relationship between BMI and mortality; the cut-off of 30 is based on the point of flexion of the curve" ("Physical Status", 1995, p. 313). No reference was provided for this statement. The expert committee defined obesity as the degree of fat storage associated with clearly elevated health risks but noted the lack of scientific consensus on exactly what level of fat this might be. They stated explicitly, "there are no clearly established cut-off points for fat mass or fat percentage that can be translated into cut-offs for BMI" ("Physical Status", 1995, p. 312). The panel did not offer any definition of obesity in terms of BMI.

In 1995, the International Obesity Task Force (IOTF, now called World Obesity Policy & Prevention) was formed by Philip James, the then director of the Rowett Research Institute (World Obesity Federation, n.d.). The object of this self-appointed task force, funded primarily by the pharmaceutical industry (Moynihan, 2006a), was to persuade the WHO to convene a special consultation in Geneva that would be solely devoted to obesity (W. P. James, 2008). The IOTF's mission was to inform the world about the urgency of the problem and to persuade governments that now was the time to act. WHO was initially reluctant but agreed to hold the consultation on the condition that it be delayed for six months. Eventually, WHO convened a three-day expert consultation on obesity in 1997, resulting in a lengthy report published in 2000 (WHO, 2000). The consultation received a substantial grant from the IOTF (W. P. T. James, 2002), and the IOTF itself prepared the draft report for the consultation, which was accepted with only minor modifications. The final WHO report largely followed the IOTF document.

The publication of the official report of the WHO consultation was delayed (W. P. James, 2008). The proposal had not been part of the WHO usual planning process nor agreed to by the WHO Executive Board. However, subsequent discussions with the then-WHO Executive Director resulted in WHO deciding to publish the report as part of the WHO Technical Report Series, "Obesity: Preventing and Managing the Global Epidemic" (2000). Due to backlogs in report preparation, the Technical Report Series publication was delayed.

However, WHO agreed to issue an interim document in 1998 ("Obesity: Preventing and Managing the Global Epidemic", 1998) that differed slightly from the final version. The IOTF sent free copies of the interim document directly to every Minister of Health in the 192 WHO member countries and to other interested persons and organizations. In the interim version of the report, WHO expressed deep appreciation for both the financial and technical contributions of the IOTF in convening the consultation.

The 1997 WHO consultation made a key terminological change from the 1995 WHO report. The section on BMI included a table on the classification and described it as being "in agreement" with the 1995 WHO report. In fact, although the BMI cut points were the same (with an additional cut point at 35.0), the terminology was not. The 1997 consultation decided to use the term "obesity" instead of "overweight" for BMI values of 30 or above, with little explanation or justification for the change. BMI, heretofore a simple indicator of weight adjusted for height, was transformed into the definition of excess fat.

In 1995, NIH had convened an expert panel to develop clinical practice guidelines for primary care practitioners, reviewing relevant scientific literature through 1997 ("Clinical Guidelines", 1998). The NIH panel overlapped with the IOTF to some degree, with the chair of the panel and several members also being members of the IOTF (International Obesity Task Force, 2000). The NIH panel adopted the same cut points for BMI and almost the same terminology as the 1997 WHO definition, citing the then as yet unpublished WHO report as the source for these definitions.

Suddenly, the US government was defining "obesity" as a BMI of 30 or above. Overnight, millions of Americans were classified into an ominous new category. The new cut points were described in the *New York Times* as providing the pharmaceutical industry with "a booming new market for diet pills for the obese, practically served to the companies on a silver platter by the government" (Stolberg, 1999). The new definitions also expanded the definition of overweight to include BMIs of 25 and 26. Some critics, including the former surgeon general C. Everett Koop, urged the panel not to broaden the definition of overweight, saying "it will confuse the public and the medical community. It needlessly stigmatizes millions of Americans and lacks a solid scientific rationale" (Squires, 1998).

Overweight is one of the conditions discussed by Schwartz and Woloshin (1999), where expanding disease definitions have increased prevalences of relatively common conditions. A later example of expanding disease definitions had to do with BMI categories for children and adolescents. The BMI range called "overweight" for children was renamed as "obese" in 2007 with little rationale (Moynihan, 2006b; Ogden & Flegal, 2010).

Reimbursement for treating obesity

In the 1990s and earlier, insurance coverage for treatment of obesity was limited (Gibbs, 1995), in part because of language in the US Medicare Coverage Issues Manual that stated bluntly: "Obesity itself cannot be considered an illness… Program payment may not be made for treatment of obesity alone since this treatment is not reasonable and necessary for the diagnosis or treatment of an illness or injury" (National Coverage Determination, n.d.). In 2001, an IOTF member who had joined the Centers for Disease Control and Prevention (CDC) organized and chaired a meeting at CDC entitled "Including Obesity Treatment in Benefit Plans" on the topic of reimbursement of health care providers for obesity treatment. Following the recommendations from this workshop, CDC put in a formal request to the Centers for Medicare and Medicaid Services (CMS) that this language be removed from the manual because it was a barrier to insurance coverage for treatment of obesity. The language was removed in 2004 ("National Coverage Determination"). Versions 1 through 4 of the coverage determination documents are accessible through CMS ("National Coverage Determination", n.d.).

This critical move opened the door for providers to get reimbursed for obesity treatments and for health insurance to cover anti-obesity medications. Stern, Kazaks, and Downey (2005) assessed the acceptance of obesity as a chronic disease and acceptance of its treatment by health management organizations, private insurers, and the government as a major reimbursement challenge. Baum et al. (2015) felt that although financial incentives and attitudes towards obesity management were changing, continuing limitations to reimbursement included perceptions of modest efficacy by patients and physicians alike, historical safety issues and regulatory obstacles. Oliver opined that "the disease characterization has less to do with the health consequences of excess weight and more with the various financial and political incentives of the weight loss industry, medical profession, and public health bureaucracy" (Oliver, 2006, p. 611).

When did obesity become a disease?

Obesity was sometimes but not always seen as a disease. Bray in 1978 asserted that "obesity is a symptom of disease, like hypertension, anemia or fever, not a disease itself" (Bray, 1978, p. 102). References to obesity as a disease began to creep into the literature. The summary of the 1985 NIH conference alluded indirectly to obesity as a disease ("Health Implications", 1985). Just over a decade later, the 1998 NIH guidelines stated forthrightly, "Obesity is a complex multifactorial chronic disease" ("Clinical Guidelines", p xi). The Obesity Society (TOS) in the US (Allison et al., 2008) and the World Obesity Federation (Bray, Kim, & Wilding, 2017) also endorsed the view that obesity should be considered a disease. In 2013, the American Medical Association (AMA) recognized obesity as a chronic disease (AMA, 2013a, p. 461), although the AMA's own Council on Science and Public Health had recommended against adopting the resolution (AMA, 2013b, pp. 335–343). European guidelines also endorsed the view of obesity as a disease (Yumuk et al., 2015; Frühbeck et al., 2019), not without some discussion (Müller & Geisler, 2017; Vallgarda et al., 2017).

Obesity becomes a disease – but what is obesity?

Discussions of obesity as a disease typically include extensive discussions of the definition of a disease but little or no discussion of the definition of obesity. According to the 1985 conference report, "Obesity is an excess of body fat frequently resulting in a significant impairment of health" ("Health Implications", 1985, p. 1073) but "because the amount of body fat… is a continuous variable within the population, all quantitative definitions of obesity must be arbitrary" ("Health Implications", 1985, p. 1074). WHO states "Overweight and obesity are defined as abnormal or excessive fat accumulation that may impair health" (WHO, 2020). But how is an excess of body fat defined? And what health impairments are involved?

Bray (1976) noted the major difficulties in identifying how much body fat should be considered obese and suggested that, as a working guideline, men with more than 20 percent fat and women with more than 28 percent fat should probably be considered obese. The report from the 1977 conference at the Fogarty Center (Bray, 1979) noted that, once a measurement of body fat was established, there was still the problem of interpreting the results because no one knew how much body fat was normal or desirable. The 1995 report from the WHO expert committee similarly noted the lack of any consensus ("Physical Status",

1995, p. 420). One set of standards was developed by Lohman, Houtkooper, & Going (1997), who estimated percent body fat with prediction equations applied to triceps and subscapular skinfold measurements in NHANES. They then presented age and sex-specific percent body fat standards based on the population distribution of the values of the estimated percent fat, although it is not clear how these standards were determined. In a comprehensive literature review of the performance of anthropometric measurements relative to body fat reference standards, Sommer et al. (2020) found that the cut-offs for the reference tests ranged from ≥ 30 percent to ≥ 43 percent body fat in women and from ≥ 20 percent to ≥ 34.6 percent in men using DXA, with most studies using a body fat percentage >35 percent in women and > 25 percent in men as the standard for defining obesity (similar but not identical to the Lohman criteria). Sommer et al. note that despite the wide use of these and other cut-offs, cut-offs were chosen arbitrarily and not necessarily with any scientific basis.

Even though it is unclear where these body fat criteria come from or why they should be considered to represent obesity, numerous articles, as reviewed by Sommer et al. (2020), have compared a BMI of 30 or above to body fat criteria and found that not only do most people with BMI of 30 meet the body fat criteria for obesity but also many people with BMI below 30 also meet these criteria, sometimes leading to the suggestion that the BMI criteria for obesity should be lowered. For instance, Blew et al. (2002) suggest that BMI >25 rather than BMI > 30 may be superior for diagnosing obesity in postmenopausal women.

In fact, it is clear that obesity considered as the degree of fat storage associated with elevated health risks does not have an exact definition. Rather, the level of body fat associated with health risks varies considerably. According to a 2011 scientific statement from the American Heart Association (Cornier et al., 2011), at a given BMI, there is a significant variability in individual body fatness and the associated risk for health conditions. This variability is related to factors such as age, sex, genetics, and ethnicity, but it is also a result of differences in body fat distribution and composition. Similarly, a 2017 statement from two professional endocrinology societies states that, scientifically speaking, BMI is a poor predictor of health and is inadequate as the sole guide for clinical decision-making. BMI at any level is not clinically sufficient as a medical diagnosis of disease for a given individual (Mechanick, Hurley, & Garvey, 2017).

Florey cautioned in 1970 that BMI and other indices should not be used as measures of adiposity. In 1972, Keys gave BMI a lukewarm recommendation and pointed out that it was "scientifically unacceptable" to use BMI to define overweight. Nonetheless, despite these early cautions, BMI came into widespread use as a measure of adiposity and was used to define overweight and obesity. Going full circle, BMI then became the target of numerous commentaries that criticized it for not measuring body composition and for being a poor measure of obesity (e.g., Ahima & Lazar, 2013; Blundell, Dulloo, Salvador, & Fruhbeck, 2014; Burkhauser & Cawley, 2008; Flint & Rimm, 2006; Franzosi, 2006; Gonzalez, Correia, & Heymsfield, 2017; Green, 2016; Kahn & Bullard, 2016; Kragelund & Omland, 2005; Müller, Braun, Enderle, & Bosy-Westphal, 2016).

Some attempts to clarify and rationalize definitions of obesity continue to use the BMI cut points of 25 and 30 but add additional criteria. These include the Edmonton Obesity Staging System developed by Sharma and Kushner (2009), the proposed definition by Garvey and Mechanick (2020) as Adiposity-based Chronic Disease (ABCD), and the European approach described by Hebebrand et al. (2017). All these approaches conserve the use of BMI as a measure of adiposity and continue to use the same BMI categories. There is little critical discussion of the cut point of 30 as opposed to other possible higher or lower cut points; rather, the value of 30 seems to be accepted uncritically, demonstrating the proposition that, once a label is established, there is a tendency to accept it rather than examine its accuracy (Foroni & Rothbart, 2013).

There is also little discussion of labelling people as having or not having a "normal weight" or "healthy weight" also simply on the basis of their BMI, although there is no clear definition of either of these terms either. In many, if not most countries in North America, Europe, and Latin America, well over half the population is above "normal" weight, calling into question what normal means in this context. In the context of BMI categories, "normal" is associated with younger people, people of white or Asian ethnicity, and wealthier people. The NIH report states, "Overweight and obesity are especially evident in some minority groups, as well as in those with lower incomes and less education" ("Clinical Guidelines", p. xi). In fact, a common finding is that people in the overweight category of BMI have the same or slightly lower mortality as those in the normal weight category (Flegal, Kit, Orpana, & Graubard, 2013). The entire concept of a single normal or healthy weight applicable across age, sex, and ethnicity groupings and even across the lifespan for a given individual has been criticized (Dixon, Egger, Finkelstein, Kral, & Lambert et al., 2015).

It would appear that the general population does not necessarily agree with the BMI categories promulgated by WHO and NIH. This is sometimes referred to as "misperception," but it might better be called "disagreement." In Denmark, 70 percent of men and 50 percent of women who self-reported a BMI of 25 or above did not view themselves as overweight (Matthiessen et al., 2014). In Mauritius, where 50 percent of adults were classified as overweight or obese, 45 percent of overweight or obese men by the WHO categories and 38 percent of women misclassified their status (Caleyachetty, Kengne, Muennig, Rutter, & Echouffo-Tcheugui, 2016). Misclassification was higher among those who reported their health as good or excellent. In England, almost 30 percent of those with BMI levels at or above 25 underestimated their status relative to the WHO categories, with higher proportions of minority groups underestimating their status (Muttarak, 2018). In a large representative Canadian sample (Herman, Hopman, & Rosenberg, 2013), 40 percent of men and 16 percent of women who reported an overweight or obese BMI classified their weight as "about right." On the other hand, 21 percent of women who reported a BMI in the "healthy weight range" classified themselves as overweight. In a qualitative study of older people in a relatively affluent rural area of the US, researchers found that participants, all with BMI levels of 30 or above, did not accept the designation of obesity as a disease, and many rejected the label of "obese" outright (Batsis et al., 2021). Researchers seem baffled by why lay people do not agree with their scientific categorizations, even suggesting in one case that perhaps misperception has increased because of improvements in fashion design for overweight women (Muttarak, 2018).

Limitations and issues with current uses of BMI

BMI is a simple way to adjust weight for height, useful for descriptive purposes and to facilitate comparisons of weight among people of different heights. It slowly became medicalized and ultimately became used as the definition of a disease. This is far from its original purpose and far from its original meaning. Because it is easy to measure and calculate, BMI creates a "streetlight effect" – a type of observational bias, whereby we look for our lost keys where the light is brightest. Attempts at international standardization have resulted in the creation and overuse of arbitrary BMI categories that don't identify the same level of health risks across individuals or populations. These categories have become used to arrive at population estimates that are in effect diagnoses of disease based solely on height and weight.

People are classified as having a disease without having ever received a diagnosis and indeed often without any medical encounter at all; yet, the estimates are treated as though they represented the prevalence of a clinically diagnosed disease. BMI is not a good measure of fat mass, but a number of studies (e.g., Han et al., 2010; Spahillari et al., 2016; Srikanthan, Horwich, & Tseng, 2016) have found that low muscle mass is more of a risk than high fat mass. Bosy-Westphal and Müller (2021) suggest that obesity should not even be considered as a question of body fat per se but should be addressed in terms of body composition, and that the use of both BMI and of body fat percentage should be avoided. They call for a new paradigm focused on fat-free mass instead and point out that, at older ages, a higher BMI may indicate more adequate fat-free mass.

Even though the many limitations of BMI are well known, and BMI is often criticized, that hasn't stopped its widespread use for purposes well beyond those for which it was intended. BMI, a simple measure of weight adjusted for height, has undergone considerable elaboration and transformation to now serve as a measure of disease, enmeshed in a complex web of medical, social, and commercial interests. The fixation on BMI may distract attention from more important aspects of health and disease.

Notes

1 **Brief explanation of Quetelet's derivation**

Let H_S be the average height of the shortest men and H_T be the average height of the tallest men. Let W_S be the average weight of the shortest men and W_T be the average weight of the tallest men. Quetelet observed that $H_S/H_T = 5/6$ and that the ratio of (W_S/H_S) to (W_T/H_T) was also 5/6. Therefore, $H_S/H_T = (W_S/H_S)/(W_T/H_T)$. Applying elementary algebra to rearrange the terms, multiplying both sides of the equation by H_S and dividing both sides by H_T show that $(H_S$ squared$)/(H_T$ squared$) = W_S/W_T$. Thus, as Quetelet observed, the ratio of weights at different heights is proportional to the ratio of the square of the heights. Now dividing both sides by H_S squared and multiplying both sides by W_T show that $W_S/(H_S$ squared$) = W_T/(H_T$ squared$)$.

References

Ahima, R. S., & Lazar, M. A. (2013). Physiology. The health risk of obesity – better metrics imperative. *Science, 341*(6148), 856–858. doi:10.1126/science.1241244

Allison, D. B., Downey, M., Atkinson, R. L., Billington, C. J., Bray, G. A., Eckel, R. H., ... Tremblay, A. (2008). Obesity as a disease: A white paper on evidence and arguments commissioned by the Council of the Obesity Society. *Obesity, 16*(6), 1161–1177. doi:10.1038/oby.2008.231

American Medical Association (2013a). Resolution 420 – Recognition of obesity as a disease. *Proceedings of the 2013 Annual Meeting.* https://www.ama-assn.org/sites/ama-assn.org/files/corp/media-browser/public/hod/a13-resolutions_0.pdf

American Medical Association (2013b). Is obesity a disease? Report of the Council on Science and Public Health. *Proceedings of the 2013 Annual Meeting.* https://www.ama-assn.org/sites/ama-assn.org/files/corp/media-browser/public/hod/a13-csaph-reports_0.pdf

Andres, R., Elahi, D., Tobin, J. D., Muller, D. C., & Brant, L. (1985). Impact of age on weight goals. *Annals of Internal Medicine, 103*(6,Pt 2), 1030–1033. doi:10.7326/0003–4819-103–6–1030

Armstrong, D. B., Dublin, L. I., Wheatley, G. M., & Marks, H. H. (1951). Obesity and its relation to health and disease. *Journal of the American Medical Association, 147*(11), 1007–1014. doi:10.1001/jama.1951.03670280009003

Batsis, J. A., Zagaria, A. B., Brooks, E., Clark, M. M., Phelan, S., Lopez-Jimenez, F., ... Carpenter-Song, E. (2021). The use and meaning of the term obesity in rural older adults: A qualitative study. *Journal of Applied Gerontology, 40*(4), 423–432. doi:10.1177/0733464820903253

Baum, C., Andino, K., Wittbrodt, E., Stewart, S., Szymanski, K., & Turpin, R. (2015). The challenges and opportunities associated with reimbursement for obesity pharmacotherapy in the USA. *Pharmacoeconomics, 33*(7), 643–653. doi:10.1007/s40273-015-0264-0

Benn, R. T. (1971). Some mathematical properties of weight-for-height indices used as measures of adiposity. *British Journal of Preventive and Social Medicine, 25*(1), 42–50. doi:10.1136/jech.25.1.42

Billewicz, W. Z., Kemsley, W. F., & Thomson, A. M. (1962). Indices of adiposity. *British Journal of Preventive and Social Medicine, 16*, 183–188. doi:10.1136/jech.16.4.183

Blanck, H. M., Khan, L. K., & Serdula, M. K. (2004). Prescription weight loss pill use among Americans: Patterns of pill use and lessons learned from the fen-phen market withdrawal. *Preventive Medicine, 39*(6), 1243–1248. doi:10.1016/j.ypmed.2004.04.040

Blew, R. M., Sardinha, L. B., Milliken, L. A., Teixeira, P. J., Going, S. B., Ferreira, D. L., … Lohman, T. G. (2002). Assessing the validity of body mass index standards in early postmenopausal women. *Obesity Research, 10*(8), 799–808. doi:10.1038/oby.2002.108

Blundell, J. E., Dulloo, A. G., Salvador, J., & Fruhbeck, G. (2014). Beyond BMI--phenotyping the obesities. *Obesity Facts, 7*(5), 322–328. doi:10.1159/000368783

Bosy-Westphal, A., & Müller, M. J. (2021). Diagnosis of obesity based on body composition-associated health risks – Time for a change in paradigm. *Obesity Reviews, 22*(Suppl 2), e13190. doi:10.1111/obr.13190

Bray, G. A. (Ed.) (1975). *Obesity in perspective*, Fogarty International Center Series on Preventive Medicine. (NIH publication 75–708.) Washington, DC: Government Printing Office.

Bray, G. A. (1976). *The obese patient* (Vol. IX). Philadelphia, PA: W. B. Saunders.

Bray, G. A. (1978). Definition, measurement, and classification of the syndromes of obesity. *International Journal of Obesity, 2*(2), 99–112.

Bray, G. A. (Ed.) (1979). *Obesity in America* (NIH Publication No. 79–359 ed.). Washington, DC: Government Printing Office.

Bray, G. A., Kim, K. K., & Wilding, J. P. H. (2017). Obesity: A chronic relapsing progressive disease process. A position statement of the World Obesity Federation. *Obesity Reviews, 18*(7), 715–723. doi:10.1111/obr.12551

Bruton, F. B. (2000, August 16). Quest for blockbuster obesity drug vexes firms. *Reuters Health eLine News.*

Burkhauser, R. V., & Cawley, J. (2008). Beyond BMI: The value of more accurate measures of fatness and obesity in social science research. *Journal of Health Economics, 27*(2), 519–529. doi:10.1016/j.jhealeco.2007.05.005

Caleyachetty, R., Kengne, A. P., Muennig, P., Rutter, H., & Echouffo-Tcheugui, J. B. (2016). Misperception of body weight among overweight or obese adults in Mauritius. *Obesity Research & Clinical Practice, 10*(2), 216–219. doi:10.1016/j.orcp.2016.02.006

Clinical guidelines on the identification, evaluation, and treatment of overweight and obesity in adults: Executive summary. Expert Panel on the identification, evaluation, and treatment of overweight in adults. (1998). *American Journal of Clinical Nutrition, 68*(4), 899–917. doi:10.1093/ajcn/68.4.899

Colman, E. (2005). Anorectics on trial: A half century of federal regulation of prescription appetite suppressants. *Annals of Internal Medicine, 143*(5), 380–385. doi:10.7326/0003-4819-143-5-200509060-00013

Cornier, M. A., Despres, J. P., Davis, N., Grossniklaus, D. A., Klein, S., Lamarche, B., … Poirier, P. (2011). Assessing adiposity: A scientific statement from the American Heart Association. *Circulation, 124.* doi:10.1161/CIR.0b013e318233bc6a.

Czerniawski, A. M. (2007). From average to ideal, the evolution of the height and weight table in the United States, 1936–1943. *Social Science History, 31*(2), 173–296.

Davenport, C. B. (1920). Height-weight index of build. *America Journal of Physical Anthropology, III*(4), 467–475.

Dixon, J. B., Egger, G. J., Finkelstein, E. A., Kral, J. G., & Lambert, G. W. (2015). 'Obesity paradox' misunderstands the biology of optimal weight throughout the life cycle. *International Journal of Obesity, 39*(1), 82–84. doi:10.1038/ijo.2014.59

Eknoyan, G. (2008). Adolphe Quetelet (1796–1874) – the average man and indices of obesity. *Nephrology, Dialysis, Transplantation, 23*(1), 47–51. doi:10.1093/ndt/gfm517

Evans, J. G., & Prior, I. A. (1969). Indices of obesity derived from height and weight in two Polynesian populations. *British Journal of Preventive and Social Medicine, 23*(1), 56–59. doi:10.1136/jech.23.1.56

Flegal, K. M., Kit, B. K., Orpana, H., & Graubard, B. I. (2013). Association of all-cause mortality with overweight and obesity using standard body mass index categories: A systematic review and meta-analysis. *JAMA, 309*(1), 71–82. doi:10.1001/jama.2012.113905

Flegal, K. M., Troiano, R. P., & Ballard-Barbash, R. (2001). Aim for a healthy weight: What is the target? *Journal of Nutrition, 131*(2S-1), 440S-450S. doi:10.1093/jn/131.2.440S

Flint, A. J., & Rimm, E. B. (2006). Commentary: Obesity and cardiovascular disease risk among the young and old – is BMI the wrong benchmark? *International Journal of Epidemiology, 35*(1), 187–189. doi:10.1093/ije/dyi298

Florey, C. d. V. (1970). The use and interpretation of ponderal index and other weight–height ratios in epidemiological studies. *Journal of Chronic Diseases, 23*(2), 93–103. doi:10.1016/0021–9681(70)90068-8

Forbes, G. B. (1999). Body composition: overview. *Journal of Nutrition, 129*(1S Suppl), 270s–272s. doi:10.1093/jn/129.1.270S

Foroni, F., & Rothbart, M. (2013). Abandoning a label doesn't make it disappear: The perseverance of labeling effects. *Journal of Experimental Social Psychology, 49*(1), 126–131. doi:10.1016/j.jesp.2012.08.002

Franzosi, M. G. (2006). Should we continue to use BMI as a cardiovascular risk factor? *Lancet, 368*(9536), 624–625. doi:10.1016/S0140–6736(06)69222-2

Frühbeck, G., Busetto, L., Dicker, D., Yumuk, V., Goossens, G. H., Hebebrand, J., … Toplak, H. (2019). The ABCD of obesity: An EASO position statement on a diagnostic term with clinical and scientific implications. *Obesity Facts, 12*(2), 131–136. doi:10.1159/000497124

Garrow, J. S. (1981). *Treat obesity seriously: A clinical manual.* Edinburgh: Churchill Livingston.

Garvey, W. T., & Mechanick, J. I. (2020). Proposal for a scientifically correct and medically actionable disease classification system (ICD) for obesity. *Obesity, 28*(3), 484–492. doi:10.1002/oby.22727

Gibbs, W. W. (1995). Treatment that tightens the belt. Is insurance part of America's obesity problem? *Scientific American, 272*(3), 34–35. doi:10.1038/scientificamerican0395-34a

Gonzalez, M. C., Correia, M., & Heymsfield, S. B. (2017). A requiem for BMI in the clinical setting. *Current Opinion in Clinical Nutrition & Metabolic Care, 20*(5), 314–321. doi:10.1097/MCO.0000000000000395

Gould, B. A. (1869). *Investigations in the military and anthropological statistics of American soldiers.* Cambridge: Riverside Press.

Graham, J. (2012, May 12). Height, weight – BMI? Doctors urged to treat body mass index as a vital sign. *Kaiser Health News.* https://www.washingtonpost.com/national/health-science/height-weight--bmi-doctors-urged-to-treat-body-mass-index-as-a-vital-sign/2012/05/12/gIQAbFbJLU_story.html

Gray, H., & Mayall, J. F. (1920). Body weight in two hundred and twenty-nine adults: Which standard is the best? *Archives of Internal Medicine, 26*(2), 133–152.

Green, M. A. (2016). Do we need to think beyond BMI for estimating population-level health risks? *Journal of Public Health, 38*(1), 192–193. doi:10.1093/pubmed/fdv007

Han, S. S., Kim, K. W., Kim, K. I., Na, K. Y., Chae, D. W., Kim, S., & Chin, H. J. (2010). Lean mass index: A better predictor of mortality than body mass index in elderly Asians. *Journal of the American Geriatric Society, 58*(2), 312–317. doi:10.1111/j.1532–5415.2009.02672.x

Harrison, G. G. (1985). Height–weight tables. *Annals of Internal Medicine, 103*(6, Pt 2), 989–994. doi:10.7326/0003–4819-103–6–989

Health implications of obesity. National Institutes of Health Consensus Development Conference Statement. (1985). *Annals of Internal Medicine, 103*(6 (Pt 2)), 1073–1077.

Hebebrand, J., Holm, J. C., Woodward, E., Baker, J. L., Blaak, E., Durrer Schutz, D., … Yumuk, V. (2017). A proposal of the European Association for the Study of Obesity to improve the ICD-11 diagnostic criteria for obesity based on the three dimensions etiology, degree of adiposity and health risk. *Obesity Facts, 10*(4), 284–307. doi:10.1159/000479208

Herman, K. M., Hopman, W. M., & Rosenberg, M. W. (2013). Self-rated health and life satisfaction among Canadian adults: Associations of perceived weight status versus BMI. *Quality of Life Research, 22*(10), 2693–2705. doi:10.1007/s11136-013-0394–9

International Obesity Task Force. (2000). Retrieved from http://web.archive.org/web/20000116082415/http://www.iotf.org/profiles/members.htm

James, W. P. (2008). WHO recognition of the global obesity epidemic. *International Journal of Obesity, 32*(Suppl 7), S120–126. doi:10.1038/ijo.2008.247

James, W. P. T. (2002). As IASO and IOTF prepare the final stages of creating a "seamless" integrated organization, Philip James reflects on progress since Paris. *Obesity Newsletter, International Association for the Study of Obesity, 4*(2), 8–9. Retrieved from http://web.archive.org/web/20050303201700/http://www.iaso.org/

Jarrett, R. J. (1986). Is there an ideal body weight? *British Medical Journal (Clinical Research Edition), 293*(6545), 493–495.

Kahn, H. S., & Bullard, K. M. (2016). Beyond body mass index: Advantages of abdominal measurements for recognizing cardiometabolic disorders. *American Journal of Medicine, 129*(1), 74–81.e72. doi:10.1016/j.amjmed.2015.08.010

Keys, A., Fidanza, F., Karvonen, M. J., Kimura, N., & Taylor, H. L. (1972). Indices of relative weight and obesity. *Journal of Chronic Diseases, 25*(6), 329–343. doi:10.1016/0021–9681(72)90027-6

Khan, L. K., Serdula, M. K., Bowman, B. A., & Williamson, D. F. (2001). Use of prescription weight loss pills among U.S. adults in 1996–1998. *Annals of Internal Medicine, 134*(4), 282–286. doi:10.7326/0003–4819-134-4-200102200-00011

Khosla, T., & Lowe, C. R. (1967). Indices of obesity derived from body weight and height. *British Journal of Preventive and Social Medicine, 21*(3), 122–128. doi:10.1136/jech.21.3.122

Knapp, T. R. (1983). A methodological critique of the 'ideal weight' concept. *JAMA, 250*(4), 506–510.

Kragelund, C., & Omland, T. (2005). A farewell to body-mass index? *Lancet, 366*(9497), 1589–1591. doi:10.1016/S0140–6736(05)67642-8

Kuczmarski, R. J., & Flegal, K. M. (2000). Criteria for definition of overweight in transition: Background and recommendations for the United States. *American Journal of Clinical Nutrition, 72*(5), 1074–1081. doi:10.1093/ajcn/72.5.1074

Kyle, T. K., Dhurandhar, E. J., & Allison, D. B. (2016). Regarding obesity as a disease: Evolving policies and their implications. *Endocrinology and Metabolism Clinics of North America, 45*(3), 511–520. doi:10.1016/j.ecl.2016.04.004

Laurent, I., Astère, M., Paul, B., Liliane, N., Li, Y., Cheng, Q., ... Xiao, X. (2020). The use of Broca index to assess cut- off points for overweight in adults: A short review. *Reviews in Endocrine & Metabolic Disorders, 21*(4), 521–526. doi:10.1007/s11154-020-09566-5

Lee, J., Kolonel, L. N., & Hinds, M. W. (1981). Relative merits of the weight-corrected-for-height indices. *American Journal of Clinical Nutrition, 34*(11), 2521–2529. doi:10.1093/ajcn/34.11.2521

Livi, R. (1898). L'indice ponderale o rapporto tra la statura e il peso [The weighting index or rapport between stature and weight]. *Rivista di antropologia, V,* 125–153.

Lohman, T. G., Houtkooper, L. B., & Going, S. (1997). Body fat measurement goes high-tech. *ACSM's Health and Wellness, 1*(1), 30–35.

Maddox, G. L., Anderson, C. F., & Bogdonoff, M. D. (1966). Overweight as a problem of medical management in a public outpatient clinic. *American Journal of the Medical Sciences, 252*(4), 394–403. doi:10.1097/00000441–196610000-00003

Maddox, G. L., & Liederman, V. (1969). Overweight as a social disability with medical implications. *Journal of Medical Education, 44*(3), 214–220. doi:10.1097/00001888–196903000-00009

Matthiessen, J., Biltoft-Jensen, A., Fagt, S., Knudsen, V. K., Tetens, I., & Groth, M. V. (2014). Misperception of body weight among overweight Danish adults: Trends from 1995 to 2008. *Public Health Nutrition, 17*(7), 1439–1446. doi:10.1017/s1368980013001444

Mechanick, J. I., Hurley, D. L., & Garvey, W. T. (2017). Adiposity-based chronic disease as a new diagnostic term: The American Association of Clinical Endocrinologists and American College of Endocrinology position statement. *Endocrine Practice, 23*(3), 372–378. doi:10.4158/ep161688.Ps

Metropolitan Life Insurance Company. (1959). New weight standards for men and women. *Statistical Bulletin, 40 (Nov-Dec),* 1–4.

Metropolitan Life Insurance Company. (1983). 1983 Metropolitan height and weight tables. *Statistical Bulletin of the Metropolitan Life Foundation, 64*(1), 3–9.

Moynihan, R. (2006a). Obesity task force linked to WHO takes "millions" from drug firms. *BMJ, 332*(7555), 1412. doi:10.1136/bmj.332.7555.1412-a

Moynihan, R. (2006b). Expanding definitions of obesity may harm children. *BMJ, 332*(7555), 1412. doi:10.1136/bmj.332.7555.1412

Müller, M. J., Braun, W., Enderle, J., & Bosy-Westphal, A. (2016). Beyond BMI: Conceptual issues related to overweight and obese patients. *Obesity Facts, 9*(3), 193–205. doi:10.1159/000445380

Müller, M. J., & Geisler, C. (2017). Defining obesity as a disease. *European Journal of Clinical Nutrition. 71*(11), 1256–1258. doi:10.1038/ejcn.2017.155

Muttarak, R. (2018). Normalization of plus size and the danger of unseen overweight and obesity in England. *Obesity, 26*(7), 1125–1129. doi:10.1002/oby.22204

National Coverage Determination (NCD) for Treatment of Obesity (40.5) – Version 1, Effective between 1/1/1966-10/1/2004; Version 2, Effective between 10/1/2004-2/21/2006. Retrieved from https://www.cms.gov/medicare-coverage-database/details/ncd-details.aspx?NCDId= 38&ver=4

National Research Council. (1989). *Diet and health: Implications for reducing chronic disease risk* Washington, DC: The National Academies Press.

Obesity: Preventing and Managing the Global Epidemic. (1998). Report of a WHO Consultation on Obesity. Geneva, 3–5 June 1997. Geneva: World Health Organization. Retrieved from WHO/NUT/NCD/98.1.

Obesity: Preventing and Managing the Global Epidemic. (2000). Report of a WHO consultation. *World Health Organization Technical Report Series, 894*, i–253.

Ogden, C. L., & Flegal, K. M. (2010). Changes in terminology for childhood overweight and obesity. *National Health Statistics Reports, 25*, 1–5.

Oliver, J. E. (2006). The politics of pathology: How obesity became an epidemic disease. *Perspectives in Biology and Medicine, 49*(4), 611–627. doi:10.1353/pbm.2006.0062

Physical status: the use and interpretation of anthropometry. Report of a WHO Expert Committee. (1995). *World Health Organization Technical Report Series, 854*, 1–452.

Puhl, R., & Brownell, K. D. (2001). Bias, discrimination, and obesity. *Obesity Research, 9*(12), 788–805. doi:10.1038/oby.2001.108

Quetelet, A. (1835). *Sur l'homme.* Paris: Bachelier.

Rohrer, F. (1908). Eine neue Formel zur Bestimmung der Körperfülle [A new formula for the determining of corpulence]. *Korrespondenz-Blatt der deutschen Gesellschaft für Anthropologie, Ethnologie und Urgeschichte, 39*(1/2), 5–7.

Rohrer, F. (1921). Der Index der Körperfülle als Maß des Ernährungszustandes [The index of corpulence as a measure of the nutritional status]. *Munchener Medizinische Wochenschrift, 68*, 580–582.

Rössner, S. (2007). Paul Pierre Broca (1824–1880). *Obesity Reviews, 8*(3), 277. doi:10.1111/j.1467–789X.2007.00303.x

Schwartz, L. M., & Woloshin, S. (1999). Changing disease definitions: Implications for disease prevalence. Analysis of the Third National Health and Nutrition Examination Survey, 1988–1994. *Effective Clinical Practice, 2*(2), 76–85.

Seltzer, C. C. (1965). Limitation of height-weight standards. *New England Journal of Medicine, 272*, 1132-1132. doi:10.1056/NEJM196505272722120

Sharma, A. M., & Kushner, R. F. (2009). A proposed clinical staging system for obesity. *International Journal of Obesity, 33*(3), 289–295. doi:10.1038/ijo.2009.2

Sharpe, L. (1999, April 27). FDA approves fat-fighting drug from Roche. *Wall Street Journal.*

Shephard, G. M. (1907). The relation of build to longevity. *Abstract of the Proceedings of the Seventeenth Annual Meeting of the Association of Life Insurance Medical Directors of America* (pp. 46–66). New York: Knickerbocker.

Simopoulos, A. P., & Van Itallie, T. B. (1984). Body weight, health, and longevity. *Annals of Internal Medicine, 100*(2), 285–295. doi:10.7326/0003–4819-100-2–285

Sommer, I., Teufer, B., Szelag, M., Nussbaumer-Streit, B., Titscher, V., Klerings, I., & Gartlehner, G. (2020). The performance of anthropometric tools to determine obesity: a systematic review and meta-analysis. *Scientific Reports, 10*(1), 12699. doi:10.1038/s41598-020-69498-7

Spahillari, A., Mukamal, K. J., DeFilippi, C., Kizer, J. R., Gottdiener, J. S., Djousse, L., … Shah, R. V. (2016). The association of lean and fat mass with all-cause mortality in older adults: The Cardiovascular Health Study. *Nutrition, Metabolism, and Cardiovascular Diseases, 26*(11), 1039–1047. doi:10.1016/j.numecd.2016.06.011

Squires, S. (1998, June 9). Pound foolish? Critics fear new weight guidelines may result in one-size-fits-all diagnoses, diet drug abuse. *Washington Post.*

Srikanthan, P., Horwich, T. B., & Tseng, C. H. (2016). Relation of muscle mass and fat mass to cardiovascular disease mortality. *American Journal of Cardiology, 117*(8), 1355–1360. doi:10.1016/j.amjcard.2016.01.033

Stern, J. S., Kazaks, A., & Downey, M. (2005). Future and implications of reimbursement for obesity treatment. *Journal of the American Dietetic Association, 105*(5, Suppl. 1), S104–109. doi:10.1016/j.jada.2005.02.048

Stigler, S. M. (1986). *The history of statistics: The measurement of uncertainty before 1900.* Cambridge, MA: Harvard University Press.

Stolberg, S. G. (1999, May 2). Ideas & trends: The fat get fatter; overweight was bad enough. *New York Times.*

Symonds, B. (1908). The influence of overweight and underweight on vitality. *Journal of the Medical Society of New Jersey, V*(4), 159–167. Reprinted: Symonds, B. (2010). The influence of overweight and underweight on vitality. *International Journal of Epidemiology, 39*(4), 951–957. doi:10.1093/ije/dyq090

Vallgarda, S., Nielsen, M. E. J., Hansen, A. K. K., Ócathaoir K, Hartlev, M., Holm, L.,... Sandoe, P. (2017). Should Europe follow the US and declare obesity a disease? A discussion of the so-called utilitarian argument. *European Journal of Clinical Nutrition, 71*(11), 1263–1267. doi:10.1038/ejcn.2017.103

Vertinsky, P. (2002). Embodying normalcy: Anthropometry and the long arm of William H. Sheldon's somatotyping project. *Journal of Sport History, 29*(1), 95–133. Retrieved from http://www.jstor.org/stable/43610055

Vertinsky, P. (2007). Physique as destiny: William H. Sheldon, Barbara Honeyman Heath and the struggle for hegemony in the science of somatotyping. *Bulletin Canadien d'Histoire de la Médecine, 24*(2), 291–316. doi:10.3138/cbmh.24.2.291

Weigley, E. S. (1984). Average? Ideal? Desirable? A brief overview of height-weight tables in the United States. *Journal of the American Dietetic Association, 84*(4), 417–423.

Weigley, E. S. (2000). Adolphe Quetelet. *American Journal of Clinical Nutrition, 71*(3), 853. doi:10.1093/ajcn/71.3.853

Weintraub, M. (1992a). Long-term weight control study: Conclusions. *Clinical Pharmacology and Therapeutics, 51*(5), 642–646. doi:10.1038/clpt.1992.76

Weintraub, M. (1992b). Long-term weight control: The National Heart, Lung, and Blood Institute funded multimodal intervention study. *Clinical Pharmacology and Therapeutics, 51*(5), 581–585. doi:10.1038/clpt.1992.68

Willett, W. C., Stampfer, M., Manson, J., & VanItallie, T. (1991). New weight guidelines for Americans: Justified or injudicious? *American Journal of Clinical Nutrition, 53*(5), 1102–1103. doi:10.1093/ajcn/53.5.1102

Wilmore, J. H., & Behnke, A. R. (1969). An anthropometric estimation of body density and lean body weight in young men. *Journal of Applied Physiology, 27*(1), 25–31. doi:10.1152/jappl.1969.27.1.25

World Health Organization (2000). *Obesity: Preventing and managing the global epidemic: Report of a WHO consultation.* https://www.who.int/nutrition/publications/obesity/WHO_TRS_894/en/

World Health Organization (2020). Obesity and Overweight – Key Facts. Retrieved from https://www.who.int/en/news-room/fact-sheets/detail/obesity-and-overweight

World Obesity Federation. (n.d.). About us – History. Retrieved from https://www.worldobesity.org/about/about-us/history

Yanovski, S. Z. (2005). Pharmacotherapy for obesity – promise and uncertainty. *New England Journal of Medicine, 353*(20), 2187–2189. doi:10.1056/NEJMe058243

Yumuk, V., Tsigos, C., Fried, M., Schindler, K., Busetto, L., Micic, D., & Toplak, H. (2015). European guidelines for obesity management in adults. *Obesity Facts, 8*(6), 402–424. doi:10.1159/000442721

4

OBESITY IN TRANSITION

A challenge in modern history

Peter N. Stearns

The fact that obesity has become a distinctive modern problem is a familiar historical finding. Traditional societies inevitably had to pay far more attention to issues of food adequacy and undernutrition than to the results of overindulgence. Obesity might be noted as a product of individual gluttony, but it was not a common threat. In Western societies, both in Europe and North America, the move toward a greater awareness of the dangers of overweight began to take shape toward the end of the 19th century and picked up momentum from that point onward. This chapter focuses on the decades of transition – into the mid-20th century – when concern about overweight and obesity began to reach not only the wider public, but also a growing array of medical practitioners (Forth, 2019).

Not surprisingly, because the problem was essentially novel, initial awareness and response were mixed. In an ideal world, people might have quickly grasped the new dimensions of their situation and adjusted expectations and behaviors accordingly (Schwartz, 1983). We can readily see, in retrospect, that it was precisely around the turn of the century that eating habits and weight issues were being transformed (along with a related shift in the balance between contagious and degenerative diseases as causes of death). Though undernutrition remained an issue for a minority, the fact was that for most people in Western societies, except perhaps in times of war, food abundance had become assured, thanks to improvements in agriculture and in transportation. More and more people were able to take advantage of improved wages not only to expand their food purchases but also to convert to growing interests in meat and dessert consumption; new commercial outlets (most obviously in the United States) sprang up to encourage additional snacking – the Nabisco company thus began its operations in the 1880s with all sorts of inducements and opportunities for eating between meals (Levenstein, 2003a; Levenstein, 2003b). At the same time, changes in work habits, and again transportation, reduced physical exertions for many people. Commuting began to transition from walking to riding (the word commuting itself is the mid-19th-century term), children increasingly shifted from work to sedentary classrooms, and the rapid growth of a white-collar class signaled less exertion from many adults. This was the point, as a cumulative result, that the basic human concern needed to shift from under- to over-consumption.

In fact, however, shifting gears proved difficult, and some of the transitional challenges survive even to our own time. This chapter deals with real indications of change from doctors' offices to beauty standards, during precisely these decades. But it also deals with some of

DOI: 10.4324/9780429344824-6

the confusions and misdirections involved, both as a matter of historical interest and because of their persistent impact in qualifying human response. The fact is, obviously, that we have yet to devise an adequate strategy to cope with the new eating and exertion experiences in contemporary society – hence the steady rise of obesity – and the transitional issues both signal and explain some of the problems involved.

Obesity was not, of course, a purely recent concern. Medical historians have highlighted Greek, and probably before them Egyptian, concern about substantial overweight as a disorder – Hippocrates wrote that "corpulence is not only a disease itself, but a harbinger of others." Early medicine in India, similarly, associated overweight with diabetes and heart disorders; the surgeon Sushruta (6th-century BCE) urged physical exertion as a means of addressing the problem (Wilkins, Harvey, & Dobson, 1995). These findings generated considerable and very sensible, advice about the importance of moderation in food and drink. Many cultures also depicted grossly fat people as figures of fun or derision, grotesque in themselves and symbols of the kinds of character flaws that led to gluttony. Christian morality considered gluttony a sin, sometimes contending that excessive indulgence in food was in fact a gateway to a host of other immoralities. The rise of medical research in Europe from the later Middle Ages onward renewed attention to cases of obesity (including diseases like the Prader–Willi syndrome that could cause obesity even in the young), and the condition was also sometimes represented in works of art.

However, concern about obesity was qualified by a number of factors. Most obviously, it was simply not a widespread condition. Only some members of the elite could regularly afford the combination of food abundance and absence of regular physical exertion that would normally generate obesity. This meant, further, that considerable obesity might, in fact, be associated with power and prosperity – as the assertive portrayals of figures like the English Henry VIII suggest. Some historians contend further that, in women, overweight might be associated with fertility, and some artists – most famously, Rubens, in the 17th century – depicted corpulent women as sexually attractive (Bray, 1995; Eknoyan, 2006; Forth, 2019).

Growing European prosperity associated with the rise of commerce from the 16th century onward may have heightened the number of people susceptible to obesity – though the condition remained uncommon, and this, along with the greater precision of scientific research more generally, may explain the rise of more precise formulations involving obesity from the 17th century onward. Growing medical interest included more frequent use of the word itself in the English language (deriving from Latin through French) and increasing awareness of the potentially fatal consequences of the condition. By the 18th century, a number of European scientists were working on more precise weight measurements, generating a greater interest as well in issues like familial predispositions. Cultural scorn for the obese may have increased as well, with literary representations associating the condition with buffoonery or worse. All the while, more traditional advice about the importance of moderation continued to be repeated – for example, in Benjamin Franklin's *Poor Richard's Almanack* in the American colonies during the later 18th century (Haslam, 2007) (Figure 4.1).

Considerable uncertainty persisted. Fat continued to be associated with health and prosperity – sensibly enough, to a point, in a period when food availability remained a crucial issue. At that time, contagious disease, not degenerative illness, continued to hold center stage. During the 1860s, for example, a spat of "Fat Men's Clubs" spread in the United States, celebrating the link between plumpness and success. And while slender (often corseted) waists were popular among young middle-class women, they also occasioned debate. Harriet Beecher Stowe, the famous crusader against slavery, attacked the new hostility to "opulence in physical proportions," while a slender French actress, visiting the United States,

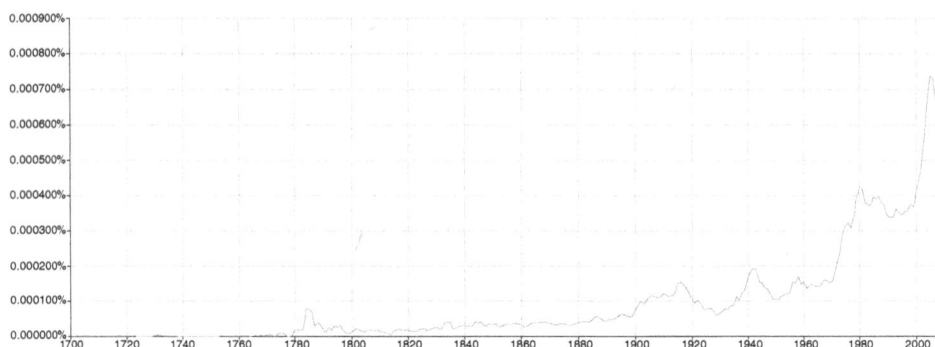

Figure 4.1   Frequency of the word "obesity" in English, 1700–2008.

was scorned for her emaciated appearance. Some early feminist leaders, like Elizabeth Cady Stanton, were valued for their comfortably expansive girth – "plump as a partridge," one commentator noted admiringly (Stearns, 2002).

While this long backdrop plays a role in the modern history of obesity, it also highlights the changes that were necessary before concerns about overweight gained more than marginal interest either in the medical community or in popular culture. This, in turn, is where developments in the later 19th century, combining still greater scientific precision with early signs of changes in actual eating patterns, ushered in a really new era.

Even here, however, it is important to be cautious. The new approaches did not, initially, feature an explicit realization that modern industrial societies had reached a turning point in which abundance replaced scarcity as a key human problem. We can look back on the later 19th century as a watershed, but the magnitude of change was, understandably enough, not realized at the time. Nor is there clear indication that the actual incidence of overweight was yet increasing – among other things because walking and other forms of normal physical exertion remained so widespread. A cultural transition did emerge clearly enough, but it was long, both somewhat vague and considerably uncoordinated.

Signs of change came from several directions. In 1863, an Englishman, William Banting, wrote a diet book that gained instant popularity throughout the English-speaking world, going through 12 editions in a few decades. Banting specifically noted his success in losing excess weight. Dieting in fact became known as "bantingism" for several years (Oxford Dictionary of National Biography, n.d.).

Medical research gained further focus, particularly, in Europe. It was in the 1870s that the word "calorie," a heat measurement, began to be applied to studies in nutrition. By the 1890s, German research specifically linked caloric intake to organic metabolism. Both in Europe and the United States, this work began to encourage specific recommendations about desirable daily calorie consumption – though the standards, as in a U.S. Department of Agriculture pamphlet that urged 3500 calories a day, remained fairly loose. On another front, researchers like Karl von Noorden in Germany also began to categorize different types of obesity and to link them more specifically to diseases such as cardiac arrest. In France, medical researchers began to generate desirable weight tables from the 1830s onward (Jones, 1897; Packard, 1897–1898; Davis, 1898; Benedict, 1902; Douglas, 1902–1903; Taussige, 1902–1903; Morrison, 1904).

In this context, actual measurements of weight began to enter diagnostic practice. Many hospitals had scales by the 1870s, along with a space for specifics as part of patient charts.

Public scales – your weight for a penny – began to proliferate by the 1890s both a sign of growing interest and a spur to greater concern (Zelizer, 1979; Schwartz, 1983).

Considerable uncertainty remained even in the more advanced medical circles. In the 1890s, French doctors extensively debated the role of water intake in obesity, some arguing that it should be curtailed. Disproportionate interest continued to apply to hereditary conditions, sometimes generating contentions that ordinary people were not really prone to any serious problem that a minor adjustment in habits could not address. Cultural prejudice might also play a distracting role, as in a brief claim by some French researchers that Jews were particularly prone to fat.

But there is no question that medical attention was increasing in ultimately constructive ways. In France, in the first decade of the 20th century, at least 12 major studies appeared, defining and categorizing obesity, indicating its role in causing a host of degenerative diseases, highlighting its indisputable contribution to shortening the lifespan, and suggesting a variety of remedies and preventives (Mathieu, 1906; Lenoir, 1909).

Along with this research, came a new set of inputs from the rising life insurance industry. Actuaries began generating standard weight tables in the final decades of the 19th century. As early as 1898, an American manual urged that anything more than 20 percent above the desired standard should be regarded as a serious health risk. In 1912, the Actuarial Society of America issued a study that attempted a precise correlation between weight levels (adjusted for height and gender) and risks of premature death. As with the growing popularity of scales, this new contribution both reflected the growing medical findings about weight and obesity and encouraged greater popular attention in turn (Stein, 1904; McLester, 1924).

Finally, and most strikingly, something of a cultural revolution occurred, particularly in the middle and upper classes and disproportionately (though not exclusively) among women. Fat, quite simply, became unpopular and unattractive, clearly losing its association with prosperity and increasingly suggesting a lack of personal competence.

On both sides of the Atlantic, a vigorous "corset debate" broke out around the turn of the century. Many leading fashion advocates now urged that beautiful women should be naturally slender, not requiring unpleasant constraints to look right – an argument that built of frequent medical arguments that corsetry was unhealthy by constraining or distorting the internal organs. New images, like the Gibson girls in American magazines highlighted slender, relaxed bodies, both male and female. (Even high art arguably picked up the shift: while early impressionists like Renoir maintained some interest in fleshy figures, the surge of Matisse and then the cubists, in emphasizing stick-figure slenderness, clearly signaled a new aesthetic.) *The Philadelphia Cook Book*, in 1914, simply noted that "an excess of flesh is to be looked upon as one of the most objectionable forms of disease." And another outlet, in the same year, simply asserted that "fat is now regarded as an indiscretion, almost as a crime" (Patten, 1897; Phillips, 1900; Banner, 1983; Schwartz, 1983; Summerville, 1916; Lowry, 1919). In the United States, the famous "fat men's clubs" closed their doors by 1907, their leaders noting that no one now wanted to be associated with this kind of terminology. A French military man, for his part, organized a chain of fitness clubs around attacks on overweight: "Obesity, source of so much suffering and also, why not say it, object of so much ridicule, is easily curable." Revealingly, new words gained currency to designate and denigrate the obese. In the English-speaking world, "porky" came into use in the 1860s, "butterball" by 1879, and "jumbo" in the 1880s. "Slob" entered the language in the 1860s from an Irish word denoting gooey mud; a London lord mayor was thus attacked as a "fat slob." Transatlantic currency for these terms emerged by the 1880s (Banner, 1983; Stearns, 2002; Fields, 2007).

And of course, on the heels of these various concerns and impulses, a huge industry began to develop, selling diet products, advice books, diet cookbooks, exercise devices – the whole panoply that quickly became part of the Western commercial scene from that point onward.

Here, then, was the turning point, clearly demarcating the turn-of-the-century decades from previous patterns in terms of medical attention and precision, popular awareness, cultural opprobrium, and commercial translations. The level and range of the transformation were truly significant, creating a new environment concerning weight and obesity with which contemporaries today can easily identify.

Beyond pinpointing and summarizing the changes, however, a further point remains: given their vigor and their association (however implicit) with fundamental shifts in health conditions in industrial societies with the growing importance of degenerative disease, why were the innovations not more quickly and uniformly successful? Why, even today, do the new findings about obesity continue to struggle against actual popular habits?

Three preliminary points are vital – and some might contend, adequate to the explanatory task. First, the advice was really new, and it would understandably take time to assimilate. We will document this obvious point in what follows.

Second, the approach was very much class specific. Life insurance was at the juncture for the middle classes, not below – when workers bought insurance, as they now eagerly did, they focused on burial costs. Doctor visits, including the inevitable office scales, became a common part of middle-class life at least by the 1920s – but again, not below the middle class (though, of course, we have no way of knowing how widely the interest in the new public penny scales applied). Fashion magazines and the great corset debate were for the fluently literate and those who could afford the subscription costs. And all of this in a situation where, for many workers, food quality and availability, not overabundance, remained the pressing issue. The Belgian worker who, around 1900, indicated that his lifestyle aspiration was to regularly be able to butter his bread, was not a target for diet advice. And even though the burdens of class stratification would moderate with greater affluence later in the 20th century, disparities in popular standards would continue to affect reactions and behaviors – as in the ongoing contemporary correlation between obesity and social status (Stearns, 1975).

Third, the new findings in advice and culture warred against the simultaneous increase in the commercial outlets for food. The woman's magazine that urged a slender body and offered diet advice featured, on the adjacent pages, succulent advertisements for the latest available cake mix. The American men who abandoned fat men's clubs also had to contend with growing middle-class interests in French-style restaurants. The parents who ultimately picked up new concerns about regulating their children's eating habits also had to register the newly available crackers and snacks (initially advertised as supporting good health) and the sugary sodas that made their appearance at this point as well. A novel contest emerged between commercial innovations in foods and the revised health standards that obviously continue to this day – it offered a fundamental complexity in the turning point from the outset.

With all this, however, there were also several features of the new medical and cultural approach itself that complicated popular response, even in the interested middle classes. Some of these features were temporary – as in the hesitations of many ordinary physicians – but some have proved more durable. Here is the final feature of the turning point itself.

Ordinary doctors were long unsure about the new concerns. Many were unaware of the cutting-edge research. Some, who picked up on simultaneous findings about the rise of nervous disorders, simply maintained different priorities. S. Weir Mitchell, who pioneered the study of neurasthenia, complacently noted that "a fat bank account tends to make a fat man" (Mitchell, 1887; Gosling, 1987). The growing popularity of new medications also competed with diet advice. As late as the 1930s, an American article noted, "The older members of the profession ... can recall with feelings of humiliation the lack of interest in the subject of dietetics in the early years of their professional life. In those days drug therapy held the center of the stage (in dealing with disease), while dietary consideration received but scant attention." Correspondingly, for many years, the scales that now adorned hospitals and doctors' offices were often ignored, the place on the patient charts for weight information left blank simply because practitioners found the subject unimportant. In some cases, overemphasis on heredity proved a deterrent, leading many physicians to wonder if most of their obese patients could really do anything about their condition. Always, as well, there was an ongoing concern about malnutrition and a worry that the new advice could actually worsen problems in this category. "I feel sure that I have several times seen persons unknowingly starve to death" because of the new standards, when they were actually suffering from an acute disease that had nothing to do with obesity (McLester, 1928; Warnshuis, 1931; Fulton, 1936).

This first set of complications would obviously ease with time, as physicians became more aware of the relevant research and the problems of degenerative disease more generally. There is no question that, from the 1930s onward, articles on the dangers of obesity and how to deal with affected patients became more common in the normal medical literature.

The second complexity, sometimes overlapping the first in the initial decades, is frankly harder to assess. There is no question that, at least for several decades, far more public attention was directed toward the new fashion standards than to relevant health advice about diet and obesity. The simultaneity of concerns was surely no accident – by whatever means the gurus of fashion and art were picking up some of the same signals that doctors and actuaries were – that new representations were vital as the implications of industrial prosperity became clearer. At the same time, we simply do not entirely understand how much the great corset debate had to do with real medical goals. And while the fashion emphasis might provide much-needed motivation for good eating habits – a connection still valid today – it could also distract.

Some doctors, for example, hesitated to address their (particularly female) patients' desire to lose weight because they found it simply frivolous. Probably, more important in the long run was the fact that fashion standards generated their own debate, independent of the health implications of overweight. Many people, men and women alike, continued to prefer fleshier partners and disputed the new aesthetic claims. And while a civil rights concern about discrimination against the overweight emerged only later (a more recent complexity), there were anticipations in the earlier fashion discussions. The French women's magazine that trumpeted the legitimacy of heavy body suggested the distraction quite clearly: "There is no ugly woman," concluded an article that praised "the big woman, with fine proportions in her lines." Aesthetic overemphasis also conduced to complaints that the new weight standards discriminated against older people, indulging a physical appearance that was only natural in the young. The whole issue of the interaction between fashion and health would obviously persist, probably on balance supporting the concern about preventing obesity but undeniably introducing some distracting considerations as well (Delbourg-Delphis, 1981; Roberts, 1993).

The transition to a new level of concern about weight and obesity also implicitly highlighted disparities in targeting, quite apart from some concern about privileging youth. While it is important to note that the new concerns embraced men as well as women – with an emphasis on slenderness and fitness for males – there was no question that women were disproportionately targeted. The assumption that women had particular responsibility for maintaining beauty sealed the disparity, and this would be widely noted later in the 20th century by second-wave feminists (Seid, 1989; Wolf, 1991; Meadows, Weiss, Cole, & Rothblum, 1993). At least as significant was the relatively scant focus on children, at least until after World War II. It was simply harder to reconceive plump children than their adult counterparts: lingering "baby fat" seemed healthy and attractive, and even many doctors agreed. Also diverting attention was the continued concern about underweight youngsters (particularly boys) that heightened during the Depression of the 1930s. To be sure, scattered comments were available. As early as 1914, the famous American government pamphlet, *Infant Care*, warned against overfeeding. Girls were occasionally singled out because of the tension between fat and beauty. European parents, less indulgent than their American counterparts, may have monitored eating habits more carefully (particularly in regulating snacks). But a substantial disconnect remained. As late as 1954, a pediatric journal noted how strange it was that parents worried so much about thin children and not much about fat ones. Polls continued to show that only a minority of American parents viewed overweight offspring as a problem compared with the larger group that saw the fat infant as the kind of "bouncy baby" that testified to good parenting. Only in the 1960s and 1970s would a consistent medical focus on childhood obesity begin to emerge, with advice reaching staple publications like *Parents* magazine by the 1980s – where, finally, the disproportionate concern with undereating began to fade (except for the understandable distraction focused on anorexia nervosa). Obviously, the childhood obesity problem remains vivid still today. While it has many components, the disparities that surfaced during the decades of transition, yet to be fully repaired, provide part of the explanation (Children's Bureau, 1914; Loomis, Reader, & Catlin, 1937; Kugelmass, 1942; Dunbar, 1949; Hughes, 1952; Holt, McIntosh, & Barnett, 1953; Ross, 1955).

Finally, the rise of new concerns about weight – particularly focused on adults – highlighted one other feature that continues to provoke debate. Depending on the commentator, the overweight individual was not only singled out as unhealthy and unattractive but also as lacking in character. As one comment noted, "Society feels we're lazy, that we have no will power, that we just don't care" (Brown, 1990). The moralistic component was particularly prominent in the United States, but it surfaced in Europe as well – though it was true that, by the 1950s, some European doctors were warning against American-style moralism as a counterproductive burden on the overweight. By the 1950s, again especially in the United States, moral opprobrium was further enhanced by references to psychological disturbance. Articles in popular magazines like *Ladies' Home Journal* made it clear: "Psychiatrists have exposed the fat person for what he really is – miserable, self-indulgent and lacking in control." "The obese woman's very dimensions reflect her need for strength and massiveness in order to deny an image of self that is felt to be basically weak, inadequate and helpless" (cited in Stearns, 2002, pp. 54, 119). While the term "fat shaming" would emerge only later, it is clear that the culture that developed during the first half of the 20th century exposed the overweight to reactions that went well beyond concerns for health or even beauty – in ways that might affect social reactions and job prospects quite directly. The results warrant continued assessment: does the moralistic or shaming component detract from the essential message, prompting some people to double down on eating simply in despair at their failure? Are there ways to cast the culture more constructively? For now, the point is that the unprecedented attention to overweight that became such a striking feature of Western society during the turn of the century decades included a fairly uncritical judgmental feature that was, at the least, debatable and that continues to complicate the health message (Wilson, 1956; Rubin, 1966; Petrie, 1968; Siegel, 1971; Farrell, 2011).

The transformation of Western culture toward new levels of concern about obesity and the relationship among body, beauty, and health was genuinely significant – reflecting, in complicated ways, the transformation of industrial society from scarcity to overabundance and from contagious to degenerative disease. The shifts were gradual, the audience uneven, but there was no question that, by the 1950s, most middle-class people were aware of the new criteria, eager to meet them at least in principle by pledges to diet or by successful restraint, open to judgments of others who failed to measure up, and not infrequently deeply ashamed of personal inadequacy. The transformation was fueled by fashion leaders, and medical popularizers enhanced increasingly by the images of movie stars held to their own demanding standards.

The new culture, at the same time, harbored a number of features that would prove questionable – though the rough edges were hardly surprising given the magnitude of the adjustments involved. Hesitations and counterargument abounded, even in the medical community so that several decades were required really to assimilate the new concerns. Emphasis on fashion was a vital part of the transition, but it might prove somewhat distracting. Disparities concerning gender and, even more, age categories raised some further questions that would be sharpened in the final decades of the 20th century, enhanced as well by debates over excessive moralism. The most important challenge remained the fact that, overall, the new culture could not keep pace with changes in popular habits of eating and exercise. The disparity was enhanced, in many cases, by some of the complexities of the new culture itself.

References

Banner, L. (1983). *American beauty: A Social history…through two centuries of the American idea, ideal, and image of the beautiful woman.* New York City: Alfred A. Knopf.

Benedict, A. L. (1902). Practical Dietetics. *Medical Standards, 26.*

Bray, A. (1995). Measurements of body composition: An improving art. *Journal of Obesity, 3*, 291–293. doi: 10.1002/j.1550-8528.1995.tb00151.x

Brown, R. (1990). Full-figured women strike back. *Ebony, 2*, 30.

Children's Bureau. (1914). *Infant care.* Washington, DC: US Government Printing Office.

Davis, N. S. (1898). Importance of regulatory dietetics in harmony with the physiological laws controlling digestion, nutrition, and waste and some of the inconsistencies in prevalent dietetic practices. *Journal of the American Medical Association, 31*, 1393–1395.

Delbourg-Delphis, M. (1981). *Le chic et le look: Histoire de la mode féminine et des moeurs, de 1890 à nos jours.* Paris: Presses Universitaires.

Douglas, C. C. (1902–1903). Starvation as a therapeutic agent. *Detroit Medical Journal, 2*, 737–741.

Dunbar, F. (1949). *Your child's mind and body: A practical guide to parents.* New York: Crown Publishing Group.

Eknoyan, G. (2006). A history of obesity, or how what was good became ugly and then bad. *Advances in Chronic Kidney Disease, 13*(4), 421–427. doi: 10.1053/j.ackd.2006.07.002

Farrell, A. (2011). *Fat shame: Stigma and the fat body in American culture.* New York: New York University Press.

Fields, J. (2007). *An intimate affair: Women, lingerie, and sexuality.* Berkeley: University of California Press.

Forth, C. (2019). *Fat: A cultural history of the stuff of life.* London: Reaktion.

Fulton, G. (1936). Evaluation of reducing diets. *Kentucky Medical Journal, 34*, 518.

Gosling, F. G. (1987). *Before Freud: Neurasthenia and the American medical community.* Urbana: University of Illinois Press.

Haslam, D. (2007). Obesity: A medical history. *Obesity Reviews, 8*, 31–36. doi: 10.1111/j.1467-789X.2007.00314.x

Holt, L. E., McIntosh, R., & Barnett, H. L. (1953). *Pediatrics.* New York: Appleton-Century.

Hughes, J. G. (1952). *Pediatrics in general practice.* New York: McGraw-Hill.

Jones, S. E. (1897). Some remarks on obesity. *Medical Brief, 25*, 1692–1695.

Kugelmass, I. N. (1942). *Superior children through modern nutrition: How to perfect the growth and development of your children from birth to maturity.* New York: E. P. Dutton & Co, Inc.

Lenoir, P. (1909). *L'Obésité et son traitement.* Paris: Baillière.

Levenstein, H. (2003a). *Revolution at the table: The transformation of the American diet.* Berkeley: University of California Press.

Levenstein, H. (2003b). *Paradox of plenty: A social history of eating in modern America.* Berkeley: University of California Press.

Loomis, H., Reader, D., & Catlin, C. (1937). Methods of treatment of obesity. *Practitioner, 138,* 95.

Lowry, E. (1919). *The woman of forty.* Chicago, IL: Ulan Press.

Mathieu, A. (1906). *L'Hygiene de l'obèse.* Paris: Masson et cie.

McLester, J. S. (1924). The principles involved in the treatment of obesity. *Journal of the American Medical Association, 82,* 2103.

McLester, J. S. (1928). Obesity, its penalties and treatment. *Southern Medical Journal, 21,* 196.

Meadows, R., Weiss, L., Cole, E., & Rothblum, E. D. (1993). *Women's conflicts about eating and sexuality: The relationship between food and sex.* Binghamton, NY: Psychology Press.

Mitchell, S. W. (1887). *Wear and tear: Or hints for the overworked.* New York: Altamira Press.

Morrison, W. F. (1904). The harmfulness of overeating. *Providence Medical Journal, 5,* 174–182.

Oxford Dictionary of National Biography. (n.d.). *William Banting.* Oxford: Oxford University Press.

Packard, F. A. (1897–1898). The prescribing of diet in private practice. *University Medical Magazine, 10,* 269–271.

Patten, S. (1897). Over-nutrition and its social consequences. *The Annals of the American Academy of Political and Social Science, 10,* 33–53.

Petrie, S. (1968). *The lazy lady's easy diet.* West Nyack, NY: Xs Books.

Phillips, D. G. (1900). *Susan Lenox: Her fall and rise.* New York: D. Appleton and Company.

Roberts, M. L. (1993). Samson and Delilah Revisited: The Politics of Women's Fashion in 1920s France. *The American Historical Review, 98*(3), 657–684. https://doi.org/10.2307/2167545

Rorer, M. S. T. (1914). *Philadelphia cook book.* Philadelphia: Arnold and Company.

Ross, M. S. (1955). *Feeding the family.* New York.

Rubin, T. (1966). *The thin book.* New York: Pinnacle Books.

Schwartz, H. (1983). *Never satisfied: A cultural history of diets, fantasies, and fat.* New York: Free Press.

Seid, R. (1989). *Never too thin: Why women are at war with their bodies.* New York: Prentice Hall Direct.

Siegel, M. (1971). *Think thin.* New York: Paul S. Eriksson.

Stearns, P. N. (1975). *Lives of labour: Work in a maturing industrial society.* London: Croom Helm.

Stearns, P. N. (2002). *Fat history: Bodies and beauty in the modern west* (2nd ed.). New York: New York University Press.

Stein, H. (1904). Who is underfed? *Medical Record, 65,* 811–812.

Summerville, A. (1916) *Why be fat? Rules for weight-reduction and the preservation of youth and health.* New York: Forgotten Books.

Taussige, A. E. (1902–1903). The treatment of obesity, or corpulence of the middle aged. *California State Journal of Medicine, 1,* 356–359.

Warnshuis, G. J. (1931). Individualizing the treatment of obesity. *Medical Review of Reviews, 37,* 676.

Wilkins, J., Harvey, D., & Dobson, M. J. (Eds.). (1995). *Food in antiquity: Studies in ancient society and culture.* Oxford and New York: Oxford University Press.

Wilson, F. J. (1956). *Glamour, glucose and glands.* New York: Vantage Press.

Wolf, N. (1991). *The beauty myth: How images of beauty are used against women.* New York: Harper Perennial.

Zelizer, V. (1979). *Morals and markets: The development of life insurance in the United States.* New York: Columbia University Press.

5

OBESITY IN BRAZIL

Between liberties and pathologies[1]

Denise Bernuzzi de Sant'Anna

Since the 1970s, a pathological root of obesity has been widely publicized in the Brazilian media. Hundreds of diets have emerged as well as a new sensitivity to body weights and volumes. Being fat ceased to be a trait of the rich. The use of scales to weigh the body has become common, while diets for weight loss have become fashionable and a recurring medical prescription. Gluttony, understood as a sin until the mid-20th century, has become a synonym of disease. Dietary habits have undergone a radical change, while the popularization of physical activity and a severe criticism of sedentary lifestyles have emerged.

However, the old valorization of large bodies has not been completely banished from Brazilian society. And the following is a frequently asked question: in a country where a myth of natural wealth feeds the dream of having a naturally healthy and lush body, how does one carry out the "keep fit trend"?

Poverty rhymed with thinness: a long history

The trend is known—in many countries, being thin has long been associated with poverty (Vigarello, 2010). Brazil did not escape the rule. In fact, until the 1950s, it was very common to associate thin bodies with malnutrition and poverty. Fat people silhouettes tended to be seen as those who could afford plenty on the table. As a matter of fact, before 1950, when the rural population was still larger than the urban population, obesity was not a commonly used word. It was more usual to speak of "strong" or "fat" people, and they were not always the target of medical diets and surgeries. Besides that, Brazilians who would be considered obese nowadays were seen as spectacular "phenomena" (Um Phenomeno, 1900). Exemplary in this regard were the eating contests for gluttons to know who ate the most. There were several reports in the press about the admirable ability with which some prodigious people devoured a kilo of bananas or a dozen eggs at once. These eating contests were not only spaces to admire how gluttons satiated their gigantic appetite but also to appreciate the largeness of bodies. In a society in which phantom of hunger was scary, the ideal body should look like an "*armazém*" [warehouse], with the capacity to store food for times of shortage. The image of this "*corpo armazém*" [warehouse body] should include a prominent belly for men and be that of a curvaceous silhouette—wide hips, thick legs—for women (Sant'Anna, 2016).

DOI: 10.4324/9780429344824-7

In line with this trend, national newspapers published sweet and savory recipes that valued fat people. The popular Brazilian cuisine-valued food considered heavy rather than light, made with lard. The idea was to leave the table with a full belly, and the gesture of dropping one's belt after a meal was seen as a sign of satisfaction and thankfulness. The boundaries between satisfaction and gluttony were not always clear. In general, gluttony suggested eating out of meal times, but it was rarely associated with anxiety, as it would be later. Fat children were the target of reprimands regarding the need to obey their parents by observing meal times. In fact, gluttony was the main suspicion that weighed on fat people. Yet, they tended to represent the promise of widely coveted abundance.

In the 1920s, this image started to change, mainly for the urban elites. The *corpo armazém* became synonymous with excessive rurality and backwardness. Instead, the ideal of a *"corpo poderoso"* [powerful body]—leaner and longer, honed with the new sports and cinematic vogue—started to emerge. Even so, for most Brazilians, the positivity of a well-nourished body with an appearance now considered "fat" prevailed. A well-known Brazilian example in this regard is the Jeca Tatu character, created by writer Monteiro Lobato (1918) in his book *Urupês* which contains stories based on rural workers from the state of São Paulo. Jeca Tatu symbolized the situation of Brazilian peasants, abandoned by public authorities to diseases, economic and educational backwardness and living in poverty. This character was thin, malnourished and always felt tired, the opposite of the healthy and robust ideal advocated by the government and by doctors. A body full of worms and other diseases that attacked the poor strata of society was an ancient specter that haunted physicians and parents.

Between 1930 and 1940, just when the science of nutrition started to gain importance in the country, the valorization of the robust, strong and often fat body—according to current standards, found a prominent place in children's robustness competitions. Hundreds of babies and kids were considered representatives of the national future based on their robustness. During the eugenic trend typical of that time, robustness competitions gave cash prizes to the parents of the most robust children. However, doctors and jury still had difficulty distinguishing the concept of "fat" from "robust". Likewise, print advertising for food and fortifiers did not differentiate these two physical types very well. In the newspapers and magazines of the time, images of "robust" and "fat" were mixed up.[2] It was also common for fat-bellied men to be looked at with a good eye. Obesity was not yet a focus of problematization as it would turn out to be later on. Before the 1960s, scales for weighing the body were not common. Knowing one's own weight was not part of one's personal imagination.

The shame of being paunchy

The first advertisements of weight loss products appeared in the 1920s. An illustrative example is that of the product called Emagrina (Zucon, 2006). In these advertisements, fat people were associated with old age, with the idea that a heavy body had lived for many years and suffered from many diseases. Scales to weigh the body were not part of everyday life, and thin people tended to represent a threat to the healthy reproduction of the species, as if they were proof of poverty and of the difficulty to get plenty of food on the table. It was still common to find advice published on newspapers and magazines designed to "cure thinness", such as the advertisement of Vikelp tablets in one of the best-known magazines in the country, O Cruzeiro (1946, p. 34). The audience devoted to food diets was still a minority, and thinning the silhouette was a demand made more on women than on men, more on young women than on women over 30.

However, the image of sportsmen and people exercising became more frequent in advertisements for the most varied types of medicines, which propagated the idea that good physical appearance could express lightness and strength. Eugenic ideas present among doctors also contributed to highlight the positivity of slender bodies and of physical exercises. In fashion magazines, the long and light silhouette appeared as a sign of modernity and of the new habits of the urban elites. While in the first half of the 20th century chubby people were considered as a model to be followed, after the 1960s, the fear of gaining weight, the censorship of prominent male bellies and the spread of weight-loss diets became evident.

Between 1955 and 1965, an old hypothesis of a "fatty heart" was updated along with the fear of cardiovascular problems caused by excess body weight. Newspapers began to publish an increasing number of articles on the relationship between fat and heart problems, and the word "paunch" became to be understood almost like a dirty word, a synonym of disease, laziness and ugliness. Progressively, the fear of gaining weight became as common in beauty councils as men's vaunted fear of getting married. In the 1960s, scales at drugstores and methods to lose weight, including physical exercise and sports, became popular across Brazil. Diets and their gurus started to become common in magazines, and for the first time, the term "cellulite" and the explanation for this "problem", considered mostly feminine, arose. At the same time, young women from Rio de Janeiro began to wear bikinis on the beaches.

In the 1960s, being fat started to symbolize the absence of modernity. An illustrative example is found in the article "*Calorias Não Engordam*" [Calories Don't Make You Fat] published in O Cruzeiro (1962). This piece, which announced the Portuguese translation of the controversial book *Calories Don't Count* written by Herman Taller in 1961, stated that controlling calorie intake was important for aesthetics and a marker of adaptation to urban life. Thus, weight control meant acquiring social status for the rising middle classes.

At the same time, national and international publications on the problems of being fat and the advertisement of weight loss drugs—such as Moderamina, Desobesi and Moderex (sold in Brazil without a prescription)—and other weight-control products flourished considerably. The first artificial sweeteners, whose ads emphasized that it was possible to consume them without getting fat, appeared in the market. For Brazilians, sweeteners looked like food as well as medicines, precisely at a time when drugstores were beginning to look more and more like supermarkets. In fact, until 1957, sweeteners were considered pharmaceutical specialties, but a decree placed them in the category of dietary supplements. It would not be long before light and diet foods celebrated a kind of merge between the pleasure of eating and losing weight. Thus, weight loss would become an experience associated with products that sold pleasure, joy and health.

However, for rural populations and for the vast majority of Brazilians, who still had difficulty having plenty on the table, the slim and lean body model was not a reference. And even in the middle and upper classes, it was still very common to limit diets to a few days a week and give them up during weekends, at parties and celebrations with friends. At the time of growing influence of the American way of life, refrigerator ads used to show them loaded with food, and the photographs published on cooking books and recipes showed the use of lots of oil, fried foods and sugar. Photographs of dishes containing more salads than pasta had not yet become commonplace in fashion magazines. Eating well was still synonymous with eating a lot. In the 1960s, fast food began to settle in Brazil, and in the late 1970s, the McDonald's chain began to be known by Brazilians, although their prices were not low enough to be considered cheap. Much later, food trucks became fashionable in big cities and a cheap way to eat on the street.

While gradually the shame of being fat began to be imposed on everyone, old habits persisted. For instance, the habit of measuring how fat or thin you were by the belt holding your pants, or the tight dress, around your waist was still common. In other words, attention was focused only on specific parts of the body.

Instead of fat or thin, "*gostoso*" and "*poderoso*"

Especially in the 1980s, a series of magazines dedicated to good shape appeared in the country. The titles of *Boa Forma* [Good Shape] and *Corpo a Corpo* [Body to Body], for instance, evoked the modern body sculpted by gymnastics and by diets, while body building became a fashion in Brazil.[3] American stars set an example, and the Portuguese language was modified by the addition of vocabulary items in English to name successful performances through jogging and body building.

However, it took a few more years for female muscles to be widely accepted. Different from being muscular, the ideal of feminine beauty that has become popular in the country is that of a woman with firm legs and prominent buttocks; strong yet sexy. This is the ideal of health and beauty that, since the 1970s, and especially in the last 30 years, has imposed itself for the various Brazilian social classes—first, a body needs to be sexy, seductive, which in Portuguese popular slang is said to be *"gostoso"* [tasty]. The old value of fat as a proof of wealth, here is invited to become well-toned. The ideal of female wide hips tended to require that the buttocks be raised and firm, indicating a new woman ideal: sexually liberated, less maternal than their mothers and more adventurous.

Tourism marketing contributed greatly to reinforce and spread the representation of women bodies as *gostosos*, especially through propaganda of the Brazilian Tourist Board [Embratur] (Pinto, 2015). Embratur helped to create and to export worldwide, the association between Brazil and young women as seductive, always available, and close to wild nature. Thus, Brazilian women were constructed as *gostosas*—invariably curvy, tanned, young and sexy. In the 1980s, one of the main images created to attract tourists to Brazil was that of *gostosas* wearing bikinis; in hundreds of travel guides and advertisements, the same kind of image represented Brazil—that of a half-naked, young and hyper-sexualized woman surrounded by forests, waterfalls or beaches. This lightness necessarily implied a fat-free body, although made of thick, muscular legs and prominent buttocks. This ideal contributed significantly to highlight the differences between fat and *gostosa* women. In the case of men, the tendency to gain muscles and reduce the belly increased exponentially with the boom of fitness centers across the country.

From the 1980s onwards, *Carioca* funk fashion from urban outskirts began to influence the lifestyle and the beauty ideal of different social groups. *Carioca* funk became popular, and it is part of a vast culture that includes Hip-Hop and Rap. Irreverence and erotic bodies are some of the elements present at dances and in their song lyrics. Brazilian Funk, while valuing the ideal of the strong and pumped body, also surpasses it and puts on the scene obese, lean and silhouettes of all kinds. Urban development, sports fashion, great appreciation of the so-called beach culture, increase of the number of cosmetic surgeries, among other factors have associated silhouettes with the concepts of sensuality, agility and even the demands of modern life (Sant'Anna, 2014).

At this point, the old idea that the body was a kind of *armazém*, started to compete with the ideal of the body as a "company for empowerment", in which everybody needs "to invest" and where everything should be transformed into more energy and self-satisfaction (Sant'Anna, 2016). Funk music started to reach a much wider audience, and the opinions about it diverged: from the grotesque to the creative, going through severe criticism and faithful adherences. Hyper-sexualized female bodies express the need to satisfy themselves and others immediately, in a reality in which postponing pleasure does not make any sense. It must be experienced here and now. Funk men and women express urgency and impatience and cannot waste any time waiting.

At the same time, Brazilian media has extensively exploited the image of the female body considered *gostosa*. A popular example was the "Miss Bumbum" competition, an annual beauty pageant to reward the owner of the best buttocks in the country.

However, Brazil shows a considerable diversity of trends and ways of expressing the body. Take, for instance, some sectors of the urban bourgeoisie, in which a "whey generation" leads a way of life that requires a lot of discipline and diets based on food supplements. Its members talk about biceps, bench press, creatine, drop sets and muscle mass with the same naturalness that their great-grandparents talked about purgatives or elixirs to cure impotence. These people embody what can be considered as "new temples of effort", displaying the "pastoral work of sweat": they condense the pleasures of belonging to a species capable of mutating from soft to hard, from weak to strong, from slow to fast and from fragile to *poderoso*. From now on, for the fat, the thin and the obese, the figure of the sedentary—real or imaginary—has become a kind of risky deficit, a pessimistic shadow in the face of gleaming images of sportspeople and "healed" bodies (Sant'Anna, 2016).

Evidently, nowadays, the ways of measuring the weight and volume of bodies have become more rigorous than in the past. Simultaneously, the habit of weighing the body has become much more integrated into the routine of Brazilians than 50 years ago. But what has come up now with great evidence is the affirmation of an ideal body assimilated as a "platform of resources" and always available to become more and more profitable (Sant'Anna, 2014).

Despite all this, obesity progressively became a worrisome topic and an increasingly evident reality. In 1986, the Brazilian Association for the Study of Obesity and Metabolic Syndrome was founded, and ten years later, it joined the International Association for the Study of Obesity, thus confirming how much the theme of obesity had given way to a huge field of scientific research and public policies. Obesity among the lower classes increased as they started to have access to a wider range of industrialized products (Ferreira & Magalhães, 2005). This change contributed to make people labeled as "obese" extremely ambivalent figures: on the one hand, they seem to be victims, extremely poor and sick, not able to afford to eat "healthy" food. On the other hand, the obese started to be seen as the only ones responsible for their bodies, the great culprits, the ones who do not know how to eat properly, do not eat healthy food and ignore elementary ways to care for their bodies.

Bodies outside the standards

In 2008, the Brazilian Society of Bariatric and Metabolic Surgery concluded that, among young Brazilians aged 18–25, two-thirds were overweight and 5 percent were obese. Obesity grew more among low-income people, who tended to eat more processed foods. Since then, the image of obesity has been overloaded with negativity and fat bodies have been seen as obese. The obese are now considered ill as well as people who don't know how to "invest" in themselves, who do not have any control over their own bodies. The negative feeling of being overweight, therefore, increased significantly in the country (Stenzel, 2002).

In fact, obesity affects all social classes as well as both sexes, but it tends to concentrate more intensely among lower income populations. As black women and men tend to make up the largest share of poor people in the country, the high prevalence of obesity among Black

Brazilians is mainly related to their eating habits and conditions. Subjected to low quality food, they tend to develop many diseases such as arterial high blood pressure, diabetes, breathing problems, among others. Around 56 percent of the Brazilian population declares itself to be black and that the majority do not have access to healthy food or to quality physical activities. Thus, in 2001, a study by the Brazilian Ministry of Health revealed that the access to health services was more limited for the black population (Ministério da Saúde, 2001). This situation leads to the worst prognosis for diseases that affect black people in Brazil.

Although racism is structural in Brazilian society, the intensity of racial prejudice varies according to "the black traits" and mainly to skin color. Racial tensions have achieved unprecedented media importance in recent years which gave visibility to a kind of apartheid (although little assumed in the country) between the poor and the rich, the black and the white. Black and mixed-race endure structural and institutional racism and therefore totally contradicting the myth of racial democracy.

However, it would be necessary to consider that, in the course of the last two decades, the context of Brazilian racism suffered a series of upheavals; yet, it was intertwined by affirmative actions that were previously unthinkable. Movements of affirmation of blackness joined those of affirmation of obesity, inside and outside social networks, drawing the attention of entrepreneurs and cultural agents who tended to include some changes in the panorama of what was considered acceptable and profitable in the mainstream.

The affirmation movements of black bodies and outside the weight standards and measures considered "healthy" and "beautiful" were also strengthened as the activism of different groups acquired public visibility. Thus, for example, attention to health vulnerabilities started to be incorporated into public management, especially after the Zumbi dos Palmares National March in 1995, which brought thousands of activists to the Brazilian capital, causing the creation of the Inter-ministerial Working Group to the Valorization of the Black Population, for the formulation of proposals for government action. Furthermore, in popular music and, in particular, in the funk universe, fat black men and women achieved an unusual role that expanded to social media and, in some cases, to the advertising of products hitherto exclusive to the thin white population.

An illustrative example is the success of MC Carol invited to appear in the advertising of a cosmetics brand. Another example is Jojo Todynho, a funk singer with thousands of followers on social media. The speed with which social media reaches thousands of people contributes to making famous individuals who would otherwise have little chance of being recognized. In this sense, Preta Gil, an activist who is promoting the aesthetics of fat black bodies through Instagram, has helped to make black fat women more visible. Tati Quebra-Barraco (2004), who is a popular singer in the funk universe, is also part of the same trend and has become famous by proclaiming the statement, "I'm ugly but I'm trendy", through one of her most famous songs.

Becoming successful in a predominantly male musical environment was a great achievement of these women and has been increasingly strong since the beginning of this millennium. The funk universe underwent important changes, thanks to the presence of black, fat women who contributed to what was called the empowerment of poor and black women. On stage and with the affirmation of what many called "sensual funk", different from the old fight funk, they have become the target of the mainstream press and some television shows. Opinions are divided between those who do not recognize funk as an artistic expression and those who, on the contrary, perceive funk—particularly that born in the poor communities of Rio de Janeiro—as a cultural experience capable of empowering its inhabitants.

Besides that, it was not long before movements in favor of the fat body produced many defenders of the plus size (Nechar, 2015). It can be noted therefore that fascination with a *corpo poderoso* remains. In a country where the population is predominantly young, there is a brutal competition in the markets of labor and of love. Thus, the fear of not seeming able to produce yourself as the owner of a powerful and youthful body reigns.

Positive views of large bodies are emerging in great numbers, at the time that advertisings of obesity as a pathology have also increased. The weight and volume of people's bodies depend, in fact, on their social and economic conditions. The old fascination with a strong and large body remains present among the various social sectors of the country, revealing that the expression of success and health for someone who lives in an extremely socially unequal, violent, yet tropical and young country, must go through to a large extent, a hyper-weighted body.

Notes

1 This chapter is part of a broader study published in 2016 in the book *Gordos, magros e obesos – Uma história de peso no Brasil [Fat, thin and obese – A history of weight in Brazil]*.
2 For example, an advertising in the *Fon-Fon Magazine* in August 1922 stated that "children will be strong, ruddy and fat by eating" the "delicious porridge" of the brand "Feculose".
3 *Boa Forma* was first published in São Paulo in 1986 by Editorial Abril. *Corpo a Corpo* was first published in São Paulo in 1987 by Editorial Simbolo.

References

Ferreira, V. A., & Magalhães, R. (2005). Obesidade e pobreza: O aparente paradoxo. Um estudo com mulheres da Favela da Rocinha, Rio de Janeiro, Brazil [Obesity and poverty: The apparent paradox. A study with women from the Rocinha slum, Rio de Janeiro, Brazil]. *Cadernos de Saúde Pública, 21*(6), 1792–1800. doi: 10.1590/S0102–311X2005000600027

Lobato, M. (1918). *Urupês*. Rio de Janeiro: Companhia ed. Nacional.

Ministério da Saúde. (2001). *Manual de doenças mais importantes por razões étnicas, na população Brasileira Afro-descendente [Handbook of most important diseases for ethnic reasons, in Afro-descendant Brazilian population]*. Brasilia, BR: Minstério da Saúde.

Nechar, P. A. (2015). *Culturas e comunicações do universo plus-size: Uma cartografia das imagens de corpo nos discursos nas redes sociais [Cultures and communications in the plus-size universe: A cartography of body images in social media discourses]*. (Master's thesis, Pontifícia Universidade Católica de São Paulo, São Paulo, Brazil).

O Cruzeiro. (1946, June 29). O vigor e a perfeição do corpo humano: Combata a causa de suá magreza e transforme-a em vigor [The power and perfection of the human body: Fight your thinness and become powerful]. *O Cruzeiro, 1946*(36), 34.

O Cruzeiro. (1962, December 15). Calorias não engordam [Calories don't make you fat]. *O Cruzeiro, 1962*(10), 97.

Pinto, R. P. (2015). *A invenção da brasileira: Uma história sobre imagem feminina e Turismo [The invention of the Brazilian woman: a history of female image and tourism]*. (Master's thesis, Pontifícia Universidade Católica de São Paulo, São Paulo, Brazil).

Quebra-Barraco, T. (2004). Sou feia, mas tô na moda [I'm ugly, but I'm trendy]. On *Boladona*. Link Records.

Sant'Anna, D. B. de. (2014). *História da beleza no brasil [A history of beauty in Brazil]*. São Paulo: Contexto.

Sant'Anna, D. B. de. (2016). *Gordos, magros e obesos. Uma história de peso no Brasil [Fat, thin and obese. A history of weight in Brazil]*. São Paulo: Estação Liberdade.

Stenzel, L. M. (2002). *Obesidade: O peso da exclusão [Obesity: The weight of exclusion]*. Porto Alegre: EDIPUCRS.

Um Phenomeno [A phenomenon]. (1900, October 26). *Jornal do Brasil*, p. 1.

Vigarello, G. (2010). *Les métamorphoses du gras. Histoire de l'obésité. Du moyen age au XXe Siècle [The metamorphosis of fat: A history of obesity. From Middle Age to the 20th Century]*. Paris, FR: Seuil.

Zucon, O. (2006). *Da corporalidade: Concepções médicas sobre a forma corporal [Corporality: Medical conceptions about body shape]*. (Master's thesis, Universidade Federal de Santa Catarina, Santa Catarina, Brazil).

6

MIDDLE-AGED BUSINESSMAN AND SOCIAL PROGRESS

The links between risk factor research and the obesity epidemic

Isabel Fletcher

Introduction

In this chapter, I will provide a brief introduction to the history of obesity research from the perspective of my interest in the 20th-century history of chronic disease epidemiology. I begin by explaining why obesity is best considered as a modern phenomenon and describe the ways in which contemporary medical knowledge about obesity and overweight derives from American and British research into the causes of coronary heart disease (CHD). I continue by describing how risk factor approaches to chronic disease were adopted by the World Health Organization (WHO) and became an important precursor to understandings of obesity as a global epidemic that developed in the 1990s. Finally, I conclude with some thoughts of what the history of medicine can contribute to debates about appropriate responses to rising rates of obesity and overweight.

Although the term obesity was first used in the early 20th century (Sobal, 1995, p. 70), large body size is not a new phenomenon. The health problems associated with excess body weight have been known to medical practitioners since the time of Hippocrates (Vigarello, 2013, p. 10). The prosperity of industrialised economies is also a relatively recent phenomenon – hunger and famine occurred in parts of Europe until the 1950s (Oddy, Atkins, & Amilien, 2009, p. 224), and in such contexts, large body size could be seen as evidence of health, and even the capacity to survive episodes of infectious disease.

However, a profound shift took place in the medical research and practice of industrialised countries after World War II. Mortality rates from infectious disease had fallen and growing concern about increasing mortality from chronic diseases, such as heart disease and cancer, led to the development of new research methods to understand the causes and treatments of these conditions. The most important of these was the large-scale prospective epidemiological study, as exemplified by the Framingham Heart Study, set up in 1948 to investigate the prevalence and development of heart disease (Dawber, 1980, p. 239). Framingham researchers developed an understanding of heart disease as a multi-factorial condition caused by a set of lifestyle-related attributes such as high blood pressure, cigarette smoking, and elevated blood cholesterol levels. These attributes quickly became known as risk factors, and this approach became a crucial element of post-war models of the causes of CHD (Aronowitz, 1998, p. 113). This model and the wider field of chronic disease epidemiology is

DOI: 10.4324/9780429344824-8

one key source of biomedical concern with excess body weight – obesity became the subject of 20th-century medical research, in large part because of its status as a risk factor for heart disease.

This case study is important to critical obesity studies because it highlights a key moment when 20th-century medical knowledge shifted its focus away from the environments in which people lived and towards the measurable effects of their behaviour on health. This narrow concern with individual behaviour and "lifestyle" continues to dominate medical and policy understanding of obesity and overweight, largely obscuring debates about the wider structural causes of ill-health and inequalities.

The epidemiological transition and heart disease

Mortality statistics collected in countries, such as the UK and the US, show a striking change in disease prevalence after the middle of the 19th century. Overall, mortality rates declined due to a decrease in death rates from infectious diseases such as cholera, typhoid, and tuberculosis. However, this decline was perplexingly associated with an increase in rates of chronic or non-communicable diseases (NCDs). Certain of these diseases, including heart disease, stroke, cancer, and diabetes, seemed to be becoming important sources of mortality and morbidity. One epidemiological textbook explained that:

> In the ageing population of an affluent society, which has mastered many of the infections and malnutrition, and has high standards of maternal and child care, these chronic diseases increasingly dominate the practice of medicine.
>
> *(Morris, 1964, p. 133)*

This change has been labelled the "epidemiological transition" (Omram, 1971; Susser, 1985, pp. 149–151; Szreter, 2007, pp. 4–5). During this transition, many countries are understood to have shifted from a pattern of high mortality and high rates of infectious diseases to one of low rates of mortality and higher rates of chronic diseases. Between the early 19th and early 20th centuries, such a shift was associated with dramatic increases in average life expectancies in the industrialising economies of the UK, USA, and Western Europe. As part of this shift, average body weight increased, and from the first decade of the 20th century, dieting for weight loss became a mass phenomenon in the US (Stearns, 2002).

As rates of infectious disease fell, widespread medical (and public) concern developed about high rates of heart disease amongst certain populations. William Rothstein argues that the diagnosis of CHD was rare in the late 19th century and only became sufficiently common to be included as a new and growing problem in medical textbooks of the 1920s (see also Lawrence, 1997; Rothstein, 2003, p. 199). By the 1950s, chronic diseases – and especially CHD in middle-aged men – were seen as a major health problem in the US, and there was a developing consensus that the British population was also suffering from rising rates of CHD (Bartley, 1985, p. 289). This new concern with heart disease led to the production of further evidence for its growing prevalence including a 1953 series of post-mortems on soldiers killed in the Korean War, which unexpectedly showed that the majority had some degree of narrowing of the arteries (seen to be a precursor of CHD) (Atrens, 1994).

From the early days of cardiology, middle-aged male businessmen had been seen as particularly vulnerable to heart disease, "Business men leading lives of great strain, and eating, and drinking, and smoking to excess, form the largest contingent of angina cases" (William

Osler [1914] quoted in Rothstein, 2003, p. 206).[1] Such accounts focused on the dangers of affluent living and the stresses of modern city life. Studies based on insurance company data (see below) from the 1920s and 1930s showed that CHD rates were higher for men than for women with a ratio that decreased with increasing age (Rothstein, 2003, p. 206). However, despite doctors' willingness to believe that CHD was a disease of the affluent, later studies in the 1950s showed that lower socio-economic groups actually had higher rates of heart disease (Rothstein, 2003, p. 208). But the stereotype meant that high mortality from heart disease was seen as an important economic problem, since it killed middle-aged men who were key wage earners.

Mid-20th-century doctors and policymakers proposed various explanations for the ep-idemiological transition. The decline in infectious disease was usually attributed to a com-bination of medical and social progress – improvements in public health and medicine and rising standards of living were all seen to have played a role (Susser, 1985, p. 150). During this period, doctors and medical scientists had developed a clear explanatory paradigm for infectious diseases based on laboratory-based scientific knowledge of the infectious and pathological role of bacteria and viruses. This new model was based on the idea of specific causes of disease rather than the environment or the patient's individual disposition. Because this "bacteriological revolution" was so successful, it eclipsed other explanations for disease for much of the next 50 years: "alternative, nonbacterial theories of infection ceased to be articulated" (Worboys, 2000, p. 280). Even in disciplines such as epidemiology, which had strong links to public health and traditions of social medicine, bacteriological explanations were dominant in this period (Amsterdamska, 2005).

By contrast, the causes of chronic diseases were not known. Because such diseases develop over several decades, researchers could not readily identify specific aetiological factors as had been the case for infectious diseases (Rothstein, 2003, p. 5). A historian of public health, Elizabeth Fee, describes the post-war situation as one of confusion and feuding between medicine and public health.

> There was little agreement or clarity about the relevance of nutritional, occupational or environmental health – or about any other aetiological factors… The chronic diseases – cancer, hypertension, diabetes and others – could neither be prevented nor cured on the older public health and medical models; at best, they could be controlled through screening, education and medical supervision.
>
> *(Fee, 1996, p. 250)*

This explanatory gap meant that doctors tended to invoke other explanations, especially the ones that involved assumptions about medical and social progress, though in often ambiva-lent or contradictory ways. The rise in chronic diseases was often attributed to the fact that, due to the decline in rates of infectious disease, people lived longer. Conditions such as heart disease and other cardiovascular diseases were simply the result of older bodies or individual organs wearing out – hence the label of "degenerative diseases". Distinguishing ageing from the diseases that often accompanied it led to the hope that these conditions might be treatable (Aronowitz, 1998, p. 122). An alternative, more pessimistic, understanding drew on narra-tives of the "pathologies of progress" (Rosenberg, 1998) to argue that diseases such as CHD resulted from changes in lifestyle due to increased wealth – hence the term "diseases of af-fluence" (Morris, 1964). Due to economic growth and increasing prosperity, the excesses of eating, drinking, and smoking that Osler described in 1914 as habits of wealthy businessman were thought to be becoming commonplace.

Obesity as a risk factor for chronic disease

Meanwhile, certain strands of research were developing new ways of investigating the aetiology of chronic diseases, especially CHD, which replaced laboratory research. A key resource was the actuarial investigations taking place within the American insurance industry. In the early 20th century, American insurance companies began to develop mortality tables, in order to be able to insure individuals at above-average risk, known as "impaired lives" or "substandard risks" (Rothstein, 2003, p. 63). Due to increasing prosperity, life insurance was a rapidly expanding industry during the late 19th and early 20th centuries. Insurance companies employed local doctors to measure and examine potential policyholders – they "systematically and effectively accumulated relevant physical examination data and related it to the health and disease potential of the largest number of people in the United States prior to World War I" (Davis, 1981, p. 394). Insurance companies, especially the Metropolitan Life Insurance Company, had the most comprehensive collection of data on trends in body weight and its relationship to health until at least the 1960s, when governments started to collect such information (Oddy, Atkins, & Amilien, 2009, p. 225).

The Joint Committee on Mortality, an insurance company body, published a series of studies between 1912 and 1939 identifying new medical factors which increased the risk of mortality. The following excerpt summarises this process for one particular risk factor, body weight:

> The most unexpected finding of the original 1903 study was the discovery of a strong relationship between mortality and "build", a construct that combined height and weight. Using industry data gathered between 1909 and 1928 for all male policyholders ages 40 to 49 and taking 100 as the average mortality rate, those who were at least 25% overweight for their height had a relative mortality rate of 141, those of average weight had a relative mortality rate of 86, and those who were 5% to 14% underweight had a relative mortality rate of 77.... The low mortality rates of slightly underweight policy holders astonished physicians who were busy treating gaunt patients sick or dying of tuberculosis, the "wasting disease". They viewed ruddy and rotund persons as the epitome of good health and underweight ones as suspect. Although the medical directors had no theory of disease etiology that explained the statistical relationship, they accepted it unequivocally and made it a key factor in selection [of policyholders].
>
> *(Rothstein, 2003, p. 64)*

Medical directors of insurance companies accepted this new and unexpected relationship between build and increased mortality. Their use of weight in medical examinations, the selection of policyholders, and the construction of mortality tables made weight – or build – one of a set of important medical risks that also included high blood pressure, diabetes, and kidney disease.

A new kind of research study

A major research effort was seen as necessary to investigate the precise causes of the epidemic of CHD and provide information on how to prevent future cases. During the 1940s, the American Heart Association (AHA) drew on fears of the growth of heart disease to raise funds and lobby politicians, leading in 1948 to the creation of the National Heart Institution (NHI) within the National Institute of Health (NIH) (Fye, 1996). This increased funding for medical research post-World War II resulting in a dramatic expansion in cardiovascular research activity, and US cardiology continued to expand throughout the 1950s and 1960s (Fye, 1996, p. 181).

Also, in 1948, the NHI and the University of Boston set up the Framingham Heart Study, a pioneering study of the risk factors for heart disease based in a small Massachusetts town. To analyse their early results, the Framingham researchers borrowed the idea of risk factors from the insurance industry, and from 1961, the terms "factors of risk" or "risk factor" were being used in study publications (Rothstein, 2003, p. 283). The first risk factors identified were age and sex; subsequently, already identified risk factors of hypertension, raised blood cholesterol, increased body weight, and smoking were also re-identified (Dawber, 1980).

The success of the Framingham researchers in identifying risk factors for heart disease led to the setting up of other large-scale prospective epidemiological studies. In 1958, Ancel Keys of University of Minnesota, with support from the WHO and the NHI, set up the Seven Countries Study. Building on his previous research, Keys and his collaborators hypothesised that "differences among populations in the frequency of heart attacks and stroke would occur in some orderly relation to physical characteristics and lifestyle, particularly composition of the diet, and especially fats in the diet" (Blackburn, n.d.). The final version of the study included 18 cohorts of men aged 40–59 from Finland, Greece, The Netherlands, Italy, Japan, the US, and the former Yugoslavia. These areas were selected for a combination of pragmatic reasons (research contacts who were willing to collaborate at low cost) and dietary or epidemiological variability – Japan had very low rates of heart disease at the time and Finland very high ones, and Greece had high levels of consumption of olive oil (Keys, 1980, p. 7).

This first group of studies were organised by American research institutions. However, in the 1970s, European bodies, such as the WHO Europe Office, began to set up their own studies. The most famous of these was the North Karelia Project, a collaboration between the Finnish government, the Finnish Heart Association, the University of Kuopio, and the WHO, which ran from 1972 to 1977. An important component of this study was an attempt to reduce the prevalence of risk factors, and therefore cardio-vascular disease, in a population chosen because they had very high rates of those diseases. The risk factors identified were smoking, blood cholesterol levels (or diet), and hypertension, and "[P]ractically none of the adult population had a 'safe' level of all risk factors" (National Public Health Laboratory of Finland, 1981, p. 18). The North Karelia Project is still routinely described as one of the very few successful health interventions in the area of cardiovascular disease.[2] The project report claims reductions in all CHD risk factors of 17.4 percent for men and 11.5 percent for women (National Public Health Laboratory of Finland, 1981, p. 303).

A final large-scale epidemiological study that falls directly in this tradition of research is the WHO MONICA project (MONitoring of trends and determinants in CArdiovascular diseases). MONICA was a European prestige project set up to rival Framingham – it was self-consciously modelled on the studies that had been running in the US since the 1950s. It began in 1978 and ran for 23 years, collecting data on 38 populations in 21 countries. Like North Karelia, MONICA had strong links with the WHO Regional Office for Europe in Copenhagen.[3] One commentator has described it as the "first global epidemiological study" (McKee, 2003, p. 613). MONICA data on average body weights in European populations was important evidence for early claims that increasing rates of obesity and overweight were becoming a public health problem (WHO, 2000).

The development of risk factor models

Risk factor analysis represented a new model for research into disease and ill-health. Its development in the UK in the 1950s has been described as a "paradigm shift" that led to the "growing acceptability of epidemiological rather than the biomedical, laboratory-based mode of proof" (Berridge & Loughlin, 2006, p. 957). Partly, this was due to wide dissemination of the "probabilistic yet 'hard' data" (Aronowitz, 1998, p. 121) produced by studies like Framingham which was important in the acceptance of risk factor approaches. Individual susceptibility to heart disease could still not be satisfactorily explained, and risk factor approaches were successful because they "gave some sense of who was at greatest risk and what one might do to decrease risk" and "embodied the cultural and medical ideals of precision, specificity and quantification" (Aronowitz, 1998, p. 125).

However, risk factor analysis, being based on the identification of statistical correlation, does not identify causes *at all* – merely associations. Moreover, a number of historians have noted that the identification of risk factors as causes has also tended to be distinctly selective. In principle, risk factor analysis is open to the possibility that multiple causes or predisposing factors – including social and environmental factors – may contribute to the production of disease and that such causes may interact holistically. Epidemiologists borrowed the concept of "risk factor" from the life insurance industry. However, life insurance risk factors were understood in terms of a gradient of risk and were related to each other and the social characteristics of the applicant, whereas Framingham risk factors were categorised as health or unhealthy, operated separately from each other, and only considered participants' medical characteristics:

> Despite some promising early findings, [Framingham researchers], disregarded social characteristics such as education, income, occupation, living conditions, usual sources of health care, marital status, place of birth, and family structure. Yet social characteristics are as important as physiological ones in clinical decisions...The narrow focus of this pioneering study established an unfortunate precedent for most subsequent studies.
>
> *(Rothstein, 2003, p. 285)*

It is not clear why this occurred. Aronowitz attributes it in part to historical accident, resulting from the initial framing of the Framingham study. The original aims of the study were far less ambitious than they subsequently became and were oriented towards identifying risks in the sense of clinically useful measurements to predict the likelihood of heart disease in particular individuals (Aronowitz, 1998, p. 120) – not larger social and environmental factors. Only subsequently was it decided to turn Framingham into a prospective study to identify risk factors more generally, but the individualised perspective was retained. He also identifies in the Framingham study a tendency towards biological reductionism, in the sense of a tendency to see risks as real only insofar as they can be explained in terms of underlying biological causal processes:

> Nonspecific and less individualistic variables, even if they could be measured and manipulated as if they were specific characteristics of the individual, have not been easily assimilated into mechanistic models of disease and mainstream clinical and public health approaches. Such variables generally lack a direct biological mechanism by which coronary artery pathology develops in the individual.
>
> *(Aronowitz, 1998, pp. 132–133)*

At the same time, this biological understanding of risk factors facilitated their incorporation, at least in certain instances, into clinical medicine, and indeed to certain risk factors coming increasingly to be seen as diseases in their own right. A case in point is hypertension, long recognised as a risk factor in heart disease. With the advent of effective drugs to treat hypertension, clinicians began to pay greater attention to the condition, and hypertension was redefined not just a risk factor, but as an occult form of pathology, defined by guideline thresholds and made visible through routine surveillance with the sphygmomanometer (Timmermann, 2006, pp. 245–246).

Ironically, this narrowing of the scope of what kinds of factors can be considered causal has actually weakened the explanatory power of the risk factor approach. As a number of epidemiologists have pointed out, risk factor analysis, as it has developed since Framingham, is only capable of explaining a certain proportion of variation in rates of heart disease within populations (Rose & Marmot, 1981). These processes of defining diseases and their causes demonstrate ways in which "medicine individualises disease and writes-out social deprivation and inequality from the description of illness" (Bartley, 1985, p. 292). Relating health inequalities to socio-economic class or race can operate a form of "black-boxing" (Berlivet, 2003, p. 52) that obscures the mechanisms creating these negative health effects. Epidemiology "renders invisible the very social relations of power structuring material and psychic conditions and life chances that contribute to the stratification of health and illness" (Shim, 2002, p. 134).

More radically, Bartley (1985) has challenged aspects of the idea of the demographic transition itself, and specifically, the ideas that there was an increase in the incidence of CHD after the World War II. She argues that the apparent post-war rise in CHD was actually due to a reclassification of forms of disease that were already prevalent among middle-aged men, and that, contrary to narrative of a post-war increase in heart disease, in the early post-war period, there was continuing uncertainty as to whether rates for heart disease were still rising (Bartley, 1985, p. 300). From her re-reading of contemporary accounts concludes that ultimately, "we can take as our problem, not the 'epidemic of heart disease', but rather, the failure of the health of men (particularly working class men) in later working life to improve appreciably in the last fifty years" (Bartley, 1985, p. 309).[4]

Such a conclusion – although not widely accepted as far as I can judge – is important because it leads to questions about the distribution of the improvements in health between different sections of the population. In arguing that the high post-war rate of heart disease among middle-aged working class men is continuous with the ill health, they suffered between the wars, Bartley is arguing, in effect, that the health improvements enjoyed by the rest of the population have largely bypassed this group. Such a conclusion is consistent with research into the wider causes of health inequalities (Wilkinson, 1996).

The role of the WHO

An international consensus about the relevant risk factors to investigate began to develop relatively fast. A 1957 WHO technical report on atherosclerosis and heart disease discussed the role of environmental factors such as calories, obesity, and overweight (labelled as dietary factors), physical activity, stress, alcohol and tobacco, and infections (WHO, 1957). In this report, the authors state that "obesity in itself is not a primary factor in producing ischaemic heart disease" (WHO, 1957, p. 17). The WHO continued to publish infrequent technical reports on heart disease, but until a 1980s publication on the prevention of CHD (WHO, 1982), these did not discuss the different risk factors in great detail. The authors of this report included body weight as one of the "life-style" risk factors for CHD referring to "the mass nature of obesity and the profound sedentariness of many modern cultures" (WHO, 1982, p. 22, p. 30). The authors of the next report which focused on prevention and control described how, "The emergence of mass CHD has accompanied the increase in affluence in industrialized societies; affluence itself is not to blame for cardiovascular disease, but only certain specific components of the affluent life" (WHO, 1986, p. 9).

However, teasing out of which aspects of the affluent lifestyle were harmful to health was proving difficult, as shown by the acknowledgement that higher mortality rates amongst the less affluent "cannot be fully explained by the standard cardiovascular risk factors" (*ibid.*). These authors framed the problem as one of "nutrient excess" and argued for the "avoidance of weight gain and obesity" by advising individuals to increase their physical activity and to reduce the energy-density of their diet (WHO, 1986, p. 14).

In the late 1960s, the WHO Europe regional office had developed a research programme into cardiovascular disease, particularly CHD (Kaprio, 1991, pp. 35–36; Lee, 1998, pp. 94–95). From the late 1980s, the Organisation as a whole began to move into the area of nutrition and health, publishing a technical report on nutrition and chronic disease (WHO, 1990) and prioritising tackling obesity and diet-related disease in the 1993 Nutrition Programme (Baggott, 2000, p. 172). This technical report contains many references to obesity, framing it as a disease in its own right resulting from rapid economic development and modernisation. This was the approach used in later reports where increasing average body weights were seen as a global health problem, an important issue in its own right (e.g., WHO, 1995, 2000). The 2000 technical report, in particular, was frequently cited in early medical and popular reporting of the obesity epidemic.

Conclusion

As I have described above, one key source of medical knowledge about the relationship between health and body weight was epidemiological and clinical research into the causes of chronic diseases and especially CHD. Historical approaches complement other analyses of medical knowledge and practice about obesity and overweight by highlighting a couple of key issues. First, risk factor models focused on individual (rather than environmental) causes of heart disease, often behavioural causes. Despite discussions of the role of "obesogenic" environments (Government Office for Science, 2007; Swinburn, 2008), the influence of these models is one reason for a continuing focus on individual behaviour in official policies around diet and health. Second, anxieties about the negative effects on health of increasing prosperity and especially modern urban life seep into debates about the causes of chronic disease and later obesity. These anxieties can make some causes of obesity and overweight – for example, sedentary lifestyles (WHO, 2000) – seem "obvious" in the absence of concrete evidence. However, combined with a focus on individual-level causes, they also obscure questions about the relationship between economic inequalities and increasing average body weights – about which groups are not benefitting from increasing prosperity.

Notes

1 These ideas fed into theories of the Type A personality that were developed by American sociologists from the late 1950s onwards (Riska, 2000).
2 It has even been regularly described as the only successful public health intervention aiming at reducing body weight, even though this was not one of the project's aims, and there is no available data to demonstrate this success.

3 One of the other members of the MONICA steering committee was Professor Jaakko Tuomilehto who was centrally involved in the North Karelia Project.
4 One of the reasons prospective studies such as Framingham were undertaken was the realisation that the positive effects of the epidemiological transition had by-passed the middle-aged (Aronowitz, 1998, p. 123).

References

Amsterdamska, O. (2005). Demarcating epidemiology. *Science Technology and Human Values, 30*(1), 17–51. doi: 10.1177/0162243904270719

Aronowitz, R. A. (1998). *Making sense of illness: Science, society and disease.* Cambridge, UK: Cambridge University Press.

Atrens, D. M. (1994). The questionable wisdom of a low-fat diet and cholesterol reduction. *Social Science and Medicine, 39*(3), 433–447. doi: 10.1016/0277-9536(94)90141-4

Baggott, R. (2000). *Public health: Policy and politics.* Basingstoke & London, UK: Macmillan Press Ltd.

Bartley, M. (1985). Coronary heart disease and the public health 1850–1983. *Sociology of Health and Illness, 7*(3), 289–313. doi: 10.1111/j.1467-9566.1985.tb00291.x

Berlivet (2003). "Association or causation?" The debate on the scientific status of risk factor epidemiology 1947 – c.1965. In V. Berridge (Ed.) *Making health policy; networks in research and policy after 1945.* Amsterdam: Rodolphi.

Berridge, V., & Loughlin, K. (2006). Smoking and the new health education in Britain 1950s to 1970s. *American Journal of Public Health, 95*(6), 956–964. doi: 10.2105/AJPH.2004.037887

Blackburn, H. (n.d., April 4, 2009). Overview: The seven countries study in brief. Retrieved from http://www.epi.umn.edu/research/7countries/overview.shtm

Davis, A. B. (1981). Life insurance and the physical examination: A chapter in the rise of American medical technology. *Bulletin of the History of Medicine, 55*(3), 392–406.

Dawber, T. R. (1980). *The Framingham Study: The epidemiology of atheroschlerotic disease.* Cambridge, MA & London: Harvard University Press and the Commonwealth Fund.

Fee, E. (1996). Public health and the State: The United States. In D. Porter (Ed.), *The history of public health and the modern state.* Amsterdam& Atlanta GA: Rodopi.

Fye, W. B. (1996). *American cardiology: The history of a speciality and its college.* Baltimore, MD & London: The Johns Hopkins University Press.

Government Office for Science. (2007). *Foresight tackling obesities: Future choices – project report.* Retrieved from https://www.gov.uk/government/collections/tackling-obesities-future-choices

Kaprio, L. A. (1991). *Forty years of WHO in Europe: The development of a common health policy.* Copenhagen: World Health Organization Regional Publications.

Keys, A. (1980). *Seven countries: a multivariate analysis of death and coronary heart disease.* Cambridge, MA & London: Harvard University Press and the Commonwealth Fund.

Lawrence, C. (1997). "Definite and material": Coronary thrombosis and cardiologists in the 1920s. In C. E. Rosenberg & J. Golden (Eds.), *Framing disease: Studies in cultural history.* New Jersey: Rutgers University Press.

Lee, K. (1998). *Historical dictionary of the World Health Organization.* Lanham, MD & London: The Scarecrow Press Inc.

McKee, M. (2003). MONICA: Monograph and multimedia sourcebook. *Journal of the Royal Society of Medicine, 96*(12), 613–614.

Morris, J. N. (1964). *Uses of epidemiology* (2nd ed.). Edinburgh: E. & S. Livingstone.

National Public Health Laboratory of Finland. (1981). *Community control of cardiovascular diseases: Evaluation of a comprehensive community programme for control of cardiovascular disease in North Karelia, Finland 1972–1977.* Copenhagen: World Health Organization Regional Office for Europe.

Oddy, D. J., Atkins, P. J., & Amilien, V. (Eds.). (2009). *The rise of obesity in Europe: A twentieth century food history.* Farnham, Surrey and Burlington: Ashgate.

Omram, A. R. (1971). The epidemiologic transition: A theory of the epidemiology of population change. *Milbank Memorial Fund Quarterly, 49*, 509–538. doi: 10.1111/j.1468-0009.2005.00398.x

Riska, E. (2000). The rise and fall of Type A man. *Social Science and Medicine, 51*(11), 1665–1674. doi: 10.1016/S0277-9536(00)00085-X

Rose, G., & Marmot, M. (1981). Social class and coronary heart disease. *British Heart Journal, 145,* 13–19. doi: 10.1136/hrt.45.1.13

Rosenberg, C. E. (1998). Pathologies as progress: The idea of civilisation as risk. *Bulletin of the History of Medicine, 72*(4), 714–730. doi: 10.1353/bhm.1998.0217

Rothstein, W. G. (2003). *Public Health and the risk factor: A history of an uneven medical revolution.* Rochester, NY: University of Rochester Press.

Shim, J. K. (2002). Understanding the routinised inclusion of race, socioeconomic status and sex in epidemiology: the utility of concepts from technoscience studies. *Sociology of Health and Illness, 24*(2), 129–150. doi: 10.1111/1467-9566.00288

Sobal, J. (1995). The medicalization and demedicalization of obesity. In J. Sobal, & D. Maurer (Eds.), *Eating agendas: Food and Nutrition as Social Problems.* New York: Aldine de Gruyter.

Stearns, P. N. (2002). *Fat history: Bodies and beauty in the modern west.* New York& London: New York University Press.

Susser, M. (1985). Epidemiology in the United States after World War II: The evolution of technique. *Epidemiologic Reviews, 7,* 147–177. doi: 10.1093/oxfordjournals.epirev.a036280

Swinburn, B. A. (2008). Obesity prevention: The role of policies, laws and regulations. *Australia and New Zealand Health Policy, 5*(12). doi: 10.1186/1743-8462-5-12

Szreter, S. (2007). *Health and wealth: Studies in history and policy.* Rochester, NY: University of Rochester Press.

Timmermann, C. (2006). A matter of degree: The normalisation of hypertension c.1940–2000. In W. Ernst (Ed.), *Histories of the normal and the abnormal.* Abingdon, Oxon & New York: Routledge.

Vigarello, G. (2013). *The metamorphoses of fat: A history of obesity* (translated by C. Jon Delogu). New York: Columbia University Press.

WHO. (1957). *Atherosclerosis and ischaemic heart disease* (Technical Report 117). Retrieved from https://apps.who.int/iris/handle/10665/40372

WHO. (1982). *Prevention of coronary heart disease* (Technical Report 678). Retrieved from https://apps.who.int/iris/handle/10665/39293

WHO. (1986). *Community prevention and control of cardiovascular diseases* (Technical Report 732). Retrieved from https://apps.who.int/iris/handle/10665/38004

WHO. (1990). *Diet, nutrition, and the prevention of chronic diseases* (Technical Report 797). Retrieved from https://www.who.int/nutrition/publications/obesity/WHO_TRS_797/en/

WHO. (1995). *Physical status: The use and interpretation of anthropometry* (Technical Report 854). Retrieved from https://www.who.int/childgrowth/publications/physical_status/en/

WHO. (2000). *Obesity: Preventing and managing the global epidemic* (Technical Report 894). Retrieved from: https://www.who.int/nutrition/publications/obesity/WHO_TRS_894/en/

Wilkinson, R. G. (1996). *Unhealthy societies: The afflictions of inequality.* London& New York: Routledge.

Worboys, M. (2000). *Spreading germs: Disease theories and medical practice in Britain 1865–1900.* Cambridge: Cambridge University Press.

7

CRISIS REVISITED

Historical notes on a modern 'obesity epidemic'

Michael Gard

Most of what follows, written slightly over a decade ago, was my attempt to characterise the scale of the 'obesity epidemic'. There are many instructing factors that one might revisit this area, particularly as the health debates and agenda has partly but steadily moved on. My purpose is first to give some historical background for the rest of the chapters in this volume and, second, to give some flavour and, in some cases, the 'heat' of these important debates.

As I have written this elsewhere, my entrance into the sociological health literature happened 20 years ago following the emergence of something called the 'obesity epidemic'. For some years, I had engaged with the fat movement and writers who their work began in the late 1960s, although there is some debate about its origins. But when the term 'obesity epidemic' was proposed in the closing years of the 20th century, it was hardly news for people who follow the health literature at that time and even less so for fat activists. The fat activists had been battling fat hatred for many years, and at least from my perspective, they must have gathered their resources for another phase of skirmishes and some bitterness for the arguments around fat.

With co-author Jan Wright in early publications (Gard & Wright, 2001, 2005) and other academics (such as Campos, 2004; Evans, Rich, & Davies, 2004; Gaesser, 2002) and commentators, we largely agreed with the fat movement, but we also saw a new turn in scientific literature, media coverage, and the generally social 'mood' around body weight around the Western world. Fat hatred and fat pride had been established for some time, but a new 'child' was born; the crisis of the 'obesity epidemic'. Entangled inside the crucial and less-so disputes, the aged differences between physical and social science surfaced again. Will not bore the reader with the many arguments and agreements, suffice to say that there are many members in scientific and public health community who agree with many critical positions similar that rehearsed across the literature and contributions to this volume. Our determination to include in this volume, for example, science, there are contributions written by Katherine Flegal, Patricia Cain and colleagues and Tim Olds and colleagues. But, at the same time, there is a historical story in which some science voices gave the most dire warnings about the rising levels of obesity.

Some years later, I conducted further research which included some media analysis. Part of what follows are my 'findings' and were published in a book (Gard, 2011). There are and is serious disagreement about this area of knowledge, but I wanted to emphasise two incontrovertible points.

DOI: 10.4324/9780429344824-9

First, I drew attention to the way a small number of specific rhetorical flourishes are endlessly recycled and, rather like viruses, passed from person to person, mutating but keeping their essential structure. Many writers have pointed out the flaws, mistakes and exaggerations of obesity science and the overheated language of the reporting mass media. In what follows, I wanted to explore we might have called 'pure rhetoric', where the truth or otherwise of certain statements is not really the point. Then and now, it is a world where language is used, more or less knowingly, not even with the intention of scientific simplification but as a tool in itself, floating free of science, in order to have an effect on readers and listeners.

Second, I wanted to show how these rhetorical viruses have become public property, untethered to temporal or geographical context. While a claim like 'America is the fattest country in the world' has repeatedly made, apparently, without much consideration of its veracity, it was still a claim about a particular place and therefore, at least asserts an empirical fact about a specific part of the world. Likewise, the idea that obesity causes heart disease, while also contentious, is still grounded in a set of scientific propositions. The kind of statements I discuss in this chapter are, in a sense, universal. They belong to no one and everyone, nowhere and therefore everywhere. As we will see, they can be used in conjunction with virtually any other obesity-related claim and offered as a justification for virtually any course of action. Taken together, it is the promiscuity and universality of these rhetorical viruses – to say nothing of their sheer perversity – that *still* demands, either in physical or social sciences, further critical attention. The present volume is a testament to that fact.

How big?

How big a problem is obesity? This is obviously a complex and probably unanswerable question. But as many public health advocates have argued, complexity and uncertainty are not of much help when it comes to raising awareness and changing minds. It is important to also remember that although the obesity epidemic has been a global news story for about ten years, there are still obesity experts and commentators who think that the problem is not being taken nearly seriously enough (e.g., Stanton, 2009; Swinburn, 2008). They see this as happening on two levels. First, at the individual level, the argument goes that we have become so inured to the sight of obese people that we no longer recognise ourselves or our children as dangerously fat. Second, Western governments are blamed for being either too short-sighted or insufficiently brave to implement rigorous anti-obesity policies (e.g., Delpeuch, Maire, Monnier & Holdsworth, 2009). Western societies are, they argue, sleepwalking into a public health catastrophe. It is not always clear what level of heightened vigilance would be enough for some obesity experts, but we can at least gain a sense of the urgency they feel by paying attention to the words they use.

Although they are quite rare, statistical comparisons of the public health challenges facing Western countries, even those intent on maximising the threat of increasing body weights, tend to place obesity below smoking. That there is an issue to be debated is at least acknowledged by some authors. Writing in the journal *Diabetes, Obesity and Metabolism*, Peterbaugh (2009, 557) says of obesity: 'This arguably has become the greatest threat to the nation's present and future health'. Amongst the more outspoken and most-quoted obesity experts, however, even a small concession to uncertainty like this is rare.

For Paul Zimmet, who, in 2008, was Director of the International Diabetes Institute, and Garry Jennings, Director of the Baker Heart Research Institute, the time for subtlety has clearly passed. In an article that appeared in the Australian newspaper *The Age*, these high-profile obesity experts warned:

> This new epidemic is our greatest public health concern and we need a population-based public health strategy to beat it… Obesity is the single most important challenge for public health in the 21st century. More than 1.5 billion adults worldwide and 10% of children are now overweight or obese.
>
> *(Zimmet & Jennings, 2008)*

Curiously, in the same article, Zimmet and Jennings go on to say that 'This *may well be* the single most important challenge for public health in the 21st century' (2008, my emphasis), raising the question of whether they think obesity really is the world's greatest health challenge or simply a contender. This could, of course, simply be an editorial error. If not, it is, I think, a small taste of the way some obesity experts employ language. Rather than aiming for precision, one senses a kind of flailing about in order to press the right emotional button and create the desired sense of urgency. So, having said that obesity is 'our greatest public health concern' and then that it 'may well be the single most important challenge for public health', they then hit on another sound-bite to conclude the article: 'We don't have the luxury of time to deal with this epidemic – it's as big a threat as global warming and bird flu' (2008).

How bad?

When new buzzwords and phrases appear, it is often impossible to know when or by whom they were first used. However, by 2010, there could surely have been few Westerners who had not at least heard that obesity would kill today's children at an earlier age than their parents. The recycling of this phrase seems to have happened in a similar fashion to the claims about obesity-related deaths I discussed above. However, there is at least one interesting difference between these two rhetorical viruses.

The idea of children dying *en masse* younger than their parents does not appear even to owe its origins to a published research paper, flawed or otherwise. Instead, it is sometimes traced to Texas Children's Hospital's William Klish, who is quoted in a 2002 edition of the *Houston Chronicle* (Ackerman, 2002). There is no clear indication that Klish meant to imply that this was a claim based on science or even that it was particularly likely. What we can say is that the idea caught on. Immediately after predicting that one-third of all children born in the United States in the year 2000 would develop Type II diabetes, the country's Surgeon General Richard Carmona told a 2004 Senate sub-committee that: 'Because of the increasing rates of obesity, unhealthy eating habits, and physical inactivity, we may see the first generation that will be less healthy and have a shorter life expectancy than their parents' (United States Department of Health and Human Services, 2004).

In one form or another, the prediction of an obesity-led decline in life expectancy was made by a string of American obesity experts and public office holders up to and including Bill Clinton. Launching the Clinton Foundation's 'Alliance for a Healthier Generation' initiative, the former president warned: 'For the first time in American history, our current generation of children could live shorter lives than their parents' (Clinton Foundation, 2005).

In time, a scholarly attempt was made to substantiate this claim. Olshansky and colleagues' article 'A potential decline in life expectancy in the United States in the 21st century' appeared in a March 2005 edition of The *New England Journal of Medicine*. The authors wrote:

An informed approach to forecasting life expectancy should rely on trends in health and mortality that may be observed in the current population. Forecasting life expectancy by extrapolating from the past is like forecasting the weather on the basis of its history. Looking out the window, we see a threatening storm – obesity – that will, if unchecked, have a negative effect on life expectancy. Despite widespread knowledge about how to reduce the severity of the problem, observed trends in obesity continue to worsen. These trends threaten to diminish the health and life expectancy of current and future generations.

(Olshansky et al., 2005, 1138)

These opening lines from the article's abstract at least acknowledge the hazards attached to making predictions, especially in light of obesity science's well-known knowledge gaps. But with this caveat out of the way, the authors move to what 'will' happen and the 'threats' that await us:

Our conservative estimate is that life expectancy at birth in the United States would be higher by 0.33 to 0.93 year for white males, 0.30 to 0.81 year for white females, 0.30 to 1.08 years for black males, and 0.21 to 0.73 year for black females if obesity did not exist. Assuming that current rates of death associated with obesity remain constant in this century, the overall negative effect of obesity on life expectancy in the United States is a reduction in life expectancy of one third to three fourths of a year. This reduction in life expectancy is not trivial – it is larger than the negative effect of all accidental deaths combined (e.g., accidents, homicide, and suicide), and there is reason to believe that it will rapidly approach and could exceed the negative effect that ischemic heart disease or cancer has on life expectancy.

(Olshansky et al., 2005, 1140–1141)

Whether conservative or not, these are quickly superseded by more pessimistic predictions:

These trends suggest that the relative influence of obesity on the life expectancy of future generations could be markedly worse than it is for current generations. In other words, the life-shortening effect of obesity could rise from its current level of about one third to three fourths of a year to two to five years, or more, in the coming decades, as the obese who are now at younger ages carry their elevated risk of death into middle and older ages.

(Olshansky et al., 2005, 1141)

In the context of this article, the proposition that obesity might lead to a decline in life expectancy of five years or more is made almost as a speculative throwaway line towards the end of the paper. It is not a claim that is based on detailed statistical analysis.

In the few years since its publication, this single paper has accrued close to 1,000 citations for two main reasons. There is, of course, the obvious value of its apparently scientific findings to those wanting to emphasise the seriousness of the obesity epidemic. However, the paper has also been extensively criticised on a number of methodological grounds, two of which may be obvious to readers from the passages quoted above. First, the paper's predictions rest on a comparison with a world where no obesity at all exists. So, even when the authors predict only a fraction of a life expectancy year lost to obesity, this is not based on a comparison between now and a United States that existed 10, 20 or 30 years ago. The comparison is with a United States that, as far as we know, has never existed.

How many?

In his book, about a year spent travelling to the strangest cultural festivals he could find, Australian writer Brian Thacker found himself at an Elvis Presley convention. He noted wryly, 'I once read that Elvis impersonators are growing at such a rate that, by the year 2050, the entire population of the planet will be Elvis impersonators' (Thacker, 2004, 10). Amongst other things, Thacker was reflecting on the way this kind of prediction appeared regularly in the media to warn of some unpleasant social or medical trend.

It is hard to know how these predictions should be viewed. Providing the upward trend really is occurring, whatever it happens to be, it stands to reason that if it continues to happen, it will one day affect everyone or be everywhere. On the other hand, since when has the rate of change of any real-world phenomenon been strictly uniform from start to finish, extending indefinitely into the future?

With this in mind, there are some grounds for puzzlement about the regularity and seriousness with which predictions about the proportion of people who will be obese at some point in the future seem to be made.

Only a small amount of systematic modelling designed to generate this kind of prediction has ever been carried out. Unlike, say, economics or meteorology, obesity is not a field of study that can call on elaborate technical procedures to make at least arguably educated forecasts about the future. For example, the field has no generally agreed upon theories or models that explain the reason for obesity rate changes. At the very least, the fact that many obesity researchers readily concede that we really do not know what has caused changes in the past should give one pause to wonder about the efficacy of any prediction concerning future obesity rates.

It is perhaps partly because of the lack of an underlying theoretical model that apparently serious obesity commentators like Paul Zimmet could feel sufficiently free to announce 'Obesity is an international scourge... This insidious, creeping pandemic of obesity is now engulfing the entire world' (CBS News, 2006). In other words, without an agreed upon system for generating or evaluating predictions, obesity experts like Zimmet may actually be free to say whatever they want. And once said, this kind of prediction – if this is what it really is – is liable to be mimicked not just by journalists, but by other researchers. Delpeuch, Maire, Monnier and Holdsworth warn that 'we are beginning to realize that no society is immune from this plague, which is rapidly engulfing the whole of the globe' (2009, xv).

Scientific consideration is no guarantee of consensus, of course, but it is interesting to speculate whether its absence contributes to the wide range of predictions about future obesity prevalence that are made. In a 2007 article for the *Nursing Standard*, Tasmin Snow draws on one set of statistical predictions in order to urge British nurses to take a proactive role in solving the obesity epidemic and thereby save the National Health Service from ruin:

> ... latest estimates predict that by 2010, around 33 percent of men and 28 per cent of women will be obese. Obesity among children is also projected to rise, with the number of obese boys rising from 750,000 in 2003 to nearly 800,000 in 2010. The largest increases are expected among girls, with a 6 per cent rise in obesity rates expected between 2003 and 2010, by which time some 910,000 are expected to be obese. This equates to more than one fifth of those aged between two and 15.
>
> *(Snow, 2007, 12)*

Perhaps, the most significant aspect of obesity forecasts, whether in the media or academic journals, is that they are not based on any theoretical model or rationale. Forecasters never attempt to construct an explanation of past trends that then feeds into predictions about the future. As I have said, this is partly because obesity experts have no theory about the past apart from a set of sweeping generalisations about 'modern lifestyles', generalisations that are mathematically inert. Future social trends are rarely factored in so that, for obesity experts, the future must always be nothing more than a pale imitation of an arbitrarily chosen moment in the past. This is much more folk superstition than it is science.

What this means, of course, is that any vaguely plausible prediction is as good as any other. As a result, obesity experts rarely, if ever, chastise each other for the rashness of each other's predictions. Instead, they have simply referenced, quoted and echoed each other to the point that obesity forecasts are now not so much scientific claims as background noise.

Predictions about the future are a fact of life, and as many obesity forecasters say, generating knowledge about the future makes planning for it at least a theoretically more precise exercise. And yet, I must admit to being bewildered by the variety of obesity predictions that are made and, even more so, the conviction with which they are sometimes delivered. Whether or not readers are inclined to put credence in them, their existence is less important than the realisation that, with a very few notable exceptions, these predictions rest on the idea of an increasing or, at best, unchanging and presumably never-ending rate of increase. This is precisely the supposition that underpins the astonishingly bold prediction, published in the *International Journal of Obesity*, that by 2030, 57.8 percent of the world's population, or 3.3 billion people, will be overweight or obese (Kelly, Yang, Chen, Reynolds & He, 2008). And it is also this logic that drives the authors of the book *Globesity: A Planet Out of Control* to ask in apparent seriousness: 'Is the whole world fated to become obese? Are we to look forward to societies in which everyone, give or take the odd exception, will be overweight?' (Delpeuch, Maire, Monnier & Holdsworth, 2009, 159).

There is, it seems, no end in sight. Or, as Gary Mason put it in Canada's *Globe and Mail* newspaper much more succinctly than I: 'In the meantime we'll just keep getting bigger and bigger and bigger and bigger' (2005, A13).

How fast?

One of the least-discussed difficulties associated with predicting future rates of obesity is that there is actually no agreement about how quickly obesity rates are changing. In the case of forecasts about whole countries or the world, the fact that different parts of the world are changing at different rates (Lobstein, Baur & Uauy, 2004) must be ignored in order to make predictions about the whole. In addition, the real rate of change for any population would depend on a long list of variables, including what definition of 'obesity' is used, the time period over which previous rates of change are calculated and, particularly important, the population's age profile.

These complexities aside, predictions based on the assumption of steady future rates of change apparently disregard assertions within the obesity research community that obesity rates are increasing at increasing rate. While I am aware of only a few obesity forecasts that have factored in increasing rates of change, it is a claim that has been regularly made.

Reporting on research into obesity rates amongst English children up to the year 1998, Lobstein, James and Cole (2003, 1136) reported an 'accelerating trend' and that 'There is a clear and urgent need for policies to be introduced to ensure that the present trends are halted and reversed' (1137, my emphasis). The idea of 'present trends' in this article is interesting because it refers to data that, by the time of the article's publication, were five years old. A couple of years later, Stamatakis, Primatesta, Chinn, Rona and Falascheti (2005, 1002) conducted a follow-up analysis of 2003 data and concluded that 'These results showed that the upward trends in overweight and obesity in children noted by other authors over the 1990s are continuing into the 2000s and, more alarmingly, that the rate of increase has accelerated over the last decade' (2005, 1002).

Generalising about European children, Jackson-Leach and Lobstein have written as recently as 2006 that 'Overweight and obesity prevalence in children is increasing. Furthermore, the significant linear trends in the annualised increments indicate that the rate of change is itself increasing: i.e., prevalence rates are not rising at a constant rate but are accelerating' (2006, 29).

In Australia, the practice of making pronouncements about the present based on old data is equally widespread. Booth and colleagues have reported in the *American Journal of Clinical Nutrition* that 'The prevalence of overweight and obesity [amongst Australian children] is not only increasing, it is accelerating' (2003, 35). Also, in 2003, Booth was quoted in the media saying 'The prevalence of overweight and obesity is not only increasing, it is accelerating' (Teutsch, 2003, 25). Similar to the Lobstein example above, Booth's claim relates to research into Australian childhood obesity between the years 1985 and 1997. In other words, Booth makes a claim about something that is going on now – 'obesity is not only increasing, it is accelerating' – when, his data concerns a period of time some six years in the past. On one level, this is understandable given the complexity of this kind of research and the length of time it sometimes takes for results to be published. However, no caveats, such as the theoretical possibility that obesity rates might have slowed or reversed in the intervening years, were reported, and I am not aware of any being offered elsewhere.

Writing more recently in the *International Journal of Pediatric Obesity*, Norton, Dollman, Martin and Harten are, if anything, more strident about the present and more alarmed about what they take to be current rates of change:

> The prevalence rate for overweight and obesity among children in Australia continues to climb and we predict it will approach adult rates within the next 30 years. [...] The increasing rate of overweight children in Australia, shown in Figure 2, is astounding. The data indicate overweight prevalence was relatively stable for much of the last century but accelerated in the early 1970s and continues to gain momentum.
>
> *(2006, 232, 237)*

More recent still is Peterbaugh's assessment of American obesity, in *Diabetes, Obesity and Metabolism*, that: 'Americans are more obese than ever, and the rates of obesity seem to be accelerating' (2009, 557).

It is interesting that as early as 2000 journalists were reporting the possibility of exponential rises in obesity rates, especially for children. From American *Newsweek* magazine:

> If the trend has continued – and many experts believe it has *accelerated* – one child in three is now either overweight or at risk of becoming so. No race or class has been spared, and many youngsters are already suffering health consequences.
>
> *(Cowley, 2000, 43, emphasis in original)*

In 2005, Philip James, Chair of the International Obesity Task Force, is reported to have told a European Union obesity conference: 'It [obesity] took off in the 1980s and looks as if it was accelerating in the last five to 10 years... It's beginning to look as if we have an exponential rise' (Smith, 2005). As with other obesity sound-bites, this is the kind of statement that could be, and in fact was, picked up and recycled in the media (e.g., see also American Health Network, 2005).

Were they right?

I want to emphasise that each of the four viral sound-bites in this chapter has been sustained by scarcely a whiff of scientific evidence. From so little, so much has grown. And while they appear to say a great deal, even gentle probing shows that each is an empty rhetorical shell, saying almost nothing and designed not to make a scientific case, but to create the impression of one.

Although I have made the point already, it is crucial to emphasise that my portrait of obesity rhetoric is not a whimsical exercise seeking simply to poke fun at people whose views I do not share. The stakes are much higher than this. My argument here it is that these sound-bites are the very substance of the obesity epidemic. They are what transforms obesity from a run-of-the-mill public health problem into a 'crisis' and what licenses its advocates to call for far-reaching, expensive and radical public health responses and policies. In other words, finishing where I began this chapter, the crime is one of gross, widespread, continuous exaggeration.

This chapter is mainly taken from the second chapter from *The End of Obesity Epidemic* (Gard, 2011) published by Routledge.

References

Ackerman, T. (2002). Study shows Houston kids getting fatter. *The Houston Chronicle*, 23 January: A19.

American Health Network. (2005). EU food industry called to battle against obesity. Online. Available at: http://www.health.am/weightloss/more/eu_food_industry_called_to_battle_against_obesity/ (accessed 11 December 2009).

Booth, M. L., Chey, T., Wake, M., Norton, K., Hesketh, K., Dollman, J. and Robertson, I. (2003). Change in the prevalence of overweight and obesity among young Australians, 1969–1997. *American Journal of Clinical Nutrition*, 77(1), 29–36. doi: 10.1093/ajcn/77.1.29

Campos, P. (2004). *The obesity myth: Why America's obsession with weight is hazardous to your health*. New York, Gotham Books.

CBS News (2006). 'Obesity an "international scourge"'. Online. Available at: http://www.cbsnews.com/stories/2006/09/03/health/main1962961.shtml (accessed 26 June 2007).

Clinton Foundation. (2005). 'Creating a healthier generation'. Online. Available at: http://www.clintonfoundation.org/050305-feature-wjc-aha-healthier-generation-initiative.htm (accessed 14 April 2008).

Cowley, G. (2000). Generation XXL. *Newsweek*, 3 July: 40–44.

Delpeuch, F., Maire, B., Monnier, E. and Holdsworth, M. (2009). *Globesity: A planet out of control?* London: Earthscan.

Evans, J., Rich, E. and Davies, B. (2004). The emperor's new clothes: Fat, thin, and overweight. The social fabrication of risk and ill health. *Journal of Teaching in Physical Education*, 23 (4), 372–391.

Gaesser, G. A. (2002). *Big fat lies: The truth about your weight and your health*. Carlsbad, Gurze Books.

Gard, M. (2011). *The end of the obesity epidemic*. London, Routledge.

Gard, M. and Wright, J. (2001). Managing uncertainty: Obesity discourses and physical education in a risk society'. *Studies in Philosophy and Education*, 20(6), 535–549. doi: 10.1023/A:1012238617836

Gard, M. and Wright, J. (2005). *The obesity epidemic: Science, morality and ideology*. London, Routledge.

Jackson-Leach R. and Lobstein T. (2006). Estimated burden of paediatric obesity and comorbidities in Europe. Part 1. The increase in the prevalence of child obesity in Europe is itself increasing. *International Journal of Pediatric Obesity*, 1(1), 26–32. doi: 10.1080/17477160600586614

Kelly, T., Yang, W., Chen, C. S., Reynolds, K. and He, J. (2008). Global burden of obesity in 2005 and projections to 2030. *International Journal of Obesity*, 32(9), 1431–1437. doi: 10.1038/ijo.2008.102

Lobstein, T., Baur, L. and Uauy, R. (2004). Obesity in children and young people: A crisis in public health. *Obesity Reviews*, 5(suppl. 1), 4–85. doi: 10.1111/j.1467-789X.2004.00133.x

Mason, G. (2005). Obesity bursting boomers' expectation of having a healthy lifestyle, expert warns. *The Globe and Mail*, 29 September: A13.

Norton, K., Dollman, J., Martin, M. and Harten, N. (2006). Descriptive epidemiology of childhood overweight and obesity in Australia: 1901–2003. *International Journal of Pediatric Obesity*, 1(4), 232–238. doi: 10.1080/17477160600962856

Olshansky, S. J., Passaro, D. J., Hershow, R. C., Layden, J., Carnes, B. A., Brody, J., Hayflick, L., Butler, R. N., Allison, D. B. and Ludwig, D. S. (2005). A potential decline in life expectancy in the United States in the 21st century. *New England Journal of Medicine*, 352(11), 1138–1145. doi: 10.1056/NEJMsr043743

Peterbaugh, J. S. (2009). The emperor's tailors: The failure of the medical weight loss paradigm and its causal role in the obesity of America. *Diabetes, Obesity and Metabolism*, 11(6), 557–570. doi: 10.1111/j.1463-1326.2009.01019.x

Smith, J. (2005). EU food industry called to battle against obesity. *Reuters Health E-Line*, 25 January.

Snow, T. (2007). Can nurses tackle the obesity crisis. *Nursing Standard*, 22(3), 12–13.

Stamatakis, E., Primatesta, P., Chinn, S., Rona, R. and Falascheti, E. (2005). Overweight and obesity trends from 1974 to 2003 in English children: What is the role of socioeconomic factors? *Archives of Disease in Childhood*, 90(10), 999–1004. doi: 10.1136/adc.2004.068932

Stanton, R. (2009). Who will take responsibility for obesity in Australia? *Public Health*, 123(3), 280–282. doi: 10.1016/j.puhe.2008.12.017

Swinburn, B. (2008). Obesity prevention: The role of policies, laws and regulations. *Australia and New Zealand Health Policy*, 5(1). doi: 10.1186/1743-8462-5-12

Teutsch, D. (2003) 'Kids pay a heavy price for lifestyle', *The Sun-Herald*, 5 January: 25.

Thacker, B. (2004). *The naked man festival and other excuses to fly around the world*. Crows Nest, NSW: Allen and Unwin.

United States Department of Health and Human Services. (2004). 'The growing epidemic of childhood obesity', *Testimony to the The Subcommittee on Competition, Infrastructure and Foreign Commerce, Science, and Transportation, March 2, 2004*. Online. Available at: http://www.hhs.gov/asl/testify/t040302.html (accessed 20 November 2009).

Zimmet, P. and Jennings, G. (2008). 'Curbing the obesity epidemic', *The Age*. Online. Available at: http://www.theage.com.au/news/opinion/curbing-the-obesity-epidemic/2008/02/21/1203467280758.html (accessed 7 March 2009).

PART C

Theory

One of the complex ways of understanding 'fat' or 'obesity' is to first know what we are talking about. Are we describing the effect of fat tissue on human health? Are we defining the rights and responsibilities of fat people? The historical emergence of the term 'obesity' as disease category and term of abuse rather than saying 'fat'? Having said all this, the construction of the word 'fat' or 'obesity' often cannot make us any wiser, other to say that we understand each beginning position before the discussion and argumentation starts.

But, in contrast, one's theory can open up intriguing and controversial area of research and theorisation. Taking this point a little further, one of the possible answers posed by having a section called 'theory' is the part of the title of this volume: 'studies'. This term portrays an intellectual defensive stance which, above all, welcomes everybody who values debate and intellectual exploration.

To begin this section, we have a chapter written by Cat Pausé, a leading scholar from fat studies. Definition is always somewhat problematic area of scholarship, and Pausé argumentation offers readers a sophisticated interpretation of where fat scholarship should be housed. She also attempts to define the areas of one's scholarship and one's thinking, emphasising that the appropriate place to study fat is from the fat studies. From the editorial position of this volume, her conclusions can often be debated, but her work is standard reading for fat and obesity readers and researchers.

The next chapter covers an obvious but important area of scholarship; poststructuralism Foucauldian theory. Like feminism and queer studies, fat studies and critical obesity studies draws intellectual theories from Foucault, Deleuze, and similar writers. Pringle describes what Foucault's ideas means to him as scholar and then gives us an example from New Zealand government public health policy. This chapter narrates the 'conversation' between policies and people who, in many different ways, are in 'dispute'. There are many ideas and strategies from this chapter that a reader may use, but perhaps, its focus on critique of policies is where Pringle's work is most useful.

The next chapter is, in some senses, a relative of Foucauldian theory and previous chapter by Pringle, although the closer relatives may be Deleuzian and Butlerian theory and materialist feminisms; that is, *new* materialist. There are many ways to approach this theory or, rather, a group of theories. Within this chapter, Fullagar and colleagues sketch out many

DOI: 10.4324/9780429344824-10

directions one could follow, but its focus on multi-species, post-humanist analysis, and their philosophical movement from what 'is' to what it 'does'. Their treatments of 'obesity' and 'fat' bodies and connecting to, say, the concept of 'disgust' and 'pleasure' steer one's attention to at least two and even more extreme directions that happened in earlier theories; the examination of '*more* than' human-centred analysis and, somewhat controversially, the ability to 'see inside' a person.

Land also wants to use new materialist theory but heads into different areas of pedagogical thinking. She argues that, in post-developmental pedagogies, we are interested in moment-by-moment educational engagements with many human and non-human species. This chapter raises more visceral moments for a reader, particularly for a reader who wants to see their fat interventions with children – or, in this chapter, a single child – that also troubles areas of 'relational activity' including '... flesh, discourses, pedagogies, logics, more-than-human others, bodies, ethics, and politics'.

The last chapter of this section is concerned with the role of an editor for a volume like this one. Written by Michael Gard, this chapter is very much a personal statement; part biographical and journalistic journey but also sketches out the over-arching editing principles for a major piece of scholarship. Whether the word 'theory' or 'philosophy' or some other term better summarising what Gard is on about it in this chapter, he believes that we are all flawed but also worthy of attention. He says that everybody, no matter where an author starts from or the arguments are of doubtful proposition, we should acknowledge our errors and our successes.

8

DEVIL PRAY

Fat studies in an obesity research world

Cat Pausé

Introduction

For the last 100 years, scholars have been turning their attention to the fat body as a site for research. Most of these scholars understand fatness as a deviance, a disease to be cured; their research is structured to address one of the most pressing problems of the 21st century: the "obesity epidemic". These obesity researchers pathologise fatness and pay little attention to the lived experiences or voices of actual fat people. From their body of scholarship, a new group of scholars emerged who ask critical questions of this thing called obesity and the science that surrounds it. These critical obesity scholars take issue with the ontological, epistemological, and methodological approaches and frameworks of obesity scholars. Then, there are weight scholars who study obesity, but with a conservative compassion; much of this work highlights the stigma and discrimination as experienced by fat people. Weight scholars often decry the very fat stigma much of their work is reproducing. Outside of these, but located within the actual subject being examined, are fat studies scholars. These scholars centre fatness and the lived experiences of fat people; many of them operate as activist scholars, working to secure civil rights for fat people. This, in turn, leads many scholars to question the voracity of the work produced by fat studies scholars. If this calls into question the validity of the work of fat studies scholars, it must also do the same for obesity scholars as they too seek to change the world through their research by eliminating fat people. This chapter presents an overview of the hallmark characteristics of these four kinds of scholarship, allowing the reader to recognise the areas in which they overlap and in which they differ. It concludes with a demonstration that fat studies scholarship is the most appropriate scholarship to study fatness.

Obesity research

The category of obesity research encompasses a range of scholarship activity. At the core though, it could be argued that any scholarship that seeks to understand obesity in order to prevent, treat, or cure obesity is obesity research. It also includes work that seeks to explain the burden of obesity. This may vary from medical research seeking to highlight a relationship between obesity and chronic health conditions, employment research seeking to

DOI: 10.4324/9780429344824-11

illustrate the negative employment impacts of obesity, or psychological research seeking to predict the factors that lead to obesity. All of this research pathologises fatness and positions it as a problem. That is the defining characteristic of obesity research. Most of what people believe about fatness stems from obesity research. Obesity is unhealthy (GBD 2015 Obesity Collaborators, 2017). Obesity contributes to global warming (An, Ji, & Zhang, 2018). Obesity is huge cost burden for society (Tremmel, Gerdtham, Nilsson, & Saha, 2017). Obesity leads to early death (Aune et al., 2016). The latter refrain, that obesity is deadly, is a common focus for obesity research.

For example, Allison, Fontaine, Manson, Stevens, and Van Itallie (1999) published a piece in the *Journal of the American Medical Association* in which they report that obesity causes between 280,000 and 325,000 deaths a year in the United States. They approached this research by asking:

> Of the people who were alive at the beginning of 1991, how many fewer would have died by the end of that year if all of the obese people alive at the beginning of the year had not been obese?
>
> *(p. 1530)*

Using data from six large publicly available prospective cohort studies, the authors determined a hazard ratio for overweight and obese persons. Applying that hazard ratio to estimates of population size and population distribution of BMI, the authors arrive at their estimate of obesity-attributable deaths between 280 and 325k. The author suggests that these are conservative estimates.

And in a special report published in 2005 in the *New England Journal of Medicine*, he claimed that obesity would be responsible for shortening life expectancy (Olshansky et al., 2005). Running a series of probabilities, the authors concluded that obesity would result in a reduction of one third to three quarters of a year from life expectancies, and they note that this is an underestimation. They suggest that, without significant interventions, to curb obesity rates would result in "the youth of today may, on average, live less healthy and possibly even shorter lives than their parents" (p. 1143).

Critical obesity studies

In-direct response to obesity research is critical obesity studies. Scholars within the critical obesity studies camp take issue with the way that obesity studies' scholars use epistemology, ontology, and methodical tools to study and shape the discourse on obesity. Critical obesity scholars focus their attention on reviewing the evidence underpinning the work of obesity researchers and exposing the flaws, errors, and erroneous assumptions present. The attention on evidence is not limited to the assumptions made about weight, behaviours, and health but also extends to the many "solutions" provided by obesity scholars to "fight obesity".

Hallmarks of critical obesity studies include the commitment to evidence-based, data-driven analysis, and a rejection of common sense, or "everyone knows" approaches to understanding fatness and how to address the "obesity" problem. A sure way to trigger a response from a critical obesity scholar is to make an assertion such as "Kids are fat today because they are less physically active than they were fifty years ago". A critical obesity scholar would identify the assumption present (that physical activity and fatness have a causal relationship) and ask for the data on physical activity in children from 50 years ago.

A key text in this field is Gard and Wright's 2005, *The obesity epidemic: Science, morality, and ideology*. In this book, Gard and Wright (2005) work to "examine the ways in which preconceived ideas and beliefs have shaped what people say about the 'obesity epidemic'" (p. 3). They work through the flaws and misleading assumptions that they believe are endemic in obesity research and present a theory about why the general public has so willingly embraced the idea of an obesity epidemic. Gard and Wright (2005) conclude by suggesting that those interested in weight and health have two possible options – to "'get over' body weight altogether" (p. 190) or at the minimal, move past the idea of the body as a machine.

Another example of this work may be found in Campos, Saguy, Ernsberger, Oliver, and Gaesser's 2006 piece in the *International Journal of Epidemiology*. In their article, the authors assert that "in our view the available scientific data neither support alarmist claims about obesity nor justify diverting scarce resources away from far more pressing public health issues" (p. 55). They build this argument by questioning the data available to support that being fat is a major contributor to mortality and morbidity, that permanent meaningful weight loss is possible, and that the current situation should be classified as an epidemic. The authors draw from evidence to illustrate holes in the often-hyperbolic language of obesity research and highlight when assumptions are taken as common sense rather than evidence-based. The authors conclude:

> Given the limited scientific evidence for any of these claims, we suggest that the current rhetoric about an obesity-driven health crisis is being driven more by cultural and political factors than by any threat increasing body weight may pose to public health
>
> *(p. 55)*

Critical obesity scholars would point to the conclusions in both the Allison et al. (1999) and Olshansky et al. (2005) as illustrations of the lack of robustness often present in obesity research. In Allison et al. (1999), the authors note towards the end, "our calculations assume that all (controlling for age, sex, and smoking) excess mortality in obese people is due to obesity" (p. 1536). Of course, this means that they arrived at their hazard ratio by taking all the deaths of overweight and obese people, regardless of reason, and attributed them to obesity.

Similarly, the Olshansky et al.'s (2005) conclusion confesses the threats to validity in this work as well. The authors note that "It is important to emphasize that our conclusions about the future are based on our collective judgment" (p. 1143). Critical obesity scholars would suggest that scientific conclusion and estimation should not be based on collective judgement but on evidence.

Weight science

Weight science scholars studying higher body weights seek to understand the relationship between weight and other factors such as social acceptance, physiological health, and engagement across the lifespan. These scholars do not accept fatness as a natural aspect of human diversity, and many seek to solve the problem of fatness. Weight science has become a more visible field of study, as the concepts of fat shaming and fat bias have become more visible. An annual Weight Stigma Conference provides an opportunity for those interested in weight science to share work and network; looking over programmes from past conferences, it appears that the conference itself usually has three main streams: a medical stream, a public health stream, and an activism stream.

Much of the scholarship in this discipline comes from the UCONN Rudd Center for Food Policy & Obesity (RCFPO). The RCFPO defines their mission to discover and promote "solutions to childhood obesity, poor diet, and weight bias through research and policy" ("What We Do"). Former Director, Kelly Brownell, and current Deputy Director, Rebecca Puhl, are well known for their work on weight bias and stigma (Pearl & Puhl, 2018; Puhl & Brownell, 2001; Puhl, Brownell & DePierre, 2014; Puhl & Heuer, 2009). Professor Puhl and her team's publications on weight bias, stigma, and discrimination are used by scholars across obesity science, critical obesity science, weight science, and fat studies. These weight science scholars appear to believe that they can both prevent and prepare for war; their work both seeks to solve the problem of obesity and reduce the stigma associated with being fat. They fail to recognise that fat stigma is reinforced by proposing that fatness is a problem to be prevented and/or solved.

Bacon and Aphramor's (2011) published review article illustrates how weight science and critical obesity studies often overlap. In the review published in *Nutrition Journal*, Bacon and Aphramor walk through the evidence that does not support the key tenets of obesity research (such as fatness posing a significant risk of death, that weight loss improves health, and that permanent weight loss is possible); they conclude by calling for a shift in the paradigm that surrounds science around weight. Their critiques of the conclusions established in obesity research and the paucity of evidence that supports these assumptions, echo much of the work done by critical obesity scholars. Bacon and Aphramor, however, have an additional goal related to social justice – they seek to promote a paradigm around weight and health that embraces body acceptance, supporting the agency of health-seeking individuals, and promotes that any person, regardless of size, can pursue health. In this social justice focus, Bacon and Aphramor echo much of the work done by fat studies scholars, as seen below.

Fat studies

The editors of the *Fat Studies Reader* (Rothblum & Solovay, 2009) define fat studies as "an interdisciplinary field of scholarship marked by an aggressive, consistent, rigorous critique of the negative assumptions, stereotypes, and stigma placed on fat and the fat body" (p. 2). Fat studies' scholars come from a range of disciplines – from history to health to business. This interdisciplinary nature of the field would suggest to some that it is, in fact, postdisciplinary. Postdisciplinary suggests that disciplines, or even fields, are an outdated idea. And, instead, scholars from a range of backgrounds converge upon a specific topic – or area – for study, regardless of their home discipline. In this way, fat studies may be a postdisciplinary field. But fat studies do not require scholars who wish to pursue this scholarship to ignore or dismiss their home fields. In fact, if we consider the organising role of academia within scholarship, as fat studies does not have an academic home – one cannot earn a qualification in fat studies, anywhere in the world – then it could be argued that there are no fat studies scholars. And, therefore, we can all be fat studies scholars. As suggested in the foreword of the *Fat Studies Reader*, Marilyn Wann (2009), "in a fat-hating society everyone is fat" (p. xv).

While fat studies' scholars may not produce diplomas or transcripts to demonstrate their pedigree or bonafides in fat studies, they can demonstrate through their scholarship whether they are, or are not, practicing fat studies. One way to demonstrate this is to "keep the actual lives of fat people at the heart of the analysis" (Rothblum & Solovay, 2009, p. 2). Fat studies scholarship centres the fat body, fatness, and the fat person in their work. Fatness and fat people are at the core. Autoethnography has been a popular methodology for fat studies scholars; providing a method to integrate literature, theory, and personal experience as a way to illustrate the impacts of structural oppression on fat people. I have used autoethnography to explore fat identity management (Pausé, 2012), physical education (Pausé, 2019b), healthcare (Lee & Pausé, 2016), pedagogy (Pausé, 2016), social media (Pausé, 2012; Pausé & Glover, 2018; Pausé & Russell, 2016), and immigration (Pausé, 2019c).

Another unique characteristic of fat studies is that it is underpinned by a belief in fat liberation. At the end of *The Fat Studies Reader* (2009), the editors printed the "Fat Liberation Manifesto" in full. This Manifesto was written by Freespirit and Aldebaran in 1973, as part of their work with the Fat Underground. Fat studies scholarship seeks to support fat activism, the fight for fat people to have the same rights and dignity as non-fat people. As I have noted in previous work, it is important that the focus of the fight for fat liberation is on those who are most in need. This means the fattest of us – fat people of colour; fat people with disabilities; those in the LGBTIAQ community – and the responsibility for fighting lies with fat people with the most privilege:

> The power transferred through white supremacy places the largest burden on white people within Fat Studies scholarship and activism to ensure that spaces are made and held for people of colour. The power transferred through capitalism places the largest burden on middle and upper class people within Fat Studies scholarship and activism to ensure that spaces are made and held for people from working and poorer classes. And the power transferred through the academy places the largest burden on those within academia to ensure that spaces are made and held for those denied entry to the Ivory Tower.
>
> *(Pausé, 2015, para 17)*

Common ground

All four of these fields seek to study and understand fatness. And while obesity research can be considered to exist on the opposite side of the spectrum from fat studies, similarities do exist across the other three. For example, both fat studies and critical obesity scholars would agree on the necessity of shining a critical lens on obesity research and the pathologisation of fatness. Fat studies and weight-science scholars would agree on the importance of understanding the stigma and discrimination associated with fatness and a commitment to eradicating both across the world. One similarity across critical-obesity studies, weight science, and fat studies is the willingness of many scholars in these areas to reflect on their own privilege and location from whence they conduct their scholarship.

Scholars in these areas recognise the role of personal position, bias, and values in the production of knowledge and the creation of scholarship. As noted by Marilyn Wann, "If you participate in the field of fat studies, you must be willing to examine not just the broader social forces related to weight but also your own involvement with these structures" (2009, p. xi). Linda Bacon gave a keynote to the National Association to Advance Fat Acceptance in which she highlighted the role of thin privilege in her scholarship and how it is received by others (Bacon, 2009). I have demonstrated through the use of Standpoint theory (Pausé, 2019a) the importance of naming and acknowledging privilege in scholarship as a key to ethical practice and a tool to avoid (re)producing fat oppression:

> All of us have a responsibility to ensure that we are checking our privilege along the way, and lifting the voices of those who may not be heard. Highlighting voices of fat people of color, voices of fat working poor, voices of super fats; these are the responsibility of those who hold power by standing outside of those identities. Being honest about

where we stand, and the privileges that we bring into our spaces, is key to ensuring that knowledge around fatness does not further oppress fat people.

(p. 10)

Just as similarities can be identified, differences exist as well. Fat studies is the only discipline that centres fatness, the fat body, and the lives of fat people. *It is the only discipline to recognise that knowledge about fat people should be created by fat people.* It is the only discipline that is dedicated to the liberation of fat people.

Unlike obesity studies, fat studies does not assume that being fat is unhealthy. Fat studies scholars do not investigate the ways that physiological fatness results in harm to the physical body. Fat studies scholars do not search for cures or treatment or ways to prevent bodies from becoming fat. Fat studies scholars may study the physiological impact of fat stigma on the health and well-being of fat people. Fat studies scholars may have an interest in understanding the diversity of human body size, but they do not pursue such questions to demonstrate the deviance of fatness. On the contrary, a fat studies scholar engaging in this kind of work would most likely begin by centering fatness as normative and extend their study from that position.

Unlike critical-obesity studies, fat studies does not focus itself on examining the soundness or robustness of obesity research. Fat studies scholars do not focus attention on highlighting the theoretical and methodological flaws and assumptions of obesity research. Fat studies scholars may seek to understand how the moral panic around obesity began, and they may seek to establish a history of fatness and culture, but the point is not to assess the validity or reliability of obesity research, but to understand the role of fatness and fat people in their own history.

Unlike weight studies, fat studies scholars do not investigate weight stigma; they investigate fat stigma. Fat studies scholars do not investigate weight discrimination; they investigate fat discrimination. These may seem to be small linguistic differences, but they represent a larger philosophical difference between the two fields. In naming the stigma and discrimination as faced by – experienced by – fat people, fat studies acknowledges that fat people are the ones who are oppressed in our current culture. There is no room for doubt in this use of language that fat people are the ones who deserve our assistance and our attention. In addition, while many weight-studies scholars seek to address weight stigma and obesity both, fat studies scholars reject the pathologisation of the fat body. Fatness is not a problem to be solved from the fat studies perspective. This is not to say that fat studies scholarship is not capable of (re)producing fat violence and oppression, but it does not begin from a place of pathologisation.

If fat studies does begin from a problem to be solved, then that problem is not with fat people, but with how fat people are treated in society. As Marilyn Wann (2009) suggests, "a fat studies approach offers no opposition to the simple face of human weight diversity, but instead looks at what people and societies make of this reality" (p. x). This work may include exploring how society separates fat and non-fat people, how society divides resources between fat and non-fat people, and how society imparts power on fat and non-fat people (Rothblum & Solovay, 2009).

The ethics of fat

Fatness will continue to be an area of interest for scholars. And most likely, research on fatness will continue to oppress fat people (Pausé, 2019a). In order to avoid reproducing the oppression of fat people, scholars interested in fatness should adopt a fat ethic. A fat ethic insists that fat people must be at the centre of research to answer questions such as these. A fat ethic insists that fat people must be at the helm of research to answer questions such as these. Nothing about us without us.

A fat ethic insists that anyone seeking to do research on fatness must recognise and acknowledge both their own privilege and attitudes about fatness, as well as recognising and acknowledging the violence that has been done against fat people in the name of research, in the name of science. Fat ethic is embedded into the field of fat studies, making fat studies the most appropriate discipline to study fatness. Fat studies scholars bring the theoretical and methodological tools needed to conduct ethical research around fatness, and it should be those voices that are amplified and prioritised when the topic of fatness arises. Scholars from outside of this area should work alongside fat studies scholars (and/or fat activists) to ensure that their work is not reproducing fat oppression.

References

Allison, D. B., Fontaine, K. R., Manson, J. E., Stevens, J., & VanItallie, T. B. (1999). Annual deaths attributable to obesity in the United States. *Journal of the American Medical Association*, *282*(16), 1530–1538. doi: 10.1001/jama.282.16.1530

An, R., Ji, M., & Zhang, S. (2018). Global warming and obesity: A systematic review. *Obesity Reviews*, *19*(2), 150–163. doi: 10.1111/obr.12624

Aune, D., Sen, A., Prasad, M., Norat, T., Janszky, I., Tonstad, S., Romundstad, P., & Vatten, L. J. (2016). BMI and all cause mortality: Systematic review and non-linear dose-response meta-analysis of 230 cohort studies with 3.74 million deaths among 30.3 million participants. *BMJ*, *353*, i2156. doi: 10.1136/bmj.i2156

Bacon, L. (2009, 1 Aug). *Reflections on fat acceptance: Lessons learned from privilege.* Keynote delivered at the National Association to Advance Fat Acceptance conference. Retrieved from https://lindabacon.org/wp-content/uploads/Bacon_ReflectionsOnThinPrivilege_NAAFA.pdf

Bacon, L., & Aphramor, L. (2011). Weight science: Evaluating the evidence for a paradigm shift. *Nutrition Journal, 10*(9), 1–13. doi: 10.1186/1475-2891-10-9

Campos, P., Saguy, A., Ernsberger, P., Oliver, E., & Gaesser, G. (2006). The epidemiology of overweight and obesity: Public health crisis or moral panic? *International Journal of Epidemiology, 35*(1), 55–60. doi: 10.1093/ije/dyi254

Freespirit and Aldebaran (1973/2009). Fat liberation manifesto. In E. Rothblum & S. Solovay (Eds.), *The fat studies reader* (pp. 341–342). New York: New York University Press.

Gard, M., & Wright, J. (2005). *The obesity epidemic: Science, morality, and ideology.* New York: Routledge.

GBD 2015 Obesity Collaborators. (2017). Health effects of overweight and obesity in 195 countries over 25 years. *New England Journal of Medicine, 377*(1), 13–27. doi: 10.1056/NEJMoa1614362

Lee, J. A., & Pausé, C. J. (2016). Stigma in practice: Barriers to health for fat women. *Frontiers in Psychology,* 7, 2063. doi: 10.3389/fpsyg.2016.02063

Olshansky, S. J., Passaro, D. J., Hershow, R. C., Layden, J. C., Bruce, A., Brody, J., Hayflick, L., … Ludwig, D. S. (2005). A potential decline in life expectancy in the United States in the 21st century. *New England Journal of Medicine, 352*(11), 1138–1145. doi: 10.1056/nejmsr043743

Pausé, C. J. (2019a). Ray of light: Standpoint theory, fat studies, and a new fat ethics. *Fat Studies.* doi: 10.1080/21604851.2019.1630203

Pausé, C. J. (2019b). (Can we) get together: Fat kids and physical education. *Health Education Journal, 78*(6), 662–669. doi: 10.1177/0017896919846182

Pausé, C. J. (2019c). Frozen: A fat tale of immigration. *Fat Studies: An Interdisciplinary Journal of Body Weight & Society,* 8(1), 44–59. doi: 10.1080/21604851.2019.1532230

Pausé, C. J. (2016). Promise to try: Teaching fat pedagogies in tertiary education. In E. Carter & C. Russell (Eds.), *Fat pedagogy reader: Challenging weight-based oppression in education* (pp. 53–60), New York: Peter Lang Publishers.

Pausé, C. J. (2015). Rebel heart: Performing fatness wrong online. *M/C Journal, 18*(3). Retrieved from http://www.journal.media-culture.org.au/index.php/mcjournal/article/viewArticle/977

Pausé, C. J. (2012). Live to tell: Coming out as fat. *Somatechnics, 2*(1), 42–56.

Pausé, C. J. & Glover, M. (2018). Exploring the threats to sociable scholarship: An autoethnographic viewing of participatory news making. *Journal of Social and Political Psychology, 6*(2), 696–710. doi: 10.5964/jspp.v6i2.904

Pausé, C. J. & Russell, D. (2016). Sociable scholarship: The use of social media in the 21st century academy. *Journal of Applied Social Theory, 1*(1), 5–25.

Pearl, R. L., & Puhl, R. M. (2018). Weight bias internalization and health: A systematic review. *Obesity Reviews, 19*(8), 1141–1163. doi: 10.1111/obr.12701

Puhl, R., & Brownell, K. D. (2001). Bias, discrimination, and obesity. *Obesity Research, 9*(12), 788–805. doi: 10.1038/oby.2001.108

Puhl, R., Brownell, K. D., & DePierre, J. A. (2014). Bias, discrimination, and obesity. In G. A. Bray & C. Bouchard (Eds.), *Handbook of obesity – Volume 1: Epidemiology, etiology, and physiopatholoy* (3rd Ed.) (pp. 461–470). London: CRC Press.

Puhl, R., & Heuer, C. A. (2009). The stigma of obesity: A review and update. *Obesity, 17*(5), 941–964. doi: 10.1038/oby.2008.636

Rothblum, E., & Solovay, S. (2009). Introduction. In E. Rothblum & S. Solovay (Eds.), *The fat studies reader* (pp. 1–10). New York, NY: New York University Press.

Tremmel, M., Gerdtham, U. G., Nilsson, P., & Saha, S. (2017). Economic burden of obesity: A systematic literature review. *International Journal of Environmental Research and Public Health, 14*(4), 435. doi: 10.3390/ijerph14040435

Wann, M. (2009). Foreword: Fat studies: An invitation to revolution. In E. Rothblum & S. Solovay (Eds.), *The fat studies reader* (pp. xi–xxvi). New York: New York University Press.

What We Do. UCONN Rudd Center for Food Policy & Obesity. Retrieved from http://uconnruddcenter.org/what-we-do

9

NOT THE MEDICINE NEEDED?

Governing fat women's bodies via exercise prescriptions

Richard Pringle

Introduction

In this chapter, I explore how a small group of self-regarded 'fat' women reflect on the process of being targeted by an exercise promotion scheme that, in Foucauldian terms, is a prime exemplar of a biopolitical technology of dominance: that is, a form of power enacted by a State to govern or control the bodies of its citizens. The nation-wide health scheme, in this case, is managed and funded by the New Zealand Ministry of Health to encourage medical doctors to prescribe exercise to 'at risk' patients via a written prescription. The patients are typically urged to make *significant* changes to their lifestyles by undertaking at least 30 minutes of moderate exercise on most days of the week forever.

The scheme is underpinned by the rationale that "the rising incidence of non-communicable diseases in western countries is being driven by *poor* lifestyle choices, including increasingly inadequate physical activity" (Hamlin, Yule, Elliot, Stoner, & Kathiravel, 2016, p. 102; *italics* added for emphasis). Ding et al. (2016, p. 1311) relatedly refer to the global levels of physical inactivity as a "pandemic" (a dubious and combative adjective) that cause "substantial economic burden" in relation to "direct health-care costs, productivity losses and disability-adjusted life years." By inference, the utility of the exercise-on-prescription (EoP) scheme rests on the assumption that select patients will act *rationally* and modify their lifestyle once they acknowledge that their current lifestyle is 'unhealthy' or poor. It is further assumed that if a collective number of patients make appropriate lifestyle changes that this will reduce population levels of morbidity and mortality and a nation's medical costs. In alignment with neo-liberal techniques of power, this mechanism of individualisation directs the dilemma of population health problems onto individuals. Thus, individuals become responsible for the success or failure of their in/actions and, indirectly, the functioning of the scheme.

The population outcome goals of the EoP scheme seem intuitively worthy. Yet, what are the individual costs that should also be considered in the process of governing physical activity? This question is pertinent to reflect on given that adherence rates to EoP schemes are low with approximately only 10 percent of patients meeting the recommended activity guidelines at 12 months post-prescription (Elley, Kerse, Arroll, & Robinson, 2003; Jones, Harris, Waller, & Coggins, 2005). This recognition of low-level intervention success, in conjunction with the acknowledgement that the EoP scheme is a corporeal disciplinary

DOI: 10.4324/9780429344824-12

technology, encouraged my desire to examine the affective response of female patients who have been prescribed exercise to primarily lose fat. I was interested to understand whether the process resulted in the interviewees becoming critical of the intervention process and/or if it produced a sense of guilt or shame about their bodies or lifestyles. My aim was inspired, in part, by recent research that illustrates how feelings of guilt have been ignored by physical activity promoters, yet guilt "as a moral and social emotion, infuses confessional practices, self-monitoring, and self-talk that women engage in as they negotiate physical activity imperatives, which inevitably link fitness with thinness" (Harman & Burrows, 2019, p. 187). In other words, exercise promotion schemes are discursively assembled in relation to notions of health, beauty and guilt: yet, the ethical workings of these assemblages are rarely considered by health promoters.

I begin this chapter by detailing Foucault's understandings of governmentality in relation to how EoP schemes work. I then describe how the interview data were collected and present the results. I conclude by suggesting that although the ethical dilemmas of the scheme may appear subtle to public health practitioners, they are deserving of greater scrutiny.

Governmentality and exercise on prescription schemes: advice from Foucault

In this section, I draw from Foucault's writings on the 'art of government' to contextualise the development, growth and management of EoP schemes. I turned to Foucault as the EoP scheme is a prime exemplar of Foucault's (1978, 1991) concepts of governmentality and bio-power. Indeed, the similarities are so overwhelming, I speculate that EoP schemes could have been drafted from Foucault's writings on how to govern a population; yet, the design of such schemes would have ignored his cautions about the ill-effects of large-scale disciplinary models.

I have long been drawn to Foucault's work as he has a gift to challenge perceptions on what we take for granted. His critical impulse was to make the strange seem familiar and the familiar strange. Foucault, for example, turned traditional understandings of power upside down (Foucault, 1980), challenged our views of madness by linking such conceptions to issues of morality and normality (Foucault, 1967), questioned the belief that our modern prison systems were more humane than the public tortures of old (Foucault, 1977), made us realise that architecture could be conceived as a form of power (Foucault, 1984a), challenged our somewhat arrogant view that humans should be conceived as the central actors in life and therefore should be the prime focus of research (Foucault, 2005) and, amongst other provocative ideas, made us realise that our own sexual desires were not necessarily natural but subject to the workings of power (Foucault, 1978).

To critically examine the world differently, Foucault developed a set of 'tools' that have proven useful for anti-humanist, post-structuralist, critical researchers. His tools revolved around relatively simple precepts: that discourses or 'ways of knowing' are influential in how we understand ourselves, abstract thoughts and other objects, and that these discourses influence how we act in the world and the relationships we develop (i.e., the workings of power in and between people and material realities). His theorising, relatedly, revolved around examinations of the relationships between discourse, knowledge, power relations and ethics. Foucault's writings and tools challenged us to see the world through different eyes and to question the authority of our assumptions and beliefs. Needless to say, it is through such reflective questioning that the genesis for social change occurs. And, it is the possibility of contributing to the possibilities of social change – in a world of injustice and inequity – that draws me to keep working with Foucault. In this project, his critical stance encouraged me to question: what existing set of power relations demanded the development of EoP schemes; what type of subjectivities and power relations evolve through the enactment of EoP schemes; and what are the ethics of such schemes?

Foucault (1982) defined 'government' as *the conduct of conduct* to encourage a recognition that governing processes are broader than the operation of state politics. In his historical writings associated with the shift away from sovereign power, Foucault (1991) nevertheless argued that new forms of power and politics developed in the late 18th century in connection with the emergence of the modern state and associated governments. These governments arose as solutions to the problem of how to manage the citizens and, specifically, "the welfare of the population, the improvement of its wealth, longevity, health ..." (p. 100). Foucault (1984b) accordingly noted that governments aim to manage the "health and physical wellbeing" of populations as "one of the essential objectives of political power," so that the "imperative of health ... (becomes the) duty of each and the objective of all" (p. 277). Hence, he identified that the contemporary obligation to health had its indirect development in the emergence of modern states and governments in the 18th century.

Foucault (1978) coined the neologism 'biopower' and its derivatives 'biopolitics' and 'anatomo-politics' to represent the proliferation of novel techniques of power that developed for governing the 'bios' or lives of individuals and the broader population. Biopolitics refers to the governance of the population in alignment with controlling the biological dimensions of life, such as attempts to control a population's rates of obesity, drug and alcohol use, sexually transmitted diseases, or physical activity levels, whereas anatomo-politics refers to the disciplinary techniques of power used to control an individual's embodied health practices, as relatedly associated with individual exercise regimes, abstinence, dieting or safe-sex practices. The government's desire to enhance the health of a population is, correspondingly, related to the disciplining or controlling of individuals. In other words, individuals are disciplined primarily for the benefit of the cost-effective management of the broader population. Although individuals may also benefit through this process, Foucault advocated that it is important to critically reflect on how governmental technologies are instituted and enacted and the associated cost for citizens.

The EoP scheme is a relatively recent technique of power aiming to govern the biological dimensions of life. The first EoP scheme in a primary health care setting was developed in Britain in the early 1990s (Iliffe, Tai, Gould, Thorogood, & Hillsdon, 1995). This scheme developed in relation to the growing scientific understanding that moderate physical activity reduces the risk of individuals developing heart disease, stroke, breast and colon cancer, high blood pressure, non-insulin diabetes mellitus and osteoporosis (Brown, Burton, & Rowan, 2007; US Department of Health and Human Services, 1996). The exercise on prescription (EoP) concept gained increased support via publication of the landmark US Surgeon General's 1996 report which concluded, from a synthesis of various epidemiological studies, that *health and quality of life* can be considerably improved by incorporating moderate levels of physical activity into everyday life (US Department of Health and Human Services, 1996). This 'health' understanding subsequently underpinned the 1998 establishment of the EoP scheme known as *Green Prescriptions* within Aotearoa New Zealand (Swinburn & McLennan, 1998).

The select health problem, in the case of EoP schemes, is the high medical costs that are assumed to occur in populations where sedentary lifestyles and high rates of obesity are deemed prevalent (Ding et al., 2016). Although the cost of converting one prescription patient from a sedentary to an active lifestyle has been calculated as NZ$1,756, this amount has been deemed cost-efficient in relation to the calculated reduction in overall health care costs (Elley, Kerse, Arroll, Swinburn, Ashton, & Robinson, 2004).

Governmentality processes involve various analyses, calculations and tactics in relation to an assemblage of institutions and individuals working to achieve a shared goal (Foucault, 1984b). The Green Prescriptions assemblage enmeshes connections between the Ministry of Health, Regional Sport Trusts, primary care health settings, physical activity counsellors, medical premises, 'patients,' and various community groups, such as walking groups and recreations centres. The Green Prescriptions process typically begins for a patient within a medical consultation. The doctor or prescriber discusses the benefits of physical activity with selectively targeted patients and provides a written prescription that identifies the type of activity and recommended duration and frequency (the dose) that should be adhered to – physical activity is patently medicalised in this process. The patient then provides informed consent for a copy of the prescription, which includes patient details such as age, weight and relevant health conditions, to be sent to a Regional Sport Trust (a government agency). An employee of the Trust then assigns an exercise specialist to make at least three telephone calls or face-to-face meetings over the next 3–4 months to the patient to provide motivation and advice concerning exercise activities.

Noted disciplinary forms of power such as surveillance and confessional techniques are used extensively in the management of governmental practices (Foucault, 1991). The monitoring and management of EoP schemes, for example, have been shaped by the results and implications of various population surveys and epidemiological studies. The New Zealand Sport and Recreation Commission, as an example, funded a random survey to identify 'target audiences' who would be more likely to become active through social marketing schemes (Sullivan, Oakden, Young, Butcher, & Lawson, 2003). A key finding from this survey found that females who were deemed overweight but who had good social support would be the most cost-effective group to target via an exercise prescription (Sullivan et al., 2003). This finding might explain why females receive a disproportionate 73 percent of the exercise prescriptions within Aotearoa New Zealand (van Aalst & Daly, 2005). Relatedly, 55 percent of all exercise prescriptions are prescribed to patients who are classified as overweight (van Aalst & Daly, 2005).[1]

Yet, the targeting of overweight women is potentially flawed for three key reasons. First, there is limited evidence of gender differences in relation to actual adherence rates to exercise advice or prescriptions (e.g. Emerenziani et al., 2018; Noon, Nwose, & Breheny, 2019; White, Randsdell, Vener, & Flohr, 2005). In other words, females appear to be no more 'cost-effective' than males in responding to exercise counselling. Second, in contrast to the common assumption that being 'overweight' is a health risk, systematic meta-analyses draw the opposing conclusion. That is, overweight individuals, as determined via BMI, have the lowest risk of major cardiovascular events in comparison with those deemed to be underweight, obese, or of normal weight (Flegal, Kit, Orpana, & Graubard, 2013). Finally, although females tend to rate their health as poorer in comparison to males, male mortality rate is higher throughout the lifespan (Case & Paxson, 2005) – which might suggest that thin males would be a better target of biopolitical schemes.

Given there is no clear medical evidence to justify why overweight females receive the majority of exercise prescriptions, I speculate that medical doctors might subjectively assume that the prescriptive task is less contentious for women. Indeed, it is likely a difficult task to tell someone that they are fat and unhealthy unless you believe that they would be receptive to such advice. Relatedly, Harman and Burrows (2019) revealed that many women have been disciplined, via various social mechanisms, to feel guilty about their varying levels of body fat and are desirous to lose weight. Yet, how do these women affectively respond to an exercise prescription that states that their bodies carry an unhealthy amount of excess fat? In the following section, I discuss how I examined this question and what I found.

Guilt, fat and the exercise prescription

The interview data presented in this chapter was originally collected from a larger qualitative study that involved critical life-course interviews to examine how 42 individuals responded to receiving an exercise prescription (see Pringle, 2008). These interviewees were purposefully selected based on ethnicity (Maori, Pasifika, European/Pakeha[2]), anatomical sex and current level of physical activity (e.g., sedentary, meeting recommended activity guidelines, or partially active). The life-history interviews typically took an hour to complete and were transcribed verbatim. The interviews were conversational and wide ranging in topic but typically began with inviting the interviewees to tell their narrative of how they received their exercise prescription, the process involved and their reaction to the prescription.

Sixty-six percent of the interviewees were prescribed exercise in relation to being overweight, 16 percent for diabetes, and 5 percent for asthma. A disproportionate percentage of females (78 percent) were prescribed exercise for weight-loss reasons. Although several of the interviewees were prescribed exercise for multiple reasons, for example, Marama was prescribed for being overweight, back pain, and high blood pressure.

This section presents evidence from 10 of the female interviewees who were prescribed exercise for being overweight yet remained sedentary post the exercise prescription. The average age of these women was 49 years, ranging from 24 to 68. Four of the interviewees identified primarily as Maori, two as Samoan, and four as having European ancestry. The research participants typically suggested that the broad prescription process was received positively, that is, the medical doctor was deemed professional, and the exercise counsellors were pleasant to talk to and attempted to be helpful. Amelia, however, found the weight-loss advice "a bit ridiculous," as she was told that, for height, she should only weigh 55 kg. Yet, Amelia knew that she would "look like a skeleton" if she only weighed 55 kg. And Rita (Samoan) thought that it was culturally inappropriate to be told that she should not eat traditional Samoan foods, such as "taro and coconut cream." In fact, immediately after receiving this medical advice, she gave up any idea of following the 'health' prescription. Sally simply believed that the process was a waste of time:

> Well, it didn't even really do nothing to me. I don't even know what it is really. All it was, was some lady that would ring me up and ask me how I was going and that was about it ... I didn't find it useful ... I guess because I didn't even know who I was talking to.

Prior to gaining their exercise prescription, the interviewees indicated that they were well aware of the health advantages of exercise and a healthy diet. Hence, the prescription did not fill a knowledge void that changed their ways of thinking. Moreover, five of the participants requested the exercise prescription as they wanted cheaper entry to a fitness centre or swimming pool in order to lose weight. Despite this desire to exercise, all five remained sedentary within two months of gaining their prescription. Angie reported that the initial exercise counselling was motivational, "cos, if you know you are going to get phoned it helps you to want to do it." Yet, as a solo mum with two boys in their late teens, she eventually found her gym routine time-consuming, boring and ineffective: "It sort of got a bit monotonous after a while cos you're just doing the same thing round and round in circles... Well actually, I didn't find the exercise beneficial anyhow." She added rhetorically: "why bother doing something boring if it does not provide any benefits?" Joc similarly reported, "I have to say the exercise all fell by the board because we were doing all this (exercise) but we weren't getting any better ... my blood pressure never changed." Amelia acknowledged that she had initially lost weight, primarily though eating less, but when she got down to 82 kg (and not the prescribed 55 kg) she had no desire to lose any more weight; she was also busy with her two young children and felt no need to be exercising for her 'health.'

All five of the women who had requested an exercise prescription were not motivated primarily by 'health' concerns but wanted to lose weight to appear more attractive. Thus, when the exercise did not result in the desired weight loss (and related appearance goal), they lost desire to exercise. They also believed that they were relatively healthy. Indeed, they appeared health conscious – none of them smoked, their alcohol consumption was reportedly moderate, and all were relatively careful with their diet. Repika concluded with a degree of healthy self-confidence, "I'm in pretty good shape for a Mum with two kids." Jane similarly reported with confidence, "I just feel that I'm active enough in what I do. I don't think that there are many women my age (68 years) that actually do what I do." Yet, all five still reported that they desired to lose weight as they had concerns about their shape and appearance.

The other five interviewees acknowledged, to a certain degree, that their health could be better. As an example, Joan, who was prescribed exercise because of her weight and chronic fatigue, was housebound, lonely, and somewhat depressed. She did want to improve her holistic health but did not believe that the exercise prescription was what she needed. Similarly, Amelia (a 19-year old solo Mum with two children under two, all sleeping in one bedroom) reported: "I'm not doing well and worried about getting depressed again. I'm sleep deprived and I'm busy… I would rate my health under average, I know my immune system is a bit down, it's a bit shot." These five interviewees, who acknowledged that their health was in need of improvement, did not believe that moderate exercise was the medicine that they needed. As such, they were not motivated to exercise for 30 minutes each day.

The interviewees further revealed that the exercise counselling process induced negative emotions. Kelly acknowledged that her reason for not exercising – a lack of time – was a "poor" excuse, and she felt relatedly guilty: "I don't really know why the exercise stopped – but they're about to start. They're always about to start." Through not following the exercise prescription, she had developed a nagging sense of inadequacy. Ariana similarly acknowledged, "I don't think I gave them (exercise counsellors) the chance to help… I might have fobbed them off or just avoided that… The only reason (for not exercising) was I got busy, which is a lame excuse." Talia similarly confessed that the prescription process had reinforced a sense of guilt: "I suppose I'm a tad lazy when it comes to exercising. Never been sport minded, never been one to get into anything really." Jane's voice was full of remorse, and negativity: "I know I won't change. Very set in my ways … I think it's in the brain. You either want to be active or you don't. And I obviously never wanted to be active. One of the lazy people I suppose." She concluded: "And now, I suppose, I'm quite happy to sit back and relax which will make it worse." Jane, accordingly, blamed her 'lazy' self for creating what she believed would be future negative health consequences.

Some concluding 'guilt-edged' words

The exercise prescription, for the ten interviewees, was not the medicine they needed – in fact, it made them feel worse. The medical process, for example, did not help the five women who requested an exercise prescription to lose weight. More specifically, the exercise prescription process blurred into to an "exercise-body beautiful complex" that left them with a residual sense of failure (Harman & Burrows, 2019, p. 197). Indeed, all still wanted to be thinner – to be more attractive rather than healthy – yet they did not blame the prescription process for their inability to lose weight. In contrast, they problematically blamed themselves for their failure in the scheme.

For the five interviewees who acknowledged that they had health issues (e.g., chronic fatigue, diabetes or arthritis), they did not believe that exercise was the best medicine for their ailments. They also recognised that they were confronted with an array of other 'social' problems associated with depression, loneliness, financial difficulty and simply being over-tired with young children to look after. In this respect, they accepted that they could benefit from some form of help but that the exercise prescription was not what they needed. Nevertheless, their stories about the prescription process were *guilt-edged* – they reported that in response to the scheme, they felt lazy, blamed themselves for not following the prescription, recognised that their excuses were "lame" and they still typically wanted to be thinner – a corporeal desire that they could not seem to achieve but was nevertheless reinforced via the EoP process.

The architects of the EoP scheme would likely *blame* these women for failing to adhere to their prescription by citing medical research to indicate that if they had followed the medical advice, this could have helped their illness conditions, reduce their 'excess fat' and problems with depression. Yet, the sizeable failure rate of this scheme (90 percent) suggests that the scheme itself is problematic. I question rhetorically: would medical authorities allow a medicine to be prescribed if it only had a 10 percent rate of adherence, let alone if its side-effects included a propensity for patients to experience guilt and poor self-esteem?

I conclude that the EoP scheme indirectly failed the 10 interviewees in this study. The interviewees were invited into the scheme via the State, were advised that their current lifestyle was poor, were told how to rectify it and how a more active lifestyle would be beneficial for them, but they did not adhere to their prescriptions and were left with residual feelings of guilt. Guttman and Salmon (2004) acknowledge that, as health increasingly signifies moral virtue, those who are deemed unhealthy are made to feel unworthy. Relatedly, the cost of being 'overweight,' as determined via BMI, is not related to cardiovascular health issues (see Flegal et al., 2013) but social stigma and body-image problems. For the interviewees in this study, the ineffectual medical process did more 'well-being' damage than good; yet, the daily cost of this harm – that is, the on-going sense of moral failure (see Harman & Burrows, 2019) – was not part of the governmental calculations in the administration of the EoP scheme. The governance of EoP schemes, as such, has escaped the scrutiny of related ethical discussions. Although public health campaigns are credited with raising awareness of the problems of chronic illness, the associated ethical dilemmas should not be dismissed as subtle, but in need of greater consideration in the governing of bios or the lives of individuals.

Through drawing on Foucault, my initial belief that EoP schemes represented a positive and potentially radical shift in the workings of medicine and health care has been challenged. Although I still like the idea of encouraging active lifestyles within health-care settings, as a potential alternative to the prescription of various medicines, Foucault's ideas have allowed me to view the EoP scheme as an extension of the biomedical model – a model that reinforces medicalised understandings of health to the potential detriment of those who do not 'measure up' to the constricted norms of what is deemed healthy (i.e., moral) and the problematic ethics of what a healthy body should look like.

Notes

1 The prime reasons for prescribing exercise are associated with weight issues (55 percent), high blood pressure (34 percent), high cholesterol (24 percent), diabetes (24 percent), arthritis (23 percent) and back pain (20 percent); these percentages do not add to 100 percent as patients can present with one or more concerns (van Aalst & Daly, 2005).
2 Pakeha is a Maori word that identifies people of European ancestry.

References

Brown, W., Burton, N., & Rowan, P. (2007). Updating the evidence on physical activity and health in women. *American Journal of Preventive Medicine, 33*(5), 404–411. doi: 10.1016/j.amepre.2007.07.029

Case, A., & Paxson, C. (2005). Sex differences in morbidity and mortality. *Demography, 42*(2), 189–214. doi: 10.1353/dem.2005.0011

Ding, D., Lawson, K. D., Kolbe-Alexander, T. L., Finkelstein, E. A., Katzmarzyk, P. T., Van Mechelen, W.,… & Lancet Physical Activity Series 2 Executive Committee. (2016). The economic burden of physical inactivity: A global analysis of major non-communicable diseases. *The Lancet, 388*(10051), 1311–1324. doi: 10.1016/S0140–6736(16)30383-X

Elley, C. R., Kerse, N., Arroll, B., & Robinson, E. (2003). Effectiveness of counselling patients on physical activity in general practice: Cluster randomised controlled trial. *British Medical Journal, 326*(7393), 793. doi: 10.1136/bmj.326.7393.793

Elley, R., Kerse, N., Arroll, B., Swinburn, B., Ashton, T., & Robinson, E. (2004). Cost-effectiveness of physical activity counselling in general practice. *New Zealand Medical Journal, 117*(1207), 1–15.

Emerenziani, G. P., Gallotta, M. C., Migliaccio, S., Ferrari, D., Greco, E. A., Saavedra, F. J.,… & Baldari, C. (2018). Effects of an individualized home-based unsupervised aerobic training on body composition and physiological parameters in obese adults are independent of gender. *Journal of Endocrinological Investigation, 41*(4), 465–473. doi: 10.1007/s40618-017-0771-2

Flegal, K. M., Kit, B. K., Orpana, H., & Graubard, B. I. (2013). Association of all-cause mortality with overweight and obesity using standard body mass index categories: A systematic review and meta-analysis. *Jama, 309*(1), 71–82. doi: 10.1001/jama.2012.113905

Foucault, M. (1967). *Madness and civilisation: A history of insanity in the age of reason.* London: Tavistock. (Original work published in 1961)

Foucault, M. (1977). *Discipline and punish: The birth of the prison* (A. M. Sheridan, Trans.). New York: Pantheon Books. (Original work published 1975).

Foucault, M. (1978). *The history of sexuality: Vol. 1. An introduction* (R. Hurley, Trans.). New York: Pantheon.

Foucault, M. (1980). *Power/knowledge: Selected interviews and other writings 1972–1977.* New York: Pantheon.

Foucault, M. (1982). The subject and power. In H. Dreyfus & P. Rabinow (Eds.), *Michel Foucault. Beyond structuralism and hermeneutics* (pp. 208–226). Chicago, IL: University of Chicago Press.

Foucault, M. (1984a). Of other spaces, heterotopias. *Architecture, mouvement, continuité, 5*(1984), 46–49.

Foucault, M. (1984b). The politics of health in the eighteenth century. In P. Rabinow (Ed.), *The Foucault reader: An introduction to Foucault's thought* (pp. 273–289). London: Penguin Books.

Foucault, M. (1991). *The Foucault effect: Studies in governmentality.* Chicago, IL: University of Chicago Press.

Foucault, M. (2005). *The order of things.* London: Routledge.

Guttman, N., & Salmon, C. T. (2004). Guilt, fear, stigma and knowledge gaps: Ethical issues in public health communication interventions. *Bioethics, 18*(6), 531–552. doi: 10.1111/j.1467–8519.2004.00415.x

Hamlin, M. J., Yule, E., Elliot, C. A., Stoner, L., & Kathiravel, Y. (2016). Long-term effectiveness of the New Zealand Green Prescription primary health care exercise initiative. *Public Health, 140,* 102–108. doi: 10.1016/j.puhe.2016.07.014

Harman, A., & Burrows, L. (2019). Leaning in while sticking out: Fat, exercise, and guilt. *Fat Studies, 8*(2), 187–202. doi: 10.1080/21604851.2019.1562838

Iliffe, S., Tai, S. S., Gould, M., Thorogood, M., & Hillsdon, M. (1995). Prescribing exercise in general practice. *British Medical Journal, 309,* 494–495. doi: 10.1136/bmj.310.6973.194c

Jones, F., Harris, P., Waller, H., & Coggins, A. (2005). Adherence to an exercise prescription scheme: The role of expectations, self-efficacy, stage of change and psychological well-being. *British Journal of Health Psychology, 10*(3), 359–378. doi: 10.1348/135910704X24798

Noon, C. T., Nwose, E. U., & Breheny, L. (2019). Evaluation of gender differences in exercise adherence for low back pain: Case reviews and survey. *European Journal of Physiotherapy, 21*(1), 49–55. doi: 10.1080/21679169.2018.1468815

Pringle, R. (2008). *Health and physical activity promotion: A qualitative examination of the effect of receiving a Green Prescription (GRx).* Report funded by Sport and Recreation New Zealand (SPARC).

Sullivan, C., Oakden, J., Young, J., Butcher, H., & Lawson, R. (2003). *Obstacles to action: A study of New Zealanders' physical activity and nutrition: Overview report December 2003.* Wellington: SPARC.

Swinburn, B., & McLennan, J. (1998). The green prescription: A novel way of increasing uptake of physical activity. *The New Zealand Public Health Report, 5*(4), 25–26. doi: 10.2105/ajph.88.2.288

US Department of Health and Human Services. (1996). *Physical activity and health: A report of the Surgeon General.* Atlanta, GA: US Department of Health and Human Services, Centers of Disease Control and Prevention, National Center for Chronic Disease Prevention and Health Promotion.

Van Aalst, I., & Daly, C. (2005). *Green prescriptions in general practice.* Wellington: Sport and Recreation New Zealand.

White, J. L., Randsdell, L. B., Vener, J., & Flohr, J. A. (2005). Factors related to physical activity adherence in women: Review and suggestions for future research. *Women & Health, 41*(4), 123–148. doi: 10.1300/j013v41n04_07

10

NEW MATERIALIST ENACTMENTS

Simone Fullagar, Emma Rich, and Niamh Ni Shuilleabhain

In this chapter, we examine the influence of new materialist theories and methodologies on emerging debates concerning obesity as a phenomenon that is entangled with the biopolitical conditions of life and knowledge production. We discuss how new materialist styles of thought draw upon various post-humanist and post-qualitative approaches to reorient the onto-epistemological assumptions of humanist critique to question *how bodies come to matter* (as fat, obese, normalised, pleasurable, disgusting, visceral, physiological, visual, mobile, and subject to intervention). The chapter explores the implications of these ideas for research, policy, and practice across health, education, and popular culture, highlighting their potential for opening new ways of thinking, doing, and being across these areas.

Introduction

A variety of theoretical and post-qualitative methodological approaches that seek to move beyond humanist assumptions are often identified under the umbrellas of new materialism, new empiricisms, and materialist feminisms (Åsberg & Braidotti, 2018; Fox & Alldred, 2016; Haraway, 2016; Taylor & Hughes, 2016; Braidotti, 2013; St Pierre, 2011; Bennett, 2010; Coole & Frost, 2010; Barad, 2007). Acknowledging the diversity of theoretical trajectories that inform the evolving practices and speculative thinking of new materialisms [and the critiques of "newness" and omissions (Ahmed, 2008)], this chapter pursues the material thread running through this work – *how does body size come to matter*? This approach moves away from the polarised debates concerning what obesity "is" (scientific fact verse ideological problem), to trace what obesity "does" to individuals and societal responses implicated embodiment configurations (such as, size, weight, appearance of (un)healthiness, aesthetic value, (dis)function, associated conditions [diseases, risk factors, disability, and mental ill health], and environmental relations [family habits, disadvantaged locales, polluted areas, childhood abuse/trauma, epigenetic expression]). How is it that fat bodies come to evoke powerful effects from shame, disgust, and aggression as well as defiance and pleasure (Probyn, 2008), while also being objects of desire that set in motion the work of obesity researchers, funding bodies, and policy makers that seeks correctives (weight loss)?

New materialists are concerned with pursuing these kinds of relational questions and an ontological politics that disrupts the normative truths circulating through the machinic

DOI: 10.4324/9780429344824-13

assemblages that constitute "obesity". These relations involve both everyday practices and the globalised flows of capitalism (food and diet products, healthy messages, wearable tech, surgical interventions, and so on). In seeking to map out the utility of new materialist styles of thought for thinking critically about obesity, we engage with work emanating from post-humanism, science and technology studies, feminist embodiment, queer, crip, critical race, and post-qualitative approaches that share a desire to move beyond the onto-epistemological assumptions of humanist thought. Recognising the complex theoretical terrain of new materialism, we provide an example of research[1] that enacts new materialist theory-methods in relation to the problem of body disaffection in English schools. Rounding off our conceptual exploration of new materialist perspectives, we discuss the implications for rethinking policy, practice, and pedagogical dilemmas.

New materialist body matters

There are a number of common assumptions that inform new materialist orientations such as the desire to undo the normative privilege afforded to (particular) humans over other forms of nature and explore co-constituted phenomena via intra-actions, relationships, assemblages, and ecologies (Åsberg & Braidotti, 2018). The orientation to an ontological politics conceives of change and causality in terms of complexity and emergence through multiple affects and intra-actions, hence agentic capacities do not reside "within" beings but are distributed relationally (Braidotti, 2013). In this sense, power is relational and works through different scales connecting the global with the micropolitics of everyday life. As an approach to theory, new materialism moves away from explanatory models or reified concepts that seek to "represent" the world as it is (supposedly) and ignoring the complex movement of material-discursive relations. Hence a different kind of analytic is mobilised as theory and method come together in research practices that attune (reading, writing, data production, etc.) to affective relations, flows of power, and the "lively" matter of material processes (Taylor & Hughes, 2016; Coole & Frost, 2010). Thinking with theory becomes a generative act, producing different, often speculative, imaginative engagements with matter as multiplicity. From her *agential realist* perspective, Barad (2003, p. 802) argues for "A *performative* understanding of discursive practices challenges the representationalist belief in the power of words to represent pre-existing things" (italics in original). For our purposes in this short exploration, we will trace certain styles of thought that have come to shape new materialist work on "obesity" and "healthy bodies" more broadly (see also Lupton, 2018; Fullagar, 2017).

Different trajectories of materialist thought turn our attention to the material, discursive, and affective relations through which fatness and obesity are produced, enacted, and circulated. Such a shift extends post-structuralist, feminist, queer, and critical approaches that have questioned the dualistic categories of human being and knowing underpinning humanist thinking: objective/subjective, reason/emotion, culture/nature, mind/body, human/non-human, and self/other mappings across social differences and inequities (colonising human and non-human bodies, perpetuating regimes of exclusion for bodies that trouble binaries). Importantly, this orientation to the *material* moves beyond the ontological assumption that fat bodies are passive *tabula rasa* upon which socially constructed meanings are inscribed either discursively, phenomenologically, or ideologically by structural power and/or individual agency.

In contrast, emphasis is placed on a *relational ontology* concerning what the matter of fat bodies "does" and how such agentic capacities are produced through entangled biopolitical relations (biological, cultural, economic, and ecological). Attention is paid to the generative force of human and nonhuman matter as an emergent relation rather than inherent property or source of agency. Fatness is the body multiple (Throsby, 2012; Mol, 2002) – gut biomes, genetic codes, fleshy substance, felt, inscribed, imagined, subjected to clinical procedures, and represented in a myriad of ways. Pushing beyond the interpretative focus on "human experience" or the assumed objectivity of measuring obesity, new materialism asks how "matter" is thought and constituted through entanglements of human and non-human bodies, forces of affect, and objects or things. Biopolitical entanglements cannot be separated from the truth-making practices of science and social science research (all methods and theories "cut" knowledge with particular effects) as well as the enactments of policy and pedagogies that are co-implicated in everyday health and body practices. Hence, new materialists make explicit the response-ability of researchers to address the entanglement of ethico-onto-epistemological matters in all aspects of knowledge production (Barad, 2007).

Permeable, multiple bodies

Barad's work as a feminist and quantum physicist raises questions about how the nonhuman acts on and through the fat body disturbing the normative assumptions of boundedness. Taking up Donna Haraway's question – why should bodies end at the skin? – Barad orients our thinking about bodies as permeable matter and to consider what is not visible in our worldly intra-actions. Considering the focus of much analysis on "human interactions" to be anthropocentric and atomistic, Barad shifts our attention to more complex "intra-actions" to examine how "phenomena" (such as fatness) materialise through entangled relations that *co-constitute* worlds. Barad helps us to see the problematic ontological assumptions that inform the categories of thought (in policy and public health research) that position fat bodies as a site of individual agentic potential that can be unleashed (by behavioural interventions) against constraints of obesogenic environments. This common discourse about obesity prevention rests upon a static notion of the subject and world as separate entities rather than entangled phenomena acted upon by multiple forces. Along with entanglement, Barad's diffractive work importantly traces "how differences get made, what gets excluded and how these exclusions matter" (Barad, 2007, p. 32). Thinking with notions of permeability, multiplicity, and entanglement also moves new materialist thinking about obesity in a post-disciplinary direction that has been taken up by science and technology study scholars.

Warin (2015) has written a compelling analysis of the science of obesity that does not simply refute claims made about the biological matter of fat bodies; rather, she troubles the assumptions underpinning disciplinary divides (see also Sanabria, 2016). In the desire to avoid essentialist biological accounts, much social constructionism (fat studies, critical health) has concerned itself with narrative, discursive, and mediated meanings that constitute obesity and fatness; yet, as Warin argues, this has ironically reproduced the Cartesian dualisms of social-biological, culture-nature. Warin's (2015, p. 48) work brings into relation the "insights of material feminism and obesity science's attention to maternal nutrition and the foetal origins hypothesis" to move beyond the existing ontological impasse. Exploring her own affective responses to obesity science (both scepticism and fascination with how biological and social matters were thought), Warin (2015, p. 62) reads for productive possibilities:

> In foetal origins work, food is a bridge or pathway that makes the uterus a social and relational space, not just a biological space. In critical periods of development (in utero, in

early years and in adolescence) the body "goes through periods of plasticity and *openness* to the environment [my emphasis]".

Her account goes on to detail how feminist insights into the conditions of women's and children's inequality materialise through food and related practices. In a move beyond the conventional parameters of critique, Warin offers a more generative analysis and proximal engagement with other disciplines that has the potential to identify biological, cultural, economic, and ecological intra-actions.

In their analysis of how obesity research enacts problems and solutions, Esmonde and Jette (2018) also identify how the continued emphasis on individual energy balance and environmental determinism points towards a paradoxical formulation of the "obesogenic environment". From a different angle, Land's (2018, p. 78) research seeks to think with feminist ethico-onto-epistemological resources (physiological knowledges) about the materialisation of fat as a problem by producing "a politicized attempt to do fat(s) differently by threading the divergent, violent, productive, and contested fat(s) enacted within, and amid critiques of, the obesity apparatus...". This approach seeks to generate critical knowledge "with physiologies" of fat in the pursuit of a more complex, entangled, biocultural understanding rather than a realist representation of materiality. Fat knowledges become subject to and also emerge from a molecular politics that troubles essentialism and reductionism. Yet, like Yoshizawa (2012), Land (2018) does not call for a transdisciplinary theory of all factors involved in obesity but rather points to an analytic focus on how knowledges continually intra-act with fat (and with particular a/effects).

Fat assemblages and flows

The writing of French philosophers Deleuze and Guattari has significantly influenced new materialist directions by opening up "the body" to thought that moves beyond the discrete, fleshy borders imagined by phenomenology and social constructionism. Fox and Alldred (2016) have drawn upon Deleuze and Guattari in their extensive writing about new materialist methodologies across health, sexuality, and sociological knowledge including obesity. Working with a flat ontology that recognises the materiality of concepts and empirical worlds occurring at once (doing away with macro/micro distinctions), Fox, Bissell, Peacock, and Blackburn (2018) explore the micropolitics of obesity that affects how adults articulate their food practices through "becoming-fat" and "becoming-slim" assemblages. Assemblage thinking in this line of thought refers to the *arrangement* of affects as pre-personal forces (power relations) that work dynamically to territorialise and deterritorialise the capacities of fat bodies and fatness. Shifting away from individualised perspectives and an anthropocentric focus on the obese body, Fox et al. (2018, p. 122) explored how:

Becoming-fat bodies were part of an assemblage that included the nutritional and sensory properties of foodstuffs, family meal preparation and consumption practices, cultural and interpersonal relations around food and eating, and contemporary approaches to food production and retailing, as manifested in outlets such as high street supermarkets and fast-food chains.

They draw out the complexity of how different material relations act upon and through the body as a dynamic biological, sociocultural, and economic formation.

Rinaldi, Rice, Kotow, and Lind (2019) move in a different direction with their research into the affective economies of fat hatred that draws together feminist, queer, and intersectional work on the materiality of power relations. They conceptualise *fatmisia* as a complex affective force, "derived from the Greek misos, meaning hatred, dislike, or contempt— refers to hatred of fat, fatness, and fat persons" (Rinaldi et al., 2019, p. 1). Exploring how fat hatred circulates as an affective economy across assemblages of health-care, transit, and exercise, these scholars draw upon interview data with queer women and trans folk to map the stickiness of feelings that connect objects and discourses in ways that erase or expunge fat bodies as intersectional assemblages (hatred of fat, racialised, gendered, and queer difference). Rather than conceive of feelings as psychologised emotion, they employ Ahmed's (2004, p. 10) notion of the in-between-ness of affective *relations*, "It is through emotions, or how we respond to objects and others, that surfaces or boundaries are made". In relation to exercising spaces, Rinaldi et al. (2019, p. 10) identify how fat bodies subject to fatmisia are rendered as matter out of place (hatred produces shameful bodies), "they function both to exclude and to prevent the existence of fat bodies" (see also Kofoed & Ringrose, 2012, on school bullying). While these scholars draw on theories of affect to explore the materiality of obesity, curiously, they do not engage with post-qualitative debates on the ontological politics of research methodology (Fullagar, 2017; Berbary & Boles, 2014; St Pierre, 2011). This theory-method shift calls for less prescriptive methods (such as the conventions of coding and thematic analysis) in the turn towards more inventive re-presentations, worlding, and activist orientations that refuse subject/object, objective/ interpretive divides.

Researching body disaffection

Rice's (2015, p. 387) "body-becoming" theory marked a generative shift in how we consider and respond to the fat body. This theory of fat that draws on constructivist and new materialist perspectives moves away from bio-pedagogical approaches that focus on what is, instead allowing us to creatively imagine how the fat body might become. Rice (2015, p. 395) demonstrates examples of how activist art communities have been able to "disrupt viewers" dominant ways of knowing "fatness". The author asks researchers to consider how to translate these insights "into actual pedagogies that expand options for becoming" that can be used in sites like schools and to explore what conditions would enable such creative imagining and body-becoming (Rice, 2015, p. 395). Niamh's work on exploring body pedagogies and body disaffection in schools sought to respond to this call.

Extensive literature explores how body pedagogies work to constitute young people's subjectivities in schools. Within this body of work, dominant conceptualisations of body pedagogy include those who, influenced by Foucault, view the body as "acted upon" (Monaghan, Colls, & Evans, 2013; Wright, 2012; Wright & Harwood, 2012; Leahy, 2009; Walkerdine, 2009; Gard & Wright, 2001). Those who influenced by Bernstein, or Durkheim and Mauss focus on "'bodies' in culture – and how culture impacts and 'matters' the body" (Evans, Davies, & Rich, 2014, p. 565), and shapes its "corporeal properties" (Shilling, 2008, p. 165). Drawing on new materialist theory, we instead conceptualise body pedagogy as an "intra-action" (of the human and non-human) through which material-discursive phenomena like the fat body emerge and become intelligible (Barad, 2007). This conceptualisation of the discursive and the material as mutually constituted and co-implicated allows for an understanding of the body and pedagogy that is neither realist nor social constructivist. An interview intra-action with Chris, one of the teachers from the Henham School, produced an orientation to the fat body that was entangled (Fullagar, 2017) with popular conceptualisations of "obesogenic environments":

> I think there is, yeah society is changing, yeah I think there is some movement happening isn't there? (…) you know there was actually a programme on recently, the truth about carbs? (…) And it was about carbs, carbohydrates and how that's clearly the major cause of obesity, just the accessibility, the cheapness and all that sort of stuff. And these kids come to school they have a monster drink right full of sugar, they have a rubbish breakfast then they just snack on, the canteen here is rubbish, the food here is rubbish, you know they get processed, like white bread, like you know, rubbish food, no good food. You know what I mean and that's, that's the issue and at home they have rubbish food as well and they come here and they get rubbish food so that's clearly where the battle should be fought, that's what I feel.
>
> *Chris (teacher at Henham School)*

This shift in focus from the individual as culpable for obesity to the "obesogenic/obesiogenic environment" has been criticised for ignoring intra-community diversities and complexities and for framing ultimate responsibility in terms of the individual once again (Evans & Rich, 2011; LeBesco, 2011; Evans, Davies, & Rich, 2008). A new materialist perspective allows us to analyse the above data to understand that we become with and through those "environments", "objects", and "practices" with which we are entangled (Fox et al., 2018). Material-discursive foodstuffs like "a monster drink right full of sugar", "a rubbish breakfast", and "white bread" cannot be separated out from the becoming of unbounded bodies. Within the above intra-action, young people's bodies are materialised as "rubbish" through their food-consumption practices that are part of broader assemblage formations like those Fox et al. (2018) identified in their analysis. When certain "pedagogical modes of address" (Giroux, 2004; Ellsworth, 1997) that "are produced through "expert" discourses of health literacy" (Fullagar, Rich, Francombe-Webb, & Maturo, 2017, p. 3) become co-implicated in pedagogical intra-actions in schools, they enact "cuts" that produce unintended affective consequences. Georgia from Henham School performatively detailed the body disaffection that can arise in pedagogical intra-actions that involve learning about healthy eating or exercise:

> I think it makes some people feel bad because like they know they aren't as good as say their friends, so they automatically just start going like really hard on themselves, like "oh I'm rubbish and really fat and don't look nice".
>
> *Georgia (student at Henham School)*

This thinking extends Rice's (2015) theory by arguing that we must consider the co-implicated non-human in body becomings. Within a new materialist conceptualisation, health problems amongst young people in schools are neither "fat fabrications" (Evans, Rich, Davies, & Allwood, 2008) nor indisputable fact (Warin, 2015). New materialist approaches call for us to attend to the emergent materialities in schools:

> (…) demand is put on us in schools to deal with a multitude of issues, including poverty and you know children coming into school not having had breakfast. You know there are families in real hardship, not being able to buy uniform, so it is, you know they are very difficult, they are very demanding environments and a frustrating thing for all teachers is how little we can do.
>
> *Alyssa (teacher at Henham School)*

While simultaneously demanding that we remain "response-able" for the ethical and affective implications of the material-discursive body pedagogies and policies, we develop surrounding the unbounded (human/non-human) becoming body in schools (Barad, 2007). This research in schools involved using creative methods with young people to explore how we may develop body pedagogies more "response-able" in relation to body disaffection.

The "fat" body within policy assemblages

These approaches can inform a more nuanced exploration of policies and the impact on bodies. We suggest that this is productive in two ways. First, these concepts lead us to ask different questions about the formation and production of policies. Second, and aligning with the idea of becoming (Rice, 2015), it might help us to reimagine policy. New materialist thinking might provide ways to respond to what is commonly framed within current obesity policy as a problem of either poor lifestyle choices or environment; paradoxically, a policy approach that positions the individual as the source and solution to a "global obesity crisis".

Rock, Degeling, and Blue (2014, p. 337) suggest that the "posthuman" turn in critical theory is "highly relevant to public health, but has yet to be articulated or interpreted for a public health audience". Anti-obesity has tended to be framed by "research evidence" which predominantly draws on what Blue, Shove, Carmona, and Kelly (2016) describe as psychological understandings and individualistic theories of human behaviour change. New materialist analyses might help illuminate how specific knowledge forms of disciplines come to "matter" (Barad, 2007), and as such, particular cuts are made in terms of "evidence" that is included or excluded in policy approaches. As such, in this final section, we argue that reading obesity policy through new materialist theories not only contributes to critical policy analysis but also provides a catalyst for thinking about obesity policy and public health in new ways.

Across multiple countries, authors have critically analysed the discourses of policy texts, but we recognise that these are only one part of a policy assemblage (Fullagar et al., 2017). Rather than being discrete from social actors and matter, policies are assembled through forces that draw into play different actors, agencies, bodies, matter. Drawing on Deleuze and Guattari (1987), Rizvi and Lingard (2011, p. 20) similarly suggest that the concept of assemblage is a useful theoretical resource through "which to understand how policy involves a complex configuration of a range of competing values". Exploring social equity within Australian higher education, they argue that policy understandings have undergone major shifts because new assemblages emerge through processes that are "contingent and affected by the changing political architecture of the state" (p. 6).

The conceptualisation of policy as an assemblage has been used elsewhere in policy research (Mulcahy, 2014; Koyama & Varenne, 2012; Mulcahy, 2011) but rather less in relation to health policy related to obesity. Such policies are shaped by onto-epistemological orientations about which "knowledge" is valid and come to inform the "evidence base" from which policies are developed or analysed; in other words, particular forms of research/research traditions have come to "matter" (Barad, 2007) within the production of obesity policy.

Such approaches differ in moving away from an understanding of policy as object to one of process and towards understanding the implementation or enactment of policy as part of a complex assemblage. The enactment of policy does not stem from the rational conduct of individuals; rather, it is formed through the relationality of material objects, levers, flows, and practices, and as such "complexity often impeded the realization of intended policy targets" (Ulmer, 2016). Such approaches might reveal what are perhaps otherwise hidden effects of policy "solutions" as they are experienced materially and relationally. The capacity to enact the recommendations of policy is limited by assemblages of consumption practices, relations of food and eating, location, and capitalist flows of food production. As such, inequalities may be silenced through these humanist notions of agency which assume that increased knowledge leads to behaviour change. In other words, this work could draw attention to what Warin (2015) describes as "tensions" between intended policies and capacities they have in particular contexts.

There is no space to examine these different policy assemblages. Instead, we flag the potential for more than human exploration of obesity and link this to policies that are recognising the food industry and environmental impacts as part of an obesity assemblage.

Presently, in many neoliberal nations, anti-obesity policies tend to endorse the idea that individuals are ultimately responsible for obesity, yet also recognise that lifestyle changes might be difficult for some, citing an "obesogenic" environment as the reason. Systemic perspectives within anti-obesity policies offer an "ecological lens addressing the "obesogenic" environment" (O'Hara & Taylor, 2018, p. 2).

Yet, while there has been increasing recognition of the impact of the food industry and the impact of environment, obesogenic environments and risky behaviours materialise through a "correctable body" as the source of agency. In other words, without a more distributed and relational notion of agency, many of these policies default to humanist assumptions that paradoxically position the individual as the source and the solution to the problem. Despite the growing evidence of policies which identify obesity as a complex systemic problem, the enactment of change most often materialises through behaviouralist practices that largely fail (Ulijaszek & McLennan, 2016).

Instead, a more-than-human approach to understanding food–body environments as biocultural productions connected to climate change, capital accumulation, and land ownership means that they are "not only discursively constituted, but also materially implicated and embodied" (Taylor, Wright, & O'Flynn, 2019, p. 916). In contrast to policies that assume a rationalist contained "agent" who can choose to act on, with or resist the environment around them (be that nature, food choices, transport options, etc.), attuning to material-discursive relations can foreground the flows of investment in technical solutions (weight loss programmes, surgery) that intra-act with a flourishing obesity research industry as well as the ways in which bodies, health, and justice come to matter as affective experiences of healthy citizenship.

Conclusion

This chapter has explored *how bodies come to matter* (as fat, obese, normalised, pleasurable, disgusting, visceral, physiological, visual, mobile, and subject to intervention) through new materialist styles of thought. Drawing upon more-than-human and post-qualitative approaches, this body of work has questioned the onto-epistemological assumptions of humanist critique to trouble the division of individuals and environments, subjects, and objects. Exploring the relational forces that produce ways of knowing and enacting "obesity" in terms of problems and solutions, we have mapped out possibilities for disrupting-doing different research, policy and practice across health, education, and popular culture.

Note

1 Niamh's PhD project as supervised by Emma and Simone.

References

Åsberg, C., & Braidotti, R. (Eds.). (2018). *A feminist companion to the posthumanities*. Cham: Springer.

Ahmed, S. (2004). *The cultural politics of emotion*. New York: Routledge.

Ahmed, S. (2008). Open forum imaginary prohibitions: Some preliminary remarks on the founding gestures of the new materialism. *European Journal of Women's Studies, 15*(1), 23–39. doi: 10.1177/1350506807084854

Barad, K. (2003). Posthumanist performativity: Toward an understanding of how matter comes to matter. *Signs Journal of Women in Culture and Society, 28*(3), 801–831. doi: 10.1086/345321

Barad, K. (2007). *Meeting the universe halfway: Quantum physics and the entanglement of matter and meaning*. Durham, NC: Duke University Press.

Bennett, J. (2010). *Vibrant matter: A political ecology of things*. Durham, NC: Duke University.

Berbary, L. A., & Boles, J. C. (2014). Eight points for reflection: Revisiting scaffolding for improvisational humanist qualitative inquiry. *Leisure Sciences, 36*(5), 401–419. doi: 10.1080/01490400.2014.912169

Blue, S., Shove, E., Carmona, C., & Kelly, M. P. (2016). Theories of practice and public health: understanding (un)healthy practices. *Critical Public Health, 26*(1), 36–50, doi: 10.1080/09581596.2014.980396

Braidotti, R. (2013). *The posthuman*. Cambridge: Polity Press.

Coole, D., & Frost, S. (Eds.) (2010). *New materialisms*. Durham, NC: Duke University Press.

Deleuze, G., & Guattari, F. (1987). *A thousand plateaus: Capitalism and schizophrenia*. Minneapolis, MN: University of Minnesota.

Ellsworth, E. A. (1997). *Teaching positions: Difference, pedagogy, and the power of address*. New York: Teachers College Press.

Esmonde, K., & Jette, S. (2018). Fatness, fitness, and feminism in the built environment: Bringing together physical cultural studies and sociomaterialisms, to study the "Obesogenic Environment". *Sociology of Sport Journal, 35*(1), 39–48. doi: 10.1123/ssj.2016-0121

Evans, J., Davies, B., & Rich, E. (2008). The class and cultural functions of obesity discourse: Our latter day child saving movement. *International Studies in Sociology of Education, 18*(2), 117–132. doi: 10.1080/09620210802351367

Evans, J., Davies, B., & Rich, E. (2014). We/you can tell talk from matter: A conversation with Håkan Larsson and Mikael Quennerstedt. *Sport, Education and Society, 19*(5), 652–665. doi: 10.1080/13573322.2013.770391

Evans, J., & Rich, E. (2011). Body policies and body pedagogies: Every child matters in totally pedagogised schools? *Journal of Education Policy, 26*(3), 361–379. doi: 10.1080/02680939.2010.500399

Evans, J., Rich, E., Davies, B., & Allwood, R. (2008). *Education, disordered eating and obesity discourse: Fat fabrications*. London: Routledge.

Fox, N. J., & Alldred, P. (2016). *Sociology and the new materialism: Theory, research, action*. London: Sage.

Fox, N. J., Bissell, P., Peacock, M., & Blackburn, J. (2018). The micropolitics of obesity: Materialism, markets and food sovereignty. *Sociology, 52*(1), 111–127. doi: 10.1177/0038038516647668

Fullagar, S. (2017). Post-qualitative inquiry and the new materialist turn: Implications for sport, health and physical culture research. *Qualitative Research in Sport, Exercise and Health, 9*(2), 247–257. doi: 10.1080/2159676X.2016.1273896

Fullagar, S, Rich, E., Francombe-Webb, J., & Maturo, A. (2017). Digital ecologies of youth mental health: Apps, therapeutic publics and pedagogy as affective arrangements. *Social Sciences, 6*(4), 1–14. doi: 10.3390/socsci6040135

Gard, M., & Wright, J. (2001). Managing uncertainty: Obesity discourses and physical education in a risk society. *Studies in Philosophy and Education, 20*(6), 535–549. doi: 10.1023/A:1012238617836

Giroux, H. A. (2004). Cultural studies and the politics of public pedagogy: Making the political more pedagogical. *Parallax, 10*(2), 73–89. doi: 10.1080/1353464042000208530

Haraway, D. (2016). *Staying with the Trouble: Making kin in the Chthulucene*, Durham, NC: Duke University Press.

Kofoed, J., & Ringrose, J. (2012). Travelling and sticky affects: Exploring teens and sexualized cyberbullying through a Butlerian-Deleuzian-Guattarian lens. *Discourse, 33*(1), 5–20. doi: 10.1080/01596306.2012.632157

Koyama, J. P., & Varenne, H. (2012). Assembling and dissembling: Policy as productive play. *Educational Researcher, 41,* 157–162. doi: 10.3102/0013189X12442799

Land, N. (2018). Fat knowledges and matters of fat: Towards re-encountering fat(s). *Social Theory and Health, 16*(1), 77–93. doi: 10.1057/s41285-017-0044-3

Leahy, D. (2009). Disgusting pedagogies. In J. Wright & V. Harwood (Eds.), *Biopolitics and the 'obesity epidemic': Governing bodies* (pp. 172–182). New York: Routledge.

LeBesco, K. (2011). Neoliberalism, public health, and the moral perils of fatness. *Critical Public Health,* *21*(2), 153–164. doi: 10.1080/09581596.2010.529422

Lupton, D. (2018). *Fat.* London: Routledge.

Mol, A. (2002). *The body multiple: Ontology in medical practice.* Durham, NC: Duke University Press.

Monaghan, L. F., Colls, R., & Evans, B. (2013). Obesity discourse and fat politics: Research, critique and interventions. *Critical Public Health, 23*(3), 249–262. doi: 10.1080/09581596.2013.814312

Mulcahy, D. (2011). Assembling the 'accomplished' teacher: The performativity and politics of professional teaching standards. *Educational Philosophy and Theory, 43*(Suppl. 1), 94–113. doi: 10.1111/j.1469-5812.2009.00617.x

Mulcahy, D. (2014). Re/assembling spaces of learning in Victorian government schools: policy enactments, pedagogic encounters and micropolitics. *Discourse: Studies in the Cultural Politics of Education, 36*(4), 500–514. doi: 10.1080/01596306.2014.978616

O'Hara, L., & Taylor, J. (2018). What's wrong with the 'War on Obesity?' A narrative review of the weight-centered health paradigm and development of the 3C framework to build critical competency for a paradigm shift. *SAGE Open,* April-June, 1–28. doi: 10.1177/2158244018772888

Probyn, E. (2008). IV. Silences behind the mantra: Critiquing feminist fat. *Feminism & Psychology, 18*(3), 401–404. doi: 10.1177/0959353508092095

Rice, C. (2015). Rethinking fat: From bio- to body-becoming pedagogies. *Cultural Studies – Critical Methodologies, 15*(5), 387–397. doi: 10.1177/1532708615611720

Rinaldi, J., Rice, C., Kotow, C., & Lind, E. (2019). Mapping the circulation of fat hatred. *Fat Studies,* pp. 1–14. doi: 10.1080/21604851.2019.1592949

Rock, M. J., Degeling, C., & Blue, G. (2014). Toward stronger theory in critical public health: Insights from debates surrounding posthumanism. *Critical Public Health, 24*(3), 337–348. doi: 10.1080/09581596.2013.827325

Rizvi, F., & Lingard, B. (2011). Social equity and the assemblage of values in Australian higher education. *Cambridge Journal of Education, 41*(1), 5–22. doi: 10.1080/0305764X.2010.549459

Sanabria, E. (2016). Circulating ignorance: Complexity and agnogenesis in the obesity 'epidemic'. *Cultural Anthropology, 31*(1), 131–158. doi: 10.14506/ca31.1.07

Shilling, C. (2008). *Changing bodies: Habit, crisis and creativity.* London: Sage.

St. Pierre, E.A. (2011). Post qualitative research: The critique and the coming after. In N. K. Denzin & Y. S. Lincoln (Eds.), *Sage handbook of qualitative inquiry* (4th ed.) (pp. 611–635). Los Angeles, CA: Sage.

Taylor, C. A., & Hughes, C. (2016). *Posthuman research practices in education.* London: Palgrave Macmillan.

Taylor, N., Wright, J., & O'Flynn, G. (2019). Embodied encounters with more-than-human nature in health and physical education. *Sport, Education and Society, 24*(9), 914–924. doi: 10.1080/13573322.2018.1519785

Throsby, K. (2012). Obesity surgery and the management of excess: Exploring the body multiple. *Sociology of Health & Illness, 34*(1), 1–15. doi: 10.1111/j.1467-9566.2011.01358.x

Ulmer, J. B. (2016). Diffraction as a method of critical policy analysis. *Educational Philosophy & Theory, 48*(13), 1381–1394. doi: 10.1080/00131857.2016.1211001

Ulijaszek, S. J., & McLennan, A. K. (2016). Framing obesity in UK policy from the Blair years, 1997–2015: The persistence of individualistic approaches despite overwhelming evidence of societal and economic factors, and the need for collective responsibility. *Obesity Reviews, 17*(5), 397–411. doi: 10.1111/obr.12386

Walkerdine, V. (2009). Biopedagogies and beyond. In J. Wright & V. Harwood (Eds.), *Biopolitics and the obesity epidemic: Governing bodies* (pp. 199–207). New York & Oxon: Routledge.

Warin, M. (2015). Material feminism, obesity science and the limits of discursive critique. *Body & Society, 21*(4), 48–76. doi: 10.1177/1357034X14537320

Wright, J. (2012). Biopower, biopedagogies and the obesity epidemic. In J. Wright & V. Harwood (Eds.), *Biopolitics and the 'obesity epidemic': Governing bodies* (pp. 1–14). New York & Oxon: Routledge.

Wright, J., & Harwood, V. (2012). *Biopolitics and the 'obesity epidemic': Governing bodies.* New York & Oxon: Routledge.

Yoshizawa, R. S. (2012). The Barker hypothesis and obesity: Connections for transdisciplinarity and social justice. *Social Theory & Health, 10*(4), 348–367. doi: 10.1057%2Fsth.2012.11

11

DOING FAT WITH POST-DEVELOPMENTAL PEDAGOGIES

Nicole Land

In early childhood education in Canada, the understandings of fat that come to matter within curriculum relations are made amid a particular political trajectory that shapes how and who children can be with – get to know, be in relation with, engage with – fat. In this chapter, I propose that children and adults are always in active relations with fat. This proposition contends that fat is a relational activity; that in each bodied moment, we participate in a relation with fat, and this relation lives within complex traffic between flesh, discourses, pedagogies, logics, more-than-human others, bodies, ethics, and politics (Land, forthcoming, 2018). To build this provocation, I think with scholars who set in motion post-developmental pedagogies, which I understand as pedagogies that create conditions (Vintimilla, 2018) for interjecting in, and nourishing alternatives to, modernist approaches to education that pivot upon Euro-Western developmental psychology (Blaise 2009, 2014; Osgood & Sakr, 2019; Pacini-Ketchabaw, 2011). The scholars who think post-developmentally that I think alongside, activate multiple theoretical propositions: common worlds (Taylor & Pacini-Ketchabaw, 2015), feminist post-humanities (Blaise & Rooney, 2020), and feminist new materialisms (Hodgins, 2019a). Importantly, I think with post-developmental pedagogies as cultivating ways of being together with children that are against perpetuating the linear, universalized, normalizing logics of developmentalism (Burman 2016; Dahlberg, Moss, & Pence 2013; MacNaughton 2003; Vintimilla, Land, Pacini-Ketchabaw, Kummen, & Khattar, 2019) *and* that bring incredible energy to creating relations and thinking with knowledges that work to be response-able (Haraway, 2012; Taylor, Blaise, & Giugni, 2013) to the political and ethical contours of everyday situated relations with children amid complicated contemporary worlds. Thinking fat with post-developmental pedagogies, I argue, is an ongoing practice oriented toward attending to relational liveliness of how fat comes to matter within our curricular decisions and intentions. In refusing the universalized curriculum practices that we create as one consequence of developmental relations with fat, I think with post-developmental propositions to intervene in pre-articulated, regulatory relations with fat by tuning to the active, participatory work of being implicated in "doing" situated pedagogical relations. To begin this chapter, I practice getting to know how fat and developmentalism become entangled amid overarching dominant logics of childhood obesity and how childhood obesity prevention and developmentalism collide in status-quo early childhood education health and physical education curriculum.

DOI: 10.4324/9780429344824-14

Quotidian relations with fat in early childhood education in Canada that come to know fat through the logics of obesity prevention and mitigation follow a particular pathway that threads neoliberalism with developmentalism with the inequalities perpetuated amid ongoing settler colonialism. Critical obesity scholars working in Canada, including Elliott (2016), Petherick and Beausoleil (2016), Rice (2007), and Ward (2016), have written extensively about the ways that the discourses and material realities of "childhood obesity" as a structure that governs bodies and subjectivities serve to maintain existing systems of power and oppression that unevenly regulate particular bodies in the name of individual responsibility, morality, and economics (LeBesco, 2004, 2011). These are relations with fat that feel, in mainstream early years, physical and health education, overtly familiar, as we understand fat as the undesirable substrate and bodied marker of childhood obesity (Land, 2015).

Logics of child development hold great power amid dominant relations that understand fat amid an overarching conception of childhood obesity, where powerful refrains like "fat children become fat adults" make visible the universalized, linear, sequential, future-oriented intentions of developmentalism (Evans, 2010; Evans & Colls, 2011). Childhood obesity and developmentalism loom over curricular relations with fats in early childhood, as curriculum works in the name of preventing and controlling a fat to be feared (Petherick & Beausoleil, 2016; Rich 2010, 2011). Obesity-preventing interventions invest in the universalized, sequential logics of child development, enacting activities for children that operate on an age and stage-based approach and encourage educators to apply developmentally appropriate activities aimed at shaping children's bodies toward a universalized developmental norm (e.g. the Canadian Society for Exercise Physiology and ParticipACTION's *24-hour Movement Guidelines for the Early Years* (2016), which outline a singular age-based sequence for increasing children's physical activity time and intensity).

In this chapter, I want to think beside critical analyses of how childhood obesity discourses create and regulate children's subjectivities and bodies by turning toward how we are in messy relations with fat that carry with them a history, life, and politic. In thinking with relations with fat, I am curious about tracing how the ways that we come to meet fat are always to encounter a particular ongoing trajectory and history of entangled knowledges, materialities, ethics, and politics. Naming the move that I want to make, in thinking alongside critical obesity scholars, is important – I want to carry with me critical analyses of the regulating and minoritizing consequences of childhood obesity discourses and pull in provocations from scholars who activate post-developmental pedagogies in order to burrow into situated, particular messy relations with multiple entangled histories and lives of fat. Thinking with post-developmental pedagogies alongside our relations with fat is, I contend, an urgent project because relations with fat in early childhood education are a site of profound, powerful, consequential tangles of developmentalism, childhood obesity, and curriculum. We, within the early childhood education project in Canada, come to know fat most often through childhood obesity discourses' affinities with developmental logics, making the spaces where obesity and development shingle together to shape relations with fat an especially high-stakes and timely site for interjecting with post-developmental pedagogies.

As I outlined at the outset of this chapter, post-developmental pedagogies are against the governing and intellectually oppressive ways that childhood development has come to be an unassailable truth in early childhood education *and* are for setting in motion other pedagogical relations that open toward non status-quo ways of being together and responding to contemporary worlds with children (Argent, Vintimilla, Lee, & Wapenaar, 2017; Hodgins & Kummen, 2018; Nelson, Pacini-Ketchabaw, & Nxumalo, 2018; Taylor & Pacini-Ketchabaw, 2018). In my project of thinking fat with post-developmental pedagogies, I am particularly inspired by Alexis Shotwell (2016), a scholar of sociology and anthropology in Canada, who offers that:

> one of my imperatives is to be against without predicting all the things there are to be for. Being against in this way – having a 'no' –...wherever we stand in relation to the world, we can scream 'no' and open the space for many yesses.
>
> *(p. 19)*

In what follows, I activate post-developmental pedagogies that "scream" no to developmental relations with fat *and* that do fat in ways that are rooted in an ethical and political desire to create more livable (Nelson, Hodgins, & Danis, 2019) – less universal, less regulatory, less already-known and more situated, more active, more lively – relations with fat with children. My intention is to agitate the grip that tangles of development and obesity prevention have on relations with fats with children while building propositions and questions and noticing entanglements that call us to respond to and relate differently with – to do in unfamiliar ways – fat in early childhood education.

The next section begins by tracing a particular shared relation with fat between developmentalism and childhood obesity prevention curriculum as it comes to matter in early childhood education. I want to be cautious to make clear that the relations of universalism that I follow are not the only resonances between developmentalism and childhood obesity discourses. I hope to investigate multiple other relations, including relations of temporality and molecularity, in work beyond the scope of this article. Then, I offer an interjection into this relation with fat by proposing how thinking with post-developmental pedagogies might orient toward alternative, imperfect, response-able (Haraway, 2012), care-full (de la Bellacasa, 2017) relations with fat. To conclude the section, I draw upon a story from an ongoing pedagogical inquiry research project with preschool and toddler-aged children in an urban child care center in Toronto, Canada. Educator co-researchers and I inaugurated this project with the question "how do we get to know movement" and work together with children to notice and sustain relations with bodies, fat, muscles and movement that live within entanglements of place, developmental and post-developmental logics, and our non-innocent ethical and political pedagogical intentions. We work to tend to small moments where we might do fat otherwise from developmentalism and childhood obesity, and I try in the story I share to center the uncertain gestures we make toward this intention. In particular, I share a story from going on walks around the quad, a public outdoor space, with children. I want to emphasize that I am not proposing post-developmental pedagogies as a "solution" to the knots of developmentalism and childhood obesity we inherit. Rather, I want to share one moment from research and the tentative thinking I have done with this moment as I try to set in motion one possibility for activating particular post-developmental propositions in one particular place. I end this chapter by proposing how we might get into the muck of the difficult post-developmental work of creating relations with fats that turn toward other logics, ethics, politics, lively more-than-human debts, and interconnections.

Doing situated fat, interjecting in universalized fat

Scholars critical of child development highlight how developmental logics work to assess all childhoods against a universalized norm (Burman, 2016; Cannella, 1997; Castañeda, 2002; Dyer, 2020; Walkerdine, 1998). As Burman (2018) argues, the referent of dominant developmental theories is a body deemed most desirable by neoliberal and capitalist logics, such that "it is now widely accepted that such [developmental] psychological modes are heir to, and in turn reinscribe, the economic and cultural privileges arising from capitalist exploitation and European colonialism" (p. 1601). In the context of ongoing settler colonialism in what is currently known as Canada, the idealized subject of developmental psychology is a white, male, heterosexual, able-bodied, thin, and fit child – a child who will become an adult with the intellectual and physical prowess to sustain existing capitalist and settler colonial systems of power. Developmental psychology, then, enacts a universalized, idealized child-body who is, and more importantly will become, the superlative subject of neoliberal humanism (Vintimilla et al., 2019): productive in economic terms; behaving through self-governance masked as individual responsibility and self-discipline; and healthy in the name of ensuring economic productivity and reducing deficits due to disease. Importantly, the systems of power that developmentalism perpetuates thread through societal discourses into everyday "racial capitalist formations" (Nxumalo, 2020, p. 165) in early childhood education. The idealized becoming-adult is taken as a universal benchmark for all children across diverse childhoods, which functions to label children who do not meet this ideal as abnormal, atypical, and in need of intervention. Curriculum, with development, becomes a practice of implementing interventions designed to shape children's bodies and behaviors toward this universalized, ideal child. Because there is singular referent of the child within developmental logic, curriculum also becomes universalized; if normative development should be a universal experience of childhood, then curriculum grounded in these developmental theories should be equally effective and meaningful for all children. There are multiple critiques of the violences of child development in early childhood education (e.g. Burman, 2016; Cannella, 1997; Castañeda, 2002; Pacini-Ketchabaw, 2011). What I want to hold on to here is one relation of developmental logic – relations of universalizing. These are relations that assume heterogeneity and declare common-ness as a tactic for brushing over situated, divergent, messy conditions and lives that do not conform to the normalizing referent centered in the act of universalizing.

Critical health and physical education scholars, as well as critical obesity and fat studies scholars, underscore the universalizing moves at the heart of childhood obesity discourses. In narratives of childhood obesity, a white, able-bodied, heterosexual, thin, and fit child is positioned as the idealized "healthy" goal or outcome of obesity and physical education curriculum (Azzarito, 2009; Evans, Davies, & Rich, 2008; Evans & Rich, 2011). This universalizing function, echoing the universalizing operations of developmental psychology, works to label as unhealthy, fat, or abnormal children who do not ascribe to the image of this idealized healthy child. Developmental logic is overtly present in childhood obesity discourses' universalized image of the child because there is a loud assertion that fat children become fat adults whereby we must take seriously a universalized healthy child as the goal of obesity interventions in order to prevent these children from diverging from this universalized norm when they are expected to make active contributions to neoliberal capitalist systems. Relations of universalizing, in childhood obesity discourses, allege their normalizing function in the name of health, where a singular vision of the healthy child serves as a moralized justification for the consequences of universalizing (Evans, Evans, & Rich, 2003; Evans, Rich, & Davies, 2004; McPhail, Chapman, & Beagan, 2011; Rich & Evans, 2012; Webb & Quennerstedt, 2010). In childhood obesity prevention curriculum, universalizing serves to center a singular vision of "the healthy child" – if we know what "counts" as a healthy child, we can study and name the conditions and behaviors that create this child, and therefore curriculum can create and maintain these practices. Childhood obesity prevention curriculum then is often assumed to be equally relevant across multiple diverse childhoods.

The universalizing function of obesity prevention discourses has been critiqued by numerous scholars (e.g. Fitzpatrick & Tinning, 2014; Rich & Evans, 2012) who outline how obesity curriculum that operates in relations of universalism serves to regulate children's bodies and perpetuate inequalities.

Universalizing then marks a shared relation between childhood obesity discourses and child development. This means that at one collision of childhood obesity and developmentalism is a relation concerned with conformity over context, compliance over complexity, and veiled governance over attuning to ethics and politics. Particular to thinking with fat in early childhood education, universalizing relations with fat assume that children have similar connections to fat (fat should be feared and regulated because it causes obesity, and obese children are not the idealized subjects of normative developmentalism nor obesity interventions) and that fat matters in the same ways across all contexts (that fat should be feared and regulated in the service of healthy development is a dictate to be carried into all the spaces and places of childhood).

Post-developmental provocation: Doing situated fat

Nxumalo (2019) offers "presencing" as a practice that aims to "create interruptive movements away from colonizing relations to place and its more-than-human inhabitants as mute sites of children's learning and discovery" (p. 160). This provocation that Nxumalo offers to attend to the situatedness of children's encounters in early childhood education activates a post-developmental provocation of interrupting universalizing relations – to attend to situatedness is to take seriously how childhoods can never be universal because it is uncommon, contextual, momentary entanglements that we are implicated in and respond within in everyday moments. Thinking with Nxumalo, to attend to how our relations are situated is to refuse colonial, capitalist, neoliberal moves toward universalizing, where universalizing is a practice of smoothing the unevenness of complex relationalities in the name of productivity. To think with situated relations is to an ongoing ethical and political practice that works to, as Nxumalo, Vintimilla, and Nelson (2018) propose, create "openings to situate early childhood curriculum within the actual, messy, highly uneven and extractive places and spaces of early childhood education" (p. 3).

Tending to these messy, uneven relations requires that we pay attention to the ways that we are implicated in relational worlds and the ways that our relational vulnerability, entanglements, and debts disrupt the conception of the idealized healthy child of universalizing developmental and obesity prevention narratives – when worlds are lively, messy, and local, what happens when we continue to implement curriculum that already knows the human, and the body, that lives within any educational space? Blaise, Hamm, and Iorio (2017) suggest that tending to situated stories "is a strategy that makes room for relationality, or the ways in which humans and more-than-humans are integral parts of the universe" (p. 39). This means that taking situatedness seriously is a proposition for unsettling how developmental and childhood obesity curriculum take as their center only an idealized, universal human child. What might we open toward if, instead of accepting the "healthy" child as the pinnacle of curricular success, we work instead to do – to get to know and respond with – fat within entangled webs of localized, contextual human and more-than-human relations?

Situated relations, or thinking about how children and educators are immersed in deeply political constellations of inequality, consumption, commodification, production, and regulation within the neoliberal worlds we inherit with children is, I suggest, one post-developmental provocation for relating differently with fat – what ways of being with fat might we orient toward when we take seriously how our relations with fat are always situated? How might tracing our situated relations with fat both refuse the universalism of child development and obesity curriculum *and* open moves toward re-creating more livable curricular relations with fat?

Doing fat with feeding "the hole"

Between two very busy sidewalks in the quad that we walk in is a small grassy 'island'. Right near the skinny end of the island is a small utility hole that is usually covered by a dark green plastic cover. For a few weeks, we have been practicing walking slowly in the quad, and each week we have paused at this island and the hole. One of the children, Luke, is very interested in caring for the caterpillars, spiders, and slugs who we think might live in the hole. We noticed, once, a caterpillar in the hole and we re-encounter the spider webs clinging to the edges of the hole on multiple weeks. Each week, Luke takes the cover off the hole, investigates the single black PVC pipe within the hole, and looks for traces of caterpillars, spiders, and slugs. Then, he collects handfuls of long grass to put in the hole because, as he tells us, the spiders and caterpillars 'need' the grass. Luke runs back and forth between the long grass area and the hole, putting handfuls of damp rich green grass in the hole. I ask him why the inhabitants of the hole 'need' grass: 'for their bodies', he tells me.

If I spend time with this moment by centering only logics made in entanglements of developmentalism and childhood obesity, I might argue that this moment is not about fat; that since we do not talk about fat, health, or exercise with Luke, our relations with fat are not relevant to thinking with Luke and the hole. From a developmental psychology perspective, I might pay attention to how Luke is hypothesizing and learning about the lifecycles and nutrition needs of bugs, or how he is showing age-appropriate responsibility as a good steward caring for the plants and animals in his place. With an obesity prevention curriculum viewpoint, I might notice how Luke runs between the long grass and the hole and is working up a bit of a sweat, and I might praise his moderate intensity physical activity as a healthy, valuable movement. This might create relations with fat where fat is seen as a substrate of health – if we take good care of the caterpillar, it will develop a healthy body with the right amount of fat; if we run our bodies enough, we will regulate the amount of fat and be healthy. This is a profoundly humanist relation with fat, where we use humanist logics (health, control, development) to get to know fat with the caterpillar and grass. Thinking with a post-developmental proposition to attend to situatedness, I want to take seriously how this moment braids together relations with more-than-human others, grass, running, fat, health, bodies, and care, and demands that we respond to these tangles of ethics, politics, and liveliness.

Attending to the messiness of a situated context as a tentative way to activate post-developmental pedagogies is a demanding proposition – one that requires I/we both notice and attend to the complexities of place, but also answer to the ways that our relations implicate us in a place (Nelson, Hodgins, & Danis, 2019; Nxumalo, 2016; Pacini-Ketchabaw & Clark, 2016; Pacini-Ketchabaw & Nxumalo, 2016). With Luke and fistfuls of grass and utility holes and caterpillars, I need to pay attention to the momentary, emplaced ways we get to know fat. As, for example, the calories Luke's body uses to nourish the cascade of muscles that tug at the grass. This might be a molecular relation with fat, one that notices how the biochemical worlds that fat participates in are entangled with the biochemical worlds of photosynthesizing grass and grass-digesting caterpillars. This is molecular relation with fat attunes to how biochemical relations implicate Luke's fingers and legs in connections of vulnerability, co-extensiveness, and mutuality with grass and caterpillars and more-than-human others. Such a relation with fat makes questions of ethics urgently palpable: if we do fat with caterpillars and grass and metabolisms, how might we answer to the multiple, layered, lively relations we are entangled in? If we tune to how we get to know fat with torn grass and not-always-visible caterpillars, we make a choice to no longer pay attention to taken-for-granted universalized humanist relations with fat required by developmentalism and childhood obesity; our easy referents of bounded, individual human bodies that want to regulate fat in service of ascribing to a universal "healthy" body do not hold up. Thinking with post-developmental pedagogies we make, in the same movement, a choice to invent other ways of doing fat together. In tuning to doing fat as situated, I propose that we need to attune do our ways of doing fat in any moment – doing fat with post-developmental pedagogies becomes a high-stakes and ongoing ethical and political practice.

Haraway (2012), a feminist science studies scholar, builds a concept and ethic of response-ability. Blaise, Hamm, and Iorio (2017), alongside other scholars who think with post-developmental provocations (Hodgins, 2019b; Otterstad, 2016) to activate unfamiliar, speculative practices of attending to place and context, think with response-ability as a way of crafting pedagogical relations that answer to how we are actively implicated in complex human and more-than-human relations. With Haraway, we are embedded in particular relationships, we nurture within those relationships a certain debt to the others (human, more-than-human others, material, discursive) that make possible that relation, and we answer to our debt through actively caring for how we are implicated in that complex relation in which not all lives are valued equally. We must, Haraway argues, act in a way that responds well to how we are intertwined in relations and with the others we are tangled with. There is nothing easy nor straightforward about response-ability – it is an ethical and political commitment to actively answer to and build livable relations.

Thinking with response-ability as we do fat requires that we ask questions of how our relations with fat respond within a context – how does thinking fat as entangled with grass and caterpillars draw our attention toward the precarious relations that enliven our worlds? How, as we think fat beyond the universalisms of developmentalism and childhood obesity, do we concurrently do fat in ways that answer well – response-ably, ethically, politically – to the messy relations we are implicated in? What happens if, for example, we notice how as Luke spills handfuls of lush green grass into the hole, he is already enmeshed within a complex relational world? We might wonder, with Luke, why picking (killing?) grass "for" caterpillar's bodies matters: where do our understandings of bodies as consumers (like how caterpillar bodies are in need of grass) come from? What logics position bodies as consumers? When we see bodies as consumers, what relations with fat do we foreground? Do we want, as a collective of children, educators, and adults implicated in the quad, to think of bodies as consumers? Perhaps, I might ask Luke why the caterpillars "need" grass and we might think together about the ideas of nutrition, wellness, utility, and demand we inherit. What happens, I might ask Luke, if we notice energy together? Maybe we will notice how grass and bodies and caterpillars do energy in complex more-than-human worlds. Maybe Luke and I might momentarily invent a response that works to answer to the relational liveliness of fat and grass and hands and caterpillars, where Luke and I do fat otherwise, as a practice of being implicated – or we might double back and focus on filling the hole with grass to provide for the caterpillars. Activating post-developmental pedagogies is always a move toward, a practice in speculation, a proposition that might fail (Vintimilla, 2018). These questions show the hard work of taking seriously our situated relations with fat because they show the non-innocence of our inherited and enacted relations with fat. It is easy, amid universalized human-centered developmental and obesity-prevention relations with fat, to think this moment with Luke is not about fat. But, I argue, in holding to a post-developmental intention to do fat as situated, this moment requires we burrow into the relations with fat we make possible and impossible in our everyday moments.

Thinking with how doing fat as situated within an intention to think with post-developmental pedagogies requires that we consider how our response-abilities entangle with our ethical, political, and pedagogical commitments. Sharing stories of children's relations with an urban forest, Woods et al. (2018) argue that

> paying close attention to others' lifeworlds also draws us into powerful modes of care that exist outside of contemporary human desires in these colonized and ecologically challenged times. Consideration of these multiplicities of care beyond the human reminds us to shift our understandings and be care-full in our practice.
>
> *(p. 54)*

I understand care as a post-developmental provocation for attuning to situatedness because, as Woods et al. (2018) argue, to paying "close attention" to more-than-human worlds requires refusing humanism, and the human, as a central referent for understanding curriculum (and life). Responding care-fully – nurturing relations of care – is a practice of noticing and answering to the complexities and liveliness of the more-than-human worlds we are implicated in. What if, as Luke uproots fistfuls of living grass and runs them over to the hole, Luke is enacting a relation of care with fat: care for the "bodies" of not-always perceptible caterpillars, spiders, and slugs? Hodgins, Yazbeck, and Wapenaar (2019) "consider how complex conceptualizations of more-than-human relationality might help educators to enact a care(ing) curriculum that responds to the material, colonial, and environmental legacies that we all live with a bequeath to children" (p. 204). Thinking this moment with the hole, ripped up grass, caterpillars, and Luke as care means wondering how we might forge relations with fat in this moment that respond well to the lived legacies and realities of the quad; how do we do fat in this place, knowing that this place is never inseparable from the systems of neoliberalism, capitalism, and ongoing settler colonialism, and entangled logics of developmentalism and childhood obesity, that we are implicated in? What possible relations with fat do we make possible, with this grass and hole and caterpillars and sweaty hands, and what relations with fat do we ignore or obscure? Why? Importantly, de la Bellacasa (2017), a feminist science scholar, argues that care is imperfect: "what as well as possible care might mean will remain a fraught and contested terrain where different arrangements of humans-nonhumans will have different and collective significances" (p. 221). This means that we do not, as we attune to situatedness, already know how to do fat. Rather, learning to attend to how do we do fat in everyday moments is an ongoing, speculative, imperfect, propositional practice.

Doing fat with post-developmental pedagogies

In this chapter, I have proposed that we do fat in everyday relations with children – and that doing fat with post-developmental pedagogies is a practice of proposing tentative, speculative ways of being in unfamiliar, response-able, care-full relations with fat. I have worked through one intersection of developmental psychology and childhood obesity discourses (relations of universalizing) while arguing how doing fat as situated within particular localized relations and entanglements might orient us toward doing fat in ways that both intervene in and propose otherwise ways of being with fat. I have argued that taking seriously our relations with fat in early childhood education as an ethical and political pedagogical question is an urgent project: what relations with fat do we want to work to enliven? Why? In doing fat with post-developmental pedagogies, I never intend to propose any one enactment of fat made within a post-developmental proposition as a "better" fat for the field to think with. Rather, I am interested in the *work* of *doing* fat with post-developmental pedagogies. I want to offer forward the provocation that we might attend to the labor of doing fat with children, taking seriously how we make possible and impossible particular non-innocent relations with fat in every moment.

References

Argent, A. L., Vintimilla, C. D., Lee, C., & Wapenaar, K. (2017). A dialogue about place and living pedagogies: Trees, ferns, blood, children, educators and wood cutters. *Journal of Childhoods and Pedagogies, 1*(2), 1–21.

Azzarito, L. (2009). The panopticon of physical education: Pretty, active, and ideally white. *Physical Education & Sport Pedagogy, 14*(1), 19–39. doi:10.1080/17408980701712106

Blaise, M. (2009). "What a girl wants, what a girl needs": Responding to sex, gender, and sexuality in the early childhood classroom. *Journal of Research in Childhood Education, 23*(4), 450–460.

Blaise, M. (2014). Interfering with gendered development: A timely intervention. *International Journal of Early Childhood, 46*(3), 317–326.

Blaise, M., Hamm, C., & Iorio, J. M. (2017). Modest witness(ing) and lively stories: Paying attention to matters of concern in early childhood. *Pedagogy, Culture & Society, 25*(1), 31–42.

Blaise, M. & Rooney, T. (2020). Listening to and telling a rush of unruly natureculture gender stories. In F. Nxumalo & C. P. Brown (Eds.), *Disrupting and countering deficits in early childhood education* (pp. 151–163). New York, NY: Routledge.

Burman, E. (2016). *Deconstructing developmental psychology* (3rd ed.). London, UK: Routledge.

Burman, E. (2018). Towards a posthuman developmental psychology of child, families and communities. In *International Handbook of Early Childhood Education* (pp. 1599–1620). Dordrecht: Springer.

Canadian Society for Exercise Physiology. (2016). *Canadian 24-hour movement guidelines for the early years (0–4 years)*. Ottawa, ON: Author. https://csepguidelines.ca/early-years-0-4/

Cannella, G. (1997). *Deconstructing early childhood education: Social justice and revolution*. New York: Peter Lang.

Castañeda, C. (2002). *Figurations: Child, bodies, worlds*. Durham, NC: Duke University Press.

Dahlberg, G., Moss, P., & Pence, A. (2013). *Beyond quality in early childhood education and care: Languages of evaluation* (3rd ed). London: Routledge.

de La Bellacasa, M. P. (2017). *Matters of care: Speculative ethics in more than human worlds*. Minneapolis: University of Minnesota Press.

Dyer, H. (2020). *The queer aesthetics of childhood: Asymmetries of innocence and the cultural politics of child development*. New Brunswick, NJ: Rutgers University Press.

Elliott, C. (2016). Find your greatness: Responsibility, policy, and the problem of childhood obesity. In J. Ellison, D. McPhail, & W. Mitchinson (Eds.), *Obesity in Canada: Critical perspectives* [Google Play eBook version] (pp. chapter 10). Toronto, ON: University of Toronto Press.

Evans, B. (2010). Anticipating fatness: Childhood, affect and the preemptive 'war on obesity'. *Transactions of the Institute of British Geographers, 35*(1), 21–38.

Evans, B., & Colls, R. (2011). Doing more good than harm? The absent presence of children's bodies in (anti) obesity policy. In E. Rich, L. F. Monaghan, & L. Aphramor (Eds.), *Debating obesity: Critical perspectives* (pp. 115–138). New York: Palgrave Macmillan.

Evans, J., Davies, B., & Rich, E. (2008). The class and cultural functions of obesity discourse: Our latter day child saving movement. *International studies in Sociology of Education, 18*(2), 117–132. doi: 10.1080/09620210802351367

Evans, J., Evans, B., & Rich, E. (2003). 'The only problem is, children will like their chips': Education and the discursive production of ill-health. *Pedagogy, Culture and Society, 11*(2), 215–240. doi: 10.1080/14681360300200168

Evans, J., & Rich, E. (2011). Body policies and body pedagogies: every child matters in totally ped-agogised schools? *Journal of Education Policy, 26*(3), 361–379. doi: 10.1080/02680939.2010.500399

Evans, J., Rich, E., & Davies, B. (2004). The Emperor's new clothes: Fat, thin, and overweight. The social fabrication of risk and ill health. *Journal of Teaching in Physical Education, 23*(4), 372–391.

Fitzpatrick, K., & Tinning, R. (2014). Health education's fascist tendencies: A cautionary exposition. *Critical Public Health, 24*(2), 132–142.

Haraway, D. (2012). Awash in urine: DES and Premarin® in multispecies response-ability. *Women's Studies Quarterly, 40*(1/2), 301–316. doi: 10.1353/wsq.2012.0005

Hodgins, B. D. (2019a). *Gender and care with young children: A feminist material approach to early childhood education.* New York: Routledge.

Hodgins, B. D. (Ed.). (2019b). *Feminist research for 21st-century childhoods: Common worlds methods.* London: Bloomsbury.

Hodgins, B. D., & Kummen, K. (2018). Transformative pedagogical encounters: Leading and learning in/as a collective movement. In S. Cheesman & R. Walker (Eds.), *Pedagogies for Leading Practice* (pp. 110–124). New York: Routledge.

Hodgins, B. D., Yazbeck, S. L., & Wapenaar, K. (2019). Enacting twenty-first century early childhood education: Curriculum as caring. In R. Langford (Ed.), *Theorizing feminist ethics of care in early childhood practice: Possibilities and dangers* (pp. 203–225). London: Bloomsbury.

Land, N. (2015). Gooey stuff, intra-activity, and differential obesities: Foregrounding agential adiposity within childhood obesity stories. *Contemporary Issues in Early Childhood, 16*(1), 55–69. doi: 10.18357/jcs.v41i3.16304

Land, N. (2018). Fat knowledges and matters of fat: Towards re-encountering fat(s). *Social Theory and Health, 16*(1), 77–93. doi: 10.1057/s41285-017-0044-3

Land, N. (2020). Tending, counting, and fitting with post-developmental fat(s) in early childhood education. *Contemporary Issues in Early Childhood.* doi: 10.1177/1463949120907383

LeBesco, K. (2004). *Revolting bodies? The struggle to redefine fat identity.* Amherst: University of Massachusetts Press.

LeBesco, K. (2011). Neoliberalism, public health, and the moral perils of fatness. *Critical Public Health, 21*(2), 153–164. doi: 10.1080/09581596.2010.529422

MacNaughton, G. (2003). *Shaping early childhood: Learners, curriculum and contexts.* Berkshire: McGraw-Hill Education.

McPhail, D., Chapman, G. E., & Beagan, B. L. (2011). "Too much of that stuff can't be good": Canadian teens, morality, and fast food consumption. *Social Science & Medicine, 73*(2), 301–307. doi: 10.1016/j.socscimed.2011.05.022

Nelson, N., Hodgins, B. D., & Danis, I. (2019). New obligations and shared vulnerabilities: Reimagining sustainability for live-able worlds. *Nordic Studies in Science Education, 15*(4), 418–432. doi: 10.5617/nordina.6407

Nelson, N., Pacini-Ketchabaw, V., & Nxumalo, F. (2018). Rethinking nature-based approaches in early childhood education: Common worlding practices. *Journal of Childhood Studies, 43*(1), 4–14. doi: 10.18357/jcs.v43i1.18261

Nxumalo, F. (2016). Storying practices of witnessing: Refiguring quality in everyday pedagogical encounters. *Contemporary Issues in Early Childhood, 17*(1), 39–53. doi: 10.1177/1463949115627898

Nxumalo, F. (2019). Presencing: Decolonial attunements to children's place relations. In B. D. Hodgins (Ed.), *Feminist research for 21st-century childhoods: Common worlds methods* (pp. 159–170). London: Bloomsbury.

Nxumalo, F. (2020). Disrupting racial capitalist formations in early childhood education. In F. Nxumalo & C. P. Brown (Eds.), *Disrupting and countering deficits in early childhood education* (pp. 164–178). New York: Routledge.

Nxumalo, F., Vintimilla, C. D., & Nelson, N. (2018). Pedagogical gatherings in early childhood education: Mapping interferences in emergent curriculum. *Curriculum Inquiry, 48*(4), 433–453. doi: 10.1080/03626784.2018.1522930

Osgood, J., & Sakr, M. (Eds.). (2019). *Postdevelopmental approaches to childhood art.* London: Bloomsbury Publishing.

Otterstad, A. M. (2016). Notes on wor (l) dly becoming with child/ren/hood (s): In the middle of small things – Writing, response-ability and be-ing-in-common-worlds-with. In A. B. Reinersten (Ed.), *Becoming earth* (pp. 99–112). Brill: Sense.

Pacini-Ketchabaw, V. (2011). Rethinking developmental theories in child and youth care. In A. Pence & J. White (Eds.), *Child and youth care: Critical perspectives on pedagogy, practice, and policy* (pp. 19–32). Vancouver: UBC Press.

Pacini-Ketchabaw, V., & Clark, V. (2016). Following watery relations in early childhood pedagogies. *Journal of Early Childhood Research, 14*(1), 98–111. doi: 10.1177/1476718X14529281

Pacini-Ketchabaw, V., & Nxumalo, F. (2016). Unruly raccoons and troubled educators: Nature/culture divides in a childcare centre. *Environmental Humanities,* 7(1), 151–168. doi: 10.1215/22011919-3616380

Petherick, L., & Beausoleil, N. (2016). Obesity panic, body surveillance, and pedagogy: Elementary teachers' response to obesity messaging. In J. Ellison, D. McPhail, and W. Mitchinson (Eds.), *Obesity in Canada: Critical perspectives* [Google Play eBook version] (pp. chapter 9). Toronto, ON: University of Toronto Press.

Rice, C. (2007). Becoming "the fat girl": Acquisition of an unfit identity. *Women's Studies International Forum, 30,* 158–174. doi: 10.1016/j.wsif.2007.01.001

Rich, E. (2010). Obesity assemblages and surveillance in schools. *International Journal of Qualitative Studies in Education, 23*(7), 803–821. doi: 10.1080/09518398.2010.529474

Rich, E. (2011). 'I see her being obesed!': Public pedagogy, reality media and the obesity crisis. *Health, 15*(1), 3–21. doi: 10.1177/1363459309358127

Rich, E., & Evans, J. (2012). Performative health in schools: Welfare policy, neoliberalism and social regulation? In *Biopolitics and the 'Obesity Epidemic'* (pp. 165–179). Abingdon: Routledge.

Shotwell, A. (2016). *Against purity: Living ethically in compromised times.* Minneapolis: University of Minnesota Press.

Taylor, A., Blaise, M., & Giugni, M. (2013). Haraway's 'bag lady story-telling': Relocating childhood and learning within a 'post-human landscape'. *Discourse: Studies in the Cultural Politics of Education, 34*(1), 48–62. doi: 10.1080/01596306.2012.698863

Taylor, A., & Pacini-Ketchabaw, V. (2015). Learning with children, ants, and worms in the Anthropocene: Towards a common world pedagogy of multispecies vulnerability. *Pedagogy, Culture & Society, 23*(4), 507–529. doi: 10.1080/14681366.2015.1039050

Taylor, A., & Pacini-Ketchabaw, V. (2018). *The common worlds of children and animals: Relational ethics for entangled lives.* New York: Routledge.

Vintimilla, C. D. (2018). Encounters with a pedagogista. *Contemporary Issues in Early Childhood, 19*(1), 20–30. doi: 10.1177/1463949116684886

Vintimilla, C. D., Land, N., Pacini-Ketchabaw, V., Kummen, K., & Khattar, R. (2019). *Offering a question to early childhood pedagogists: What would be possible if education subtracts itself from developmentalism?* Retrieved from https://ceeycc-cepege.ca/provincial-en/2019/12/12/scholarly-reflection/#more-688

Walkerdine, V. (1998). Developmental psychology and child-centred pedagogy. In J. Henriques, W. Hollway, C. Urwin, C. Venn, & V. Walkerdine (Eds.), *Changing the subject: Psychology, social regulation, and subjectivity* (2nd ed.; pp. 153–202). Abingdon: Routledge.

Ward, P. (2016). Obesity, risk, and responsibility: The discursive production of the 'ultimate at-risk child'. In J. Ellison, D. McPhail, & W. Mitchinson (Eds.), *Obesity in Canada: Critical perspectives* [Google Play eBook version] (ch. 8). Toronto, ON: University of Toronto Press.

Webb, L., & Quennerstedt, M. (2010). Risky bodies: Health surveillance and teachers' embodiment of health. *International Journal of Qualitative Studies in Education, 23*(7), 785–802. doi: 10.1080/09518398.2010.529471

Woods, H., Nelson, N., Yazbeck, S. L., Danis, I., Elliott, D., Wilson, J., Payjack, J., & Pickup, A. (2018). With(in) the forest: (Re)conceptualizing pedagogies of care. *Journal of Childhood Studies, 43*(1), 44–59. doi: 10.18357/jcs.v43i1.18264

12

A PERSONAL REFLECTION ON EDITING

'Unmasking' the critical obesity researcher against itself

Michael Gard

1

Steve Fuller's scholarship, at least for me, is not for the faint-hearted reader. As a 'science and technology studies' sociologist, he draws on diverse and somewhat surprising areas of work. He is also a very quotable writer: '… the unmasker presumes that the mind is a house divided against itself, so that to address knowledge claims simply as expressed is to ignore the conflicting motives that remain unexpressed in the claims' (Fuller, 2006; p. 19).

2

Most people probably have a similar experience to this; as a young person, I would wander outside and look upwards; see constellations of stars, black spaces and think about the unending circle of time and space without me. Of course, some years later, I realised that many, perhaps, a majority of people have had this comparable experience, dissimilar reactions notwithstanding. On reflection, the meaningless of existence and my endless western day-to-day trials is just a sign of the irritation of life's comings and goings. After all, I have to live a life rather than continually getting bogged down in philosophical niceties. And, besides, there are so many important social issues to consider and interesting books to read. Like the notice to students on the door of one of my former academic colleague's office (perhaps like the moon saying quietly to us or, at least, to me): 'Stop staring at the stars, put your skates on and, for God's sake, read'.

3

What does 'critical' mean for obesity researchers? Having been one of the editors of this present volume, to define 'critical' is a usual, significant and, in many ways, crucial job. Through this chapter, and with theoretical and methodological issues in mind, I want to describe a path through critical obesity research that I tried to follow, explicitly emphasising the word 'I'. A reader might not agree with some or all of the material that I have covered here, but they should at least understand my approach to the writing and editing of this volume. I also want to underscore that I have worked and negotiated with and enjoyed the

DOI: 10.4324/9780429344824-15

company of Darren Powell and José Tenorio as we got down to the serious job of editing this volume together. All three editors have stamped their influence on this volume in their own way particularly, but not only, selecting, discussing and working with our authors.

But, on the other hand, I do not want to camouflage myself behind 'editorial decisions'. For me, this short chapter is both an academic text and also a personal narrative. Of course, personal narrative can be a huge nuisance, particularly when one wants to focus on a body of ideas developed by a famous academic or theorist. I can see the arguments for or against the mixing of personal narratives and ideas, but, in general, it depends on what one wants to achieve through a piece of writing. In this particular chapter, I want to describe many and linked ideas; an apology, a confessional tale, a reasoned argument and even a call to arms. Despite the many directions that this chapter may seem to take, for me, the tangled arguments within come from the same source; how to be a critical obesity researcher? A researcher may not agree with me or is not ready to make this move – from a position where the factors are theatrically separated to a land where the differences are blurred – but the ideas that I want to develop in this chapter illustrate my position. Following many thinkers who stated this point more elegantly than me, my position boils down to an appreciation that one's ideas and one's narrative are important, interchangeable and performative as each other. In other words, my position is that difference between two things is mostly a language 'problem', although I probably would not use the term in this way. After all, the engine of life's 'problems' often emerges from the same source. Most obvious is that any narratives can be told in any number of ways, and therefore, narratives can be represented by ideas or even through 'theory'. More than this, though, is that a theory can be built on one's life experience: reading, acting, interacting, reflecting, researching, writing, staring at the stars and changing one's mind.

There is much to say about the connection between narrating and ideas about one's experience but, for now, I want to remind the reader of the two opening points of this chapter. First, this text is focused on *editing of this present volume* rather than other areas of academic work such as writing and researching. Editing is hard to define partly because people chose to do it with divergent and contrasting reasons. For example, some academics do their editing quickly or leave it to junior colleagues. On the other hand, some academics will want more control on what is said in each contribution.

Second, and building on this previous point, critical obesity studies, at least for me, is not a discipline or movement or even a politic. This point is especially important for, say, contrasting critical obesity studies with fat studies. For example, fat studies are often defined as movement for empowerment and pride regardless of one's body dimension. Fat studies researchers are also working against anti-fat bias wherever it occurs. On a good day, critical obesity studies researchers might share this belief but, on a bad day, we might ask for the entrance fee back. Critical obesity studies are an idea rather than an academic field of inquiry. In some senses, critical obesity studies are larger than fat studies (e.g., school practice and food marketing) but, also in contrast, in this area, the material can be swapped and discussed. There has to be boundaries for critical obesity studies although it is not for me or anybody else to say. I am for social justice but what I mean by 'social justice' for fat people is always open to interesting questions. This volume is partly compiled by me, with all those biases and blank spaces it entails.

I want to emphasise that there were many authors who were approached to contribute to this volume. There are many reasons that potential authors refused this invitation; being busy, close to retirement, their research was not close enough to critical obesity studies or just had not received the invitation. But there were authors who had ideological doubts about critical obesity studies. By contrast, there were many other authors who eagerly wanted to contribute to the debates about fat and obesity. That was especially true for authors from Latin America and Europe. At this point, I want to argue that critical obesity studies are, at present, a possible area for those ideas to be circulated without engaging with fat studies. There are unfortunately negative reasons but, then again, there are ambiguous and positive reasons these ideas should be read and discussed. This is why critical obesity studies exist.

4

I also want to tell a personal story as well as an important line of argument for *critical* obesity research. Of course, often when one makes a rather ambitious set of arguments, one expects some resistance. As a writer, one needs to inspect oneself, and for me, there are many issues to own up to. When I first started my academic career, more senior colleagues asked me to 'position' myself with my work. To understand where my developing sense of self and my arguments come from was always a challenging and problematic process. How far back should one go? Is it necessary in all cases? Are there any academic and disciplinary fences that, in the end, one should not jump over? Speaking generally, I want to say that my gender, my socio-economic status and my sexuality and many others are always 'in play'. I warmly welcome those debates about my direction and the politics of my work. My life's background and my academic research work are, like everybody's, always 'problematic'.

In the speed of today's academic life, these 'position' debates are somewhat sidelined by academic talk about one's 'impacts' and one's 'outputs'. Although I have written quite extensively about my 'position' as a researcher, I would ask the curious readers to consult other publications. For now, my early academic education was in teacher education, which was happily dominated by 'critical' feminists and post-structural colleagues in which one cannot escape uncomfortable interactions. But, in jumping to one's conclusions, I (do I need to say 'we'?) need to be able to think in many directions carefully. As an academic and teacher, I have to be able to understand where, for example, Marxist or post-structuralist or free-market or biological thinking comes in, perhaps whether we are considering obesity or not. Of course, I may be completely wrong about the applicability of thinking to an issue, but I stand by this position. One might not be interested in a particular theory or an issue, but this does not make it wrong.

In fact, I want to emphasise two guiding principles that led my thoughts about my research and, therefore, my editing of this volume. First, my position is that, most and perhaps, all writers, no matter what area of scholarship they are in, are both wrong and right. For example, there are many academics writing who wear their faith proudly. They might call themselves a devotee of a particular thinker or call themselves an academic follower of particular writers or movements. My biases are multiple. In fact, I find it hard to call myself anything, which may be the dividend of being not sinned against. On the other hand, one bias of mine is to emphasise the *gaps* between different ways of thinking. For example, although my understanding can be easily critiqued, I have some understanding of post-structural feminism having been academically raised by them. But, as a listener to conference presentations and a reader of academic work, one of the first questions that comes to my mind is: where are the gaps? In other words, where are the 'black spots' in one's theory and one's thinking? By reading and listening to this work, this 'black spot' point should not become the main subject of discussion. I am keenly interested in the direction they (the writer/presenter) are following. But, when I ask (mentally or in-person) about the gaps in their thinking, often, the response is half-hearted or misses the point. Of course, my question may be hard to understand, but it can also be a chance for reflection in what else.

Second, in following this previous point, my case is not really about 'academic' gap filling *per se* or endlessly 'philosophising'. Rather, my argument is that the gaps are where productive thinking regularly happens. Again, I am not claiming a major lack in modern obesity research. Rather, my argument here is a point of emphasis; every theory covers up. Putting it somewhat poetically, there is a room in the back where one puts one's garbage (Bauman, 2004), intentionally or not. It can be difficult to locate this room, but it can be also be productive.

There are many reasons to adopt this way of thinking, researching and, with this volume in mind, editing. For many years, I have studied the 'reproducibility crisis' in many fields of study, including the work of Ioannidis (2013, 2016) in biomedical research and Makel and Plucker (2014) in educational research. Those who are involved in this area of research are interested in the explosive effect of 'bloated' research 'findings'. To put it simply, once the research system rewards over-production, then the 'real' findings can get crowded by research 'chatter'. But there is also the 'ideological' effect in which the politics of one's area can cloud one's thinking. Of course, who I am to state the truth about anything but when the conversations veer to another territory it can build new and controversial thinking.

5

My relationship with religion was never close although what I mean normally by the term 'religion' amounts to a grab-bag of religious items such as churches, Easter and Christmas services, people and culture. Like a family friend, religion was always *there*. There were times when the relationship was felt intimately, and then where times when it inched to a more icy cold, but there was never as major interruption. I went to boarding school in 1970s where I spent many unsettled years, but I loved singing and enjoyed being in the choir for chapel. It took a few years to find myself in boarding school, partly because of the bullying that I often received, and one of the few positive factors at school was singing in church. I hated modern hymns or what they called 'popular' songs. My taste stretched across early Gregorian chants to late Victorian hymns. Sometimes, I thought I was born way too late, and if I was being completely honest, I think there was an old-fashioned high-protestant spirit lurking in the wings.

Some years later, I travelled. After reflecting on these experiences, one of the main reasons for these journeys was my interest in history, particularly medieval to Victorian. In fact, many of my destinations were also the main story: steeples, catholic domes, decaying country churches and non-conformist meeting houses. Standing in the buildings, I also became aware of the transformative effects of these quiet and simultaneously grand spaces. By this time, my official religious faith had never returned, but the connection between historical curiosity and the religious buildings, art and music was obvious, at least for me.

But it was not the churches that mattered most, although these buildings started my journey. I especially was also drawn to religious writers about history. Although one might have diverse understandings of 'what actually happened', I was always interested in curious and even radical interpretations. My background in post-modernist and post-structural history (e.g., Jenkins, 1991; Wesseling, 1991) collided and reverberated with religious theorists and historians (Buber, 1952; Bickermam, 1998; MacCulloch, 2010; McAleese, 2012). I read and was radically changed by Elise Wissel who became known as a NAZI concentration camp survivor, a teacher and Nobel Peace Prize winner (e.g., Wissel 1960, 2011; see also Burger,

2019, for a tribute to Wissel's life). This created new directions of reading for me and, in particular, the way Jewish – observant or at least flavoured – writers can often look at the world slightly or starkly differently. My mind goes back to Amos Oz (2005, 2011) and Hillel Schwartz (1986) who has contributed a chapter in this volume.

In this section, I have quickly marched through many areas of writing and thinking from English country churches to Schwartz's thoughtful accounts of fat anxiety throughout history. For me, the connection here is the way space – in buildings or in people's thinking – invites us to rest, to listen to the echo and to think again. How can one's view on, say, 'identity' or, closer to the material of this chapter, one's ideas about bodies and obesity, be challenged without seeing new paths or hearing somewhat unfamiliar voices? As all areas of critical thinking, science, physical or social, about obesity is often wrong or at least limited (Gard and Wright, 2005; Gard, 2011). I am also not talking about one's faith partly because I do not have any faith left. But, like Schwartz's writing which makes demands on a reader's rational and imaginative capabilities, critical obesity thinkers are always traveling.

6

To state the obvious, the background of my thinking is partly connected to fat studies and, more generally, to the fat movement. From my perspective, many of the most important and even daring writers are the fat activists and later, academics. Of course, when I ask when did the fat 'movement' begin, this invites one's arguments to be critiqued; 1,000 years, 1950s, post-2000? Each fat term – 'activists', 'movement', 'studies' – leads one to further debates which are all potential areas of discussion and disagreement. There are many takes on the historical fat movement but, following radical re-readings of their situation, feminism, black liberalism and the rest, the 'fat movement' began in the late 1960s. My reading began with early writers (Louderback, 1967, 1970; Schoenfielder & Wieser, 1983) who created new ways of engaging with fat bodies and western 'hatred' towards fat people. Of course, the radical turn of 'fat' behaviour, attitudes and even the law has touched everyone, whether we understand it or not, but, for me, the pure skill of thinking by activists was a special case. Yes, I was interested, excited and in awe of their writings and their actions, and it also inspired me to take this path as a researcher. I also learned a great deal from my contemporaries such as Samantha Murray (2008) and, a contributor in this volume, Cat Pausé (2012). In other words, it was their intellectual and physical 'hutzpah' that took my breath away.

But people, which include researchers, came to talk about fat in many ways. When I originally wrote a book with Jan Wright, I had just completed my PhD on dance, narrative and masculinity studies. At the same time, the 'obesity epidemic' was everywhere, and Sydney Olympics committee were preparing for the 'best Olympics'(!) in history. Many commentators were worked up about the 'obesity generation', the implication for the Australia's medal tally, and looking to schools to do something about it. Of course, the obvious solution was to improve physical education.

Like many education researchers, there are times when you have to speak out, particularly for the students in schools and universities. Moreover, as an early career academic, the ripples of fat hatred become more obvious the more you looked. So where to start? At that time, fat activists were fairly well known across English speaking countries, and certainly, I understood and respected their achievements. I also read and listened with eagerness to the experiences of fat activists and fat studies scholars. Working with Jan Wright, who has a background in post-structural feminism and critical language analysis, we drew heavily from fat history. On the other hand, engagement with 'obesity' also called for emerging and perhaps radical ways of researching fat. This included, but was not limited to, critiques of evolutionary science and 'evidence-based' medicine. Thinking back on it now, the idea was to bring many disciplines together in conversations and debates rather than splitting disciplines or provoking needless arguments.

In other words, we wanted new answers for new questions. Once fat studies became established and, amongst other things, a 'movement', there also emerged strengths and limitations. I will not convince you of the strengths of fat studies because the average reader of this volume may know better than me, but once a field of studies emerges, the politics and blind-spots become more obvious. This statement is no more or less true of any other fields.

We understood the politics of fat but, at some point, we had to talk with and teach to people who, for whatever reasons, did not buy 'fat liberation'. We wanted to discuss this issue with doctors, students and the public as well as social, science and medicine academics. And there were times when I just had to use 'obesity' and 'overweight'. Many times, the audience would not let me in the door unless I was using the same language as them. I needed to bring as *many* 'languages' with me as I could if I wanted to make a difference.

Take science. To discuss fat movement and fat hatred with my students, I need to use different and potentially conservative arguments. In fact, I often start my courses with physiology, public health and epidemiology evidence, graphs and ways of thinking. Fat studies often start with a fat position, but this can be difficult for some students (especially those studying exercise science and physical education). This is an important point because a fat 'position' blocks other productive paths with my students and the public. The world is full of very different ideas about fat, and there are many routes to salvation including, amongst others, science. This means that writers such as Katherine Flegal, Timothy Olds, Gyorgy Scrinis and others were warmly invited to contribute to this volume. For me, these 'science' (a term which can be hotly debated) writers have a position that can be constructive for researchers, depending of course on one's material. At the risk of repeating myself, my approach here is not being epistemology right or wrong, although there are always some ideas who should generally be discounted. Rather, my argument is that writers are *always* right and wrong at the same time. Sometimes, I often find myself agreeing with some science writers, particularly when discussing where fat tissue becomes a serious risk for human health. But after a period of deep reflection, often, I accuse myself of being on some weird drugs. The point is that it is often hard to take a firm position on basically anything, including 'fat' debates, with contradictory and compelling arguments competing for attention.

7

The purpose of this brief chapter is to say exactly what 'critical' means to me as a scholar. Of course, I have attempted to explain what I am doing through my research and editing. This purpose of this chapter and, therefore, my purpose of my research career may seem quite unusual for some readers and may strike some readers as exercise in self-deception. In fact, I can hear the sounds of voices accusing me of being a bad poet-*poseur* but, as scholar, I wanted readers to see the stars differently every day or, more to the point, every night. So be it.

But returning to being a normal academic, I have chosen a short passage to begin this chapter, written by Steve Fuller, a sociologist and, as my understanding of his output record, a very hard worker indeed. This extract is focused on the lengthy scientific and sociological debates between Karl Mannheim and Karl Popper during the early part of the 20th century. But, for this chapter, I am drawn to the image of the 'unmasker'; the scholar who is struggling against an academic foe but, closer to the main point, also against her/himself.

Fuller's argument can be seen as the 'motives' of one's thinking, a fairly simple idea but worth repeating it; whether the material is fat, obesity or anything else, we have to find ways to understand *ourselves*. For me, one strategy – and it is one suggestion amongst many others – is to be to read against one's thinking, even engage with unfashionable positions. This is why I and my colleagues have tried to shape this volume.

From my perspective, the world is very confusing. To get good evidence is hard work, and most research can often be average or worse. I have also seen crimes committed on every side of the fat and obesity debate, critical or not. My agreement of being one the editors of this volume is, first and foremost, that the readers of this area of research should find complicated and many-sided. Certainly, there are many authors who I would probably agree with. But the main underlying point is that the 'critical' in the title of this volume is not for the contributors but for the reader, and an alert reader can already see the embers of disagreement fires.

References

Bauman, Z. (2004). *Wasted lives: Modernity and its outcasts*. Cambridge, Polity.

Bickermam, E. J. (1988). *The Jews in the Greek Age*. Cambridge, Harvard University Press.

Buber, M (1952) *Eclipse of God: Studies in the relation between religion and philosophy*. New York, Harper and Brothers.

Burger, A. (2019). *Witness: Lessons from Elie Wiesel's classroom*. Boston, Mariner Books.

Fuller, S. (2006). *The philosophy of science and technology studies*. London, Routledge.

Gard, M. (2010). *The end of the obesity epidemic*. London, Routledge.

Gard, M. and Wright, J. (2005). *The obesity epidemic: Science, morality and ideology*. London, Routledge.

Ioannidis, J. P. A. (2013). Implausible results in human nutrition research, *British Medical Journal*, 347 (f6698). doi: 10.1136/bmj.f6698

Ioannidis, J. P. A. (2016). The mass production of redundant, misleading, and conflicted systematic reviews and meta-analyses, *The Milbank Quarterly*, 94(3), 485–514. doi: 10.1111/1468–0009.12210

Jenkins, K. (1991). *Re-thinking history*. London, Routledge.

Louderback L. (1967). More people should be fat. *Saturday Evening Post*. Nov 4, pp. 10–12.

Louderback, L. (1970) *Fat power*. New York, Hawthorn Books.

McAleese, M. (2012). *Quo vadis? Collegiality in the code of canon law*. Dublin, Columba Press.

MacCulloch, D. (2010). *A History of Christianity: The first three thousand years*. London, Penguin.

Makel, M. C. and Plucker, J. A. (2014). Facts are more important than novelty: Replication in the education sciences. *Educational Researcher*, 43(6), 304–316. doi: 10.3102/0013189X14545513

Murray, S. (2008). *The 'fat' female body*. London, Palgrave-Macmillan.

Oz, A., (2005). *A tale of love and darkness*. Houghton, Mifflin Harcourt.

Oz, A. (2011). *How to cure a fanatic*. Princeton, Princeton University Press.

Pausé, C. (2012). Live to tell: Coming out as fat. *Somatechnics*, 2(1), 42–56.

Schoenfielder, L. and Wieser, B. (eds.) (1983). *Shadow on a tightrope: Writings by women on fat oppression*. San Francisco, Aunt Lute Book Company.

Schwartz, H. (1986). *Never satisfied: A cultural history of diets, fantasies, and fat*. New York, Free Press.

Wesseling, E., 1991. *Writing history as a prophet: Postmodernist innovations of the historical novel*. Amsterdam, John Benjamins Publishing.

Wissel, E. (1960) *Night*. Trans. Stella Rodway. New York, Hill and Wang.

Wiesel, E. (2011). *From the kingdom of memory: Reminiscences*. New York, Schocken Books.

PART D

Food

The fourth theme in the Handbook focuses on the role of food in debates about obesity. Certainly, public and political discourses tend to focus on food as part of the problem of, and solution to, obesity. It would be difficult to imagine an article or blog or social media post or news story about obesity that did not connect fatness to food through taken-for-granted assumptions about energy imbalance, gluttony, junk food advertising, 'Big Food', low carb-high fat (LCHF) diets, a lack of food education, ultra-processed food, school meals or arguments for or against implementing a 'sugar tax' (or other forms of regulatory and legislative controls).

The chapters which follow explore food in a myriad of ways and in disparate contexts: how children experience food in Australian schools; the role of workplace food and eating in Britain and France; how Chinese international students understand food and health in relationship to Chinese and Australian 'norms'; the influences on food in schools in Mexico; how capitalism in the United States relating to agro-food capital has increased people's body sizes and developed the diet industry; the relationships between the 'war on sugar' and the 'war on obesity' in the United Kingdom; and the uncertain connection between junk food marketing and childhood obesity. Despite their diversity, the chapters in this section are bound by an important thread: food is central to life and to living; it is more than just a means to create a particular body size, weight or shape. How we eat, why we eat, what we eat, who we eat with and where we eat is shaped by a range of powerful social, historical, cultural, political, individual, familial, environmental and economic factors. To understand 'obesity', we need to develop a deeper understanding of how food and eating 'works'. This is a significant contribution that the following authors make in this section.

Karen Throsby begins this section by exploring the social meanings and practices of sugar in the context of the broader 'war on obesity'. In this chapter, Throsby argues that while the contemporary attack on sugar has some similarities with earlier iterations of the 'war on obesity', it also constitutes a 'crisis' of its own entangled with changing understandings of the body, the moralisation of health and the socio-political context of austerity. Throsby's close examination of 'anti-sugar' and 'anti-obesity' campaigns in the United Kingdom demonstrates how the 'war on obesity' should not be understood as a fixed phenomenon,

DOI: 10.4324/9780429344824-16

but as flexible and adaptable, one that is reconfigured with the socio-cultural environment in which it needs to remain meaningful. Crucially, Throsby illustrates how the capacity for the 'war on obesity' to be reinvented highlights the ways in which anxieties around sugar are never 'just' about either sugar or obesity, but act as a relay point for public and political anxieties about citizenship, individual responsibility and belonging.

Julie Guthman examines how capitalism has helped to create obesity as a material phenomenon and then has made it a moral problem that must be resolved in a 'capitalist' way. Using the concept of the socio-ecological fix, Guthman suggests that the so-called problem of obesity exists through efforts of agro-food capital to overcome a particular limit of accumulation. Specifically, the author argues that the tendency towards over-production of food creates problems of profitability – a problem worsened by Engel's Law. Guthman discusses how efforts to overcome the limits of agro-food capital have resulted in increased body sizes – through marketing that encourages people to eat more, and through the use of substances used in food production that contribute to obesity. However, Guthman also points out how the 'obesity crisis' has created new opportunities for accumulation, namely in the form of the myriad diet programs, foods, medications, and surgeries that are bought and sold in the interest of weight loss; socio-ecological fixes that have their own limits and health problems.

Next, José Tenorio looks at schools in Mexico as 'gastro-political spaces', where various organisations attempt to be part of the solution to childhood obesity by 'educating' children to eat healthy food. By using short fieldwork stories – based on observations and interviews in two primary schools in Veracruz, Mexico – Tenorio demonstrates the key tensions between a nutrition-focused understanding of food and the day-to-day practices and meanings associated around food in schools; tensions often resulting from culturally, politically and economically decontextualised public health goals. In this chapter, Tenorio also illuminates that although food in schools is significantly shaped by culture, taste and the economy, the healthy/unhealthy classification of food has created space for the stigmatisation of meals that are culturally significant. Tenorio further argues that these gastro-political spaces are porous, where schools act as a connection point between the broader political projects of the state and corporations, the beliefs and knowledges of the school staff, and the private lives of families.

Bonnie Pang examines Chinese international students' relationship with food and how this contributes to their navigation of the 'norm' in their construction of a healthy lifestyle. Informed by research focusing on the health-related experiences of ten Chinese international students attending higher education institutions in New South Wales, Australia, this chapter explores how the students engaged with discourses about food in relation to health, physical activity and culture, and how, in a Foucauldian sense, they become a subject to particular positions. Using key themes of 'Chineseness and food habits', the binary of 'healthy/unhealthy foods and lifestyles' and 'drinking cultures', Pang highlights how these students navigated the 'norm', those related to typical Western subjectivities of health and food practices, with discourses of healthism, nutritionism and obesity. At the same time, however, Pang demonstrates how students' food practices consisted of an 'in-betweenness' – a constant negotiation between the (Western) 'norm' position and their Chineseness as they compared, contrasted and reflected on their lived food and health experiences.

Deana Leahy, Jan Wright, Jo Lindsay, Claire Tanner, JaneMaree Maher and Sian Supski's chapter offers new insights from children and parents about the effects of contemporary policy approaches to schooling food in Victoria, Australia. Drawing on research about children as health advocates, the authors investigate how children and their families experience school food programs. Their research not only reveals how food was an integral part of everyday schooling but also how schools were rather haphazard and inconsistent in their attempts to regulate food consumption and were perceived to provide little, if any, formal food education. Critically, Leahy and colleagues interrogate and illustrate several food programs and spaces that worked to create multiple points of contradiction and confusion about food for both students and parents: the canteen, 'nude food' lunchboxes, 'brain food' programs and fundraising activities. The authors' findings provide significant 'food for thought' for both policy makers and policy actors alike, especially when school foodscapes continue to be transformed in response to concerns about the 'childhood obesity epidemic'.

Jean-Pierre Poulain and Cyrille Laporte take a socio-historical perspective to investigate how food systems are institutionalised at the workplace, and how technical solutions devised by professional stakeholders take into account a 'real meal' or a 'proper meal'. By comparing French and British workplace food contexts through concepts of the 'food day' and 'food synchronisation', the authors demonstrate how these technical systems influence eating practices by allowing and facilitating a number of key changes. More so, Poulain and Laporte suggest that this research opens up possibilities to understand the relationship between dietary practices and the prevalence of obesity, specifically how food cultures and food support systems in the workplace shape individual's health in ways that is beyond the control of the individual.

Finally, Darren Powell critically examines how certainty about the relationship between childhood obesity and the marketing of 'junk food' is (re)produced through expert knowledge and the unquestioning acceptance of the 'junk food marketing=childhood obesity' discourse. By analysing key public health documents (in particular, those by the World Health Organization) alongside academic articles about food marketing and childhood obesity, Powell demonstrates how the alleged 'unequivocal evidence' that junk food marketing exacerbates the 'childhood obesity crisis' is based on uncertain evidence. Furthermore, this chapter also sheds light on how 'cherished beliefs' about fat children and food marketing enables public health scholars to (re)produce the certainty that there is a childhood obesity crisis, that junk food marketing is a significant cause and that reducing marketing will provide a solution in spite of the lack of certain evidence.

13

SWEETENING THE "WAR ON OBESITY"

Karen Throsby

In the second decade of the 21st century, the familiar enemy in the "war on obesity" – dietary fat – has been increasingly supplanted by sugar. Against a background of international policy interventions encouraging sugar reduction (World Health Organisation, 2015), in the UK, sugar has been the subject of national policy (Public Health England, 2015; Scientific Advisory Commission on Nutrition, 2015), including the 2018 implementation of the Soft Drinks Industry Levy (SDIL), or "sugar tax" (HM Treasury, 2018), as well as attempts to limit the sales of sugary foods in locations such as hospitals and schools and to control advertising, particularly to children. In January 2014, the anti-sugar campaigning organisation, *Action on Sugar*, was launched with the headline-grabbing claim that "sugar is the new tobacco" (Action on Sugar, 2014), and the obesity-focused public health campaign *Change4Life* (Change for Life, 2017) urges consumers to be "sugar smart" and substitute sugary foods for low-sugar alternatives. The alarm surrounding sugar has opened up a burgeoning anti-sugar market for popular science tracts (Gillespie, 2008; Lustig, 2009; Moss, 2013; Taubes, 2017), TV and film documentaries (Cooper, 2015; Gameau, 2014), autobiographies (Mowbray, 2014; Schaub, 2014) and self-help guides (Carr, 2018; DeFigio, 2013; McKenna, 2016). Collectively, these policy interventions, campaigns and published texts sound the alarm, leaving no space for doubt about the "wrongness" of sugar and its culpability in the obesity "crisis", intensifying the urgency that characterises all anti-obesity discourse and practice that *something must be done* (see Mayes, 2016, p. 1).

Using the UK context as a case study, this chapter asks what the elevation of sugar to dietary enemy *du jour* can tell us about the contemporary "war on obesity" and the social context within which it continues to make sense. I argue that, while the contemporary attack on sugar shares many continuities with earlier iterations of the "war on obesity", it also constitutes a "crisis" of its time, eliding with changing understandings of the body, the intensification of the moralisation of health and the social and political context of austerity. This elision shores up public consent not only for the attack on sugar (and by extension, obesity) but also for the widening inequalities within which a "war on obesity" continues to make sense in spite of its ongoing failures to warrant its core empirical claims (Gard, 2011). As such, the "war on obesity" should be understood not as a fixed phenomenon, but as flexible and adaptable, reconfiguring itself in line with the social and cultural environment in which it needs to remain meaningful and revivifying itself in the face of its own failures.

DOI: 10.4324/9780429344824-17

The next section of the chapter briefly sets out the research on which this chapter is based and then addresses, in turn, the three dimensions that render the attack on sugar a crisis of its time: (1) changing understandings of the body; (2) the intensification of healthism; and (3) the context of austerity.

Sugar rush

The chapter is based on a wider research project called *Sugar Rush: Science, Obesity, and the Social Life of Sugar*,[1] which begins from the question: "What are the social meanings and practices of sugar in the context of the 'war' on obesity?" At the core of the project is database of almost 500 newspaper articles from 2013 to 2018, gathered from nine UK newspapers, including both tabloids and broadsheets. This was foregrounded by a preliminary search from 2000 to 2018, which demonstrated a dramatic rise in newspaper reporting of sugar from 2013, informing the parameters of the final dataset. For example, from 2010 to 2012, there were only 11, 16 and 27 articles, respectively, jumping to 43 in 2013 and peaking at 120 in 2016. This core dataset was then expanded to include key research papers, popular science tracts, campaign press releases, websites and other sources that had triggered news stories, along with other texts encountered along the way including lifestyle guides, autobiographical accounts and campaign materials. This assemblage of texts has been analysed using a critical discourse analytic approach (Fairclough, 2010; Richardson, 2007), treating texts as both active and productive and asking what those texts are *doing*, *how* and to what *effects*.

Sugar and the molecular body

One of the key factors that makes sugar an ideal target in the current moment is the shift towards the molecularisation of the body – that is, the move away from "molar" conceptualisations of bodies "at the scale of limbs, organs, tissues, flows of blood, hormones and so forth" towards molecules such as DNA, which can only be seen and "known" via new biomarkers made legible only via technologies of measurement and visualisation (Rose, 2007, p. 5). Without question, (anti-)obesity still operates on a molar scale, with its focus on internal and external fat, "clogged arteries" and fat-suffocated organs, but it is also increasingly imagined in terms of metabolic disorder, which can only be "known" via clinical and laboratory measurements (Hatch, 2016; see also, Throsby, 2018). Sugar has been a long-standing (albeit contested) concern in relation to health and obesity (Yudkin, 1972), but its recent rise to prominence can be accounted for in part by the ease with which it aligns with this molecularised understanding of the body. Understood as acting imperceptibly *in* the body, it constitutes an unseen and insidious threat to health that *can* be signalled by fatness but may also be at work menacingly within *any* body, meaning that no-one is exempt from the sugar's metabolic impacts and the demands of anti-sugar vigilance. For example, in a 2013 article in the *Daily Mail* about the manifold harms of sugar consumption, cardiologist and anti-sugar activist, Aseem Malhotra, observed:

> What people don't realise is that you can develop [cardiac] problems and have a normal body mass index (BMI). I see it all the time in my clinic. People aren't overweight and don't have diabetes, yet they've had a heart attack. I think sugar is one of the main culprits.
>
> *(Lambert, C., 2013)*

More melodramatically, popular anti-sugar author and paediatric endocrinologist, Robert Lustig, warns: "You think you are safe? You are SO screwed. And you don't even know it" (Lustig, 2014, p. 7).

This molecularised understanding of the insidious action of sugar on the body is exemplified by neuroscientific discourses of addiction that attach so easily to sugar (Throsby, 2020). In spite of long-standing uncertainties about what constitutes "addiction" (Fraser, Moore, & Keane, 2014; Keane, 2002) and a profound lack of scientific consensus around neuroscientific models of addiction (Heim, 2014), sugar is widely conceptualised as "hijacking" the brain's hedonic pathways. For example, in an article in the *Daily Telegraph* about the unseen toxicity of dietary sugar, journalist Victoria Lambert cites warnings from rodent studies that "the intense stimulation of these [sweet] receptors by our 21-st century sugar-rich diets must generate a supra-normal reward signal in the brain, with the potential to override self-control mechanisms and thus lead to addiction" (Lambert, V., 2013; see also Throsby, 2020). Paralleling discourses of illicit drugs, this conceptualisation of sugar gains common sense purchase from the familiar experience of craving more of a sweet food, with the fat body functioning as collateral evidence of sugar-induced havoc within. The focus on sugar, therefore, extends and intensifies the reach of the "war on obesity" to the unseen structures and systems of the body, ramping up the urgency of the twin "crises" of sugar and fatness and the need to *do something* about it (Throsby, 2020).

Importantly, while the rhetorics of addiction may appear at first glance to offer means of minimising the stigma that attaches to both obesity and the derogated habits of consumption associated with it, neuroscientific models of addiction are embedded in assumptions of brain plasticity (Pitts-Taylor, 2010). This can be seen in the repeated exhortations to remove dietary sugar and retrain the body as a response to addiction. For example, in the same *Daily Telegraph* article cited above, David Gillespie (author of the popular anti-sugar book *Sweet Poison* (2008)) offers reassuring words about the ease of breaking a sugar addiction:

> you are breaking an addiction, so you need to stop consuming all sources of the addictive substance. They are all hard to give up because they are addictive – but they are all easy to give up once you understand what you are doing and why.
>
> *(Lambert, V., 2013)*

This renders the brain as much a site of self-intervention and bodily discipline as a fat stomach or an untoned muscle, insisting on the possibility (and necessity of) remedial action and locating it firmly within contemporary neoliberal ideologies of self-management that already characterise the "war on obesity" (LeBesco, 2011; Pitts-Taylor, 2010). As such, we can understand the rush to blame sugar not as a simple switch from one dietary enemy to another, but rather, as the means through which the "war on obesity" can be revivified, extended and intensified in line with changing understandings of the body. This signals the next dimension of the contemporaneousness of the attack on sugar – the intensification of healthism (Crawford, 1980, 2006).

Healthism and the "hidden sugar shock"

At first glance, we can understand the attack on sugar simply as the continuation of the imperative to health (Lupton, 1995), both in general, and specifically in the case of the "war on obesity". But as Crawford argues (2006), this has intensified in the 21st century, bringing with it the potent demand to "achieve" health and manage risk as a matter of moral obligation. He argues that insecurities around health have been aggravated by the commercialisation of health products and services, the growth of risk factor detection technologies and the rise of personal biosensing technologies (Mort, Roberts, & Mackenzie, 2019), reinforcing the conviction that health is a matter of individual responsibility. This intensification provides fertile ground for the attack on sugar, which is increasingly imagined not only as dangerously "empty" of nutritional or health-giving properties but also as *hidden*, demanding new levels of surveillance both of the body and of the foods that we consume.

The epitome of this can be found in what I have called the "hidden sugar shock" stories that are a stock-in-trade for anti-sugar campaigns and their associated news stories. This genre of stories follows a predictable pattern of, first, selecting a particular type of food and second, using product nutritional information to detail its sugar content across different outlets and formulations. Surveys include foods branded as "healthy" but revealed to contain high levels of sugar (e.g., cereal bars, breakfast biscuits, coffee shop drinks, and pasta sauces) and foods already coded as "unhealthy" but revealed to contain even more sugar than expected. For example, in 2018, the campaigning organisation and determined purveyor of "hidden sugar shock" stories, *Action on Sugar*, issued a press release following a survey of supermarket and coffee shop muffins with the headline: "Warning over blueberry muffin hidden sugar content – with leading brands containing up to 10 teaspoons of sugar; more than a can of Coke" (Action on Sugar, 2018a). A similar survey of cakes and biscuits later that year focused its reporting on Battenberg cake, whose pink and yellow-chequered sponge squares wrapped in an outer layer of jam and marzipan ranked highest for sugar content (Action on Sugar, 2018b). The story was taken up enthusiastically in the newspapers: the *Daily Mail* reported its "shocking sugar content" (Pike, 2018); *The Sunday Times* reported its newfound status as a "public health risk" (Peake, 2018); and *The Guardian* covered the story by offering a low sugar recipe using Medjool dates and sugar-free jam as an alternative to the "dangerously sugary" real thing (Holland, 2018). Even when hidden in plain sight, as in a cake or biscuit, the key element in these stories is sugar's *hidden* nature. Just as the effects of sugar on the body are hidden from view, so is the sugar itself, especially given that it is rarely eaten in isolation and instead is combined with other foods to add taste, mouth-feel and act as a preservative (Moss, 2013). The management of the risks of sugar, therefore, demands constant vigilance from consumers.

This demand for vigilance is embodied in the Department of Health-funded public health campaign, *Change4Life*, which urges consumers to be "Sugar Smart" and to make "sugar swaps" that exchange high sugar items for their lower sugar equivalents (Change for Life, 2017). This was exemplified in an animated campaign ad launched in January 2019, which showed angry sugar cubes pouring out of food packets and cupboards, threatening to overwhelm the household's two children and their father, who desperately tries to fight the cubes off with a frying pan (Change4Life, 2019). Danger here lurks in everyday foods, constituting a threat that undermines the safety of the home itself. The family is only saved by the entry of a woman into the kitchen battle zone – presumably, the children's mother – laden with bags of "sugar smart" shopping. The angry cubes eventually flee the scene, defeated by her shrewd consumption; no room is left for doubt that it is women who are responsible for rooting out hidden sugar on behalf of the family and managing its effects.

The normative gendering of the work of being "sugar smart" is further illustrated by a sub-genre of "hidden sugar shock" stories – the "mortified mother" news story. These stories are primarily, but not exclusively, tabloid staples and typically take the form of an "expert" who assesses a family's diet and then delivers a verdict and a series of recommendations, often focusing on products which are commonly coded as "healthy", but which contain large quantities of "hidden" sugar – a concealed threat to the health of the family which the expert teaches the mortified mother to detect and remove. For example, in February 2017, *The Sun* published an article headlined "The hidden risks of a spoon of sugar", where stay-at-home mother of three, Gemma, responded to a nutritionist's evaluation of her children's daily diet:

> I'm really surprised and shocked by how much sugar all the children have been eating. It's been a real eye-opener. I always thought cereal bars were a good option for breakfast but I've already started making Findlay toast and porridge instead. I was told to put Macie on a high-calorie diet when she was a baby, but it's my fault she's ended up on a high-sugar one as well. I'm going to make sure she eats a lot more nutritious foods. All the kids love spaghetti Bolognese, but since doing this diary, I've started making my own pasta sauce [...]. I've also started shopping online as the nutritional information is much easier to see and add up, which is making a difference.
>
> *(Earle, 2017)*

The shame of failed motherhood is countered by her confession and renewed attention to the details of her children's consumption – a process that generates significant additional labour for her that is cast as part of her maternal responsibilities and is therefore never coded as work. This is all performed against a background of burning maternal guilt and without any discussion of the distribution of domestic and reproductive labour in the household. This highlights the ways in which the labour generated by intensified healthism embodied in, and sustained by, the attack on sugar, falls heavily and mundanely onto women. This compounds the already-gendered division of labour in the planning and preparation of household food (Charles & Kerr, 1988; DeVault, 1991) and the burden of responsibility for family health that already weighs so heavily on women. The "hidden" nature of sugar, therefore, and the (unevenly distributed) need for constant vigilance against it, makes it a perfect target for the escalating expectations of the healthism in which the "war on obesity" is embedded.

Austerity

The final dimension to the timeliness of the attack on sugar is the context of austerity. As mentioned earlier in the paper, newspaper coverage of sugar began to rise in 2013 after creeping up slowly in the previous few years. The beginnings of the rise coincide with the establishment of the Conservative-Liberal Democrat coalition UK government in 2010, which, as a response to the 2008 financial crisis, set about a programme of public spending cuts resulting in a raft of austerity policies that were entrenched in the 2012 Welfare Reform Act. These policies have shrunk the welfare state, enacted punitive sanctions against those unable to conform to the proliferating demands of the welfare system and created conditions of profound precarity and poverty in some of the most disadvantaged sections of UK society (Cooper & Whyte, 2017; Evans & McBride, 2017; Garthwaite, 2016; O'Hara, 2015; Ryan, 2019). This occurred alongside, and was facilitated by, a hardening of attitudes towards those dependent on the welfare system, sedimenting a binary between the feckless "scroungers" who are seen as irresponsibly over-consuming and the deserving "strivers" who work hard and take responsibility for themselves and dependent others. Austerity provides the context through which the attack on sugar has gained purchase, particularly via narratives of irresponsible over-consumption (of sugar, of health services). Conversely, the attack on sugar shores up the figure of the feckless and abject Other, who Imogen Tyler (2013) argues is central to securing public consent for the cruelties of austerity (see also, Jensen, 2018; LeBesco, 2011).

In this context, a "war on obesity", spearheaded by an attack on sugar, is able to thrive with an intensity that dietary fat cannot achieve, highlighting anti-obesity's capacity for situationally responsive strategic renewal (although as with the attack on sugar's alignment with the interests of healthism, this should be seen as an intensification rather than a fresh departure).

One of the key features of the mutually supporting relationship between the attack on sugar and austerity is the authority that austerity grants to the targeting of socially and economically disadvantaged people and communities. Running counter to claims discussed earlier in this chapter that sugar poses an equal threat to all, this exposes the unevenness of the attack on sugar and the foundational inequalities on which it is quietly premised. One of the most common claims about sugar, usually via the proxy of obesity, is that those in poorer areas are more likely to consume an unsustainably high sugar diet and to be fat than those in wealthier areas. By extension, they are therefore identified as more likely to experience the expensive non-communicable diseases commonly presumed to be caused by sugar and fatness. Following Tracey Jensen's work on parent-blaming (2018), these framings of "the poor" address a presumed *culture of poverty* rather than poverty itself, and this is evident in repeated assumptions about the imperviousness of the poor to dietary and health advice as an explanation for obesity. For example, a *Daily Telegraph* editorial in August 2015 about the possibility of introducing a tax on sugary drinks argued that "...if those [poorer households] most prone to obesity simply won't listen and the costs to the NHS continue to soar, a fat tax might be the only answer" (Johnston, 2015). The poor are defined here by their poor choices rather than their poverty, making them targets for coercive intervention and placing them firmly in the frame for the erosion of the NHS, shifting attention away from the relentless government retreat from adequate funding. This is, in many ways, a familiar story for the "war on obesity", whose classed, raced and gendered effects have been well documented (e.g., Herndon, 2005; Murray, 2008). But sugar brings an added dimension, since the poor are figured not only as impervious to dietary advice but also as dietarily incontinent, particularly in the face of sugar and its seductive false promises.

This is exemplified by another *Action on Sugar* "hidden sugar shock" story from November 2018, launched to mark Sugar Awareness Week. The story focused on the sugar content of milkshakes sold in high street restaurant and fast food chains, settling on the "freakshake" as the target of its ire (Action on Sugar, 2018c). Freakshakes are spectacularly excessive concoctions of milkshake, ice cream, sweets, cookies and cake, containing well over 1000 calories and over 30 teaspoons of sugar in some cases. The campaign whipped up salacious media coverage, focusing on products sold by the Harvester and Toby Carvery chains, both of which cater to a working-class demographic. Without providing any evidence of who was consuming the freakshakes, in what circumstances and with what prevalence, *Action on Sugar* cultivated a vision of greedily incontinent consumption and called out for regulation to protect the feckless consumers from their own failure to manage their sugar-filled shake intake. In a similar vein, the anti-sugar campaigner and celebrity chef, Hugh Fearnley-Whittingstall, launched a vociferous campaign as part of a BBC documentary, *Britain's Fat Fight*, focusing on the high street store, WHSmiths, which targets a primarily working-class customer demographic. Under the hashtag #WHSugar, Fearnley-Whittingstall's campaign protested the arrays of cheap chocolate displayed around the checkouts, arguing that customers would be unable to resist temptation and should therefore be protected from it by the replacement of the displays with "healthy" alternatives. Fearnley-Whittingstall, however, remains secure in his white, middle-class, masculine command over his impulses and never displays the vulnerability to the lure of the sugary treats laid before him that he presumes governs the store's customers.

Fundamentally, both the focus on freakshakes and the #WHSugar campaign are founded on the assumption that working-class people simply cannot be trusted with sweet treats and won't be able to stop. This demonstrates that, for all the claims that we are *all* at risk from sugar, not all bodies (and brains) are treated as equally vulnerable to its addictive allure. This elides easily with the rhetorics and practices of austerity, which demand the relentless policing of the welfare system in the certainty that claimants will always incontinently take more than their share if left unmonitored. This is not to argue that austerity has *caused* the attack on sugar, but rather, that it has provided the conditions for its rise to prominence, while the attack on sugar reciprocally shores up the figure of the abject over-consuming Other that sits at the heart of austerity campaigns (Tyler, 2013).

Conclusion

While there are many continuities with the ongoing "war on obesity" – for example, the (uneven) contempt for the fat body, the certainty of its "wrongness" and the need to *do something about it* – its current articulation through the attack on sugar also marks it out as a phenomenon of its time. Sugar elides with the molecularisation of the body, the intensification of healthism and the context of austerity to create the conditions through which the "war on obesity", mired in its own failures, can be revivified and intensified. This not only highlights the flexibility and adaptability of the "war on obesity" to reconfigure itself but also, more importantly, illustrates the ways in which the attack on fatness thrives not as a result of its own unassailable logics, but rather, through strategic and mutual alliances with other contexts and interests that enable it to exercise common-sense appeal. This capacity for reinvention highlights the ways in which anxieties around sugar are never straightforwardly about either sugar or obesity, but act as a vector for public anxieties about deserving citizenship, individual responsibility and belonging in ways that should give pause for thought in our encounters with both anti-sugar campaigns and the anti-obesity campaigns in which they are embedded.

Note

1 This research was funded by a Leverhulme Trust Research Fellowship (RF-2017-382).

References

Action on Sugar. (2014). Worldwide experts unite to reverse obesity epidemic by forming "Action on Sugar" [Press release]. Retrieved from http://www.actiononsugar.org/news-centre/press-releases/2014/items/worldwide-experts-unite-to-reverse-obesity-epidemic-by-forming-action-on-sugar.html

Action on Sugar. (2018a). Warning over blueberry muffin hidden sugar content – with leading brands containing up to 10 teaspoons of sugar; more than a can of Coke [Press release]. Retrieved from http://www.actiononsugar.org/news-centre/surveys/2018/2018/warning-over-blueberry-muffin-hidden-sugar-content---with-leading-brands-containing-up-to-10-teaspoons-of-sugar-more-than-a-can-of-coke.html

Action on Sugar. (2018b). New BMJ Open study reveals wide variation in sugar and calories in cakes and biscuits, as industry accused of not complying [press release]. http://www.actiononsugar.org/news-centre/surveys/2018/2018/new-bmj-open-study-reveals-wide-variation-in-sugar-and-calories-in-cakes-and-biscuits-as-industry-is-accused-of-not-complying.html

Action on Sugar. (2018c). Call for ban on excessively high sugar and calorie milkshakes sold in high street and restaurant food chains [Press release]. http://www.actiononsugar.org/news-centre/

press-releases/2018/call-for-ban-on-excessively-high-sugar-and-calorie-milkshakes-sold-in-high-street-restaurants--fast-food-chains-.html

Carr, A. (2018). *Good sugar, bad sugar: Eat yourself free from sugar and carb addiction.* Arcturus.

Change for Life. (2017). Sugar. https://www.nhs.uk/change4life-beta/food-facts/sugar - Pcuzm XCo5dPZZK2y.97

Change4Life. (2019). Smart swaps. https://www.youtube.com/watch?v=PWE_UMno5P8

Charles, N., & Kerr, M. (1988). *Women, food and families: Power, status, love and anger.* Manchester University Press.

Cooper, V. (Writer). (2015). Jamie's sugar rush [TV]. Channel 4.

Cooper, V., & Whyte, D. (Eds.). (2017). *The violence of austerity.* Pluto Press.

Crawford, R. (1980). Healthism and the medicalization of everyday life. *International Journal of Health Services, 10*(3), 365–388. https://doi.org/10.2190/3H2H-3XJN-3KAY-G9NY

Crawford, R. (2006). Health as a meaningful social practice. *Health, 10*(4), 401–420. https://doi.org/10.1177/1363459306067310

DeFigio, D. (2013). *Beating sugar addiction for dummies.* John Wiley and Sons, Inc.

DeVault, M. (1991). *Feeding the family: The social organisation of caring as gendered work.* University of Chicago Press.

Earle, C. (2017, 14 February). Hidden risks in a spoon of sugar. *The Sun*, pp. 22–23.

Evans, B., & McBride, S. (Eds.). (2017). *Austerity: The lived experience.* Toronto, ON: University of Toronto Press.

Fairclough, N. (2010). *Critical discourse analysis.* Routledge.

Fraser, S., Moore, D., & Keane, H. (2014). *Habits: Remaking addiction.* Palgrave.

Gameau, D. (Writer). (2014). *That sugar film* [DVD]. Madman Production Company.

Gard, M. (2011). *The end of the obesity epidemic.* Routledge.

Garthwaite, K. (2016). *Hunger pains: Life inside foodbank Britain.* Policy Press.

Gillespie, D. (2008). *Sweet poison: Why sugar makes us fat.* \ Penguin.

Hatch, A. R. (2016). *Blood sugar: Racial pharmacology and food justice in black America.* University of Minnesota Press.

Heim, D. (2014). Addiction: Not just a brain malfunction. *Nature Reviews: Neuroscience, 507*, 40.

Herndon, A. M. (2005). Collateral damage from friendly fire? Race, nation, class and the "war against obesity". *Social Semiotics, 15*(2), 127–141. https://doi.org/10.1080/10350330500154634

HM Treasury. (2018). Soft drinks industry levy comes into effect [Press release]. https://www.gov.uk/government/news/soft-drinks-industry-levy-comes-into-effect

Holland, M. (2018). How to stop your Battenberg being a health risk. https://www.theguardian.com/lifeandstyle/shortcuts/2018/aug/06/how-to-stop-your-battenburg-being-a-health-risk

Jensen, T. (2018). *Parenting the crisis: The cultural politics of parent-blame.* Policy Press.

Johnston, P. (2015, 8 August). Is a fat tax the only way to combat our growing obesity epidemic? *The Daily Telegraph*, p. 16.

Keane, H. (2002). *What's wrong with addiction?* Melbourne University Press.

Lambert, C. (2013). From dementia to liver damage, the real toll of too much sugar. https://www.dailymail.co.uk/health/article-2524962/From-dementia-liver-damage-real-toll-sugar-diet.html

Lambert, V. (2013). Sweet poison: why sugar is ruining our health. https://www.telegraph.co.uk/foodanddrink/healthyeating/9987825/Sweet-poison-why-sugar-is-ruining-our-health.html

LeBesco, K. (2011). Neoliberalism, public health and the moral perils of fatness. *Critical Public Health, 21*(2), 153–164. https://doi.org/10.1080/09581596.2010.529422

Lupton, D. (1995). *The imperative of health: public health and the regulated body.* Sage.

Lustig, R. (2009). Sugar: The bitter truth. https://www.youtube.com/watch?v=dBnniua6-oM

Lustig, R. (2014). *Fat chance: The hidden truth about sugar, obesity and disease.* Fourth Estate.

Mayes, C. (2016). *The biopolitics of lifestyle: Foucault, ethics and health choices.* Routledge.

McKenna, P. (2016). *Get control of sugar now! Great choices for your health future.* Transworld Publishers.

Mort, M., Roberts, C., & Mackenzie, A. (2019). *Living data: Making sense of health bio-sensing.* Chicago University Press.

Moss, M. (2013). *Salt, sugar, fat: How the food giants hooked us.* Random House.

Mowbray, N. (2014). *Sweet nothing: Why I gave up sugar and how you can too.* Orion.

Murray, S. (2008). *The "fat" female body.* Routledge.

O'Hara, M. (2015). *Austerity bites.* Policy Press.

Peake, J. (2018, 9 August). Battenberg's show stopping sugar content branded a public health risk. *The Sunday Times*, p. 9.

Pike, M.R. (2018). How unhealthy are YOUR favourite treats? Nutritionist reveals the shocking sugar content of Battenberg cakes (and just a slice contains your ENTIRE recommended daily intake). https://www.dailymail.co.uk/femail/food/article-6028725/Nutritionist-reveals-shocking-sugar-content-Battenberg-cakes.html

Pitts-Taylor, V. (2010). The plastic brain: Neoliberalism and the neuronal self. *Health, 14*(6), 635–652. https://doi.org/10.1177/1363459309360796

Public Health England. (2015). *Sugar reduction: The evidence for action*. Public Health England.

Richardson, J. (2007). *Analysing newspapers: An approach from critical discourse analysis*. Palgrave.

Rose, N. (2007). Molecular biopolitics, somatic ethics and the spirit of biocapital. *Social Theory and Health, 5*, 3–29. https://doi.org/10.1057/palgrave.sth.8700084

Ryan, F. (2019). *Crippled: austerity and the demonization of disabled people*. Verso.

Scientific Advisory Commission on Nutrition. (2015). *Carbohydrates and health*. The Stationery Office.

Schaub, E. (2014). *Year of no sugar: A memoir*. Sourcebooks, Inc.

Taubes, G. (2017). *The case against sugar*. Portobello Books.

Throsby, K. (2018). Giving up sugar and the inequalities of abstinence. *Sociology of Health and Illness, 40*(6), 954–968. https://doi.org/10.1111/1467-9566.12734.

Throsby, K. (2020). Pure, white and deadly: Sugar addiction and the cultivation of urgency. *Food, Culture and Society, 23*(1), 11–29. https://doi.org/10.1080/15528014.2019.1679547

Tyler, I. (2013). *Revolting subjects: Social abjection and resistance in neoliberal Britain*. Zed Books.

World Health Organisation. (2015). *Guideline: Sugars intake for adults and children*. World Health Organisation.

Yudkin, J. (1972). *Pure, white and deadly: How sugar is killing us and what we can do to stop it* (2012 ed.). Penguin Life.

14

OBESITY AND ITS CURES AS SOCIO-ECOLOGICAL FIXES FOR AGRO-FOOD CAPITALISM

Julie Guthman

On the October 14, 2009 *Colbert Report* (a now defunct faux news/comedy television show), Stephen Colbert was poking fun at former US Senator John Ensign for his proposed amendment to what was then the still-being-formed health care bill (so-called Obamacare) that would have mandated lower premiums for those who lost weight. To that, Colbert said, "The government is really sending mixed messages here. First, they subsidize corn, making it so cheap we can gorge on subsidized corn syrup, and then they charge us more for health insurance just because our organs have caramelized … . Well, I'm sorry," he quipped, "but our bodies are the only growth industry America has left." With one quick barb, Colbert captured what I believe is an essential truth about the so-called obesity crisis, especially as it has played out in the US: contemporary US capitalism has helped to create obesity as a material phenomenon and then has made it a moral problem that must be resolved in a way that is equally kind to capitalism.

In this chapter, I will elaborate on the capitalist underpinnings of obesity and its cures. Specifically, and without conceding that fatness results in an entirely straightforward way from eating, I will use the concept of the socio-ecological fix as a way to suggest that the so-called problem of obesity in some sense exists by efforts of agro-food capital to overcome a particular limit of accumulation. This limit stems from the problem of inelastic demand for food, otherwise known as Engel's Law. I will also apply this concept to commodified means to address the problem capital helped create. Here, metabolism-defying diet foods present the example par excellence. Finally, I will suggest that there are limits to these fixes because there are limits, albeit ones always being tested, of what substances humans can eat and digest. As such, capitalism's involvement in food production is not only persistently crisis-prone but also unhealthy in the worst of ways. To work through this argument, I begin with recapitulating both the spatial and socio-ecological fix as resolutions to capitalism's persistent crises.

Capitalism and its fixes

The notion of the spatial fix is most associated with the work of geographer David Harvey. In his ground-breaking book *Limits to Capital* (1982), Harvey systematically attempted to make geographical Marx's theories of capital. The limits to capitalism, Harvey noted,

DOI: 10.4324/9780429344824-18

revolved on its persistent tendencies toward crises of over-accumulation, referring to moments of too much capital in circulation and not enough profitable investment opportunities. During such crises, capitalism stagnates, sometimes profoundly, and thus begins to lose value. Historically, such crises were often resolved (if temporarily) through geographical expansion. Pretty much all rounds of global capitalist expansion, whether classic colonialism, 'development,' or 'globalization,' created the conditions for capitalism to develop in regions less subsumed by capitalist relations. The production of infrastructure – roads, dams, communication software – have been particularly important in absorbing excess capital and thus resolving the problem of over-accumulation, while laying anew conditions of production. Harvey thus dubbed such expansion a spatial fix.

Yet, as Harvey was clear to point out, spatial fixes never fully resolve crises of accumulation but displace them elsewhere, making them temporary at best. In addition, spatial fixes are not seamless, as evident in the many regions in the world that contain undeveloped markets, non-waged work, and non-commodified assets. In light of what are effectively (geo-) political limits on various expansionary fixes, more recent theorizations of the spatial fix suggest that they can be more involuted – involving the reworking of internal subdivisions (Katz, 1998, p. 45). Here, space is not appropriated anew but reworked in ways that allows new rounds of accumulation. Capitalist restructuring of industries and regions can be seen in this vein.

Others have argued that spatial fixes are limited by the earth's ability to sustain capitalist growth, given accelerating crises of waste, soil erosion, climate disaster, and much else. When so-called natural resources are degraded, they, in effect, harm and even destroy the conditions of production and consumption and therefore interfere quite profoundly with the circulation of capital. For O'Connor (1989), the tendency for capitalism to destroy its own conditions for reproduction is so pronounced as to be the second contradiction of capitalism. Moore (2015) characterizes this problem as the end up cheap nature, which amounts to the same thing – a potentially major crisis of capitalism. For Harvey, however, such crises present opportunities, as evident in his response to O'Connor's second contradiction of capital (1996) and his discussion of ecological limits to growth (2010). Although he certainly acknowledges the problems of resource depletion and degradation, one of his points is that there is accumulation potential in at least some attempts to resolve these contradictions. Ecological crises, that is, may serve as platforms for further capital investment, what have been dubbed as socio-ecological fixes (Ekers & Prudham 2015). Consider all manner of recent "eco-modernization" projects – from geo-engineering to clean energy technologies to soilless farming in which degraded nature serves as an accumulation strategy (cf. Katz, 1998). Yet, socio-ecological fixes have their limits, too, although when and how they are reached is not always evident. How, then, might these ideas be applied to human bodies?

Bodies as an accumulation strategy

To consider how human bodies are sites of socio-ecological fixes (and their limits), it is useful to consider other ways in which bodies have been conceptualized as part of capitalism's dynamics. And they have been through and through. Even in classical political economy formulations, human bodies are central to capitalist accumulation. As workers, bodies operate machines, pick fruit, and type at consoles, ostensibly creating the value through which profits are made. As consumers, these same workers buy and use the cars, fruit, and software programs, allowing profits to be realized. Neither production nor consumption are abstract processes; bodies must do them.

In addition, bodies are immersed in circuits of capitalism through processes known as social reproduction. For bodies to produce commodities central to capitalist accumulation, that is, they must themselves be produced, even though many aspects of social reproduction are not fully subsumed in capitalist markets (Bakker, 2007; Laslett & Brenner 1989). These days, bodies are also enrolled in capital flows in ways beyond their routine roles in production and reproduction – such as through the creation of property rights around the human genome as well as the increased use of bodies for drug transportation (mules), for organs, sperms, eggs, and genetic material, and for various forms of sexual and reproductive surrogacy (Harvey & Haraway, 1995, p. 511).

To claim the body as a site of a socio-ecological fix, however, means something different again. For the point of the fix is not simply one of an appropriation or dispossession, as is selling a body part or patenting a gene, but opening up a space or site for the circulation, production, and absorption of capital in an ongoing way. A socio-ecological fix is at work when bodies become integral to the *circulation* of capital, when, for instance, they absorb surplus production or when bodily processes become sites of capital investment (Cooper, 2008), particularly in relation to a specific limit or crisis. This, I want to argue, is where food comes in, given the limits that food production poses for capitalist production and accumulation. To this, I now turn.

Limits to agro-food capital

The importance of food in this analysis begins with the axiom that food is essential for social reproduction. It is through the ingestion, digestion, and metabolism of food (and medicine) that commodities most intimately interact with bodily processes and ultimately make or remake the body. Food thus literally grows and energizes workers and thus is an essential ingredient for capitalist labor processes from which profits are amassed. It is bodily consumption that produces the material laboring body, which in turn transforms materials into commodities.

That food is both socially necessary and intimate lays the ground for a host of arguments around agro-food exceptionalism under capitalism. For instance, food must be abundant and cheap enough that people can afford it with wages that capital is willing to pay. At the same time, it cannot be so cheap as to compromise its status as food. As a contributor to biological processes, food must be palatable, digestible, and provide at least a minimum amount of nutrition and energy (Fine, 1994). Yet, while food is crucial for capitalist production, the production of food itself poses particular problems for capitalist accumulation. Indeed, a huge literature in the political economy of food discusses how and why particular elements of food production, especially agriculture, have been slow or resistant to be subsumed in capitalist logics (see, e.g., Fine, 1994; Goodman et al., 1987; Mann, 1989). More generally, much of the way that food provision is organized and regulated to overcome these limits lends itself to systematic over-production, particularly in the US (Cochrane, 1993; Winders, 2009).

This persistent tendency toward over-production creates problems of profitability and thus poses a first cut limit on accumulation in the manufactured food sector – which is where most agro-food capitals operate. The problem is worsened by what is known as Engel's Law, the idea that, as income increases, the proportion of income spent on food falls. Also referred to as the problem of inelastic demand, it is that with increased income people do not buy and eat more food, as they might with other commodities, although they may well eat different food. With inelastic demand, only population growth offsets the declining rate of expenditures on food associated with rising incomes. Essentially, then, surplus food production runs up against the limits of food consumption, ironically so considering that millions of people do not get enough food and amidst more generalized fears of food scarcity. In any case, over-production of crops, coupled with Engel's Law, makes food manufacturing a highly competitive business, and it is prone to slow and even flat growth rates (Guptill & Wilkins 2002). So, this imbalance of food production over food consumption poses a limit to capitalist accumulation in food production, posing a recurrent obstacle that must be overcome for agro-food capital not to stagnate. And it is in trying to overcome this obstacle that capital contributes to obesity.

Binging – the body as fix I

While farmers perennially face low prices, it is generally food processors, manufacturers, and, increasingly, food service operators that confront the limits of the market as capitalists. The main strategy for addressing a competitive market has been cannibalization – attempts to take market share from others in the same business – thus the tremendous emphasis the food industry has placed on food marketing, advertising, and product placement since its florescence in the early part of the 20th century (Levenstein, 1988). In the last three or so decades, food marketing has charted a different path not only geared toward taking markets away from others but also inducing people to eat more (Nestle, 2002). So-called value meals, supersizing, big-box packaging, and a variety of other means, many of which play on consumers' desires to get a 'good deal' while costing the food manufacturer very little on a marginal basis, clearly sell more food. Presumably, much of this food is eaten, although food waste works equally well for agro-food capitalism.

The transubstantiation of this increased food intake into greater muscle or body fat is the most literal way in which the body is the site of a social-ecological fix. That said, it is somewhat debatable how and whether eating more calories has made people fatter since 1980, the beginnings of the so-called obesity epidemic. Gard and Wright (2005) have provided a good deal of evidence that calls into question widespread increases in caloric intake and decreases in physical activity since that time. Others have suggested that it is not how much people are eating but what they are eating that has contributed to larger body sizes. Taubes (2007), for example, has attributed weight increases to the increased intake of carbohydrates relative to fats and proteins, ironically so given that reduced-fat food came on the market as a preventative to weight gain. Indeed, based on codified US dietary guidelines, in a classic cannibalizing move, certain agro-food capitalists formulated high-carb, low-fat recipes into many manufactured foods (e.g. Snackwells), no doubt with the hopes that consumers would not only switch brands but also buy more. To the extent that people have come not only to buy more but also to eat more, whether calories or carbohydrates, the body in effect has accommodated a faster turnover of commodities, helping capital to circulate (Guthman & DuPuis 2006). The marketing of snack foods more generally, also indicted for the rise in obesity, has provided a related fix for agro-food capitalism. Many of the snack foods are made from overproduced crops and thus also help absorb surplus agricultural production (Drewnowski & Specter 2004).

Another way that the food industry has confronted the limits of agro-food profitability is through a trend known as 'substitutionism,' As formulated by Goodman et al. (1987), substitutionism refers to processes that move food production from the farm into factories where food can be produced in more predictable, less risky, and ultimately cheaper ways than it can be on farms. In theorizing substitutionism, Goodman et al. first discussed the substitution of farm commodities that could be grown in temperate rather than tropical zones, such as beet sugar for cane sugar, or corn oil for palm oil. This sort of substitutionism was largely geopolitical, often pursued in the interest of national food security. Substitutionism has also involved substituting farm-based commodities with those that could be further processed or even produced *ab initio* within factory walls. So, for example, margarine was substituted for butter or latex for rubber (an agricultural product if not a food product) to cheapen and industrialize the production of each. Substitutionism then came to play a larger role in facilitating factory-based food processing through the introduction of ever more flavoring additives, preservatives, nutrient fortification, and so forth. In the last few decades, this last sort of substitutionism has been taken to entirely new levels. Chemically derived artificial flavorings substitute for real plant extracts, a range of emulsifiers, gums, and transfats produce the mouth feel that used to come from both plant and animal fats, and chemically altered high fructose corn syrup (HFCS) substitutes for even beet sugar. Substitutionism can make food very cheap – in quality and cost – and thus lends itself to higher margins until competition erodes such margins.

Substitutionism has had all manner of effects on bodies – in ways scientists are just beginning to understand. Margarine, once touted as a healthier alternative to butter, has in more recent years come under attack for containing transfats, associated strongly with heart disease. Transfats are produced as a side effect of partial hydrogenation, itself a process aimed at eliminating rancidity (and thus extending shelf-life) in making vegetable oils into solids. One study found that monkeys that fed transfats gained more weight and visceral fat than control monkeys given non-transfats of the same caloric constitution. They also exhibited heightened insulin resistance (Kavanagh et al., 2007). HFCS, once claimed to be no different than table sugar, is now understood to act quite differently than glucose, the other sugar that comprises sucrose-based sugars. Fructose does not stimulate either leptin or insulin secretion. Therefore, ingesting a particular dose of fructose will produce a less robust insulin response than the same caloric dose of glucose and will insufficiently signal satiety, conceivably encouraging more eating (Power & Schulkin, 2013). Even if not, one study of overweight or obese adults that compared the effects of beverages sweetened with glucose and sucrose found similar overall weight and fat gain, but the group that had consumed the fructose-sweetened drinks had substantially greater increases in the more health-threatening visceral fat than in subcutaneous fat (Stanhope & Havel, 2010). In affecting fat creation, fat disposition, and otherwise interfering with metabolism, substitutionism is effectively altering bodily processes. To the extent that these ingredients only exist to resolve a particular limit to capitalism implicates them in a socio-ecological fix.

As it happens, however, substitutionist ingredients do not only transform bodies through direct transubstantiation (or metabolism). They have been shown to transform them through endocrine disruption and other epigenetic processes which alter developmental pathways by interfering with genetic and, hence, protein expression (Crews & McLachlan, 2006; Krimsky, 2000). Several aspects of food production have been associated with such epigenetic processes, and substances with estrogen-mimicking properties are especially implicated in obesity in a range of studies (Grün & Blumberg, 2009). Soy, for example, is a plant-based estrogen and has been demonstrated to increase the production of fat cells in the offspring of lab animals exposed to it during gestation (Newbold et al., 2008). Soy, it should be noted, is not only a major source of livestock feed but it is also a micro-ingredient in many processed foods. Another study found that certain synthetic food additives have estrogen-mimicking properties (Amadasi et al., 2008). The use of hormones in livestock, several different pesticides, and a number of substances used to transport and contain food, most notably bisphenol A, have also been associated with increased body fat, with these transformations occurring regardless of dietary intake (Grün & Blumberg, 2009). These all suggest additional ways in which the efforts to fix problems of profitability in food production manifest at the site of the body.

At the same time, there are limits to substitutionism as a way to resolve capitalism's obstacles in food production. Too much substitutionism tests the boundaries of food, notwithstanding that the boundaries of what constitutes food are being plied all the time (think algae based shrimp, *in vitro* meat, cricket flour cookies). Many of the limits of what can be substituted for food or in food turn on issues of edibility, digestibility, safety, and the highly important, albeit difficult to quantify 'yuck factor' that makes certain food inventions unacceptable. There are limits to the body as fix as well. At the most basic level, there are limits to how much food any one person can eat, certainly at a sitting and possibly over time. We may not know what those limits are, but we can imagine they exist. And again, to the extent that some products impair bodily functionality, they may limit food consumption as well. In addition to these material limits, obesity-inducing substances find their limit in the social and moral reprobation that fat people are unremittingly subject to as well as the more generalized culture of thinness. This is where the limits create possibilities.

Purging – the body as spatial fix II

What I have suggested thus far is that efforts to overcome the limits of agro-food capital created by Engel's law have resulted in increased body sizes – in the first instance in marketing food that explicitly encourages people to eat more – a more intentional fix and in the second instance through the use of many substances used in food production that inadvertently contribute to obesity through altering insulin response or processes that affect protein synthesis. But, as is patently evident to anyone paying attention, the so-called obesity epidemic is an enormous cultural crisis, if not necessarily a public health crisis, and this too has created new opportunities for accumulation, namely in the form of the myriad diet programs, foods, medications, and surgeries that are bought and sold in the interest of weight loss. And these are sold not only to those who are evidently fat but also to those who feel themselves too fat owing to the constant drumbeat of an obesity crisis (Campos 2004).

It is well established that the diet industry is enormously profitable (Austin, 1999; Fraser 1998). What is less known is the role that industry itself plays in hyping an obesity epidemic. A great deal of obesity research is sponsored by the International Obesity Task Force, itself funded by the pharmaceutical industry (Saguy & Riley, 2005). Such investment in research is founded on the expectation that the research will result in effective, reasonably safe, and profitable drugs to 'cure' obesity. Owing to the ways that selling drugs and other weight loss programs have become a fix to the limit imposed by the construction of obesity as a problem, the entire phenomenon can be seen as a political and cultural economy of bulimia (Guthman & DuPuis, 2006).

Here again, the more interesting fix is through other substitutionist products: food products that are lower in calories (or fats or carbohydrates) than their counterparts are designed to defy metabolism altogether, by, for example, engineering ingredients to inhibit absorption and utilization of fats and carbohydrates (Scrinis, 2013). Of those that substitute for fat, the most noted of these have included Simplesse, an egg, and dairy whey protein product used as a low calorie fat substitute in low-calorie food; Z-Trim, which is made from the hulls of oats, peas, soybeans, and rice, or bran from corn or wheat, and thus not only reduces calories but as fiber is not digested; and Olestra, a substance similar to fat in terms of molecular structure to provide 'mouth-feel' of fat but in is 'bulkiness' is not digested and absorbed by the body at all. Substitutes for sugar include Splenda which contains sucralose, a 'zero-calorie' artificial sweetener that is not broken down by the body, in addition to aspartame, saccharin, and other 'zero-calorie' sweeteners. Using several such ingredients, Walden Farms is a manufacturer that offers a range of zero-calorie foods that ostensibly contain no calories, fats, carbohydrates, or sugars – including dressings, sauces, and even peanut spread! Many of these are designed to break right through the problem of inelastic demand enshrined in Engel's Law. The commodity simply passes through enabling the product to be consumed with no weight-gaining effect, at least allegedly. Some of the new pharmaceuticals (e.g., Xenical) and nutritional supplements (e.g., garcinia cambogia, derived from tamarind) are designed to reduce the body's absorption of fat and thus fulfill a similar function.

However, as with some of the substitutionist products that are unwittingly obesogenic, it may be the case that these substances do not actually have these intended effects. One possible reason is that calories may not be a good indicator of how the body transubstantiates food. Calories, after all, are fictive. They are not molecules found as constituents of food but only come into being through the literal burning of food, derived from the early experiments of Atwater and his 'bomb calorimeter' (Mudry, 2009). So, at best, calories are an approximation of energy intake, and not all energy taken in is necessarily absorbed (Prentice, 1995). Moreover, it appears that the key mechanism in the actual production of fat is insulin response, not caloric intake (Taubes, 2007). That being the case, zero calorie diet sodas may actually be contributing to weight gain by instigating an insulin response (Power & Schulkin, 2013). So, while diet foods may do well as a socio-ecological fix for capital in terms of commodities they sell, their efficacy in regard to their intended effects is questionable.

Of course, there are other kinds of limits to these fixes, too, because they do act with less than salubrious effects. Olestra, for example, dissolves other fat-soluble substances, including vitamins A, D, E, and K and thus depletes bodies of these essential vitamins. In addition, there are undesirable side effects such as diarrhea, abdominal cramping, and anal leakage. Sucralose, according to one study, reduces the amount of good bacteria in the intestines, increases the pH level in the intestines, and affects a glycoprotein in that can counteract the benefits of certain medications (Abou-Donia et al., 2008). Other artificial sweeteners, notably Aspartame, have been associated with carcinogenesis (Whitehouse et al., 2008). The bodily degradation caused by these fixes may not be amenable to medicalized and commodified cures, at least at this point in history.

In sum, agro-food capital faces recurring crises of profitability, much having to do with over-production of crops and limited demand for food, given Engel's Law. Yet, it appears that both efforts to sell more debilitated food, as well as efforts to sell thinness as socio-ecological fixes to these crises, have their limits, as well, as many products being sold severely compromise bodily function. So, there may be limits to these fixes. Nevertheless, to the extent that human bodies are bearing the burden of capitalism's necessity to fix its perennial crises through less salubrious fixes, we might ask ourselves exactly what is unhealthy.

References

Abou-Donia, M. B., El-Masry, E. M., Abdel-Rahman, A. A., McLendon, R. E. & Schiffman, S.S. (2008). Splenda alters gut microflora and increases intestinal p-glycoprotein and cytochrome p-450 in male rats. *Journal of Toxicology and Environmental Health, Part A,* 71(21), 1415–1429. https://doi.org/10.1080/15287390802328630

Amadasi, A., Mozzarelli, A., Meda, C., Maggi, A. & Cozzini, P. (2008). Identification of xenoestrogens in food additives by an integrated in silico and in vitro approach. *Chemical Research in Toxicology,* 22(1), 52–63. https://doi.org/10.1021/tx800048m

Austin, S. B. (1999). Commodity knowledge in consumer culture: The role of nutritional health promotion in the making of the diet industry. In J. Sobal and D. Maurer (Eds.) *Weighty issues: Fatness and thinness as social problems* (pp. 159–181). Aldine De Gruyer.

Bakker, I. (2007). Social reproduction and the constitution of a gendered political economy. *New Political Economy,* 12(4), 541–556. https://doi.org/10.1080/13563460701661561

Campos, P. (2004). *The obesity myth: Why America's obsession with weight is hazardous to your health.* Gotham Press.

Cochrane, W. W. (1993). *The development of American agriculture.* University of Minnesota Press.

Cooper, M. (2008). *Life As surplus: Biotechnology and capitalism in the neoliberal era.* University of Washington Press.

Crews, D. & McLachlan, J. A. (2006). Epigenetics, evolution, endocrine disruption, health, and disease. *Endocrinology,* 147(6), s4–10. doi.10.1210/en.2005-1122

Drewnowski, A. & Specter, S. (2004). Poverty and obesity: The role of energy density and energy costs. *American Journal of Clinical Nutrition,* 79, 6–16. https://doi.org/10.1093/ajcn/79.1.6

Ekers, M. & Prudham, S. (2015). Towards the socio-ecological fix. *Environment and Planning A: Economy and Space,* 47(12), 2438–2445. https://doi.org/10.1177/0308518X15617573

Fine, B. (1994). Towards a political economy of food. *Review of International Political Economy,* 1(3), 519–545. https://doi.org/10.1080/09692299408434297

Fraser, L. (1998). *Losing it: False hopes and fat profits in the diet industry.* Penguin.

Gard, M. & Wright, J. (2005). *The obesity epidemic: Science, morality, and ideology.* Routledge.

Goodman, D., Sorj, B. & Wilkinson, J. (1987). *From farming to biotechnology.* Basil Blackwell.

Grün, F. & Blumberg, B. (2009). Minireview: The case for obesogens. *Molecular Endocrinology,* 23(8), 1127–1134.

Guptill, A. & Wilkins, J. (2002). Buying into the food system: Trends in food retailing in the US and implications for local foods. *Agriculture and Human Values,* 19(1), 39–51. https://doi.org/10.1023/A:1015024827047

Guthman, J. & DuPuis, E. M. (2006). Embodying neoliberalism: Economy, culture, and the politics of fat. *Environment and Planning D: Society and Space,* 24(3), 427–448. https://doi.org/10.1068/d3904

Harvey, D. (1982). *Limits to capital.* University of Chicago.

Harvey, D. (1996). *Justice, nature, and the geography of difference.* Blackwell.

Harvey, D. (2010). *The enigma of capital and the crisis of capitalism.* Oxford University Press.

Harvey, D. & Haraway, D. (1995). Nature, politics, and possibilities: A debate and discussion with David Harvey and Donna Haraway. *Environment and Planning D: Society and Space,* 13(5), 507–527.

Katz, C. (1998). Whose nature, whose culture: Private productions of space and the 'preservation' of nature. In N. Castree, N. & Willems-Braun (Eds.), *Nature at the end of the millennium: Remaking reality and the end of the twentieth century* (pp. 46–63). Routledge.

Kavanagh, K., Jones, K. L., Sawyer, J., Kelley, K., Carr, J. J., Wagner, J. D. & Rudel. L. L. (2007). Trans fat diet induces abdominal obesity and changes in insulin sensitivity in monkeys. *Obesity,* 15(7), 1675–1684. https://doi.org/10.1038/oby.2007.200

Krimsky, S. (2000). *Hormonal chaos: The scientific and social origins of the environmental endocrine hypothesis.* Johns Hopkins University Press.

Laslett, B. & Brenner, J. (1989). Gender and social reproduction: Historical perspectives. *Annual Review of Sociology,* 15, 381–404. https://doi.org/10.1146/annurev.so.15.080189.002121

Levenstein, H. A. (1988). *Revolution at the table: The transformation of the American diet.* Oxford University Press.

Mann, S. A. (1989). *Agrarian capitalism in theory and practice.* University of North Carolina Press.

Moore, J. W. (2015). *Capitalism in the web of life: Ecology and the accumulation of capital.* Verso Books.

Mudry, J. J. (2009). *Measured meals: Nutrition in America.* SUNY Press.

Nestle, M. (2002). *Food politics: How the food industry influences nutrition and health.* University of California Press.

Newbold, R. R., Padilla-Banks, E., Jefferson, W. N. & Heindel, J. J. (2008). Effects of endocrine disruptors on obesity. *International Journal of Andrology,* 31, 201–208. https://doi.org/10.1111/j.1365-2605.2007.00858.x

O'Connor, J. (1989). Capitalism, nature, socialism: A theoretical introduction. *Capitalism, Nature, Socialism,* 1(1), 11–38. https://doi.org/10.1080/10455758809358356

Power, M. L. & Schulkin, J. (2013). *The evolution of obesity.* Johns Hopkins University.

Prentice, A. M. (1995). Are all calories equal? In R. Cottrell (Ed.) *Weight Control* (pp. 8–33). Springer.

Saguy, A. C. & Riley, K. W. (2005). Weighing both sides: Morality, mortality, and framing contests over obesity. *Journal of Health Politics, Policy and law,* 30(5), 869–923. https://doi.org/10.1215/03616878-30-5-869

Scrinis, G. (2013). *Nutritionism: The science and politics of dietary advice.* Columbia University Press.

Stanhope, K. L. & Havel, P. J. (2010). Fructose consumption: Recent results and their potential implications. *Annals of the New York Academy of Sciences, 1190,* 15–24. https://doi.org/10.1111/j.1749-6632.2009.05266.x

Taubes, G. (2007). *Good calories, bad calories: Fats, carbs, and the controversial science of diet and health.* Anchor.

Whitehouse, C. R., Boullata, J. & McCauley, L. A. (2008). The potential toxicity of artificial sweeteners. *Aaohn Journal,* 56(6), 251–261. https://doi.org/10.1177/216507990805600604

Winders, B. (2009). *The politics of food supply: U.S. agricultural policy in the world economy.* Yale University Press.

15

ENCOUNTERING 'HEALTHY' FOOD IN MEXICAN SCHOOLS

José Tenorio

Schools as gastro-political spaces

In 2006, the results of the National Health and Nutrition Survey 2006 (ENSANUT 2006) reported that Mexicans, particularly women and children, had considerably increased their body weight since the late 1980s (Olaiz-Fernández et al., 2006). This report positioned obesity as a burning public health problem resulting from an "imbalance" between "energy intake"—food and calories—and "energy expenditure"—physical activity—(Olaiz-Fernández et al., 2006, p. 85). Since then, various organisations have proposed and launched "urgent" responses to the so-called problem. Underpinned by the energy balance idea, these responses have sought to 'educate' people to eat 'healthy' food and to be more physically active. Similar to the global trend (Story, Nanney, & Schwartz, 2009), schools in Mexico have been depicted as the space to promote healthy eating *par excellence* (Safdie et al., 2013) for their capacity to bring people together and their alleged educational nature (for a critique, see Gard & Pluim, 2014).

For this reason, after the discussion of myriad policy proposals to change eating habits in and through schools (Orozco-Gómez, 2007; Sosa-Govea & Moreno-Valle, 2008), in 2010, the Mexican government released the *Guidelines 2010*, a national policy to regulate food in schools. Through the same years, food corporations launched a variety of school-based programs promoting 'healthy' eating through the primary education curriculum (Plazas, 2010). Simultaneously, non-government organisations (NGOs) started to lobby for banning "junk food" from schools (Fuentes, 2007). With slight differences, these strategies either ask teachers to teach students to make informed food choices or regulate the practices of cooking, selling food and eating in schools with the purpose of offering the 'healthiest' possible food options to students (Gerardo Rodríguez, 2010).

Promoting healthy eating in schools has been seen as a sound strategy against obesity because these spaces are considered to be part of the problem. In line with the global obesity discussion (Swinburn, Egger, & Raza, 1999), for instance, schools in Mexico have been depicted as "obesogenic environments", because they facilitate the conditions for children to gain body weight, mainly, due to the high amounts of 'junk food'—a problematic category that is used to narrowly encompass foods rich in fats and sugars—that are available to, and consumed by, students in these spaces (*Agreement, 2010; Strategy, 2013*).

DOI: 10.4324/9780429344824-19

The idea that what is prepared, sold and eaten in schools can be classified as healthy or unhealthy and regulated in the name of 'fighting' obesity rests upon the assumption that food is, above all, nutrients, calories and energy with specific biological functions. This idea is significantly influenced by a reductionist nutritional perspective, or what Scrinis (2013, p. 2) calls "nutritionism", an approach to food characterised by a focus on nutritional and biological dimensions of foods and by a "reductive *interpretation* of the role" of nutrients in health [original emphasis]. As someone who has worked and done research in schools in Mexico for about ten years, I acknowledge that some of the foods offered in these spaces are, from a strictly nutritional point of view, not always the ideal. However, from these experiences, I also learned that, far from being an exclusively nutritional object, food in Mexican schools plays multiple, many times competing, roles, a fact that is commonly overlooked in the making of healthy eating strategies.

Through the discussion of a series of observations while food was being produced, sold and eaten in two public primary schools located in the central region of the state of Veracruz, Mexico and with interviews with diverse actors involved in these processes[1], in this chapter, I show the tensions between the nutritionist understanding of food underpinning healthy eating initiatives and the day-to-day practices and meanings associated around food in schools. Following Appadurai's (1981, p. 494) conceptualisation of food as a "highly condensed social fact" and a "marvelously plastic kind of collective representations", I argue that food in Mexican schools is more than a simple form of 'energy' that is always there, waiting to be consumed. As a social fact, for instance, food is produced across diverse spaces and the integration of practices. Ingredients do not appear in schools magically; either cooks or teachers themselves source them from a range of local stores or warehouse-format supermarkets, which many times is done under a tight budget.

Drawing on this broader understanding of how food become to exist, I show how food options in these schools are not determined by public health guidelines but shaped by culture, taste and, notably, the economy. For this endeavour, I also draw on Appadurai's (1981) notion of gastro-politics—understood as the cultural and economic competitions that emerge as food is produced and eaten—to explore the multiple and competing roles that food plays in schools. To complement my analysis, I draw on Solomon's (2016)—who has combined gastro-politics and political geography to discuss the political and economic contests that take place as street food in Mumbai is made object of public health regulations—elaborations to argue that rather than as 'obesogenic environments' schools need to be seen as complex gastro-political spaces, where food is in constant tension with what many times are culturally, politically and economically decontextualised public health goals.

In what follows, I, first, use short fieldwork stories to describe the broad contexts surrounding the schools to illustrate the intrinsic relationship between what I refer to as school food practices and the Mexican economy, 'state education policies' for government policies and local cultural traditions. Second, focusing on the multiple meanings that food acquires and is assigned as it is prepared, I discuss how the healthy/unhealthy classification of food has opened space for the stigmatisation of meals that are culturally significant and, more importantly, economically viable for schools. Then, I show how the language used by cooks in one school to speak about food competes against the technical language underpinning regulatory strategies. I end this chapter claiming that a broader perspective on food, and its relation to health, needs to be considered anti-obesity strategies are to really address any of the negative effects that free-market policies have had on the health of the Mexican population (Chavez, 2002; Clark et al., 2012; Gálvez, 2018; Otero, 2011; Reardon & Berdegué, 2002; Wise, 2009).

Food in schools: between culture, needs and health

On a hot morning in April 2016, I drove from Veracruz City to Santa Rosa, the small town where Emiliano Zapata Primary School[2] is located. The route follows 25 kilometres of highway and 15 kilometres of an entertaining backroad covered in speed bumps. After exiting the highway, a child and an adult were next to a speed bump selling bundles of white fishes recently caught in the river behind us. Ahead, food in multiple forms was found at almost every speed bump. Makeshift stalls provided shade for people selling small plastic bags with fresh coconut meat, peeled sugar canes, bottled water and sugary drinks among other products. I arrived at Emiliano Zapata Primary School at around 9 am. I went to the kitchen, where Martha, Beatriz, Moni and Angela, the four school cooks, were industriously cooking *tostadas* (handmade and deep-fried tortillas topped with black beans, lettuce, cheese, cream and *salsa*). At 10:30 am, students stormed into the kitchen through the front door, lining up behind the plastic table. "*¡Tostadas!*", one student shouted delightedly. Knowing that, for some kids, the *tostadas* were their first, and perhaps only, meal of the day, Beatriz served as many *tostadas* as the students asked for. With their *tostadas* and cheerful faces, students went through the rear door to a covered patio with corrugated roofing being used for dining. About half of the student population had the school meal. The rest received food through the school fence near the dining area. Similar to the foods on offer from the school kitchen, with a few exceptions, most of the students received meals made out of *masa* [corn dough], a vital food for many Mexicans.

The next day, I went to Benito Juárez Primary School, located in Paso de Leones, a suburb in Veracruz City's metropolitan area. During my 30-minute bus ride from my place to Paso de Leones, I observed indigenous women sold candies, teenagers cleaned windscreens and children offered freshly squeezed orange juice in plastic bags at traffic lights. At about 8:30 am, I arrived at the school and went to the kitchen. Elena, the school kitchen's manager and her employees were making *empanadas* (deep-fried pockets of *masa* stuffed with cheese) and a bunch of handmade tortillas to be used in *quesadillas* (a folded tortilla filled with cheese). She grabbed a piece of *masa* and said, "I also add plantain to the *masa*, so the meals on offer are not only *masa*-based, but they also contain a fruit". To convince me of the quality, taste and nutritious content of her foods, Elena offered me a product. I chose a *quesadilla*. She personally grabbed one of the tortillas being kept warm under a cloth, put it on the griddle, added shredded Oaxaca cheese on top and then folded the tortilla. "This is how we prepare *quesadillas*. No fat is added", Elena claimed proudly.

Multiple forms of *masa* and fats[3] of different kinds have been central ingredients in Mexican's day-to-day cooking and eating practices. A study of food consumption in 1970s Mexico, for example, showed that products made out *masa*, lard and vegetable oil were among the most-consumed food products among a large segment of the population (Lustig, 1980). The preference for these foods prevailed in Emiliano Zapata and Benito Juárez primary schools and around in the broader contexts where they were located. From a cultural point of view, for example, Emiliano Zapata Primary School's principal, Andrés, who had worked in the school for more than 10 years and lived in a nearby town, considered that people in town "love" *masa*-based foods because they are "a tradition, a deeply rooted eating habit". Beyond its cultural roots, however, the students' affinity for *masa*-based foods can also be explained, as Andrés remarked, by their energetic contribution to, or their utility in, students' diets. "If our little kids don't have foods with the basic ingredients—*masa*, *salsa*, cheese and beans—during the school breakfast, they will be hungry and asking for food at noon".

However, in the midst of the 'fight' against obesity in Mexico, the relevance of *masa* and fats, and its derived foods, in Mexican's diets has become contentious. From the bio-logically reductionist perspective that constructs food exclusively as nutrients and calories, *masa*-based meals such as *tostadas*, *empanadas* and *quesadillas* are seen as nutritionally unhealthy products which negatively impact students' health and body weight and therefore have to be banned from schools (García-García et al., 2008; Treviño Ronzón & Sánchez Pacheco, 2014). This reflects the tensions between the nutritional advice encouraging students to eat 'healthy' and the centrality of *masa* and fats in the particular context of these schools and their communities.

The nutritious content of foods that combine *masa* and fats has been questioned to a point where their consumption has been stigmatised by people within the school communities. Some of the teachers I interviewed, for instance, included homemade *masa*-based foods in the 'junk food' category, together with ultra-processed products such as chips, cookies and candies. For example, Carla, a young teacher at Benito Juárez Primary School, constantly spoke of homemade *masa*-based foods and junk food as synonyms. From her perspective, kitchen offered only "unhealthy" foods, but she justified this issue because these foods were convenient and profitable.

Convenient and profitable, but inconveniently 'unhealthy'

The above stories show that the place and functions of food within Mexican society are rather complex. Beyond its cultural significance, food in Mexico has a central role in the economy. Bakić Hayden (2014), Long-Solís (2007) and Roever (2010), for instance, have shown that the market-oriented economic policies launched from the 1990s have considerably increased the size of the informal economy, making many people reliant on street food selling. The food stalls and the people selling food along my trips to the schools are an example of how families who were excluded from the 'formal' economy, make a living. In a similar way, the preparation and sale of food in schools also represent a source of income for multiple families. In Benito Juárez Primary School, for example, the kitchen was run privately by Elena and her husband, who employed two more women as cooks. The provision of food to students in Emiliano Zapata Primary School followed a cooperative mode, under which the price for each breakfast was only intended to cover expenses, but still the four cooks received a salary.

The local economy also had a significant role in shaping food in schools. Beyond culture, the preference of cooks to prepare and students to consume *masa*-based foods was significantly shaped by the prices of ingredients, the convenience of foods and families' economies. For example, many of the people that I interviewed coincided that there is not cheaper and tastier food to students in Emiliano Zapata and Benito Juárez primary schools than *empanadas*, *tostadas* and *quesadillas*. These foods were by far the preferred option of most of the members of both schools. However, this food preference also embodied a socioeco-nomic dimension. As Andrés mentioned, "*masa*-based foods, together with *salsas* and beans" were widely and frequently consumed by children from worse-off families because they "are cheap ingredients". This association between *masa* consumption and social class distinction was further reinforced by teachers in both schools.

Unlike teachers in Emiliano Zapata Primary School, whom almost all had a high appre-ciation for the cultural and economic significance of *masa*-based foods in the community, most of the school staff at Benito Juárez Primary School had low esteem for them. Like Carla, Susana, the school's principal, also considered that all *masa*-based foods were "unhealthy" and also justified the presence of these products because they were the students' preference and profitable, both for Elena and for the school. Elena paid a daily share for the right to operate the school kitchen. The school used this income to pay for multiple expenses that were not covered by government funding. However, there was also controversy among the school staff about who benefited more from food sales, Elena or the school. As one teacher put it during our interview, "I cook, and I know that cooking with *masa* is very profitable!", implying that Elena was gaining more.

Through my research, I perceived that the association of *masa*-based foods as 'junk food' had been positioned in schools through multiple healthy eating strategies implemented since 2010. Emiliano Zapata and Benito Juárez primary schools, for example, had been trying to incorporate the *Guidelines 2010* to change the eating habits of students. Also, these two schools had participated in SUMA-Nutrir, a healthy eating program launched jointly by local education authorities and Nestlé, the global food corporation. Through this policy and program, schools were constantly reminded about the need of avoiding *masa*-based foods to curb the energy intake of students in schools. Nevertheless, the accessible price of these foods, their energetic content and their cultural significance contested the energy balance hypothesis. This premise assumes that food, or 'energy in', is already *there*, available for people to consume it. Therefore, under the simplistic energy balance equation, people can be held responsible for either not choosing the 'right' food or for not expending enough energy.

However, students' affection for *masa*-based in Benito Juárez and Emiliano Zapata primary schools tells us that the kind of energy consumed is not always a choice, but a need that is culturally and, of course, economically shaped. Also, as I spoke to people, particularly cooks, in the schools, I noticed that they barely assigned the healthy category to food. The language, for example, that cooks used with food differed vastly from the language made material in policy documents. In their own way, cooks were also conscious of the adverse effects that frequent, high consumption of fats represents for human health. Therefore, instead of quantifying portions or counting calories, they drew on their own cooking knowledges acquired during years to procure students' health.

Food as a collective representation

In Emiliano Zapata Primary School, no one was more aware of the students' fondness for *masa*-based foods than the women who devoted their lives to satisfying stomachs that craved the perfect combination of *masa* and fats. Martha, Beatriz, Moni and Angela knew perfectly that students loved *masa*-based foods, and they prided themselves on satisfying this desire. Paradoxically, while all the school foods were made from scratch and involved hard work, the preparation of *empanadas*, *tostadas* or *quesadillas* demanded even more. For the cooks, this posed no problem. Indeed, they happily engaged in the production of labour-intense *masa*-foods because, in their own words, cooking what students liked was their form of expressing care. This can be read more vividly in the cooks' own words. During one of our conversations, I asked what their main challenges had been while cooking. They responded:

BEATRIZ: What has been most difficult for us is when we have to prepare *masa*-based foods
MONI: And that is what children like the most!
BEATRIZ: And what they eat most of!
MONI: What the kids eat most of!
BEATRIZ: And what they waste the least... because the students like *masa*-based foods, they eat everything and there isn't any food waste... But when we cook spaghetti or

something like that, there's more food waste, because many children fill their plates but do not eat much. However, when *masa*-based foods are served they do not waste them!

MONI: Like today, we had *empanadas* and the waste was minimal.

JOSÉ: So, children do not waste *masa*-based foods ...

MONI: *Enchiladas, empanadas, picadas, tostadas* ...

JOSÉ: All the *masa*-based foods.

BEATRIZ: Yes, exactly.

MARTHA: All the foods prepared with *masa*.

To gain the cooks' insights into the nutritional value of these foods, however, I asked them whether all the *masa*-based foods had to be fried and whether they were 'healthy'. Martha answered that sometimes they cooked *masa*-based foods too often and added lard, which was not "healthy". Therefore, if the school's finances could afford it, they tried to make *masa*-based foods no more than three days a week. Retaliating, Beatriz said that only *empanadas* and *tostadas* were deep-fried, but that in other foods, only "a little bit of lard" was added to give foods more "flavour!".

In Mexico, the consumption of vegetable oil, a form of fats, has increased steadily since the 1950s. In a country where a large section of the population used lard in food preparation, advertising played a central role to transform this practice particularly through pushing the idea that vegetable oil was a 'healthier' option—still debatable (see Scrinis, 2013; Willet, 1994, e.g.)—and a product that was 'classier' than lard (Aguilar-Rodríguez, 2009). From the mid-1990s, the agribusiness transformations introduced by the North American Free Trade Agreement have also helped to increase the availability and consumption in Mexico of vegetable oil produced in the United States (Torres-Torres and Aguilar-Ortega, 2003; Yunez-Naude and Barceinas, 2002). However, in spite of these changes, the use of lard has remained a common practice among cooks to potentiate flavours.

In the strategies regulating food in schools in the name of health, people, specifically women, who cook are presented as de-politicised and mostly passive subjects who lack the skills required to prepare 'healthy' food. However, cooks in schools are the owners of cooking knowledges that enable them to prepare tasty food under a tight budget and, at the same time, also take care of students' health. One day in Emiliano Zapata Primary School, for example, I observed Beatriz poking tortillas with a toothpick. Intrigued by this unknown technique, I asked why she made the holes. "If we don't puncture the tortillas, they absorb more oil when they're fried", she answered. Martha organised the punctured tortillas in pairs, threw a piece of *masa* into the large, shallow metal frying pan of oil. Bubbles rose around the small piece of *masa*, which meant the oil temperature was right. Martha submerged the first two tortillas, spreading oil around them with a slotted metal spoon. Less than a minute later, she removed the deep-fried tortillas from the frying pan and stood them vertically over a metal bowl with holes at the bottom.

The four cooks never talked about food in any term associated to health. I can say that they were, instead, guided by an understanding of food from where cooking was seen as the process through which an expression of care materialised in an edible object. Knowing that ingredients were scarce, for example, the cooks at Emiliano Zapata Primary School cautiously used them in cooking, trying to make the most out of them. However, when it came to pleasing the students' stomachs, they never minded giving more than was stipulated, in the 'rules' or the budget. Similarly, the cooks considered that hand-making complex, tasty foods was a form to express care for the students. "I think we have given our best... we care for the kids", Beatriz emphasised, when I asked what could be done for children to access 'healthier' food at school. "We have given our best", Martha seconded. "Many times, we even make *miracles!*". Every single day during my fieldwork, I witnessed miracles being achieved in the kitchen. There were never enough ingredients, but the cooks always made miracles.

The competing economic, political and cultural roles that food has in Mexican schools, I argue, show the inoperability of an understanding of food that has been proposed in school food regulations. One explanation for this, though simplistic, would be that, in some schools and their communities, the economic dimension of food is so strong that simply telling them to eat 'healthy' without actually doing broader actions to enable the access to food, becomes empty words. However, with this idea, I am diminishing both the agency of the various actors and the positive contributions that healthy eating strategies can have in schools. Therefore, I prefer to stand by the idea that the cooks integrated into their practice something from the myriad programs they have been exposed to. But they did so by adapting them to their own needs and for the students' benefit. While it appears to be a romantic language that contradicts, or diminishes, public health goals, I consider that the language used by cooks and other women that I talked to as part of my research, needs to be listened if more contextually informed healthy eating strategies are to be developed.

School food and obesity: a broader perspective

As part of the research supporting this chapter, I also interviewed people in Mexico City whose voices have been heard in the obesity discussion. I wanted to grasp why and how schools had been positioned both as part of the problem of, and as a solution to, obesity. Based on his more than 20 years as a nutrition researcher at a national health research institute, Dr Gómez told me during our interview that food sales in Mexican schools are a "model of the free market", where students can buy as much food as their budget allows. In a more direct link between school food and obesity, Ernesto, the director of the non-governernment organisation (NGO) Obesity Coalition, considered that Mexicans schools were "factories for obese people". Adolfo, the director of the NGO Obesity Action, claimed that schools are "closed", "controled", spaces where kids spend long hours, which make them "fundamental" places to promote healthier diets.

To expand the conversation, however, in this chapter, I proposed an analysis that pays attention to the cultural, economic and political dimensions of food (Appadurai, 1986; Solomon, 2016) to argue that food in Mexican schools cannot be reduced to a quantifiable biological object that needs to be regulated to achieve health. Therefore, the idea that schools are, at the same time, "factories for obese people" and the spaces to 'fight' obesity par excellence, I suggest, needs to be reconsidered and critically debated (Gard & Pluim, 2014). The fieldwork stories offered above contradict, or at least open space to debate, the conceptions that policymakers have about the food practices in schools and their relation to health, showing the tensions between ideas. Through showing how food is cooked, sold and eaten in schools, I challenged the dominant narrative that blames teachers and families for their unwillingness to make students to adopt a healthy diet. Mexican schools, as Adolfo suggested, are physically delimited by either fences or walls, depending on what a school can afford. Yet, far from being "closed and controlled", they are porous gastro-political spaces where discourses and material objects flow outwards and inwards. Schools are the point of encounter between the broader political project of the state and corporations, the beliefs and knowledges of the school staff and the private and intimate life of families.

Nothing exemplifies this better than teachers', parents', students' and cooks' practices around food. When a lunchbox or a plastic bag with homemade food is brought inside the school, a whole system of household ideas regarding food and cooking crosses the school's physical boundaries. Corporations penetrate the life of schools through material discourses, such as Nestlé's program SUMA-Nutrir, which display their perspectives on how to eat 'healthy'. The state made its way into the community's, families' and students' lives through curriculum content and policies like the *Guidelines 2010*. Mothers' cooking knowledges enter schools to compete with the ideas about 'nutrition' and 'health' presented within the materials of national curriculum and health-promotion programs. This is the complexity that should be considered when trying to develop any policy or program to promote 'healthy' eating. In their making, therefore, food needs to be seen as a politically, economically and culturally shaped artefact that takes multiple, many times competing, forms as it is produced, sold and eaten.

Notes

1 This chapter is part of a broader research project conducted as part of my doctoral training, funded by the Australian Research Council Discovery Project: DP140102607. More methodological details about this research can be found in the thesis entitled, "Cooking 'healthy lifestyles' as a *dispositif*: Obesity policies, school food politics and corporations in neoliberal Mexico".
2 The names of people, places and organisations have been changed for anonymity purposes. In Mexico, the majority of public schools are named after famous personages in Mexican history. I have followed this same pattern to choose a name for the schools that were part of my research.
3 Fats is a complex term. My use here refers to vegetable oil and lard.

References

Aguilar-Rodríguez, S. (2009). La mesa está servida: Comida y vida cotidiana en el México de mediados del siglo XX [The table is served: Food and daily life in mid-twentieth century Mexico]. *HIB: Revista de Historia Iberoamericana, 2*(2), 52–85.

Agreement 2010, (Acuerdo Nacional para la Salud Alimentaria. Estrategia contra el Sobrepeso y la Obesidad [National Agreement for Nutritional Health. Strategy against overweight and obesity]), Secretaría de Salud, México (2010).

Appadurai, A. (1981). Gastro-politics in Hindu South Asia. *American Ethnologist, 8*(3), 494–511.

Bakić Hayden, T. (2014). The taste of precarity: Language, legitimacy, and legality among Mexican street food vendors. In R. D. C. Vieira Cardoso, M. Companion, & S. R. Marras (Eds.), *Street food: Culture, economy, health and governance* (pp. 83–98). London: Routledge.

Chavez, M. (2002). The transformation of Mexican retailing with NAFTA. *Development Policy Review, 20*(4), 503–513. https://doi.org/10.1111/1467-7679.00186

Clark, S. E., Hawkes, C., Murphy, S. M. E., Hansen-Kuhn, K. A., & Wallinga, D. (2012). Exporting obesity: US farm and trade policy and the transformation of the Mexican consumer food environment. *International Journal of Occupational and Environmental Health, 18*(1), 53–64. https://doi.org/10.1179/1077352512Z.0000000007

Fuentes, F. (2007, June 22). Fundación Mídete inicia guerra contra obesidad [Mídete Foundation starts war against obesity]. *El Universal*. Retrieved from https://archivo.eluniversal.com.mx/articulos/40853.html

Gálvez, A. (2018). *Eating NAFTA: Trade, food policies, and the destruction of Mexico*. Oakland: University of California Press.

García-García, E., De la Lata-Romero, M., Kaufer-Horwitz, M., Tusié-Luna, M. T., Calzada-León, R., Vázquez-Velázquez, V., … Sotelo-Morales, J. (2008). La obesidad y el síndrome metabólico como problema de salud pública. Una reflexión [Obesity and metabolic syndrome as public health problems. A reflection]. *Salud Pública de México, 50*(6), 530–547. Retrieved from https://www.scielosp.org/article/spm/2008.v50n6/530-547/

Gard, M., & Pluim, C. (2014). *Schools and public health. Past, present and future.* Plymouth: Lexington Books.

Gerardo Rodríguez, P. (2010). La nueva fábula de las abejas. En torno a la regulación de los alimentos chatarra en las escuelas [The new fable of the bees. A discussion on the regulation of junk food in schools]. *Revista Latinoamericana de Estudios Educativos, 40*(3), 9–54.

Guidelines 2010, (Acuerdo mediante el cual se establecen los lineamientos generales para el expendio o distribución de alimentos y bebidas en los establecimientos de consumo escolar de los planteles de educación básica [General Guidelines for the Distribution or Sales of Food and Drinks by Retailers within Basic Education Schools]), Diario Oficial de la Federación: Órgano del Gobierno Constitucional de los Estados Unidos Mexicanos 1–28.

Long-Solís, J. (2007). A survey of street foods in Mexico City. *Food and Foodways, 15*(3–4), 213–236. https://doi.org/10.1080/07409710701620136

Lustig, N. (1980). Distribución del ingreso y consumo de alimentos en México [Income distribution and food consumption in Mexico]. *Demografía y economía, 14*(2), 214–245. Retrieved from http://www.jstor.org/stable/40602232

Olaiz-Fernández, G., Rivera-Dommarco, J., Shamah-Levy, T., Rojas, R., Villalpando-Hernández, S., Hernández-Avila, M., & Sepúlveda-Amor, J. (2006). Encuesta Nacional de Salud y Nutrición 2006 [2006 Mexican National Health and Nutrition Survey]. Cuernavaca, México: Instituto Nacional de Salud Pública.

Orozco-Gómez, J. (2007). *Proyecto de decreto por el que se reforman diversas disposiciones de la Ley General de Salud y de la Ley General de Educación. [Proposal to reform the Health General Law and the Education General Law].* Senado de la República, October 16, 2007. Gaceta del Senado LX/2PPO-136/14273. Retrieved from https://www.senado.gob.mx/64/gaceta_del_senado/documento/14273

Otero, G. (2011). Neoliberal globalization, NAFTA, and migration: Mexico's loss of food and labor sovereignty. *Journal of Poverty, 15*(4), 384–402.

Plazas, M. (2010). Juego y Comida dan salud a tu vida [Eat and Play make you healthy]. *Revista Latinoamericana de Estudios Educativos, 40*(2), 153–164.

Reardon, T., & Berdegué, J. A. (2002). The rapid rise of supermarkets in Latin America: Challenges and opportunities for development. *Development Policy Review, 20*(4), 371–388. https://doi.org/10.1111/1467-7679.00178

Roever, S. (2010). Street trade in Latin America: Demographic trends, legal issues and vending organisations in six cities. In S. Bhowmik (Ed.), *Street vendors in the Global Urban Economy* (pp. 208–241). New Delhi: Routledge.

Safdie, M., Jennings-Aburto, N., Levesque, L., Janssen, I., Campirano-Nunez, F., Lopez-Olmedo, N., … Rivera, J. A. (2013). Impact of a school-based intervention program on obesity risk factors in Mexican children. *Salud Pública de México, 55*(3), 374–387.

Scrinis, G. (2013). *Nutritionism: The science and politics of dietary advice.* New York: Columbia University Press.

Solomon, H. (2016). *Metabolic living, food, fat, and the absorption of illness in India.* Durham, NC: Duke University Press.

Sosa-Govea, M., & Moreno-Valle, R. (2008). *Proyecto de decreto por el que se reforman y adicionan diversas disposiciones de la Ley para la Protección de los Derechos de Niñas, Niños y Adolescentes; de la Ley General de Educación y de la Ley General de Salud. [Project to reform different dispositions in the Law to Protect the Rigths of Children and Adolescents; in the General Education Law and in the General Health Law].* Senado de la República, November 11 2008. Gaceta del Senado LX/3PPO-292/18591. Retrieved from https://www.senado.gob.mx/64/gaceta_del_senado/documento/18591

Story, M., Nanney, M., & Schwartz, M. (2009). Schools and obesity prevention: Creating school environments and policies to promote healthy eating and physical activity. *The Milbank Quarterly, 87*(1), 71–100. https://doi.org/10.1111/j.1468-0009.2009.00548.x

Strategy 2013, (Estrategia Nacional para la Prevención y el Control del Sobrepeso, la Obesidad y la Diabetes [National Strategy for the Prevention and Control of Overweight, Obesity and Diabetes]), Secretaría de Salud, México (2013).

Swinburn, B., Egger, G., & Raza, F. (1999). Dissecting obesogenic environments: The development and application of a framework for identifying and prioritizing environmental interventions for obesity. *Preventive Medicine, 29*(6), 563–570. https://doi.org/10.1006/pmed.1999.0585

Torres-Torres, F., & Aguilar-Ortega, T. (2003). Aspectos externos de la vulnerabilidad alimentaria de México [External negative aspects on food security in Mexico]. In F. Torres-Torres (Ed.), *Seguridad alimentaria: Seguridad nacional* (pp. 87–123). México: UNAM, Plaza y Valdés.

Treviño Ronzón, E., & Sánchez Pacheco, G. (2014). La Implementación de los Lineamientos para Regular el Expendio de Alimentos y Bebidas en dos Escuelas Telesecundarias de Veracruz. Análisis desde la Perspectiva de los Sujetos [The implementation of the Guidelines to Regulate Food and Drinks Sales in two secondary schools in Veracruz: The perspective of the participants]. *CPU-e: Revista de Investigación Educativa 19*(julio–diciembre), 60–85.

Willet, W. C. (1994). Diet and health: What should we eat? *Science, 264*(5158), 532–537. https://doi.org/10.1126/science.8160011

Wise, T. A. (2009). Agricultural dumping under NAFTA: Estimating the costs of U.S. agricultural policies to Mexican producers. *Global Development and Environment Institute, Working paper*(09-08), 1–38. Retrieved from https://ageconsearch.umn.edu/record/179078

Yunez-Naude, A., & Barceinas, F. (2002). Lessons from NAFTA: The case of Mexico's agricultural sector. *Final Report to the World Bank*.

16

NAVIGATING THE 'NORM' IN FOOD EXPERIENCES AND HEALTHY LIFESTYLES OF CHINESE INTERNATIONAL STUDENTS IN AUSTRALIA

Bonnie Pang

Introduction

This chapter examines how Chinese international students discuss their relationship with food and how this discussion contributes to their navigation of the 'norm' in their construction of a healthy lifestyle. It is informed by research focusing on the health-related experiences of ten Chinese international students attending higher education institutions in New South Wales, Australia. Controversy exists in public health about the approach and key messages that should be adopted in regard to body size, body mass index (BMI), and food-related behaviours when seeking to promote 'health' (Fitzpatrick, Leahy, Webber, Gilbert, Lupton, & Aggleton, 2019; Wright & Harwood, 2012). Healthism (Crawford, 1980) contributes to a pervasive message reinforcing the construction of 'good' and 'bad' bodies and an ideal health practice. The pedagogical message is that a good body is achieved through regimented exercise and food intake. Food-based dietary guidelines, such as the food pyramid, are often used to communicate nutritional information to the general population (Davis, Britten, & Myers, 2001). Those who do not conform to the Western ideal and neoliberal rationality of healthy citizenship are 'othered' and labelled as 'bodies at risk' (Gard & Wright, 2001).

Foucault's discursive practice and subject positions

For Foucault, discourse contributes an important role in (re)producing subjectivities as it embodies meanings. Discourses are 'practices that systematically form the objects of which they speak' (Foucault, 1972, p. 49). Discourses about food are embodied by those who engage with them. As these students engage with discourses about food in relation to health, physical activity and culture, they become a subject to particular positions, as Foucault described as 'discursive practice' and 'subject position'. Foucault asserts that each culture has its own social and cultural values considered to be 'true' (Foucault, 1981). In the context of food-related practices, healthism is often taken as the regimen of truth in contemporary Western society. Hanganu-Bresch (2019) discussed the impact of healthism on people's eating habits. He critiqued the preoccupation with consuming healthy food (e.g., vegan food) in the context of neoliberalism as well as the notions of 'health' and 'purity' that have contributed to

DOI: 10.4324/9780429344824-20

orthorexia (unhealthy obsession with eating healthily) as a form of neoliberal cultural pathology. To become a 'healthy' subject, one must know how to eat 'properly'; eating properly is understood as knowing the kind of food to eat, the manner of preparing and serving food, and the order and timing of eating. Most importantly, knowing how to eat properly signals that you are an insider within a society. From a Foucauldian perspective, normalisation is a contemporary form of disciplinary power which aims to govern by homogeneity/sameness rather than direct repression. Normalisation is therefore a powerful instrument for people to conform to an ideal body and/or an ideal food practice. While conforming to this ideal/norm is not necessarily problematic, it is important to note that these dominant discourses could undermine voices that are different and therefore could position people at 'at risk' due to their differences in values and practices (Lupton, 1999).

In other words, food is never 'just food', and its importance is more than just nutrition. It is closely associated with social relations, discourse, power, emotions, cultural values, the human body, and health experiences (Caplan, 2013; Lupton, 1996). Arguably, the dominant health and dieting discourses can have an impact on people's understanding of what constitutes an ideal diet, body, and health practice, and therefore, such discourses may have silenced alternative perspectives and created 'docile bodies' (Foucault, 1981). To this end, the relationship between food and identity, as well as food studies more broadly, has been extensively explored in anthropology, sociology, cultural studies, and education (Albala, 2013; Ashley, Hollows, Jones & Taylor, 2004; Flowers and Swan, 2016). We eat not just because of our physiological needs or because we are hungry; we have a relationship with food. It is also a social need; meals are almost always shared, as people eat together, and thus food creates belongingness and security (Neely, Walton, & Stephens, 2014). While food is material, it is also discursive and emotional. To move beyond the current silencing of Chinese international students' voices that might have created 'docile bodies', this chapter focuses on the different discursive practices these students take on in relation to their food-related experiences.

Chineseness, university students, and food experiences

Food is a meaningful part of the Chinese experience, as historically exemplified through the establishment of Chinese restaurants by immigrants in Chinatowns (Liu & Lin, 2009). Chinese international students represent a significant social, cultural, and economic force in Australian society. In 2015, there were 136,097 Chinese students studying in Australia, which accounted for 27 percent of the total international student population (Department of Education and Training, 2016). Despite the large numbers of Chinese international students coming to Australia, many of whom stay on permanently post-study, very little is known about the health-related practices, such as food experiences, of this Chinese diaspora population. There has been little research on the role of these new diaspora formations in international higher education and knowledge production. In this chapter, the focus is on Chinese international students' relationship to food.

Recent studies on 'Asian' international students examined their food consumption, drinking behaviours, food security, and food experiences. For example, Lee, Contento, and Gray (2018) described East Asian international students' changes in food consumption after arriving in the United States (US). The students consumed more processed food, water, raw vegetables, meat, dairy, as well as Asian foods, and ate fewer cooked vegetables and foods from their home countries. The main reasons given for these changes were concerns about health, weight, availability, convenience, taste, and price. Concerns about food sustainability were mentioned the least. Research on alcohol use among Asian students showed that they drink less often than European students (Wicki, Kuntsche, & Gmel, 2010) and that they are more able to refuse alcohol when under social pressure (Oei & Jardim, 2007). Chinese international students who have become more integrated into the American lifestyle are more likely to be drinkers than non-drinkers (Cai, 2015).

Arguably, these studies tend to overlook the complexity of Asian cultures and Chineseness and the students' experiences with food, which are discreetly but sharply different between ethnic groups. This 'groupism' effect (Brubaker, 2002) continues to reify and racialise their drinking, eating, and other food-related practices. As Sen (2007) noted, this creates an othering through the 'cheap classification' of identities. Ang (2014) highlighted that a more processual and flexible understanding and analysis is needed to move beyond the groupness of Chinese experience. This chapter, therefore, provides a multifaceted understanding of Chinese international students' relationships with food and explores their experiences by going beyond the pervasive reductionist approach of ethnic understanding, and health promotion, healthism, 'at risk' bodily discourses. The methods that were used to collect and analyse the data are outlined.

Methods

This chapter looks at data from research examining ten Chinese international students studying in higher education in NSW (Australia), who were interviewed about their health-related experiences. The student participants, two males and eight females, differed by their country of origin (Mainland China and Hong Kong), years of residency (recent arrivals to those who had been residents for 10 years), levels of study (Undergraduate, Master, and PhD), socioeconomic status, and mobility trajectory. Using purposive sampling, students were recruited through professional connections in NSW universities and organisations, and emails were sent by agreed contacts to their respective students' networks. Each of the participants was invited for two one-hour semi-structured interviews to talk about their physical activity and health-related experiences in NSW.

All interviews were conducted in both English and Chinese (Mandarin and Cantonese) by the author and a research assistant who assisted with notetaking during the discussions. The first interview was a photo-elicitation interview, and the second was a walking interview. These two methods help to evoke the sensory, emotional, and material aspects of their food experiences whilst also offering participants flexibility and time for reflection, which are usually absent when using standalone methods such as interviews or survey research (Power, 2003). This chapter will report the qualitative interview data only.

The interview data were analysed using content analysis, as described by Saldaña (2009). The first reading of the data was used to gain an understanding of how the students talk about their overall health-related experiences. The second reading was done to explore the students' food experiences in relation to people, places, lifestyles, and Chineseness. The third reading was done to examine discourses demonstrating the commonalities as well as the differences in the students' food experiences. Ethical clearance for the research was gained through the university and from participating students. Pseudonyms have been used throughout to ensure anonymity.

The three main themes that resulted from this analysis include *Chineseness and food habits*, *healthy/unhealthy foods and lifestyles*, and *drinking cultures*. While this chapter risks presenting a false dichotomy between the East (Chinese) and the West (Australians) and acknowledges that the participant's experiences are diverse, the findings provide insights into the possible differences that might have been silenced in our understanding of food experiences with diverse ethnic populations. The discussion will highlight how the students navigate the 'norm', meaning those related to typical Western subjectivities of health and food practices, with discourses such as healthism prevailing strongly.

Results and discussion: navigating the 'norm'

Chineseness and food habits

Most of the students commented on how food practices, including cooking habits, food choices, daily dietary intake, grocery habits, and their own experiences, differed between China or Hong Kong and Australia. They were impressed by foods that are found only in Australia, such as kangaroo meat, and by those that are rarely found in their home cities in China, such as fresh seafood.

Food safety, price, and accessibility have an impact on the students' dietary habits. Lily (a PhD student who came to Australia in 2017) believes that food in China is not very safe to eat because there are many food accidents, such as the use of toxic chemicals in milk production. Therefore, she tends to consume more food while she is in Australia. The discourses of food safety constitute a form of bio-power aimed at taking the body as its focus of subjectification. In *The History of Sexuality* (1978), Foucault writes of 'a power that exerts a positive influence on life, that endeavours to administer, optimize, and multiply it, subjecting it to precise controls and comprehensive regulations' (p. 137). As the students compare the food safety between China and Australia, they take on a subject position that privilege Australia's food production and safeguarding process alongside disciplining their own food consumption as they navigate the food terrains of both countries. William (a Master's student who came to Australia from Shanghai in 2008) talked about the food markets in China, which he said are more accessible and sell more varieties of vegetables and fruits than Sydney's supermarket stores. He said that food in China is generally much cheaper, and therefore he preferred consuming it there. Yet, he agreed that fast food in China is quite expensive and said that he therefore usually consumes more meat and fewer vegetables while in Australia:

> I definitely have much more protein here, since the meat is cheaper here, but vegetables are relatively more expensive here. Back in China, fast food is not actually at a lower price. In China, we do have our diet largely based on vegetables, which seems like a healthier option than based on red meat.
>
> *(William)*

Because William lived and studied in Greater Western Sydney (GWS), he seldom travelled to the Sydney Central Business District (CBD) for food because of the cost and distance of traveling. He felt that, despite the range of food choices in Penrith, the food quality is poor while the price is still high:

> Here the restaurants are, you do get a variety of things, you get Middle Eastern food, Thai food, Chinese food, Korean food, and you've got hamburgers, but they often are, most of them I would say are very poor quality but still expensive.
>
> *(William)*

This comment is not surprising as research has shown that there is an increasing need to improve neighbourhood environments and address the underlying inequalities in the social aspects of health rather than merely modifying individuals' dieting behaviours, and GWS is a typical context for such work to be done (Barosh, Friel, Engelhardt, & Chan, 2014). Although William highlighted the poorer quality of food in Penrith and his preference and ability to pay for such food in Sydney, his way of eating is confined to the social space. He further explained that he has no intention of moving to the city because the rent is too high. Those who live near Sydney's CBD usually do their groceries in Asian supermarkets and the Paddy Markets in Chinatown, while those who live further away, such as Penrith or Burwood, go to their local supermarkets. Foucault noted in *Discipline and Punish* (2012a), 'discipline proceeds from the distribution of individuals in space' (p. 141). The students' spatial practices of food consumption are considered as deployed as governmental techniques by limiting their action. The students' subject positions in food practices are confined to their living spaces underpinned by the cost of living, including rent and traveling, their proximity to their study place, and the quality of food provision within these spaces. And in William's case, he has taken up a subject position that is associated with a multicultural food practice that is of low quality but overly priced.

Most of the participants chose Chinatown and other ethnoburbs (Li, 1998), such as Burwood, for their walking interview. Their accounts testify to the importance of Chinatowns and ethnoburbs which offer a sense of home and belongingness within a multicultural landscape (Ang, 2016). As William noted:

> If I'm talking to my friends who are back in China, we talk about my lifestyle in Australia, we definitely talk about things like the restaurants here. Here is a location, it's like a small alley in Burwood. It's filled with Chinese street food stalls. It's really fun talking about it, like my friends, I can actually enjoy relatively authentic food here. So it feels like maybe they would probably create a sense of belonging to be here. I do feel like I don't really miss my home that much, since I do enjoy the food here.
>
> *(William)*

The 'authenticity' of food (Lu & Fine, 1995) is discussed in relation to the students' cultural expectations, which are influenced by the dynamic of fixity and flow. William's opinion of taste changed depending on where he was. On the contrary, Linda (a Master's student who came to Australia from China in 2013) commented that she missed the 'original' taste of food and that some of the restaurants in Chinatown are not authentic enough:

> Chinese cuisine is really special, when foreign food comes to China I think they make adjustments to the Chinese here, like the taste, but I don't like it because I want food to be in their original taste.
>
> *(Linda)*

Linda continued to say that Chinese people have stronger taste buds and therefore add more flavour to their food. She commented that China is such a diverse country, and different cities have their own specific tastes:

> I come from a south-east city, and generally we like food a bit sweet, and very light. My family, my grandfather and my father love tea, so I think I grew up in that family and I started to know about it. Green tea keeps you awake, and in China we would say black tea is really good for women because it warms you from inside out. And warm water is good for the body.
>
> *(Linda)*

The discourses of the 'authenticity' of food highlight the two different subject positions which are influenced by the student's perceptions of space – the 'real' space and food from China (e.g., Linda); and the symbolic space of China Town/Burwood that (re)produced authentic food taste and memories (e.g., William). Indeed, food brings back nostalgic memories, reveals relationships between the past and the present, and reflects changing identities across different places (Chan, 2010). The description of black tea as warming the body resonates with Qin's (2014) discussion on the Chinese belief that food has hot and cold properties that generate different sensations in the human body.

In order to remember and record memories and experiences with food, Linda has a food blog and she enjoys taking pictures and writing comments on the foods and restaurants she visits. She also said the blog is primarily written for Chinese audiences in China:

> I'm a food blogger; I like to take food pictures, and I think food is really a big part of my health and wellbeing… Because life's boring, but the food looks fancy. There's a social media platform in China, and I post on Instagram as well. I would write where is it, and how does it taste, and how much I would rate it. And people would respond to me like, 'That looks yummy', and ask me the detail location, and they would ask me to recommend some signature food from that restaurant.
>
> *(Linda)*

Linda's experiences resonated with Pennell's (2018) study, which examined university students' food photography. As students take pictures and post on social media, they are given new and changing ways to investigate, document, and produce food-related issues, emotions, experiences, and material. The students further anchored their memories and belongingness through consuming 'home' foods in familiar places and connecting with familiar people to gain a sense of security. During the walking interview, a few students talked about hot pot as their favourite food and pastime at home or in Chinatown. Others related hotpot to Chineseness but rejected the dining experience. Wendy (Master's student who came to Australia from China in 2008) worked in a Chinese public relations company whose boss owned a hotpot restaurant in Chinatown. Although she identified herself as a Chinese person who often went to hotpot restaurants, she did not enjoy the food:

> I think pretty much all the Chinese students or students from Chinese backgrounds, they like hot pot or barbecue. But I don't like the food, because I'm really sick of hot pot. My boss has a hot pot restaurant and I have to go there for business meetings every time. (Wendy)

Healthy/unhealthy foods and lifestyles

Most of these students gathered information about food from online sites using Google search as well as from fitness magazines and celebrity accounts on social media. Their experiences with healthy food include organic food, which is healthy and clean but expensive, and food that contains less sugar and salt. Others who commented on unhealthy food behaviours stated that they do not eat breakfast in the morning due to oversleeping, and that they cook unnutritious food due to their lack of cooking abilities and time. Some said that they consume too much fast food late at night. Others were more ambivalent about their experiences and said that their friends ate food with no oil at all, because it is healthier, but were obsessed with exercising, which they said was unhealthy. William stated that he thought the taste of food is important to health and especially to bodybuilders who are improving their fitness:

> If you try to get fit, you choose food based on a diet that pretty much is more natural, less flavour adding to it. Let's say chicken breast is really healthy, bodybuilders eat them, tasteless.
>
> *(William)*

This is exemplified by Linda, who is on a fitness training regimen. She uses her mobile phone scanner application to plan her meals each day so that she meets the diet standards set by her fitness coach. She also travels to an organic store to buy groceries in the city because the food is more natural and healthier. This purchase of organic food products demonstrates how contemporary health-conscious citizens are persuaded by health promotion discourses to follow a certain lifestyle that seeks to minimize risk and maximise prudent food choices (Ayo, 2012). It seems that Linda's subject position of a healthy citizen reflects body surveillance that cuts across ethnic difference.

While trying to live healthier, Gilian (Master's student who came to Australia from China in 2013) stated that she thought that learning how to cook healthily signified becoming an independent adult. However, at the moment, she seemed to be focused on coping with the reality of taking care of herself in other aspects of her life such as academic studies. Others have learned to become more independent through taking care of their health, and therefore, they are more aware of their dieting habits in Australia. Sally (undergraduate student who came to Australia from China in 2016) said that her diet in Australia is different from that when she is in China. In China, she ate whatever her father cooked, while in Australia, she deliberately eats less fat, sugar, and salt:

> I'll deliberately eat healthier while I'm here because I find the fat and sugar amount here with the same food is higher than those we have in China. I think I have a more strong sense of health, developing a healthy lifestyle after I came to Australia because I only started an independent life here. Before that, my parents takes care of me, including the diet, so I like didn't pay attention to that. But after I came to Australia I have to take care of all of these things by myself so I initially put on a lot of weight, and then I realised that okay, I need to lose weight.
>
> *(Sally)*

As Carol recalled her lifestyle back home, she noted that her irregular meals in Hong Kong were not really healthy:

> I get a little bit better here in Australia than Hong Kong, because in Hong Kong life is just really busy all the time, even though it's very convenient to get food in Hong Kong, but because of work we just don't have regular meals all the time. I finished work at 7:30 at night, so after I went back home it's already 9:00, so it was quite late and I don't eat healthily.
>
> *(Carol)*

Wendy noted that, in addition to being able to cook, take care of one's academic studies and eat regular meals, being an adult means being financially independent. She noted that some of her friends would choose to save money rather than eating healthily:

> We have to stay within the budget, to go shopping every time is kind of expensive in Sydney. You have to watch the budget more often than in living in other countries.

And you have to manage to cook the healthy food. To eat healthy is much about the cost of the food.

(Wendy)

Submitting to the healthism discourses, Sally felt pressure to lose weight when she compared her body to those of her peers in Australia and took up the discursive position to exercise and eat healthily (Foucault, 1981):

I realised just how seriously fat I am, and when I compared myself to other friends, their bodies, I realised that I need to lose weight. I began to pay attention to healthy dieting and have a balance between an appropriate amount of activities.

(Sally)

William was the only participant who moved beyond the binary of healthy/unhealthy food discourses and stated the importance of having a balanced diet:

My idea about healthy, I mean I wouldn't call it healthy food, I'd call it a balanced diet because it's not like one food that is really bad, even for example, doughnut, they are rich in sugar and the fat. You need sugar and fat; you just don't want to eat too much of it I think. So I was having a, I think our diet is pretty balanced although I probably eat too much, I confess.

(William)

William's account resonates with Welch, McMahon, and Wright (2012) who challenge the orthodoxy of meanings afforded to foods that draw a distinct binary between 'good' and 'bad' or 'healthy' and 'unhealthy'. As William accepted the need for a balanced diet, he also felt that he had to confess his actual eating behaviours. This suggests that he admits his own neglect over his body and sees overeating as a reason for guilt, resonating with Foucault's (1978) notion of the 'confessing subject' that one is difficult to escape when operating within the governing technique of a society.

Drinking culture

Some of the students started drinking only after arriving in Australia. The change of environment provided them with the freedom that they did not previously have in China. For example, in China, Gilian had to be back at home at 9:00 pm, while in Australia, her parents were not able to restrict her life. Because they are in university, these students have opportunities to meet friends and socialise through drinking. Those who socialised with other international students felt more inclined to adopt a drinking culture. As Linda explained, the international student cohort has a culture of drinking and clubbing due to loneliness:

A lot of international students, when they are lonely, they just go clubbing and drinking, and socialising with other people, like I can see a lot of Chinese international students don't have a friend that they can really talk to here in Australia.

(Linda)

Others compared their drinking to the 'wine culture' of their Australian peers. Some of the Chinese students do not have this culture and are not used to drinking in China. As Gilian noted, drinking can have different meanings; it symbolises maturity in Australia, while in China, drinking is a gendered practice:

> It's different, like in China, the girl age of me, if you don't drink wine it's normal, I think. If you don't drink wine here it's fine, but they think, 'Oh, you're 23 or so and you still don't drink wine'.
>
> *(Gilian)*

Wendy, who spent a lot of time doing part-time work, felt obliged to drink with her boss at work. She also talked about being aware of her drinking limits:

> I don't like that. I think drinking with my friends, I can express myself more to talk more about myself or what I'm feeling. But to go out with colleagues or my boss, I don't like it. And they like drinking a lot.
>   *Interviewer: Do you feel you have control over how much you drink?* I definitely am not going to drive after I consume the alcohol. I am quite aware how much I can drink and what type of drinks I can do.
>
> *(Wendy)*

Yet, others who drank for social purposes perceived that some of their friends developed binge drinking habits at house parties and did not know their limits. Some of the students highlighted the importance of education surrounding safe drinking, including knowing one's boundaries, knowing how to protect one's self, and looking after one another at parties.

Drinking, to these students, means more than the wine culture that is common among their Australian peers. The Chinese students used drinking to help navigate with their work environments, socialise with peers, and cope with their sense of loneliness. Drinking with others is not merely an individual choice or responsibility; rather, this group membership strengthens their self-identity and social acceptance, especially in an overseas country (Borsari & Carey, 2001). As Jiang (2011) noted, in China, alcohol is used as a tool for communication and developing rapport, whereas in Western cultures, it is associated with appreciation and enjoyment, and the taste of wine is of importance.

Conclusion

Adequate and nutritious food is conducive to good health. However, the food experiences of Chinese international students are influenced by more than nutrition. Students' food choices and dietary practices are influenced by structural, social, cultural, and economic factors. The students' food practices and experiences point to Foucault's 'care of the self' (2012b), a cultivation of the self through self-knowledge and techniques of living. In the international educational experiential process, these students are becoming an independent healthy subject, developing a set of practices, rituals, lifestyles by way of negotiating with both the 'norm' position and their Chineseness as they compare and contrast their past and present-lived experiences as well as food terrains. Their discursive food practices suggest an in-betweenness that is influenced by an array of factors related to the price, belongingness, authenticity, balanced diet versus healthy/unhealthy diet, and drinking cultures. The temporal and spatial nature of these students' reflexive food discourses (e.g., choosing to skip breakfast, comparing the different pace of life between Hong Kong and Australia) provided further insights into their food 'rhythms'. The students do not seem to feel othered in their food choices or normalised in their food practices through contemporary western public health discourses or through traditional Chinese values. Instead, there are ongoing reflexive practices that these students (re)create in response to the differences and diversity they experience in everyday food practices.

What is positive to note is that these students' narratives suggest that most of them did not use food as a way of coping with stress and everyday challenges. The research findings indicate that these students were addicted to drinking, and they were not performing at-risk behaviours such as driving under the influence (Chang, Shrake, & Rhee, 2008). Their experiences are also different from those found in some other studies, in which students identified negative feelings as a primary emotional trigger for engaging in emotional eating behaviours (Evers, Marijn Stok, & de Ridder, 2010). Generally, the students in this study seemed to have food security, unlike many other university students who lack money to buy food on campus, struggle to pay for both tuition fees and food, and suffer from poor overall health, mental health, and high stress (Hughes, Serebryanikova, Donaldson, & Leveritt, 2011). Interesting to note is that these Chinese international students often associated food security with becoming an independent adult, and so they sought to consume cheaper food in order to save money for leisure and academic purposes.

This chapter extends current food studies and discourses aiming to promote health focused on nutrition and diet. It offers a panoramic view of how different Chinese international students, who come from various sociocultural backgrounds and locations in NSW, relate to food in their everyday experiences, some of which may be similar to their Australian peers. Chinese international students experience ongoing negotiations in regard to their healthy lifestyles, including when to eat in relation to their work/study time; what to eat based on the price and accessibility of restaurants and supermarkets, their need for exercise, and their transnational context; how to cook food as they develop their cooking skills and learn to be independent; and how to protect themselves from and educate themselves about the dominant drinking culture. It provides the impetus for further studies related to a whole range of food experiences. This includes food, Chineseness, and belongingness; food safety, accessibility, choices, and security; food pedagogies with internationals students; food, memories, and authenticity; food and healthy lifestyles; food photography and social media; and drinking culture, isolation, and freedom.

Acknowledgements

The author would like to thank Ms Sophia Li for the bilingual interview and research assistant work during this project.

References

Albala, K. (Ed.). (2013). *Routledge international handbook of food studies*. Oxon: Routledge.

Ang, I. (2014). Beyond Chinese groupism: Chinese Australians between assimilation, multiculturalism and diaspora. *Ethnic and Racial Studies, 37*(7), 1184–1196. doi: 10.1080/01419870.2014.859287

Ang, I. (2016). At home in Asia? Sydney's Chinatown and Australia's 'Asian century'. *International Journal of Cultural Studies, 19*(3), 257–269. doi: 10.1177/1367877915573763

Ashley, B., Hollows, J., Jones, S., & Taylor, B. (2004). *Food and cultural studies*. London and New York: Routledge.

Ayo, N. (2012). Understanding health promotion in a neoliberal climate and the making of health conscious citizens. *Critical Public Health, 22*(1), 99–105. doi: 10.1080/09581596.2010.520692

Barosh, L., Friel, S., Engelhardt, K., & Chan, L. (2014). The cost of a healthy and sustainable diet—who can afford it? *Australian and New Zealand Journal of Public Health, 38*(1), 7–12. doi: 10.1111/1753-6405.12158

Borsari, B., & Carey, K. B. (2001). Peer influences on college drinking: A review of the research. *Journal of Substance Abuse, 13*(4), 391–424. doi: 10.1016/s0899-3289(01)00098-0

Brubaker, R. (2002). Ethnicity without groups. *European Journal of Sociology, 43*(2), 163–189. doi: 10.1017/S0003975602001066

Cai, S. (2015). *Acculturation and alcohol drinking behavior among Chinese international university students in the midwest*. Nebraska: University of Nebraska-Lincoln. (Master's Thesis).

Caplan, P. (Ed.). (2013). *Food, health and identity*. London and New York: Routledge.

Chan, S. C. (2010). Food, memories, and identities in Hong Kong. *Identities: Global Studies in Culture and Power, 17*(2–3), 204–227. doi: 10.1080/10702891003733492

Chang, J., Shrake, E., & Rhee, S. (2008). Patterns of alcohol use and attitudes toward drinking among Chinese and Korean American college students. *Journal of Ethnicity in Substance Abuse, 7*(3), 341–356. doi: 10.1080/15332640802313346

Crawford, R. (1980). Healthism and the medicalization of everyday life. *International Journal of Health Services, 10*(3), 365–388. doi: 10.2190/3H2H-3XJN-3KAY-G9NY

Davis, C. A., Britten, P., & Myers, E. F. (2001). Past, present, and future of the Food Guide Pyramid. *Journal of the Academy of Nutrition and Dietetics, 101*(8), 881. doi: 10.1016/S0002-8223(01)00217-6

Department of Education and Training (2016). *Research snapshot: International student numbers 2015*. Canberra: Australian Government.

Evers, C., Marijn Stok, F., & de Ridder, D. T. (2010). Feeding your feelings: Emotion regulation strategies and emotional eating. *Personality and Social Psychology Bulletin, 36*(6), 792–804. doi: 10.1177/0146167210371383

Fitzpatrick, K., Leahy, D., Webber, M., Gilbert, J., Lupton, D., & Aggleton, P. (2019). Critical health education studies: Reflections on a new conference and this themed symposium. *Health Education Journal, 78*(6), 621–632. doi: 10.1177/0017896919860882

Flowers, R., & Swan, E. (Eds.). (2016). *Food pedagogies*. London and New York: Routledge.

Foucault, M. (1972). *The archaeology of knowledge and the discourse of language*. New York: Pantheon.

Foucault, M. (1978). *The will to knowledge: The history of sexuality Vol. 1*. New York: Vintage.

Foucault, M. (1981). History of systems of thought, 1979. *Philosophy & Social Criticism, 8*(3), 353–359. doi: 10.1515/9781501741913-010

Foucault, M. (2012a). *Discipline and punish: The birth of the prison*. New York: Vintage.

Foucault, M. (2012b). *The history of sexuality, Vol. 3: The care of the self*. New York: Vintage.

Gard, M., & Wright, J. (2001). Managing uncertainty: Obesity discourses and physical education in a risk society. *Studies in philosophy and education, 20*(6), 535–549. doi: 10.1023/A:1012238617836

Hanganu-Bresch, C. (2019). Orthorexia: Eating right in the context of healthism. *Medical Humanities*. Retrieved online: doi: 10.1136/medhum-2019-011681

Hughes, R., Serebryanikova, I., Donaldson, K., & Leveritt, M. (2011). Student food insecurity: The skeleton in the university closet. *Nutrition & Dietetics, 68*(1), 27–32. doi: 10.1111/j.1747-0080.2010.01496.x

Jiang, L. (2011). Comparison of the difference between Chinese and Western drinking culture. *Asian Social Science, 7*(5), 251. doi: 10.5539/ass.v7n5p251

Lee, J. M., Contento, I., & Gray, H. L. (2018). Change in food consumption and food choice determinants among East Asian International Students in New York. *Journal of Hunger & Environmental Nutrition, 15*(3), 418–441. doi: 10.1080/19320248.2018.1555071

Li, W. (1998). Anatomy of a new ethnic settlement: The Chinese ethnoburb in Los Angeles. *Urban Studies, 35*(3), 479–501. doi: 10.1080/0042098984871

Liu, H., & Lin, L. (2009). Food, culinary identity, and transnational culture: Chinese restaurant business in Southern California. *Journal of Asian American Studies, 12*(2), 135–162.

Lu, S., & Fine, G. A. (1995). The presentation of ethnic authenticity: Chinese food as a social accomplishment. *The Sociological Quarterly, 36*(3), 535–553. doi: 10.1111/j.1533-8525.1995.tb00452.x

Lupton, D. (1996). *Food, the body and the self*. London: Sage Publications.

Lupton, D. (1999). *Risk*. London: Routledge.

Neely, E., Walton, M., & Stephens, C. (2014). Young people's food practices and social relationships. A thematic synthesis. *Appetite, 82*, 50–60. doi: 10.1016/j.appet.2014.07.005

Oei, T. P., & Jardim, C. L. (2007). Alcohol expectancies, drinking refusal self-efficacy and drinking behaviour in Asian and Australian students. *Drug and Alcohol Dependence, 87*(2–3), 281–287. doi: 10.1016/j.drugalcdep.2006.08.019

Pennell, M. (2018). (Dis)comfort food: Connecting food, social media, and first-year college undergraduates. *Food, Culture & Society, 21*(2), 255–270. doi: 10.1080/15528014.2018.1429074

Power, E. M. (2003). De-centering the text: Exploring the potential for visual methods in the sociology of food. *Journal for the Study of Food and Society, 6*(2), 9–20. doi: 10.2752/152897903786769670

Qin, J. (2014). Food and binary oppositions in the Chinese meal system. *Society, 51*(1), 35–39. doi: 0.1007/s12115-013-9735-0

Saldaña, J. (2009). Popular film as an instructional strategy in qualitative research methods courses. *Qualitative Inquiry, 15*(1), 247–261. doi: 10.1177/1077800408318323

Sen, A. (2007). *Identity and violence: The illusion of destiny.* India: Penguin Books.

Welch, R., McMahon, S., & Wright, J. (2012). The medicalisation of food pedagogies in primary schools and popular culture: A case for awakening subjugated knowledges. *Discourse: Studies in the Cultural Politics of Education, 33*(5), 713–728. doi: 10.1080/01596306.2012.696501

Wicki, M., Kuntsche, E., & Gmel, G. (2010). Drinking at European universities? A review of students' alcohol use. *Addictive Behaviors, 35*(11), 913–924. doi: 10.1016/j.addbeh.2010.06.015

Wright, J., & Harwood, V. (Eds.). (2012). *Biopolitics and the 'obesity epidemic': Governing bodies* (Vol. 3). New York and London: Routledge.

17

SCHOOL FOOD IN AUSTRALIA – A DOG'S BREAKFAST?

Deana Leahy, Jan Wright, Jo Lindsay, Claire Tanner, JaneMaree Maher and Sian Supski

A dog's breakfast: UK informal for something or someone that looks extremely untidy, or something that is very badly done.

(Cambridge Dictionary)

Introduction

As we sat down to come up with a focus and title for this chapter, we were in the midst of data analysis for our Australian Research Council Discovery project, *Children as health advocates: assessing the consequences.* At that particular stage, our team had been tallying up the many school food programs that Victorian families had told us about. We had also been coding our data in an attempt to understand what kinds of messages children and their families were receiving about food via the various school programs. The picture that was emerging was that school food was in a bit of a mess. Through our many interviews, we had heard about a multitude of programs being delivered differently both across different schools and also within schools. Families were also commenting on the confusing and contradictory messages they were receiving. From the many family stories we heard, it really did sound like a dog's breakfast. In some ways, we expected to see "messiness" as governmentality scholars have, for some time, told us that contemporary approaches to governing the population that are made up of ad hoc arrangements of agencies, actors, knowledges and practices ultimately result in a broad range of heterogeneous and fragmented approaches (Dean, 2010; Moore and Valverde, 2000; O'Malley, 2004; Rose, 2000). With specific reference to school health programs, ethnographic research had also revealed some of the troubling effects that neoliberal governmental assemblages have for school health and food programs (see Leahy, 2012, 2014; Powell, 2015). This chapter offers new and much-needed insights from children and parents about the effects of contemporary policy approaches to schooling food in Victoria, Australia. And even though we were fully expecting some policy and program messiness, we were surprised by what we found. The chapter begins by providing a brief overview of the role that school food programs are expected to play within public health agendas via a review of the critical scholarship that has emerged over time. We then provide an overview of our project and findings about school food programs and practices. We conclude by suggesting that we need to take stock of the current state of school food policy and programs before

DOI: 10.4324/9780429344824-21

amplifying further efforts. We also suggest that critical scholars may need to develop some new engagement tactics in order to ensure that we are (more) welcome at the policy table given the obesity "crisis" is going to be with us for the foreseeable future.

Schooling food

For public health advocates, both old and new, schools provide an important platform for dealing with the various health crises of the day (Gard & Pluim, 2014). So, when the World Health Organisation announced, in 1996, that we were in the midst of an obesity epidemic, it came as no surprise that schools were called upon to act as key sites for intervening in the crisis. For those of us who were in schools at the time, either teaching, researching or both, the effects of the obesity epidemic on programs were tangible. It was clear that health teachers had heard the call to duty, and they had to do something to halt the crisis (Leahy, 2012). Researchers at this time, unsurprisingly started to report on the different ways teachers were changing their programs so as to curb the epidemic. Critical scholars from Australia, New Zealand, the United Kingdom, Canada and the United States began to draw attention to the problematic effects of school responses. Specifically, they were finding that programs fuelled by obesity prevention imperatives adopted highly individualized approaches that ignored the social determinants of health. This meant that programs tended to be characterised by instrumental approaches and thus embraced a narrow focus on physical activity and eating, including weighing children and insisting students kept food diet diaries (Burrows, Wright, & Jurgensen, 2002; Gard & Wright, 2001; Leahy & Harrison, 2004; Wright & Burrows, 2004). Research that examined broader school food programs revealed that teachers had begun surveilling lunch boxes via lunchbox inspections. These inspections continue today in Australia, New Zealand, the US (Pluim, Powell, & Leahy, 2018) and in the UK (Harman & Cappelini, 2015) as a way to reinforce healthy eating messages. Implicitly, and sometimes quite explicitly, lunchbox inspections provided teachers and health promoters with an opportunity to "reach into" the family in an attempt to change family food practices. Teachers were doing this via sending notes home to parents about the poor state of their child's lunchbox and/or by publicly shaming particular kinds of lunch box contents either at assemblies, parent meetings or at lunchtimes during overt or covert lunch box inspections (see Burrows & Wright, 2020; Harman & Cappelini, 2015; Pike & Leahy, 2012). At the same time, a myriad of other biopedagogies were being developed by policy writers, program workers and teachers. Whilst we do not have space in this present chapter to detail them all, we do want to draw particular attention to health advocacy as a key biopedagogical tactic in the fight against obesity. Health advocacy has been a mainstay of the new public health since the early 1980s (Peterson & Lupton, 1996), and in 2003, it was identified as a key approach that could be harnessed in the fight against obesity. Specifically, the *Healthy Weight 2008: Australia's Future* report argued for children and teenagers to become advocates of healthy eating within families as an intervention method directed towards curbing obesity (Commonwealth of Australia, 2003). In order to realise this, schools were expected to get involved in order to develop the requisite knowledge and skills required for children's health advocacy work.

It is within this context that the *Children as Health Advocates* study was conceived. We had noted that there was very little literature that had explored how school health messages were taken up by children and young people and whether or not they were being transported home. We also wondered about how families, particularly mothers, would respond to calls from their children to change family food practices. Our study involved interviewing 50 families who had primary school-aged children in school, across a range of demographics

Table 17.1 Number of school food programs and practices nominated by families

Program	No. of families (n = 50)	Program	No. of families (n = 50)
Nude food	38	Birthdays, celebrations	34
Brain food	35	Family cooking program	3
Canteen	39	School cookbook	5
Life Education	20	Kitchen and cooking activities	21
Food fundraisers	19	School gardens	34
Food themed days	15	Breakfast club	11

and family types in rural and urban areas in Victoria, Australia. One child in each family was provided with an iPad at the initial interview and invited to photograph or film food events in the family context. A second follow-up interview involved interviewing the child using the iPad videos and photographs as prompts and asking general questions about food and school. Both interviews also involved talking with the parents and asking questions about their experiences of school food policies and practices and how and when these were communicated to the family. Data were analysed in a number of ways. An excel spreadsheet was used to organise the photographs and video material into themes – for example, lunchboxes, celebrations and fridges. QSR Nvivo was used to manage the large data set and to code across the interviews; many of these codes overlapped with the themes identified in relation to the visual material. In this chapter, we focus specifically on the codes related to school food programs. We were interested in the different programs and practices that children and families experienced at school and when and how health advocacy was a part of the programs. Our findings reveal that schools tend to do food in a myriad of ways and often have multiple program offerings. These programs and approaches and the number of families who mentioned them are listed in the table below (see Table 17.1). An important proviso to the material we discuss below is that this was not a study of the schools per se but of the 50 families' experiences of school programs; schools were not the units around which data were organised, rather we were interested in a diversity of family experiences of everyday day school food programming.

The many ways schools do food

Our research revealed that food is an integral part of the everyday of schooling. The infographic in Figure 17.1 below visualises the different families' accounts of the way food was addressed in their primary schools (based on Table 17.1). Each numbered segment represents a single family and the different school food programs and events they said they experienced. The pattern of shading indicates that for some children and their families there is a lot going on in relation to school food, and for others, there were very few programs. Whilst it is clear from the diagram that there is variation across schools, what is not obvious in Figure 17.1 is the variation in offerings within individual schools. We discovered this variation by talking to families who had children at the same schools. Also, families with more than one child at the school talked about the different experiences and offerings based on their child's year level and teacher and time at the school. For example, some parents pointed out how different food programs and initiatives had started and then stopped over the time that their children attended the school.

A common theme throughout discussions was how haphazard schools were in their attempts to regulate food choice and consumption. Participants discussed different examples

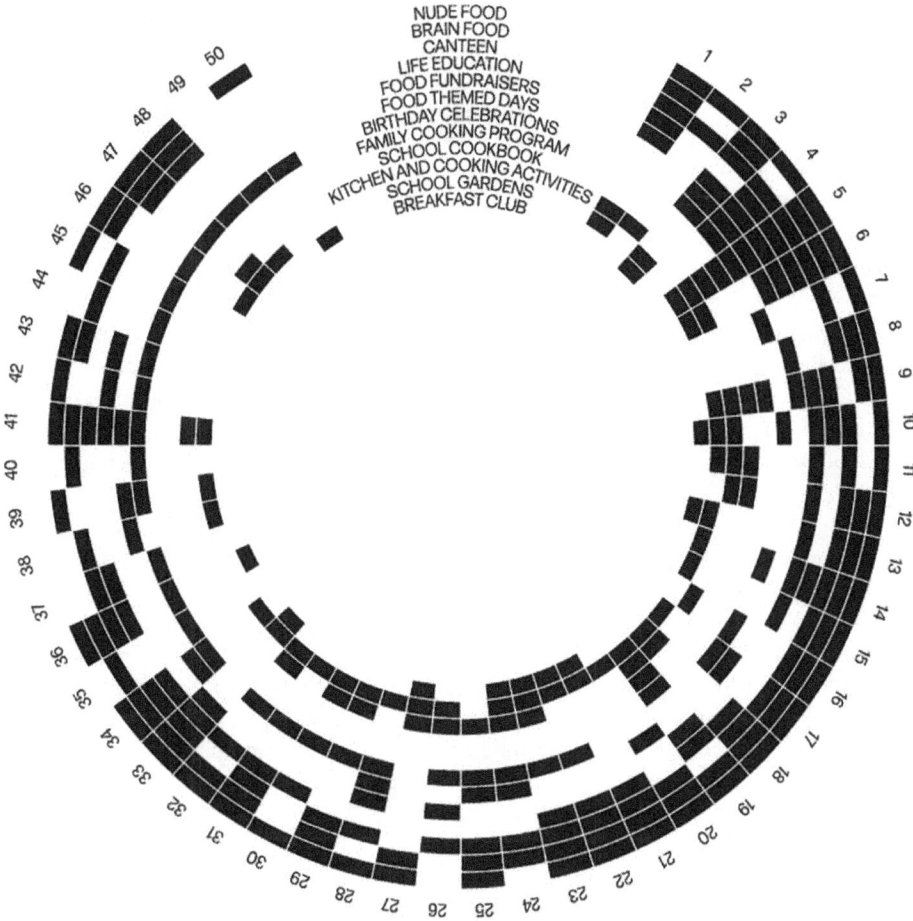

Figure 17.1 How food is addressed in primary schools.

to highlight the inconsistencies they experienced. For example, some talked about how the attention that was paid to lunchboxes and healthy eating seemed to have little bearing on the fact that they were often asked to sell chocolate or soft drinks as fundraisers for the school. Others talked about how their children at the same school experienced very different rules about lunch boxes depending on what grade they were in and what teacher they had. Different teachers effectively meant that children were exposed to different regulations around places where they could eat, the amount of time they had to eat and the monitoring of food brought to school.

Throughout our many discussions about the multitude of school food programs and activities, families reported an overall lack of ongoing formal nutrition or food education (see Maher et al., 2020). Some children and families (*n* = 20) did however talk about the Life Education Program, an external health education provider that has been visiting primary schools in Australia and New Zealand for over 40 years. Exposure to this program seemed to be something that was more present for children in the early years of schooling. Despite being involved in the program, children's knowledge about health and food rarely extended beyond simple understandings of what are considered to be healthy and unhealthy foods. In contrast to formal curriculum, references to nude food, brain food, canteens, garden and cooking programs were common. It was too clear that the programs impacted on children's understanding of food. For example, they could tell us what was considered to be brain food or nude food according to their school. Overall, we found that the schools in our study were replete with programs and practices targeting food consumption more broadly, and as a result, these programs acted in lieu of any formal ongoing quality health, food or nutrition education.

In addition to the above-mentioned programs, families also talked about food events and activities that were a part of the children's school day. Some schools, for example, hosted themed days that encouraged the children to celebrate food from "other cultures" ($n = 15$). Many of the schools permitted birthday celebrations ($n = 34$). Though within each school, there was variation across classrooms as some teachers did not allow birthday celebrations. Where celebrations were permitted children could bring a variety of foods, depending on the individual school or classroom rules. Some schools, for example, allowed cakes, and others celebrated with hummus and carrot sticks, while elsewhere, it was sushi. At schools where food was not permitted for birthday celebrations, families talked about being allowed to take stationery items as gifts instead of cakes or other celebratory food. Below, we provide further discussion about the main programs and activities children and their families talked about in our interviews. Each program or activity can be understood as either a formal or informal site of learning, which form part of a constellation of school food pedagogies that have emerged and/or transformed over time because of the "obesity epidemic" (see Flowers and Swan, 2015). Often, these sites are understood in policy to function in quite simplistic ways; however, our data illustrate how the enactment of each of the programs is characterised by complexity and contradictions. Many families we spoke to expressed uncertainty about which guidelines to follow and indicated that they were perplexed at the obvious contradictions in approaches to managing food at schools.

The canteen

In the primary schools in our study, most of the children brought lunch from home, but many schools also had a canteen or "tuck shop", open between one day to all week, from which the children could order lunch. In their comprehensive policy document on Canteens and Other School Food Services, Victoria Health states that "School canteens and other school food services are important educational resources. ... The school canteen should reflect the educational goals of the school and support and complement student learning" (Department of Education and Early Childhood Development, 2012, p. 2). The document goes on to state that "A healthy school food service should provide foods that reflect the Dietary Guidelines for Children and Adolescents in Australia" (p. 6). The kit utilises a traffic light system (green, amber, red categorizations of "everyday", "select carefully" and "occasionally") as a guide. The policy also states that:

> From 2007, high sugar content soft drinks should not be supplied through school food services.... This includes energy drinks and flavoured mineral waters with high sugar content ... From 2009, no confectionery should be supplied through school food services.
>
> (p. 9)

As indicated by student descriptions and our collection of school canteen menus from families, the canteens to which they had access varied from those which had "homemade food" and baked goods (with restrictions) made by parents to those with very diverse menus covering a wide range of types of food (including soft drinks) and catering to cultural and religious requirements (e.g. Halal). Some canteens were online, and food needed to be ordered via an app. Food that was ordered online was either prepared at school or off site and delivered at lunch time.

Most families seemed to use canteens about once a week if they were available. Parents generally had some idea of what was available and supervised to a greater or lesser degree what children bought. Spending money at the canteen was often viewed as a treat, an alternative to "good" food brought from home. Nine-year-old Ava's comments about the canteen at her inner metropolitan public school reveal both her knowledge about the categorisations of food (healthy and unhealthy foods) and illustrate fairly typical food available at most of the canteens. They also reflect how canteen food was considered to be a treat and different to regular lunch. Elizabeth's (Ava's mother) comments reflect the "trust" and belief that there are limits on what is available, a trust commonly shared by other parents. However, like Elizabeth, parents were sometimes surprised about what was actually available in the canteen and also what their children ordered:

AVA: Yeah. So our canteen has a mix of healthy and unhealthy food so that provide things - people might have an allergy to so they don't provide those things, like nuts and coconut. They started selling fruit drinks and soft drinks. Nearly all the food there has sugar on them. There's natural sugar and processed sugar so they don't have fruit bits. Mainly like cupcakes, jellies and things like that.

ELIZABETH (MOTHER): I didn't know they started selling soft drink. Because you can do your lunch order online and so obviously I can see what they order or sometimes I just give them two dollars just to get something. But I didn't realise - they had, what do they call it, juices, they're sort of like fruit juice thing?

AVA: Yeah, they're like frozen juice.

ELIZABETH: Yeah, frozen juice or once frozen milk, sort of like that. But yeah, I've never seen soft drink so that's just a new thing.

AVA: They got it like last year but yeah, I guess relatively new.

INTERVIEWER: So do you order your lunch once a week or once a month?

AVA: Maybe every fortnight. Not once a week.

INTERVIEWER: Do you have favourite things that you like to order?

AVA: Mainly, I get hot food because they have a lot of pies and just a few other things.

INTERVIEWER: Is that because you don't have them at home or that's a favourite food?

AVA: Yeah, probably because I don't have them at home and because if you're spending money and if you can make it at home there's not really any point of getting it.

INTERVIEWER: That's good?

ELIZABETH: It's when it's really cold generally, isn't it?

AVA: Yeah.

ELIZABETH: You get something hot but they'll never order a sandwich or anything like that. There's no point, unless I've absolutely got nothing (Interview 2, Family 6)

Nude food lunch boxes

Lunch boxes, in general, have been a contentious area of regulation and informal site of school food knowledge (Harman & Cappelini, 2015; Pike & Leahy, 2012; Pluim, Powell,

& Leahy, 2018). In our study, photos of videos of children proudly demonstrating how they packed their lunch boxes were more evident than any other photos of food-related incidents and occurred in 30 out of our 50 families, with multiple photos within particular families (see Figure 17.1 under Nude Food). References to "Nude Food" were often a feature of talk around lunchboxes – the provision of food to school without packaging – but also in reference to school "Nude Food" programs. Nude Food programs are connected to Nude Food Movers, a product range produced by Smash Enterprises, an Australian lunch box manufacturer (https://www.nudefoodmovers.com.au). In 2010, Smash Enterprises partnered with *Nutrition Australia* to launch Nude Food Day, as a way to encourage healthy lunches and minimise waste. Adopted by many of the schools in our study, Nude Food was implemented in different way. Some schools were Nude Food schools, that is, all food brought to school needed to be "nude", that is unpackaged (not in single use plastic) every day. Some ran the program once a week (Nude Food Tuesday), some once a term and others once a year. Some even held "surprise" Nude Food Days, where children and parents were only told the day before that "tomorrow is Nude Food Day".

Parents said they found the actual Nude Food lunch boxes useful, with their tiny compartments and containers convenient for "brain food" and snacks. However, parents also described the tireless "hunt" for many lost small containers and lids. When components went missing, parents had to replace whole lunch boxes. Nude Food Day also sparked anxiety in some parents, spurring trips to school lost property and last-minute runs to the grocery store, tearing packaging off at home before packing food into containers in order to meet the Nude Food standards.

Some children and parents described the fear of turning up to school with food in wrappers when it was Nude Food Day. During our interviews, we met six-year-old Emily who attended a Nude Food school. When Emily was in prep, her mother packed a wrapped muesli bar in her lunch box. Emily realised her mother's mistake as soon as she opened her lunch. Terrified that she would be told off, she ran outside and buried the offending muesli bar in the school garden. We heard several stories like Emily's from other children and families.

While some of the talk around appropriate food to be included in lunchboxes engaged with food knowledge about healthy and unhealthy foods, the school information around nude food seemed to draw primarily on an environmental discourse of sustainability (that is the avoidance of single use plastic). In contrast, the children's talk about nude food programs was more likely to be characterised by references to regulatory practices – the desire to reduce the amount of rubbish at school and also punishments and rewards for individuals and school classes for their compliance.

Brain food

Thirty-five families in our study reported that their children had experienced or were currently involved in a brain food program. In the following excerpt, seven-year-old Lara describes her morning snack as brain food, which would be consumed in the classroom. Lara was an only child who lived with her mum and dad in an affluent south eastern Melbourne suburb. She attended a Catholic school. In the following excerpt, Lara reveals her feelings about brain food and also her understanding of what brain food is and does:

LARA:... for brain food, I used to have celery and hummus... I love celery and hummus.
INTERVIEWER: And when you have brain food, what time do you have that?

LARA: In the morning ... And then it sort of gets our brains ready, so that's why it's called brain food.

As we mentioned above, this taken-for-granted association of particular foods with brain activity was common throughout our data and provides a fascinating example of how "knowledge" about food becomes an accepted truth through constant and widespread recitation. While we can see no problem with providing children with an additional opportunity to have a break and a snack, it is the apparently arbitrary specification of particular kinds of foods, none of which seem to be related to the complex science around foods and brain function (see, e.g., Gómez-Pinilla, 2008) that is both fascinating and troublesome. Like many of the practices associated with school food, the kind of food children brought to school as "brain food" was also sometimes policed in ways that were more related to arbitrary ideas about vegetables and fruit (and sometimes yoghurt and hummus) as healthy than any contribution to brain development or activity. Like other school food sites, they also had the potential for regulatory practices that singled out individual children for "shaming".

Food and school fundraising

Whilst families were subject to one set of rules about what food they could pack in school lunchboxes, there seemed to be a different set of rules for many schools when it came to fundraising efforts. And whilst school fundraising may not be understood to have the same function as nude food and brain food programs, it can be understood to be a pedagogical site that teaches children and parents "something about food". In our study, parents and children reported that they were required to buy or sell fundraising items such as pies and sausage rolls, hot cross buns, sandwiches and coffee. Food and beverage companies played an active role in fundraising efforts. For example, Cadbury chocolates, Subway sandwiches and products from soft drink manufacturers often appeared alongside sausage sizzles and bake sales. Some families talked about school efforts to raise money via the sale of healthier foods, but overall, it seemed that a different set of rules applied to food at school when funds were sought.

School food for thought

The many school food programs coupled by the lack of any ongoing formal curriculum and assessment served to create multiple points of contradiction and confusion about food for both students and parents. This is not to say that individual programs are failing. Rather, our findings reveal that understandings about food were produced across multiple sites via different programs, regulations and events. Given this, it is important to consider the multiple food pedagogies that are operating within a school rather than focusing on one program and its intended or real effects. We found that children talked largely about good (healthy) and bad (unhealthy) foods – with the distinction between them being the degree to which they contained sugar and fat. This simplistic binary, in large part, has been and continues to be motivated by popular, political and medical anxieties about overweight and obesity. What this means, as Welch and her colleagues point out, is that other meanings associated with food are "socially and pedagogically marginalised" (Welch, McMahon, & Wright, 2012, p. 213).

Our research findings provide significant food for thought for both policy makers and policy actors (Ball, Maguire, Braun, & Hoskins, 2011), including principals, teachers, public health workers and organisations that contribute to the (re) transformation of school food-scapes in response to the ongoing obesity epidemic. In suggesting this, we are not pointing the finger of blame at any specific policy actors for the "dog's breakfast" that we witnessed from our data across 44 schools and 50 families. Rather, we see complexity as an inevitable part of what it is to intervene in any health problem (see Warin & Zivkovic, 2019). Part of that complexity can be attributed to the prevailing neoliberal policy conditions that enable and constrain how school food is thought about and addressed. For example, schools and teachers are required to respond to a serious crisis, with very little, if any, funding. Additionally, schools find themselves in a position where they have to fundraise and so canteens and other fundraising efforts have to make a profit for them and so they find themselves having to balance profits with health. Teachers also have a lack expertise (content and peda-gogic), and this has significant consequences for the uptake of particular programs and their implementation. Our research points to the need for us to develop more sophisticated and nuanced insights into the everyday policies and practices of schools from multiple viewpoints including teachers, canteen workers, principals, children, parents and community partners and stakeholders.

Our research also provides ample food for thought for critical obesity scholars. We started the chapter by drawing attention to the early impact of the obesity epidemic on school pro-grams and research. In concluding the chapter, we want to draw attention to the changing nature and significance of the "epidemic" for those interested in researching school food and for critical obesity studies moving forward. In January 2019, The Lancet Commission acknowledged that the current approach to obesity prevention is failing and that obesity needs to be looked at in a much wider social and political context. It proposed the idea that we are now in a Global Syndemic that consists of a triplex of crises: obesity, malnutrition and climate change (Lancet, 2019). The report urged a radical rethink of business models, food systems, civil society involvement and national and international governance to address the syndemic. Alongside this, in Australia, we have had yet another inquiry into obesity which highlighted further increases in the prevalence of overweight and obesity (Commonwealth of Australia, 2018). The constant failure to make any headway in changing these statistics has resulted in calls for "amplification" of programs. Schools are, as expected, viewed as an integral component in any strategy moving forward. So, for those critical obesity scholars who secretly (or not so secretly) want schools to be left out of public health efforts to curb obesity, we would suggest that the reality of this happening is unlikely; as we type, this work has already begun in various school food policy forums to strategize how best to set about amplifying efforts.

In the context of the multiple pressures on schools to perform on numerous indicators and on the basis of our research (and that of others in this collection), we suggest that gov-ernments and those involved in efforts related to food and schools take stock before further amplifying current school programs. For critical obesity researchers, now might be the time to adopt some new tactics and to think about what, if any, opportunities the new global syndemic might offer us to reframe the problem and develop new approaches that take into account insights derived from critical obesity studies. For example, in relation to schools and education, we think that there is both an opportunity and a pressing need to include critical obesity studies in the formal curriculum as a way to broaden the study of food to enable more sophisticated understandings to emerge (Leahy et al., 2016; Welch & Leahy, 2018). We realise that, given the lack of formal curriculum opportunities identified in our research, the desire for a more educative study of food in schools – which takes into account the complex interaction of personal, social and cultural contexts – might be perceived to be wishful thinking. But we have examples already of where Food Studies has been introduced as a senior subject area in Victoria, and the new Australian Curriculum provides opportunities for critical inquiry in the focus area of food and nutrition. The new global syndemic is not going to go away anytime soon, and we do desperately need to transform school food programs and nutrition education to be able to respond adequately to the crises. Given this, we follow Warin and Zivkovic (2019) in suggesting that, perhaps, it is time for us to think about ways we might "assemble all knowledge practices and compare them, without privileging one over the other [and this could mean], a very useful way may emerge for us to reimagine obesity, and to find new ways to address it" (p. 215). Insights from critical obesity studies are crucial to informing future iterations of school food programs, and we need to find ways to ensure we have a seat at the table.

References

Ball, S., Maguire, M., Braun, A., & Hoskins, K. (2011). Policy subjects and policy actors in schools: some necessary but insufficient analyses, *Discourse, 32*(4), 611–624. doi: 10.1080/01596306.2011.601564

Burrows, L., & Wright, J. (2020). Biopedagogies and family life: A social class perspective. In D. Leahy, K. Fitzpatrick, K., & J. Wright (Eds). *Thinking with theory in health education* (pp. 19–32), London: Routledge.

Burrows, L., Wright, J., & Jurgensen-Smith, J. (2002). "Measure your belly" New Zealand children's constructions of health and fitness, *Journal of Teaching in Physical Education, 22*(1), 39–48.

Commonwealth of Australia. (2003). *Healthy Weight 2008: Australia's Future*. Canberra. http://www.healthyactive.gov.au/publications.htm

Commonwealth of Australia. (2018). *Obesity epidemic in Australia: Final report*. Retrieved from https://www.aph.gov.au/Parliamentary_Business/Committees/Senate/Obesity_epidemic_in_Australia/Obesity/Final_Report

Dean, M. (2010). *Governmentality: Power and rule in modern society* (2nd ed.). London: Sage.

Department of Education and Early Childhood Development. (2012). *Healthy canteen kit: School canteen and other school food services policy*. Retrieved from https://www.education.vic.gov.au/Documents/school/principals/management/gfylpolicy.pdf

Flowers, R., & Swan, E. (Eds.) (2015). *Food pedagogies*. Surrey: Ashgate.

Gard, M., & Pluim, C. (2014). *Schools and public health: Past, present, future*. Lanham, MD: Lexington Books.

Gard, M., & Wright, J. (2001). Managing uncertainty: Obesity discourses and physical education in a risk society. *Studies in Philosophy and Education, 20*(6), 535–549. doi: 10.1023/A:1012238617836

Gómez-Pinilla, F. (2008). Brain foods: The effects of nutrients on brain function. *Nature Reviews Neuroscience*, 9(7), 568–578. doi: 10.1038/nrn2421

Harman, V., & Cappelini, B. (2015). Mothers on display: Lunchboxes, social class and moral accountability. *Sociology, 49*(4), 764–781. doi: 10.1177/0038038514559322

Lancet. (2019). The global syndemic of obesity, undernutrition, climate change: The Lancet Commission Report. Retrieved from https://www.thelancet.com/commissions/global-syndemic

Leahy, D. (2012). *Assembling a health[y] subject*. PhD Thesis. Deakin University: Geelong.

Leahy, D. (2014). Assembling a health[y] subject: risky and shameful pedagogies in health education. *Critical Public Health, 24*(2), 171–181 doi: 10.1080/09581596.2013.871504

Leahy, D., & Harrison, L. (2004). Health and physical education and the production of the 'at risk self'. In J. Evans, B. Davies and J. Wright (Eds.), *Body knowledge and control: Studies in the sociology of physical education and health* (pp. 130–139). London: Routledge.

Leahy, D., McCuaig, L., Burrows, L., Wright, J., & Penney, D. (2016). *School health education in changing times: Policies, pedagogies and partnerships*. London: Routledge.

Maher, J., Supski, S., Wright, J., Leahy, D., Lindsay, L., & Tanner, C. (2020). Children, 'healthy' food, school and family: The '[n]ot really' outcome of school food messages, *Children's Geographies*, doi: 10.1080/14733285.2019.1598546

Moore, D., & Valverde, M. (2000). Maidens at risk: 'Date rape drugs' and the formation of hybrid risk knowledges. *Economy and Society, 29*, 514–531. doi: 10.1080/03085140050174769

O'Malley, P. (2004). *Risk, uncertainty and government*. London: Glasshouse Press.

Peterson, A., & Lupton, D. (1996). *The new public health: Health and self in the age of risk.* St Leonards, NSW: Allen & Unwin.

Pike, J., & Leahy, D. (2012). School food and the pedagogies of parents. *Australian Journal of Adult Learning, 52*(3), 434–459.

Pluim, C., Powell, D., & Leahy, D. (2018). Schooling lunch: Health, food, and the pedagogicalization of the lunch box. In S. Rice & A. G. Rud (Eds.), *Educational dimensions of school lunch: Critical perspectives* (pp. 59–74). Cham: Palgrave Macmillan.

Powell, D. (2015). *"Part of the solution"? Charities, corporate philanthropy and healthy lifestyles education in New Zealand primary schools* (Doctoral dissertation, Charles Sturt University, Bathurst, NSW).

Rose, N. (2000). Government and control. *British Journal of Criminology, 40,* 321–339. doi: 10.1093/bjc/40.2.321

Warin, M., & Zivkovic, T. (2019). *Fatness, obesity and disadvantage in the Australia suburbs: Unpalatable politics.* Cham: Palgrave Macmillan. doi: 10.1007/978-3-030–01009-6

Welch, R., & Leahy, D. (2018). Beyond the pyramid or plate: Contemporary approaches to food and nutrition education. *ACHPER Active and Healthy Magazine, 25*(2/3), 22–31.

Welch, R., McMahon, S., & Wright, J. (2012). The medicalisation of food pedagogies in primary schools and popular culture: A case for awakening subjugated knowledges. *Discourse, 33*(5), 713–728. doi: 10.1080/01596306.2012.696501

Wright, J., & Burrows, L. (2004). "Being healthy": The discursive construction of health in New Zealand children's responses to the National Education Monitoring Project. *Discourse, 25*(2), 211–230.

18

OBESITY AND THE PROPER MEAL AT WORKPLACE

French and English at the table and (or beyond) the culturalist explanation

Jean-Pierre Poulain and Cyrille Laporte

Introduction

When comparing the distribution of daily food intakes of the British population to those of the French studies reveal strong transformations of the former between 1960s and to-day (Cheng, Olsen, Southerton & Warde, 2007; Southerton, Diaz-Méndez & Warde, 2012; Warde & Martens, 2000) as opposed to a rather stable situation for the latter (Fischler & Masson, 2008; Poulain, 2017; Saint Pol, 2006). That is, while the French meal structure has indeed been simplified, the time frames as well as the level of socialization (i.e. the act of eating with others) have remained almost the same (Poulain, 2017; Poulain, Guignard, Michaud & Escalon, 2010; Riou, Lefèvre, Parizot, Lhuissier & Chauvin, 2015; Saint Pol, 2016)[1].

Relying on a socio-historical perspective supported by a review of literature besides qualitative and quantitative empirical data resulting from the authors' research programs carried out since 1995 (Poulain, Delorme, Gineste, & Laporte, 1996), this chapter investigates the methods used to institutionalize food systems at the workplace (Laporte & Poulain, 2014) and how technical solutions (e.g. catering types from enterprises and public authorities) devised by professional stakeholders take into account a 'real meal' or a 'proper meal' as Douglas (2002 [1984]) would have put it. The chapter also analyses how these technical systems influence eating practices by allowing (or not) and facilitating (or not) a number of changes. Finally, it considers to what extent the technical systems might have impacted a higher or lower prevalence of obesity in France and in the United Kingdom. A massive amount of data is definitely emerging that tends to relate the development of obesity to food practices damaging socialization (Fischler, 2011; Fischler & Masson, 2008; Poulain, 2009; Poulain et al., 2003).

Eating out of home: theoretical and practical issues

In this chapter, the word 'technique' is understood within the approach defined by Haudricourt (1987) who mentioned that technological choices depend on the cultural frames which give them meaning and help to legitimate their usage. The socio-cultural contexts within the food system devised at work have led the players involved in the process (e.g. human

DOI: 10.4324/9780429344824-22

resources managers, heads of works councils, and staff restaurants professionals) to define the contents and services included in a 'proper' and 'acceptable' meal for people at work. This process, which they openly rely on systems of social norms, is different in France and in the United Kingdom, according to Durkheim (1982). These norms account for the choice of some technical catering set-ups/systems against others as well as the way they have been or will be implemented. Referring to this, 'proper' meal is more important than what people eat. But it shows the particular context of the workplace. Therefore, our approach focus on the way these technical systems are being institutionalized through political ideas, the balance of power between the states and trade-unions, and management which all shaped by the economic social and political history of these two areas.

In addition, while there are a large number of studies focused on family-based daily diet or on the top quality food in gastronomic restaurants, few studies have been done on food at workplace whether in collective catering or in restaurants in the vicinity of the workplace (Corbeau, 1986; Dubuisson-Quellier, 1999; Grignon, 2001; Jacobs & Scholliers, 2003; Lambert & Bassecoulard-Zitt, 1987; Maho & Pynson, 1989; Poulain, 1993; Poulain et al., 1996; Wanjek, 2005). For some social and age groups, the eating environment may cover a significant part of their food intakes. Dealing with family diet, it is known that the type of family, the number of people, their sex, and the distribution of the house chores influence individual practices and decisions. However, in the case of out-of-home catering, other variables such as catering services, individualized methods of payment, company or government contribution to the costs, the forms of socialization provided and the existence of alternative solutions should be considered. The number of meals taken outside the home and the related expenses incurred vary from one country to the other, which cannot solely be accounted for by economic factors, such as the purchasing power, the price of services, or the level of economic development. Countries like Poland and Denmark display similar budgetary percentages assigned to out-of-home food (3 percent), while their gross domestic product (GDP) per inhabitant differs widely (less than EUR 10,000 per inhabitant for Poland and almost EUR 40,000 for Denmark). The outbreak of meals consumed in canteens or in restaurants also varies.

We have to make the distinction between collective catering services, what the hospitality managers call the 'cost sector', and the restaurants called 'profit sector' (Laporte, 2017). This second category regroups all the restaurants open to everybody, while the first one concerns food and beverage outlets set up by companies or organizations. In France, the foodservice cost sector is over 50 percent of the meals, while in the United Kingdom, it only adds up to 35 percent (Gira Foodservice, 2011).

In addition, eating at the workplace has undergone one of the highest levels of development in Western Europe since the 1970s. Corporate social policies, sometimes encouraged by government tax incentives, have been geared towards contributing to employees' lunches either by providing staff restaurants or by meal vouchers. In both cases, employees' lunch expenses are partly paid for by the company, also by the state through tax exemptions, because catering services are tax-free up to a given threshold for both employees and companies. In staff restaurants, a great number of meals can be served within short time-slots to optimize commute times. Their goal in France was to provide with a 'starter, main dish and dessert' type of service. But, to what extent, they contributed to slow down the evolution towards simplified meals? This context leaves eaters with little freedom when choosing their meals, which already overdetermined by decisions regarding the types of menus and dishes or their turnover, or decisions made by rather distant actors such as human resources managers, catering providers, works councils, or restaurant managers in an organizational system (Poulain, 2002a).

Moreover, there are three main types of catering management systems at the workplace: (1) providing special premises where employees may have their lunch, (2) implementing a staff canteen restaurant, and (3) providing meal vouchers. Depending on the choice employers have made, both their investment and the focus on catering is part of their corporate social policy. Both in France and the United Kingdom, labour legislation requires companies to provide their employees with a lunch area[2]. However, they may also set up a staff canteen where 'a real meal' can be eaten at little cost. Many services and industrial companies have adopted this approach.

Furthermore, employers may opt for meal vouchers. Smaller enterprises have particularly selected this system, as a means to contribute to their employees' meals at little cost. Because, they are entitled to deductions from the employers' social contributions and to some tax benefits. It also saves them from investing into a restaurant. In the French Labour Code, meal vouchers are defined as payment documents to be used by employees to fully or partly pay for their restaurant meals[3]. The system had been initiated at the beginning of the 1950s by Dr Winchendron who devised vouchers for using by his clinic staff in the restaurants which he had passed an agreement with whether true or highlighted as a milestone, this story is everywhere in the professional literature to reveal the age-old medical approach over 'eating well'.

In France, vouchers were used in the early 1960s for the first time. Nevertheless, that policy, which improves employees' purchasing power indirectly, was devised in a state of full-employment and has become a source of inequality in times of growing unemployment now.

In addition, restaurants in the vicinity of companies offer more individualized schedules and lunch breaks. Regarding the meal vouchers, they give employees freedom of choice for the restaurant, the date, the time, and even partly, the recipient employees may choose to use them for what they were devised. That is to say, for their own lunches in the company commercial environment on workdays, or for other occasions, for example, on their own, or with family and friends on weekdays[4]. The vouchers can also be used for buying food. What impact do the development and differentiated use of these catering systems have on the actual implementation of food practices and schedules? We study these differences by gearing our research towards the social and cultural phenomena that may account for them, first. Next, we attempt to analyse their impact on the various forms of food sociability.

French and British eaters

In a socio-historical perspective and in line with Elias' work (1982), Mennell, Murcott, and Van Otterloo (1992) suggested the differences in the gastronomic cultures of France and the United Kingdom, and more generally, the relation of two areas to food originated from curialization[5]. In his analysis of food temporalities and of their evolution, Cheng et al. (2007) highlighted that French spent more time eating which it shrunk significantly in the United Kingdom over the last 20 years. This time has remained stable in France over the same period. In the following section, we compare the budget devoted to food as well as the number and types of meals in two areas first. Next, we focus on the meals eaten inside and outside of home and how they are distributed between community catering and catering businesses.

Meals and 'food days'

For a closer look at the types of meals and to describe food practices, five dimensions have been listed by Herpin (1988): (1) concentration (i.e. complex organization of food intakes in the form of meals), (2) time-framing (i.e. keeping fixed times for meals and snacks), (3) synchronization (i.e. sharing meals with the whole family), (4) localization (i.e. the place where meals are eaten in the kitchen or in the dining room), and (5) ritualization (i.e. 'everyday meals' alternating with 'festive meals').

To explain how some of these dimensions such as concentration time framing and synchronization interact, the concept of 'food days' has been suggested by Poulain (2001, 2002b). Food days is defined as the distribution of the various food intakes in meals and outside meals in the course of a day. The time frame of intakes gives the day its food tempo with highlights dedicated to this activity by a significant part of the society. The socialization of meals and other intakes outside the meals imply that schedules are being co-ordinated. Analysing the consumption places enables to identify the limits between the domestic work and catering worlds on a macrosociological scale.

The concept of 'food days' also highlights another dimension of 'food synchronization' which reports on the fact that the individuals belonging to the same social group or same society eat at the same time. Also, the great number of possible combinations between meals and outside meals make up the day profiles (Holm, 2001; Mäkelä, 2000; Mäkelä et al., 1999; Poulain, 2001; Poulain et al., 1996). In regard to the United Kingdom, the structures of the British meals have been throughly studied in valuable qualitative research work; however, unlike France, quantitative data are few and fragmentary. Douglas (1972) and Murcott (2012) identified the 'proper meal' by studying the differentiation in the forms of days in the social hierarchy. Douglas (1972) underlines that identical names hide different types of meals. She also mentions that the meal time schedules depend on social classes. For example, tea is a ritualized snack among the aristocracy, but in other social classes, there may also be a large meal which may not include any tea (tea or high tea have little to do with tea time). In addition, considering the evolution of meal times during the 'food days' in 1961–2001 in the United Kingdom shows that food intakes were spaced out over the day which resulted into social desynchronization and probably into decreasing community meals. Data from BBC, ONS, and nVision have a grey literature status that has not been published academically. However, published research based on the United Kingdom Time Use Survey for the year 2000 shows an identical daily food intake distribution (Southerton, 2009; Southerton et al., 2012). The analysis of temporal rythms between 1937 and 2000 shows desynchronization.

According to Figure 18.1, there is a move from four distinct peaks in 1961 during which a high proportion of the population ate at the same time to slight regroupings into three points and spaced out intakes over the day in 2001, which reflects strong desynchronization. Although the data available for France do not cover quite the same time span, they show a clear breakdown of the time frames allocated to the three main meals and small snacks. (i.e. '[insert Figure 18.2]').

In 1999, the French curve is close to that of 1961 for the United Kingdom and remains stable for over seven years. As opposed to the evolution in the United Kingdom, the data highlight the permanence of a strong synchronization of meals while the structure of meals has been changed in France. The comparison of types of meals through the Health and Food barometer number 3 of the French National Institute of Health Promotion and Education (INPES, Intitut national de promotion et d'éducation pour la santé) (Baudier, Rotily, Le Bihan, Janvrin & Michaud, 1997; Guilbert & Perrin-Escalon, 2004; Poulain et al., 2010)

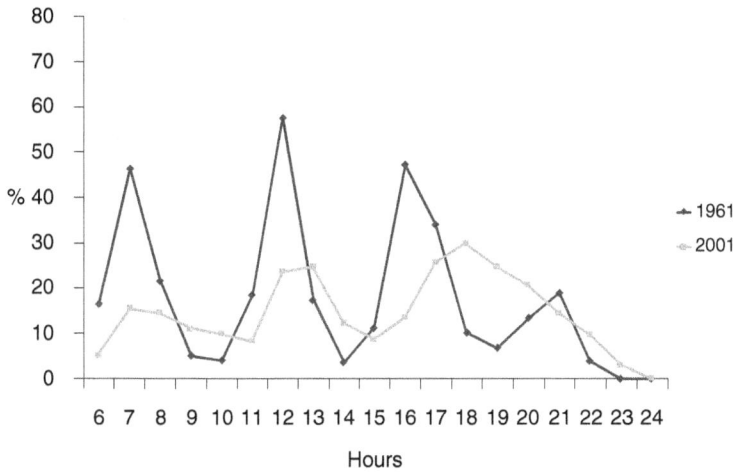

Figure 18.1 Time framing and synchronization of daily food intakes in % – England/Britain (1961 & 2001).

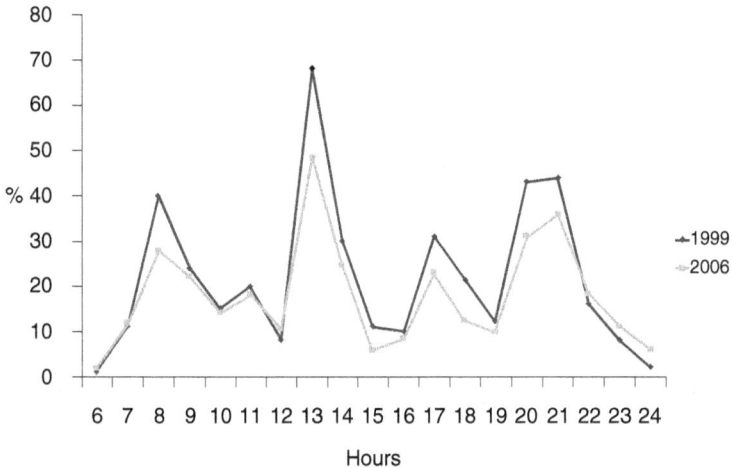

Figure 18.2 Time framing and synchronization of daily food intakes in % – France (1999 & 2006).

shows that the percentage of meals with four components has moved down from 25 percent to 17 percent. For those with three components, it has moved down from 37.8 percent to 33 percent (Poulain et al., 2010). Therefore, there are both a move towards meal simplification and at the same time a continued synchronization due to remaining identical times.

Furthermore, the evolutions in types and times of meals in the British world are different from what are found in the French world. The impacts of these transformations are significant because British eat more often outside their homes (21 percent, 2011) than French do (13.6 percent, 2006) which increases the desynchronization of meals in the United Kingdom.

Considering corporate catering in France, it shows that the greater number of company canteens has reinforced the synchronization of food intakes by setting lunch during the midday break. Also, more than one out of five British people does not have a meal at lunch time (Eurest, 2006). What may account for such a significant difference between two countries enjoying very similar living standards? Our hypothesis is that the level of out-the-home consumption and the differentiated development of catering technical solutions, more or less, impact the individualization of food decisions and consumption. However, this differentiated development can only be understood by referring to the value systems which allow such practices. That is, cyclical causalities could have been at work in that case.

In addition, beyond the divergences in the way corporate catering management systems have been mobilized, the cultural differences in defining what a 'proper meal' is tend to increase desynchronization in the United Kingdom, on the one hand, and synchronization in France on the other hand.

Views and norms underlying technical catering systems

In France, the establishment and stabilization of 'food days', including three meals, was the outcome of several combined factors originating back to the French Revolution. The *Bourgeoisie* chose to follow the rules of the *Service à la Russe* rather than the one's of the *Service à la française* (Flandrin & Montanari, 1999) to serve dishes, which reflects the social hierarchy very much. This time could be counted as the starting point of the development of the French meal national model. Its dissemination to other social groups was slow and gradual. The peasants' food still depended on local resources and seasons just as the craftsmen's eating organization followed their work schedules. The institutionalization of the model stems from the French taste for ruling inherited from the *Ancien Régime* monasteries and convents as well as the hold of the Catholic religion which believes that the spirit should control the body. The dissemination and stabilization of the three-meal model are the outcome of a wider and deeper process which contributed to the building up of French identity. The use of the French language or the creation of institutions responsible for staging the big egalitarian myth (e.g. school, army, and hospital) supported the homogeneization and dissemination of the national model. Also, because it was accompanied by the dissemination of the universal values, the ideology of hygienics supported this ideal model as well.

In addition, the development of biology found favour with 'ways of eating well', the three-meal model became the norm (Aymard, Grignon & Sabban, 1993; Poulain, 2001, 2017). In the United Kingdom, the structures of dishes, menus, and meal times rely on three elements: (1) cooked dinner, (2) fish and chips, and (3) tea (Murcott, 1982). As mentioned earlier, each of these elements is not given the same meaning according to the social class the one belongs to. For example, tea is the main meal among the working class, while it may refer to a snack or dinner (high tea) for the middle and upper classes. Therefore, it is more difficult to duplicate homogeneous technical catering systems to fragmented expectations. Besides, according to Murcott (2012), the evening meal is seen as the highlight of Anglo-Saxon daily food intakes. This is one of the strongest divergences with the French model in which lunch is central to 'food days'.

In addition, the differences in the number of daily meals schedules and meal structures are part and parcel of the social representations of the stakeholders in charge of defining the catering systems. That is, the stakeholders have to provide the patterns of thought presiding over the choice of catering forms, the definition of the offer, or the valorization of financial support for lunch at work. In view of this, the homogenization of the post-war French meal, emerging as a model and a symbol of social progress, led to seeking the systems and formulas that would be suitable for everybody. Another difference in the way of implementing the systems is the average cash value of meal vouchers, which expresses how important catering at work is to decision-makers and corporate catering managers (e.g. the state, enterprises, and institutions) in two areas. In France, EUR 6.50 enables recipients to buy a multi-component meal, whereas EUR 4.18 in the United Kingdom only cover one simple food intake or a snack (Wanjek, 2005).

From catering technical systems at workplace to addressing the issue of obesity

In the United Kingdom, meal synchronization has significantly decreased over the last few decades, while it has remained more or less stable in France. These phenomena reveal differences in food budgets, the number of meals outside the home, and their distribution between collective catering and restaurants. These differences are due to the transformations in job structures and the cultural approaches of technical systems, which help to meet the need for eating at work. The arguments developed in this article open up avenues for research to understand the relations between food practices, their correlated catering technical systems providing meals at the workplace, and the prevalence of obesity. The big differences in the ways corporate catering management systems are used, and the different conditions of lunchtime socialization do prompt to consider whether there may be links to be established with the highly differentiated growth of obesity in these two areas. According to the report of International Association for the Study of Obesity (IASO) in 2007, the prevalence of obesity is higher in the United Kingdom than in France. That is, 23.1 percent of British males and 24.3 percent of British females are obese (BMI over 30), whereas only 11.8 percent of French males and 13 percent of French females are obese. The same applies to overweight (BMI between 25 and 29.9), which is 43.4 percent for males and 32.1 percent for females in the United Kingdom, but 35.6 percent for French males and 23.3 percent for French females.

Moreover, Qvortrup (2005) has provided an explanation at the macrososiological level. According to him, the successive social changes from a traditional industrial society to a deregulated and globalized economy have led to the emergence of new life and work structures, which have had negative impacts on food consumption and physical exercising by growing up the epidemic of obesity. Relying on the United Kingdom's data, Qvortrup (2005) shows that the development of a neoliberal economic policy deeply influenced employment because there was a rapid increase in temporary jobs with negative consequences on household income. The introduction of job flexibility has contributed to changing meal times and developing out-of-home eating, in addition to the compelling people to use pre-processed products often. This may be seen as undermining the social supervision of people's ways of life, and above all, of their foodways.

In addition, Fischler and Masson (2008) have emphasized on the process of food decision-making, which has undergone greater individualization in the 'anglo-saxon world' than in France. They also suggest that the persistence of synchronized meals could be one of the factors accounting for the rather low rate of obesity in the United Kingdom. Drewnowski and Darmon (2005) have shown that the lower the share of food in a population's budget (such as the case in the United Kingdom), the more highly nutrient food is purchased.

Furthermore, this chapter examines how the technical catering systems, selected to organize meals at work on either side of the channel, may have contributed to the growth of desynchronization and social marginalization of eating practices to increase the individualized situations which tend to favour obesity. This approach endorses the culturalist-biased hypothesis of 'the more individualistic British' and of 'the more commensal French', as supported by fact-finding observations. The cultural views of what the 'real meal' is have determined the ways that technical catering systems are viewed and set (e.g. the amount of the meal voucher which is supposed to meet a worker's needs for lunch). The other way round is that the systems are influencing concrete food practices by making some types of practices available and more or less lasting. If one goes in line with the idea that a shared meal helps good nutritional practices by positioning the individual under the supervision of others, it means that the French systems facilitate the socialized and synchronized meals, which could have slowed down the development of obesity in France. Even if non-domestic catering only concerns the working population and only for one-third of the week meals, there is still evidence to suggest that it influences the organization of 'food days'.

As a result of this study, the notion of food synchronization emerges as an indicator to analyse the consequences of social contexts over food practices. Friendliness and conviviality, in addition to the accompanying shared pleasure of eating (Dupuy, 2013; Fischler, 2011), support the idea that it may have a positive influence on people's health. This is what the case of obesity tends to suggest. However, socialized meals should not be naively over-idealized. In other contexts, such as people who suffer from hypercholesterolemics, the influence seems to be much more ambivalent (Fournier, 2012).

The arguments developed in this chapter open up avenues of research to understand the relationship between dietary practices and the prevalence of obesity. They show that the determinants are not only at the level of individuals and their decisions (Poulain 2020; Warde, 2016). They show that the organization of food support systems in the workplace (collective restaurants, luncheon vouchers, etc.) overdetermines choices, making certain types of eating behaviour possible or not. It also shows how food cultures correlated providing meals at the workplace.

The design of the systems is the result of social interactions between several categories of actors (HRDs, staff representatives, tax authorities, catering professionals, etc.) who think of their action within a food culture. Through the consensus that is established on the means and devices (and periodically redefined), cultural conceptions of what is a real meal, a decent meal, are expressed. More broadly, we see here how individuals' decisions are embedded in social and cultural phenomena that predetermine them. Actions to prevent obesity are likely to be ineffective if they do not take into account these levels which are beyond the individual. Worse, by designating individuals as responsible and making them feel guilty, they are likely to be counterproductive. Obesity is a scientific and social problem requiring the mobilization of researchers, of industrial actors (food, catering and pharmacy), of public health stakeholders, but also of fashion, and the media. This is a problem which involves shared responsibilities (Gard & Wright, 2005; Poulain, 2011).

Notes

1 Other works have compared the French and British situations; Mennell (1996) in a historical perspective and from the point of view of gastronomic styles; Darmon and Warde (2014) from the point of view of culinary and alimentary practices of Anglo-French couples; and Lhuissier (2014) from the point of view of the criteria for organizing national surveys.
2 French Labour Code: articles R4228-19, R4228-22 and R4228-23.
3 Article L3262-1 of the French Labour Code.
4 However, as the staff working on weekends may use meal vouchers, few establishments control this aspect, which means that their utilization goes beyond the limits of meals at work.
5 The process of curialization refers to the organization of relations between a king and the aristocratic élites. Court manners were accompanied by some particular forms of civility Mennell accounts for the differences between English/British and French gastronomes by resorting to the major difference existing between the two aristocracies, that is, the latter's permanent residence in the capital or at Versailles, whereas the former travelled back and forth between London and their regional settlements. Elias has demonstrated how, within the French curialization, the continuous renewal of culinary forms as well as of fashion aimed at keeping at a distance the emerging groups from the bourgeoisie and at ensuring the élites' legitimate domination.

References

Aymard, M., Grignon, C., & Sabban, F. (1993). *The time to eat: Food time and social rhythms*. Editions MSH-INRA.

Baudier, F., Rotily, M., Le Bihan, G., Janvrin, M.P., & Michaud, C. (1997). *Baromètre santé nutrition 1996 [Nutritional Health Barometer]*. CFES.

Cheng, S.L., Olsen, W., Southerton, D., & Warde, A. (2007). The changing practice of eating: Evidence from UK time diaries 1975 and 2000. *The British Journal of Sociology. 58*(1), 39–61. doi: 10.1111/j.1468-4446.2007.00138.x

Corbeau, J.P. (1986). L'avaleur n'attend pas le nombre des années ou l'éducation alimentaire [The swallower does not wait for the number of years or the food education]. *Les Cahiers de l'iforep. 49*, 15–19.

Darmon, I., & Warde, A. (2014). Under pressure – learning from the culinary and alimentary practices of Anglo-French couples for cross-national comparison. *Anthropology of food*. https://journals.openedition.org/aof/7649.

Douglas, M. (1972). Deciphering a Meal. *Daedalus. 101*(1), 61–81.

Douglas, M. (2002 [1984]). *Food in the social order. Studies of food and festivities in three American communities*. Routledge.

Drewnowski, A., & Darmon, N. (2005). Food choices and diet costs: An economic analysis. *The Journal of Nutrition. 135*(4), 900–904. doi: 10.1093/jn/135.4.900

Dubuisson-Quellier, S. (1999). Le prestataire, le client et le consommateur. Sociologie d'une relation marchande [The provider, the client and the consumer. Sociology of a market relationship]. *Revue française de sociologie. XL*(4), 671–688.

Dupuy, A. (2013). *Plaisirs alimentaires. Socialisation des enfants et des adolescents [Food pleasures. Socialization of children and adolescents]*. Presses Universitaires de Rennes.

Durkheim, E. (1982). *The rules of the sociological method*. The Free Press.

Elias, N. (1982). *The civilizing process* (Vol. 2). Pantheon books.

Eurest. (2006). *Eurest Lunchtime*. Uxbridge.

Fischler, C. (2011). Commensality society and culture. *Social Science Information. 50*(3–4), 528–548. doi: 10.1177/0539018411413963

Fischler, C., & Masson, E. (2008). *Manger: Français Européens et Américains face l'alimentation [Eating: French Europeans and Americans face food]*. Odile Jacob.

Flandrin, J.L., & Montanari, M., (Eds.). (1999). *Food: A culinary history*. Columbia University Press.

Fournier, T. (2012). Suivre ou s'écarter de la prescription diététique. Les effets du "manger ensemble" et du "vivre ensemble" chez des personnes hypercholestérolémiques en France [Follow or stay away from dietary prescription. The effects of "eating together" and "living together" in French people with hypercholesterolemics]. *Sciences sociales et santé. 2*(2), 35–60. doi : 10.3917/sss.302.0035

Gard, M., & Wright, J. (2005). *The obesity epidemic: Science, morality and ideology*. Routledge.

Gira Foodservice. (2011). *The contract catering market in west Europe*. Paris.

Grignon, C. (2001). Commensality and social morphology: An essay of typology. In M. Jacob & P. Scholliers (Eds.), *Food drink and identity: Cooking, eating and drinking in Europe since the Middle Ages* (pp. 23–33). Berg Publishers.

Guilbert, P., & Perrin-Escalon, H. (2004). *Baromètre santé nutrition 2002 [Nutritional health barometer 2002]*. Editions Inpes.

Haudricourt, A.G. (1987). *La technologie science humaine. Recherches d'histoire et d'ethnologie des techniques [Technology as a human science. Research on the history and ethnology of technology]*. Editions de la Maison des Sciences de l'Homme.

Herpin, N. (1988). Le repas comme institution. Compte rendu d'une enquête exploratoire [The meal as an institution. Report of an exploratory survey]. *Revue française de sociologie. 29*(3), 503–521.

Holm, L. (2001). Family meals. In L. Holm & U. Kjaernes (Eds.), *Eating patterns: A day in the lives of Nordic peoples* (pp. 199–212). National Institute for Consumer Research.

IASO. (2007). *Prevalence of obesity in European Countries*. International Association for the Study of Obesity.

Jacobs, M., & Scholliers P (2003). *Eating out in Europe: Picnics gourmet dining and snacks since the late eighteenth century*. Berg Publishers.

Lambert, J.L., & Bassecoulard-Zitt, E. (1987). La place de la restauration dans la consommation alimentaire en France [The place of the restaurant industry in food consumption in France]. *Cahiers de Nutrition et de Diététique 22*(3), 210–219.

Laporte, C. (2017). Restauration collective [Foodservice cost sector]. In J.P. Poulain (Ed.), *Dictionnaire des cultures alimentaires [Dictionary of food cultures]* (pp. 1231–1236). Presses Universitaires de France.

Laporte, C., & Poulain, J. P. (2014). Restauration d'entreprise en France et au RoyaumeUni. Synchronisation sociale alimentaire et obésité [Meal at the workplace in France and the United Kingdom. Social food synchronization and obesity]. *Ethnologie française, 44*(1), 93–103. doi: 10.3917/ethn.141.0093

Lhuissier, A. (2014). Anything to declare? Questionnaires and what they tell us. *Anthropology of food.* http://journals.openedition.org/aof/7625.

Maho, J., & Pynson, P. (1989). Cantines comment s'en débarrasser? [Canteens how to get rid of them]. In F. Piault & R. Louis (Eds.), *Nourritures plaisirs et angoisses de la fourchette [Food pleasures and anxieties of the fork]* (pp. 200–205). Autrement.

Mäkelä, J. (2000). Cultural definitions of the meal. In H. L. Meiselman (Ed.), *Dimensions of the meal: The Science, Culture, Business and Art of Eating* (pp. 7–18). Springer.

Mäkelä, J., Kjærnes, U., Ekström, M.P., Fürst, E.O., Gronow, J., & Holm, L. (1999). Nordic meals: Methodological notes on a comparative survey. *Appetite 32*(1), 73–79. doi: 10.1006/appe.1998.0198

Mennell, S. (1996). *All manners of food: Eating and taste in England and France from the Middle Ages to the present.* University of Illinois Press.

Mennell, S., Murcott, A., & Van Otterloo, A.H. (1992). *The sociology of food: Eating, diet and culture.* Sage.

Murcott, A. (1982). On the social significance of the "cooked dinner" in South Wales. *Social Science Information 21*(4–5), 677–696. doi: 10.1177/053901882021004011

Murcott, A. (2012). Royaume-Uni [United Kingdom]. In J.P. Poulain (Ed.), *Dictionnaire des cultures alimentaires* [Dictionary of food cultures] (pp. 1186–1196). Presses Universitaires de France.

Poulain, J.P. (1993). Les nouveaux comportements alimentaires [The new food behaviours]. *Revue technique des hôtels et des restaurants, 521,* 49–57.

Poulain, J.P. (2001). *Manger aujourd'hui. Attitudes normes pratiques [Eating today. Attitudes, norms and practices].* Paris: Privat.

Poulain, J.P. (2002a). Les pratiques alimentaires de la population mangeant au restaurant d'entreprise [Food practices of the population eating at the workplace]. *Consommations et sociétés, 2,* 97–110.

Poulain, J.P. (2002b). The contemporary diet in France: "De-structuration" or from commensalism to "vagabond feeding". *Appetite, 39*(1), 43–55. doi: 10.1006/appe.2001.0461

Poulain, J.P. (2009). *Sociologie de l'obésité [Sociology of obesity].* Presses Universitaires de France.

Poulain, J.P. (2011). Sociologie de l'obésité : déterminants sociaux et construction sociale de l'obésité [Sociology of obesity: Social determinants and social construction of obesity]. In A. Basdevant (Ed.), *Traité de médecine et chirurgie de l'obésité [Treaty of medicine and surgery of obesity]* (pp. 35–47). Lavoisier.

Poulain, J.P. (2017). *The sociology of food. Eating and the place of food in society.* Bloomsbury Academic.

Poulain, J.P. (2020). Towards a sociological theory of eating: A review of Alan Warde's The Practice of Eating. *Anthropology of food.* https://journals.openedition.org/aof/10866

Poulain, J.P., Delorme, J.M., Gineste, M., & Laporte, C. (1996). *Les nouvelles pratiques alimentaires entre commensalisme et vagabondage [The new food practices between commensalism and vagrancy].* French Ministry of Agriculture and Food, Research Programme "Aliments Demain". Paris, February.

Poulain, J.P., Guignard, R., Michaud, C., & Escalon, H. (2010). *Les repas: Distribution journalière, structure, lieux et convivialité [Meals: Daily distribution, structure, location and conviviality].* In H. Escalon, C. Bossard & F. Beck (Eds.), *Baromètre santé nutrition 2008 [Nutritional Health Barometer 2008]* (pp 187–211). Paris: Editions Inpes.

Poulain, J.P., Romon, M., Jeanneau, S., Tibère, L., Barbe, P., Prigent, S., & Serog, P. (2003). *Alimentation hors repas et corpulence: Rare-Nutrialis [Off-meal feeding and weight: Rare-Nutrialis].* French Ministry of Research.

Qvortrup, M. (2005). Globalisation and obesity. *Obesity in Practice. 1*(2), 50–59.

Riou, J., Lefèvre, T., Parizot, I., Lhuissier, A., & Chauvin, P. (2015). Is there still a French eating model? A taxonomy of eating behaviors in adults living in the Paris metropolitan area in 2010. *PLOS ONE. 10*(3). doi. 10.1371/journal.pone.0119161

Saint Pol, T. (2006). Le dîner des Français: un synchronisme alimentaire qui se maintient [The French dinner: A food synchronicity that is maintained]. *Economie et statistiques. 400,* 45–69.

Saint Pol, T. (2016). Les habitudes alimentaires des Français: une institution sociale entre constance et renouveau [French food habits: A social institution between constancy and renewal]. *Esprit 425,* 111–120.

Southerton, D. (2009). Temporal rhythms: Comparing daily lives of 1937 with those of 2000 in the UK. In E. Shove, F. Trentmann & R. Wilk (Eds.), *Time, consumption and everyday life: Practice materiality and culture* (pp. 49–63). Berg.

Southerton, D., Diaz-Méndez, C., & Warde, A. (2012). Behavioural change and the temporal ordering of eating practices: A UK-Spain comparison. *International Journal of Sociology of Agriculture and Food. 19*(1), 19–36. doi: 10.48416/ijsaf.v19i1.233

Wanjek, C. (2005). *Food at work: Workplace solutions for malnutrition obesity and chronic diseases.* International Labour Organization.

Warde, A. (2016). *The practice of eating.* Polity.

Warde, A., & Martens, L. (2000). *Eating out: Social differentiation consumption, and pleasure.* University Press.

19

JUNK FOOD MARKETING, CHILDHOOD OBESITY, AND THE PRODUCTION OF (UN)CERTAINTY

Darren Powell

Introduction

In the global 'war on childhood obesity', so-called junk food marketing is frequently positioned by politicians, public health experts, media, and the public as a key battleground. The rationale is fairly simple and frequently articulated as follows: "Marketing affects what children want, buy and eat, which in turn affects their health and contributes to the increasing levels of childhood obesity" (World Cancer Research Fund, 2020, para. 2). While there is much research that demonstrates how marketing practices shape 'what children want, buy and eat'– after all that is the point of marketing – the relationship between food marketing, children's health, and childhood obesity is far less clear or certain.

The point of this chapter is to disrupt the 'truth' that food marketing contributes to childhood obesity by critically examining how *certainty* about this relationship is (re)produced through expert knowledge and the unquestioning acceptance of the 'junk food marketing = childhood obesity' discourse. My aim here is to illuminate how dominant obesity discourses work to produce 'regimes of truth' (Foucault, 1980) about the relationship between food marketing and childhood obesity; how expertise, power, knowledge, and discourses congeal and cohere to (re)produce the taken-for-granted assumption that junk food marketing = childhood obesity. In a similar vein to Gard and Wright's (2001, 2005) critique of 'certain' obesity discourses in physical education, my central concern is how scholars – particularly in the field of public health – contribute to the dismantlement of uncertainty (with respect to knowledge about the relationship between 'junk' food advertising and fatness) and the concomitant construction of certainty "where none seems justified" (2001, p. 535).

Junk food marketing and childhood obesity: joining two discourses

Although there are numerous critiques of obesity science that demonstrate how the causes, consequences, measurements, prevalence, and solutions to childhood obesity are complicated and uncertain (e.g., see Ellison et al., 2016; Evans & Colls, 2009; Gard, 2011; Wright & Harwood, 2012), articles written by public health researchers articles (and accompanying media releases) tend to conclude with a strong air of certainty that (a) being fat is unhealthy, (b) there is a childhood obesity crisis, (c) exposure to junk food marketing is a vital part of

DOI: 10.4324/9780429344824-23

the 'problem' of obesity, and (d) removing junk food advertising is a key 'part of the solution'. The way this knowledge is discursively produced can be illustrated, in part, by an interrogation of the introductions of academic journal articles on 'junk food' marketing and its impact on childhood obesity.

In the next section, I critically analyse a handful of journal articles by public health researchers that focus on the alleged dangers of food marketing for children's fatness and health. As I endeavour to demonstrate, the 'certain' relationship between junk food marketing and childhood obesity is achieved by drawing on and connecting together two dominant discourses, a narrow selection and understanding of particular studies, and communicating research through a now rather familiar argument.

Childhood obesity discourses

In introduction to journal articles on the alleged health effects of junk food marketing, authors tend to begin by outlining global and/or national childhood obesity statistics, such as "Over the past three decades the global prevalence of childhood overweight and obesity has increased by 47%" (Signal et al., 2017, p. 2) or "New Zealand's rates of childhood obesity are unacceptably high" (Vandevijvere et al., 2017a, p. 3029). Often, these statistics are accompanied by 'alarming' rhetoric that positions childhood obesity as a crisis, such as the first line of Vandevijvere and colleagues' (2017b, p. 32) article which reads: "The prevalence of childhood obesity has increased dramatically worldwide since the 1980s, and is considered one of the most serious public health issues of the 21st century". This claim is immediately backed by statistics: "The most recent New Zealand Health Survey (2015/2016) showed that one in three children are overweight or obese; a two percentage point increase since 2006/2007" (p. 32). Even though there is an effortlessness in which these statements are accepted as being certain 'truths', the interconnected ideas that childhood obesity is the "most serious public health issues of the 21st century" and is increasing globally in epidemic proportions are also assumptions that have been contested, critiqued, and challenged (e.g., see Gard, 2011; Gard & Wright, 2005; Powell, 2020a).

The work of critical obesity scholars is valuable here because it recognises that "definitions of the problem of overweight and obesity as well as suggested interventions are not as simplistic, straightforward, or as ideologically neutral as they appear" (Vander Schee & Boyles, 2010, p. 170). For example, the 'truth' that there *is* a childhood obesity crisis, that rates of childhood obesity are not only increasing but also increasingly increasing, was challenged by Gard over a decade ago, (2011, p. 66) providing strong evidence "that overweight and obesity prevalence amongst Western children had flattened and, in some cases, begun to decline even before the world-wide alarm about spiralling childhood obesity had been raised". However, when 'expert' biomedical knowledge, fear of the fat body, and alarming rhetoric of an obesity crisis are assembled together (see Evans et al., 2004), dominant obesity discourses are strengthened and "help create cultural environments where the claims themselves are treated as uncontestable truths, void of any ambiguities and uncertainties" (Vander Schee & Boyles, 2010, p. 170).

The 'uncontestable truth' that there *is* a childhood obesity crisis in New Zealand is demonstrated through Vandevijvere et al.'s (2017b, p. 32) introductory paragraphs, where the authors draw on an official report from the Ministry of Health (2016) to state that "one in three children are overweight or obese; a two percentage point increase since 2006/2007". These statistics, however, do not tell the full story. For example, the use of the "one in three children are overweight or obese" was a deliberate rhetorical device that combined two body mass index (BMI) categories, making the 'problem' of fat children seem larger than only reporting childhood obesity statistics (which the government report stated was 11 percent at the time). In addition, although Vandevijvere et al. reported a significant increase in the prevalence of 'obese' children reported between 2006/2007 and 2015/2016, there was no significant increase in waist to height ratios or a significant increase in the prevalence of 'overweight' children. Over this same period, there was a significant increase in the prevalence of 'thin' children; yet, this was not raised as an 'alarming' increase, a serious public health issue, or even a cause for concern. If the authors had decided to select two different points in time, such as the period from 2011/2012 to 2015/2016, this may not have supported their argument of obesity as increasing 'dramatically'. During this particular period, there was *no significant increase* in the prevalence of overweight or obese children, and even the Ministry of Health (2016, para. 5) reported in their overview of key findings that "Child obesity rates have stabilised to 2011/12 rates".[1]

It is through this type of research and writing that dominant obesity discourses circulate and are (re)produced as the 'truth' about children, bodies, and health. As Foucault (1980) also argued, every society has 'regimes of truth' – particular discourses that are accepted by society and allowed to function as true. Although, in this chapter, I am not attempting to substitute one set of obesity 'truths' with another, what I am trying to point out is how certain discourses of childhood obesity 'work'; how they may produce certain truths, subjugate other knowledges, and are fused with junk food marketing discourses to become even more undeniable and unquestionable.

Attaching 'junk food marketing' discourses to childhood obesity discourses

After authors have set the familiar scene that childhood obesity is a crisis, they then draw on expert knowledge – most often through citing from a select few systematic reviews and World Health Organisation (WHO) reports – to state clearly that 'junk' food advertising does indeed make children fat/ter. For example, immediately following their first introductory paragraph outlining the 'dramatic' increase in childhood obesity, Vandevijvere et al. (2017b, p. 32) state: "Unhealthy food marketing to children is one risk factor for childhood obesity". Similarly, Signal et al. (2017, p. 2) begin the second paragraph of their article with the decisive sentence: "Marketing of energy-dense nutrient-poor (EDNP) foods and beverages contributes to the worldwide increase in childhood obesity". The language used in both these claims makes the evidence seem certain: junk food marketing *is* a risk factor and *does* contribute to a global childhood obesity epidemic. So where does this certain evidence come from?

The expert and official evidence base that these types of assumptions are based on come from several key documents that are continually recycled and recited to (re)produce the 'junk food marketing = childhood obesity' discourse. One central document is the WHO's (2016) *Report of the Commission on Ending Childhood Obesity* (cited over 600 times, including by Signal et al., 2017; Vandevijvere et al., 2017b). The first line of this report, predictably, reinforces dominant obesity discourses: "Childhood obesity is reaching alarming proportions in many countries and poses an urgent and serious challenge" (p. vi). Among the WHO Commission's many recommendations for governments, schools, private sector groups, and philanthropists is Recommendation 1.3: "Implement the *Set of Recommendation on the Marketing of Foods and Non-alcoholic Beverages to Children* to reduce the exposure of children and adolescents to, and the power of, the marketing of unhealthy foods" (WHO, 2016, p. 18). The official rationale for this recommendation is as follows: "There is *unequivocal evidence* that the marketing of unhealthy foods and sugar-sweetened beverages is related to childhood obesity" (WHO, 2016, p. 18, emphasis added). Upon closer examination, however, this 'unequivocal evidence' about food marketing's relationship with childhood obesity is *solely* based on two publications: *Review of research on the effects of food promotion to children* (Hastings et al., 2003) and *Food Marketing to children and youth: Threat or opportunity?* (Kraak et al., 2006). As I illustrate next, these two publications – and the research their conclusions are based upon – are far from unequivocal.

Food Marketing to children and youth: Threat or opportunity? (Kraak et al., 2006, cited over 800 times) was an Institute of Medicine (IOM) study in the United States of America, which at the time was described by *Food Politics* author Marion Nestle (2006, p. 2527) as providing a "chilling account" of how marketing affects children's health, especially in a context where "everyone knows that American children are getting fatter". However, the 'chilling' evidence provided by Kraak and colleagues of the relationship between marketing and childhood obesity was also laced with uncertainty. Without delving into the methodology and statistical analyses used in their research (which is beyond the scope of this chapter), the authors found that even though there was strong evidence that television advertising influences the food and drink preferences and requests of children (aged 2–11 years), there was insufficient evidence about its influences on the food and drink preferences and requests of young people aged 12–18 years. The authors further reported that there was weak evidence that television advertising influences the usual dietary intake of children and young people aged 6–18 years. Critically, in terms of the relationship between advertising and childhood obesity, the authors concluded that "current evidence is *not sufficient to arrive at any finding about a causal relationship* from television advertising to adiposity among children and youth" (p. 292, emphasis added). In short, the authors could find no evidence of any *causal* relationship between food marketing and childhood obesity.

The other piece of research that provided 'unequivocal evidence' for WHO's Commission on Ending Childhood Obesity was Hastings and colleagues (2003) *Review of research on the effects of food promotion to children*; a report that has been updated several times over the past two decades (see Cairns et al., 2009, 2013; Hastings et al., 2006). In their initial report, Hastings et al. (2003, p. 2) were forthcoming with some of the significant methodological issues when attempting to understand the relationship between food marketing and childhood obesity:

> … trying to establish whether or not a link exists between food promotion and diet or obesity, is extremely difficult as it requires research to be done in real world settings. A number of studies have attempted this by using amount of television viewing as a proxy for exposure to television advertising. They have established a clear link between television viewing and diet, obesity, and cholesterol levels. It is impossible to say, however, whether this effect is caused by the advertising, the sedentary nature of television viewing or snacking that might take place whilst viewing.

The authors of this report were relatively open about some of the methodological constraints which made it 'impossible' to articulate the link between a child's fatness and food advertising. They added:

> … the literature does suggest food promotion is influencing children's diet in a number of ways. This does not amount to proof, as … with this kind of research, incontrovertible proof simply isn't attainable. Nor do all studies point to this conclusion; several have

not found an effect. In addition, very few studies have attempted to measure how strong these effects are *relative* to other factors influencing children's food choices.

(p. 3)

So, to reiterate: WHO's (2016, p. 18) *Report of the Commission on Ending Childhood Obesity* statement that: "There is unequivocal evidence that the marketing of unhealthy foods and sugar-sweetened beverages is related to childhood obesity" is based on one review that concluded that there was insufficient evidence of any causal relationship (Kraak et al., 2006) and another review that stated "incontrovertible proof simply isn't attainable" (Hastings et al., 2003).

Aside from methodological issues making proof not possible for Hastings and colleagues, there was also the significant problem that they could only find one article that claimed to illustrate the impact of food marketing on childhood obesity: Dietz and Gortmaker's (1985) *Do we fatten our children at the television set? Obesity and television viewing in children and adolescents.* This article (cited over 2000 times) was described by Hastings et al. (2003, p. 16) as finding "significant relationships between television viewing and obesity". What this research *did not do* though was analyse or report on the effects of *advertising* – food or otherwise – on obesity, just television watching *in general.* There were other aspects that the Hastings et al. report appears to be flawed. For instance, their claim that food marketing was important in determining children's food knowledge, preferences, and behaviours was based on two studies (Bolton, 1983; French et al., 2001); studies which found that the influence of food advertising exposure was small and certainly in comparison to other variables. Bolton's (1983) study, for instance, reported that the influence of parental behaviour was 15 times greater than that of television advertising, while French and colleagues (2001) research (focused on promotional signs on snack vending machines in secondary schools) reported that the price of food was more influential than marketing. As Ashton (2004, p. 52) wrote shortly after the release of Hastings et al. (2003) review: "The claim that food advertising is a major contributor to children's food choices and the rising tide of childhood obesity has obvious appeal, but as an argument it does not stand up to scrutiny".

Despite the lack of 'equivocal' proof or evidence, since the Hastings et al.'s (2003) report was originally published, the same authors – and other researchers drawing on this report as evidence – appear to have become even more certain of the 'junk food marketing = childhood obesity' relationship. For instance, only two years later, McDermott et al. (2006) claimed that *their own* 2003 report had "identified commercial food marketing as a possible contributory factor to childhood obesity" (2006, p. 252), although later admitted that "the review did not directly examine the link between food promotion and *obesity*" (p. 262, italics in original). The authors again noted the difficulties in conducting research that could conclusively demonstrate how food marketing actually impacts children:

> Food knowledge, preferences, and behavior are influenced by a wide range of complex and dynamic factors. Unpicking these is difficult, and isolating the possible influence of just one variable—in this case promotion—particularly so. Moreover, social science research of this ilk can never provide final incontrovertible proof.
>
> *(2006, p. 262)*

Even though the authors acknowledged that their research "reduces uncertainty rather than produces certainty" (2006, p. 262), they concluded that due to the nature and extent of food promotional activity (and its ability to influence young people), *it would be reasonable to conclude* that the current promotional climate is encouraging children to make unhealthy rather than healthy choices. It is also *likely that this will be having an impact* on their dietary health.

(2006, p. 264, my emphasis)

There was no specific mention of the relationship between junk food marketing and childhood obesity.

In 2006, yet another report was published by WHO: *The extent, nature and effects of food promotion to children: a review of the evidence* (Hastings et al., 2006). This time, only one more article had been added to the evidence base to provide 'proof' of a relationship between food marketing and obesity: *Children's food consumption during television viewing* (Matheson et al., 2004). However, like Dietz and Gortmaker (1985), this research did not provide *any* evidence of the connection between food marketing and obesity, only a "speculation that eating while watching television is a potential mechanism linking television viewing to obesity" (Matheson et al., 2004, p. 1094). This also contradicted their results which stated that the "amount of food consumed during television viewing was not associated with children's BMI" (p. 1088). In fact, the only mention of advertising in their entire article was that their "results do not support the hypothesis that children consume more highly advertised foods while watching television" (p. 1093).

To summarise, by the time the last systematic review of the evidence on the nature, extent, and effects of food marketing to children was published (Cairns et al., 2013), there were a grand total of two articles that provided WHO's 'unequivocal evidence' (i.e. Dietz & Gortmaker, 1985; Matheson et al., 2004), and critically, *neither of these* provided any evidence about an evidence-based relationship between food marketing and childhood obesity.

Reproducing the 'junk food marketing = childhood obesity' discourse

By framing their arguments with the dual 'truths' about childhood obesity and junk food marketing, public health scholars transform the uncertain evidence – essentially an assumption about the relationship between junk food marketing and childhood obesity – into a certain conclusion that their research on children's 'exposure' to advertising will shape government policy and make a significant difference to the 'war on childhood obesity'.

The first two paragraphs of Signal et al.'s (2017, p. 2) article[2] on children's exposure to food marketing are a useful illustration of how these discourses are joined and to what intended effect:

Over the past three decades the global prevalence of childhood overweight and obesity has increased by 47% [1]. Excess adiposity during childhood and adolescence is associated with an increased risk of many serious health conditions and has lifetime consequences for children's health, well-being, and productivity.

[2–4]

Marketing of energy-dense nutrient-poor (EDNP) foods and beverages contributes to the worldwide increase in childhood obesity [WHO, 2016] by encouraging the repeat purchase and consumption of foods that do not meet nutritional guidelines [Cairns et al., 2009; Cairns et al., 2013; Hastings et al., 2003] .... The World Health Organization

(WHO) Commission on Ending Childhood Obesity (ECHO) recommends reducing children's exposure to, and the power of, marketing of unhealthy foods.

[WHO, 2016]

A number of rhetorical devices are used in this article to re-construct uncertain knowledge as a certain 'truth'. As Gard and Wright (2001) demonstrated in other obesity literature, the use of the past tense 'has', and the present tense 'is' in the first two sentences of the quotation, combined with the word 'contributes' "leaves few spaces for contestation – grammatically the statement is constructed as 'truth'" (p. 544). Likewise, the first paragraph uses phrases like "the global prevalence of childhood overweight and obesity has increased by 47%" and "lifetime consequences for children's health, well-being, and productivity" work to "make invisible the conflicting and complex research that would challenge the assumptions about obesity on which these phrases rely" (Gard & Wright, 2001, p. 544). In addition, the final sentence draws on official policy, as if by attaching this research to WHO recommendations adds *gravitas* to the importance of this research – and the ability to 'fight' childhood obesity.

For instance, Signal et al. (2017) used wearable cameras on children to measure the types and frequency of exposure to food advertisements across multiple media and settings. One hundred and sixty-eight children (aged 12 years) wore a wearable camera for four days, capturing images every seven seconds, and images were coded as either recommended (core) or not recommended (non-core) to be marketed to children by setting, marketing medium, and product category. The researchers reported that the children in their study were exposed to non-core food marketing 27 times a day (although this did not necessarily mean that the children saw any or all this advertising), more than twice their average exposure to core food marketing. There was no evidence that children 'saw' any of these advertisements or any data on these children's health or fatness. Researchers did not draw on any evidence about what children understood or how they experienced these types of marketing practices. Yet, the authors drew a bold conclusion: "This research suggests that children live in an obesogenic food marketing environment that promotes obesity as a normal response to their everyday environment". They then provided the following conclusion (in full):

> The Commission [on Ending Childhood Obesity] is right to call for the reduction of children's exposure to marketing of unhealthy foods [WHO, 2016]. This research provides further evidence of the need for action and suggests both settings and media in which to act. Urgent action is required if the vision of the Commission on Ending Childhood Obesity is to be achieved.
>
> *(Signal et al., 2017, p. 9)*

In this type of research, the 'food marketing = childhood obesity' duplex is impossible to prove, so scholars continue to create and maintain a 'junk food marketing = unhealthy eating = fat/unhealthy child' triplex, whereby a child's fatness is 'proof' of ill-health, the result of unhealthy eating that has undoubtedly been shaped by an 'exposure' to junk food marketing. This triplex was reinforced by the media release from the researchers:

> The researchers are calling for urgent Government action to clean up the junk food advertisements surrounding children to help reduce obesity.
>
> "The findings are a real concern given high rates of obesity amongst NZ children and the known influence of marketing on children's food choices," says the overall programme director Professor Cliona Ni Mhurchu from the University of Auckland.

....

Junk food marketing contributes to the worldwide increase in childhood obesity by en-couraging the repeat purchase and consumption of unhealthy foods. The World Health Organization (WHO) Commission on Ending Childhood Obesity (ECHO) recom-mends that such marketing should be reduced and that 'settings where children and ado-lescents gather (such as schools and sports facilities or events) should be free of marketing of unhealthy food and sugar-sweetened beverages'.

(University of Otago, 2017, para. 7–10)

'Cherished beliefs' about childhood obesity and food marketing enables scholars to (re)con-struct 'expert' knowledge in and through academic literature, policy documents, and the media, further re-producing the certainty that there *is* a childhood obesity crisis, that junk food marketing *is* a significant cause, and that reducing marketing *will* provide a solution.

Conclusions

Of course, the absence of 'unequivocal' proof does not constitute proof in itself that there is no relationship between junk food marketing, children's health, or childhood obesity. How-ever, the taken-for-grantedness of dominant marketing and obesity discourses, combined with the methodological difficulties in establishing the precise nature of the relationship, has resulted in a dearth of quality research that explains how marketing actually shapes children's bodies or wellbeing. This is not only a methodological issue but also an ethical one. The uncritical acceptance of these particular discourses as 'true' may help legitimise particular academic fields of research and public health imperatives, but it does little to help us under-stand or challenge this complex phenomenon (see Gard, 2004).

More so, the reproduction of certainty when there is none may have unintended, even 'unhealthy', consequences. One such repercussion is a narrowing of what 'health' means in research on the impact of marketing on children. While there is a gamut of research that centres on childhood obesity, there continues to be relatively little consideration paid to how marketing tactics shape emotional, mental, spiritual, social, and spiritual wellbeing. The privileging of Western, biomedical notions of health, where health is defined according to mostly physical dimensions, especially the removal of fatness through the promotion of healthy lifestyles, may result in 'other' understandings, beliefs, knowledges, and embodi-ments of health (including those of indigenous peoples) being dominated and ignored (see Powell, 2020b). For instance, indigenous understandings of 'health' are often inextricably interconnected with the natural world (e.g., see Harmsworth & Awatere, 2013; Panelli & Tipa, 2007; Sangha et al., 2015); yet, the devastating impact of consumerism and 'extreme materialism' on our environment (Santa Barbara, 2021) receives little attention in marketing to children research.

Relatedly, the myopic attitude of public health research towards particular products or industries deemed to be inherently 'unhealthy' (such as ultra-processed food high in fat, salt and sugar, tobacco, alcohol, and breastmilk substitutes) acts at the expense of broader, critical research; studies that could and should interrogate the global 'corporate assault' on children and childhood (e.g. Bakan, 2011; Boyles, 2008; Kenway & Bullen, 2001, Powell, 2018a). For decades, activists, advocates, and scholars have demonstrated how children have become insidiously and increasingly commercialised and commodified, not just through junk food marketing but also a seemingly endless array of advertising techniques that attempt to shape the child-consumer (e.g. Powell, 2018b; Spring, 2003).

However, there still appears to be little appetite from researchers and policymakers to look at the big picture of how *all* marketing may be harmful for people and the planet. As Costello et al. write: "It will be hard enough to tackle opposition from corporations promoting health-harming products. Imagine trying to fight opposition from a large coalition of companies that range from toys and games to technology and household products" (Costello et al., 2020, p. 1735). And herein lies the problem: the 'chilling effect' from corporations and the advertising industry (as well as governmental partners, including WHO) is perceived to be difficult enough from 'certain' unhealthy products, never mind those which are seen as innocuous (or even 'health-promoting'). The reproduction of the healthy/unhealthy binary – both in terms of consumable products and consuming bodies – assists the production of this 'impossible' task of challenging the global advertising industry and its corporate funders. And, at the same time, researchers and policymakers continue to put all of their eggs into the 'junk food marketing basket', despite there being far more influential factors that shape children's health, such as poverty, social inequality, colonisation, food insecurity, welfare policy, housing, parent's education, and access to healthcare and early childhood education, to name just a few.

Finally, I am not trying to argue that there necessarily needs to be 'unequivocal proof' of the harm of marketing – junk food or otherwise. The issue of marketing to children is an ethical issue as much as (if not more than) a scientific one. Should children be targeted by junk food advertisers in ways that may shape their food and eating preferences, behaviours, and desires? No, of course not. But should we continue to focus research and policymaking on uncertain evidence that it makes children fat or fatter? In my view, no. Collectively, we need to re-imagine the 'dangers' of marketing to children as being more than a matter of fatness and critically interrogate how the commercial exploitation of children may work to insidiously (whether deliberately or accidently) re-shape children's health, behaviours, knowledge, and identities. In this way, it does not matter so much whether the product being marketed is 'healthy' or 'unhealthy' in a physical sense, but how marketing encourages forms of consumption that are potentially harmful for the whole child, the planet, and children's futures.

Acknowledgements

Thank you to Kristy Telford for collating and analysing the vast gamut of literature that was cited in the key documents in this chapter. This research was made possible through a Royal Society Te Apārangi Marsden Fund Fast-Start Grant.

Notes

1 At the time of writing, the latest figures on the prevalence of childhood obesity in New Zealand – taken from 2019/2020 – showed that only 9.4 percent of children were classified as 'obese' (down from 10/7% on 2011/2012) (Ministry of Health, 2020).
2 Although in the original article, endnotes are used for citations, I have replaced the endnote numbers with the citation in brackets to show which articles are being cited.

References

Ashton, D. (2004). Food advertising and childhood obesity. *Journal of the Royal Society of Medicine, 97*(2), 51–52. https://doi.org/10.1177%2F014107680409700201
Bakan, J. (2011). *Childhood under seige: How big business ruthlessly targets children.* Vintage.

Bolton, R. N. (1983). Modeling the impact of television food advertising on children's diets. *Current Issues and Research in Advertising, 6*(1), 173–199.

Boyles, D. R. (2008). *The corporate assault on youth: Commercialism, exploitation, and the end of innocence.* Peter Lang.

Cairns, G., Angus, K., & Hastings, G. (2009) *The extent, nature and effects of food promotion to children: A review of the evidence to December 2008.* World Health Organization. https://www.who.int/dietphysicalactivity/Evidence_Update_2009.pdf

Cairns, G., Angus, K., Hastings, G., & Caraher, M. (2013). Systematic reviews of the evidence of the nature, extent and effects of food marketing to children. A retrospective summary. *Appetite, 62,* 209–215. https://doi.org/10.1016/j.appet.2012.04.017

Costello, A., Dalglish, S. L., Banerjee, A., Shiffman, J., & Clark, H. (2020). Harmful marketing to children – Authors' reply. *The Lancet, 396*(10264), 1735. https://doi.org/10.1016/S0140-6736(20)32471-5

Dietz, W. H., & Gortmaker, S. L. (1985). Do we fatten our children at the television set? Obesity and television viewing in children and adolescents. *Pediatrics, 75*(5), 807–812.

Ellison, J., McPhail, D., & Mitchinson, W. (Eds.). (2016). *Obesity in Canada: Critical perspectives.* University of Toronto Press.

Evans, J., Rich, E., & Davies, B. (2004). The emperor's new clothes: Fat, thin, and overweight. The social fabrication of risk and ill health. *Journal of Teaching in Physical Education, 23*(4), 372–391.

Evans, B., & Colls, R. (2009). Measuring fatness, governing bodies: The spatialities of the Body Mass Index (BMI) in anti-obesity politics. *Antipode, 41*(5), 1051–1083.

French, S. A., Jeffery, R. W., Story, M., Breitlow, K. K., Baxter, J. S., Hannan, P., & Snyder, M. P. (2001). Pricing and promotion effects on low-fat vending snack purchases: The CHIPS Study. *American Journal of Public Health, 91*(1), 112–117.

Foucault, M. (1980). The confession of the flesh. In C. Gordon (Ed.), *Power/knowledge: Selected interviews and other writings, 1972–1977* (pp. 194–228). Pantheon Books.

Gard, M. (2004). An elephant in the room and a bridge too far, or physical education and the 'obesity epidemic'. In J. Evans, B. Davis, & J. Wright (Eds.), *Body knowledge and control: Studies in the sociology of physical education and health* (pp. 68–82). Routledge.

Gard, M. (2011). *The end of the obesity epidemic.* Routledge.

Gard, M., & Wright, J. (2001). Managing uncertainty: Obesity discourses and physical education in a risk society. *Studies in Philosophy and Education, 20*(6), 535–549. https://doi.org/10.1023/A:1012238617836

Gard, M., & Wright, J. (2005). *The obesity epidemic: Science, morality, and ideology.* Routledge.

Harmsworth, G. R., & Awatere, S. (2013). Indigenous Māori knowledge and perspectives of ecosystems. *Ecosystem services in New Zealand—conditions and trends.* Manaaki Whenua Press.

Hastings, G., Stead, M., McDermott, L., Forsyth, A., MacKintosh, A. M., Rayner, M., Godfrey, C., Caraher, M., & Angus, K. (2003). *Review of research on the effects of food promotion to children.* Food Standards Agency.

Hastings, G., McDermott, L., Angus, K., Stead, M., & Thomson, S. (2006). *The extent, nature and effects of food promotion to children: A review of the evidence.* World Health Organization.

Kenway, J., & Bullen, E. (2001). *Consuming children: Education-entertainment-advertising.* Open University Press.

Matheson, D. M., Killen, J. D., Wang, Y., Varady, A., & Robinson, T. N. (2004). Children's food consumption during television viewing. *The American journal of clinical nutrition, 79*(6), 1088–1094. https://doi.org/10.1093/ajcn/79.6.1088

McDermott, L., Stead, M., & Hastings, G. (2006). Does food promotion influence children's diet? A review of evidence. In N. Cameron, N. G. Norgan, & G. T. H. Ellison (Eds.), *Childhood obesity: contemporary issues* (pp. 252–265). Taylor & Francis.

Kraak, V. I., Gootman, J. A., & McGinnis, J. M. (Eds.). (2006). *Food marketing to children and youth: Threat or opportunity?* National Academies Press.

Ministry of Health. (2016). *Annual update of key results 2015/16: New Zealand Health Survey.* https://www.health.govt.nz/publication/annual-update-key-results-2015-16-new-zealand-health-survey

Ministry of Health. (2020). *Annual data explorer.* https://minhealthnz.shinyapps.io/nz-health-survey-2019-20-annual-data-explorer/_w_1ea6ecac/#!/

Nestle, M. (2006). Food marketing and childhood obesity—a matter of policy. *New England Journal of Medicine, 354*(24), 2527–2529. https://doi.org/10.1056/NEJMp068014

Panelli, R., & Tipa, G. (2007). Placing well-being: A Maori case study of cultural and environmental specificity. *EcoHealth, 4*(4), 445–460. https://doi.org/10.1007/s10393-007-0133-1

Powell, D. (2018a). Governing the (un)healthy child-consumer in the age of the childhood obesity crisis. *Sport, Education and Society, 23*(4), 297–310. https://doi.org/10.1080/13573322.2016.1192530

Powell, D. (2018b). Culture jamming the 'corporate assault' on schools and children. *Global Studies of Childhood, 8*(4), 379–391. https://doi.org/10.1177/2043610618814840

Powell, D. (2020a). *Schools, corporations, and the war on childhood obesity: How corporate philanthropy shapes public health and education.* Routledge.

Powell, D. (2020b). Harmful marketing to children. *The Lancet, 396*(10264), 1734–1735. https://doi.org/10.1016/S0140-6736(20)32403-X

Sangha, K. K., Le Brocque, A., Costanza, R., & Cadet-James, Y. (2015). Ecosystems and indigenous well-being: An integrated framework. *Global Ecology and Conservation, 4*, 197–206. https://doi.org/10.1016/j.gecco.2015.06.008

Santa Barbara, J. (2021). *How extreme materialism is killing the climate.* Newsroom. https://www.newsroom.co.nz/page/extreme-materialism-is-killing-the-climate

Signal, L. N., Stanley, J., Smith, M., Barr, M. B., Chambers, T. J., Zhou, J., Duane, A., Gurrin, C., Smeaton, A. F., McKerchar, C., Pearson, A. L., Hoek, J., Jenkin, G. L. S., & Mhurchu, C. N. (2017). Children's everyday exposure to food marketing: An objective analysis using wearable cameras. *International Journal of Behavioral Nutrition and Physical Activity, 14*(1), 1–11. https://doi.org/10.1186/s12966-017-0570-3

Spring, J. (2003). *Educating the consumer-citizen: A history of the marriage of schools, advertising, and media.* Routledge.

University of Otago. (2017, October 9). *Kiwi kids see 27 junk food ads a day on average.* https://www.scimex.org/newsfeed/kiwi-kids-see-27-junk-food-ads-a-day

Vander Schee, C., & Boyles, D. (2010). 'Exergaming,' corporate interests and the crisis discourse of childhood obesity. *Sport, Education and Society, 15*(2), 169–185. https://doi.org/10.1080/13573321003683828

Vandevijvere, S., Soupen, A., & Swinburn, B. (2017a). Unhealthy food advertising directed to children on New Zealand television: Extent, nature, impact and policy implications. *Public Health Nutrition, 20*(17), 3029–3040. doi:10.1017/S1368980017000775

Vandevijvere, S., Sagar, K., Kelly, B., & Swinburn, B. A. (2017b). Unhealthy food marketing to New Zealand children and adolescents through the internet. *New Zealand Medical Journal, 130(1450),* 32–43.

World Cancer Research Fund. (2020). *Governments failing to protect child rights by not restricting junk food marketing.* https://www.wcrf-uk.org/uk/latest/press-releases/governments-failing-protect-child-rights-not-restricting-junk-food

World Health Organization. (2016). *Report of the commission on ending childhood obesity.* World Health Organization. https://apps.who.int/iris/bitstream/handle/10665/204176/9789241510066_eng.pdf

Wright, J., & Harwood, V. (Eds.). (2012). *Biopolitics and the 'obesity epidemic': Governing bodies.* Routledge.

PART E

Bodies

This section focuses on different types of bodies: fat bodies, overweight bodies, obese bodies, and skinny bodies. Importantly though, the chapters in this section demonstrate how corporeality extends beyond the physical body and its size, shape, and weight. Our bodies are an essential aspect of our lived experiences *as people* – as children, parents, women, young people, pregnant people, and brown people. The authors in the following chapters draw on a range of perspectives to illuminate how the fat body – fat people – is entangled with and shaped by a complex assemblage of discourse, culture, politics, and power.

The section begins with Aimee Simpson's exploration of the terms 'fat', 'overweight', and 'obese'. This chapter draws upon interview research conducted with 18 self-identifying fat people on the issues of health, body size, and identity. Simpson demonstrates that the labels of 'fat', 'overweight', and 'obese' take on diverse meanings for people which are informed by their histories as fat individuals as well as wider discourses relating to health and body ideals. Simpson raises important questions regarding which labels people are able to 'choose', how this process is impacted by the ascription of (and being ascribed) labels by others, and the extent to which these labels are universally applicable. By illustrating how complicated the issue of fat identity formation is, Simpson highlights the need to look deeper into both language use and language *in* use.

In the next chapter, Susan Greenhalgh draws on material and expands on arguments made in her book *Fat-Talk Nation: The Human Costs of America's War on Fat* (Cornell University Press, 2015) by interrogating how the 'war on fat' has not only worsened stigma and discrimination against fat people, but for those deemed 'underweight' or 'skinny' too. This chapter focuses on the narratives of 'skinny persons', how they are subjected to 'skinny talk', and how skinniness and fatness are constituted in the same moment and in relation to one another. Greenhalgh demonstrates how the 'war on obesity' attempts to turn all Americans into virtuous biocitizens, thus also producing 'thin, fit biocitizens' that must take responsibility for their diets, exercise, and weight, and at the same time, ensure that others do the same.

Eva Barlösius turns to the concept of 'typifications' in order to analyse the social realities of young fat people in Germany, and how their actions, clothing, eating behaviours, how they spend their free time, and so forth are typified according to whether they are considered thin or fat. The author examines in detail the ubiquitous experience of young people being considered 'too fat': the somewhat unconscious hints and reaction from others as well as the

DOI: 10.4324/9780429344824-24

more conscious staring, provocative comments, and condemnations. Barlösius demonstrates how these social interactions significantly shape relationships between young people and society, moulding their view of themselves and the social world.

George Parker's chapter explores the emergence of maternal obesity as a problematising discourse and its effects. This chapter charts the rise of maternal obesity as a contemporary health crisis that has significantly altered reproductive health care policy and practice, along with contemporary understandings of fat reproductive bodies. Using a critical feminist intersectional lens to view empirical evidence, Parker disrupts the certainty of problem discourses about pregnancy fatness by revealing their harmful discursive and material effects in the lives of fat women and gender diverse people who birth babies. Further, Parker argues for critical obesity scholarship to provide a counter-knowledge of pregnancy fatness that works to de-centre body weight as the determining force of health during pregnancy; to draw on more holistic and arguably non-Western epistemological views of pregnancy health that takes into account the social, political, and cultural contexts of health, body weight, and mothering.

Lisette Burrows provides an in-depth examination of the ways school-based health messages reach into family homes, and how school food education may (or may not) shape families, relationships, and children's everyday lives. Burrows provides evidence that, contrary to prior research that has demonstrated the propensity for schools to 'teach' children about food, fatness, and health in highly problematic ways, the 20 New Zealand families in her research demonstrated "spectacular amnesia" about what is taught about food in schools. Rather, Burrows demonstrates how the children in these families experience food in ways that were not 'tainted' by schools. The children were highly engaged in food practices at home, notions of pleasure were at the forefront of their understanding of food and eating, and the words 'fat' or 'obesity' were not mentioned at all.

Tim Olds, Dorothea Dumuid, and Melissa Wake employ the novel concept of optimal activity composition or the "best day" to question how children can best use their time to optimise fatness, and whether that optimal mix is also optimal for other important outcomes such as mental health and academic achievement. The researchers describe how low levels of fatness (in Australian children) are characterised by a specific amount (or activity composition zone) of sleep, sedentary behaviour, and physical activity, a zone which is quite different from other outcomes, such as academic performance (which is characterised by much higher sedentary time and very low levels of light physical activity). The findings in this chapter are significant as they challenge current government guidelines that tend to promote a 'one-size-fits-all' approach to physical activity; guidelines that are based on the desire to 'fight obesity', yet ignore other important outcomes for children and society.

Jenny Ellison's chapter acknowledges two historic and contemporary problems with fat activist groups: a limited engagement of activist groups with questions of gender, race, and ability and a tendency to homogenise all 'fat women'. Ellison focuses on aerobics classes organised by Canadian activist group Large as Life (LAL) and demonstrates how aerobics for fat women reflected a fluid approach to fat activism, one which drew on feminist and feminine popular culture of the 1980s and focused on pleasure, clothing, and personal experience. This chapter sheds light on the potential for playful forms of activism to respond to the needs of particular groups and shows how fat women in the LAL aerobics programmes were able to draw from feminist discourses of liberation and contemporary popular culture to create physical activity experiences tailored to their needs, interests, bodies, and lives.

Finally, Fetaui Iosefo provides a powerful account of her aversion to, and rejection of, the 'O word'. This chapter is grounded in the Samoan Indigenous Reference, namely, the Va', where Iosefo uses Critical Autoethnography and Critical Beauty to 'wayfind' (navigate) the meaning of 'obesity'. Using poetry and stories, this chapter wayfinds through the author's experience with a 'skinny white guy', the ambiguity of the 'O word' (especially when there is no equivalent in the Samoan language), and two Victorian fetish archetypes of Pacific women: the dusky maiden and the noble savage. Iosefo closes this chapter – and this section – with ten important reminders for scholars engaging in critical obesity research.

20

(RE)DEFINING LANGUAGE

'Fat', 'overweight', and 'obese' identities

Aimee B. Simpson

The language used to describe and discuss fat bodies within contemporary societies is under-pinned by a complex network of social signifiers of physical size. For instance, mainstream understandings of fatness are profoundly informed by discourses of 'obesity', wherein dom-inating networks of language, ideology, and power work to designate fatness as a health risk and/or a disease (Rich, Monaghan, & Aphramor, 2011). Critical scholarship has notably taken issue with this, highlighting how terms such as 'overweight' and 'obese' medicalise bodies and rely on the notion that there is an 'ideal weight' that one is in excess of (e.g. An-derson, 2012; Bacon, 2008; Wann, 2009). For these reasons and others, there has been an activist and scholastic push to avoid these 'O' words in favour of 'fat' as a more size-inclusive and non-medical term. Yet, the 'O' words remain popular in academic and mainstream settings due to their accessibility and the perception that they are 'value-free' descriptors, unlike 'fat' which can be taken as inflammatory or derogatory by some audiences (Dickins, Thomas, King, Lewis, & Holland, 2011). Consequently, what constitutes 'appropriate' lan-guage to use when discussing bodies of size remains contested and awkward ground.

Debates around language use exist in conjunction with 'language in use', that is, to say, how these terms are co-opted, transformed, challenged, and thus (re)defined by those who embody fatness. As Cooper (2010, p. 1021) suggests, fatness is a "fluid subject position rel-ative to social norms, it relates to shared experience, is ambiguous, has roots in identity politics and is thus generally self-defined". From this position, the terms 'fat', 'overweight', and 'obese' carry diverse meanings and, as identity markers, are deeply rooted in lived expe-riences of labelling. Thus, it is important to examine how people choose to identify them-selves and the meanings they ascribe to such labels. This chapter draws upon interview research conducted with 18 self-identifying fat people living in Aotearoa/New Zealand on the issues of health, body size, and identity. Specifically, it collates and dissects the most common responses given to the question "how would you refer to yourself?" in conjunction with related excerpts from my research diary. As both a researcher of fat and one who *is* fat, introspective conversation with participants about their fat identities often brought my own lived experience to the fore. While this work is by no means auto-ethnographic, the process of exploring the subject of identity was undoubtedly framed by, but importantly also altered, my own fat identity.

DOI: 10.4324/9780429344824-25

'Fat'

Participants who self-identified as 'fat' did so as they felt that it was the most 'generic' word and liked that it felt inclusive and non-medical. One participant, Cheryl, described it as the 'least offensive' word. For many, to self-identify as fat involved reclaiming and thus neutral-ising a formerly pejorative term, in a similar vein to the reuptake of the word 'queer' in the LGBTQIA+ community. Queer theorist, Eve Sedgwick, refers to this as 'coming out as fat' which can be thought of as "a way of staking one's claim to insist on, and participate actively in, a renegotiation of *the representational contract* between one's body and one's world" (Moon & Sedgwick, 2001, p. 306, *original emphasis*). In this sense, to self-identify as 'fat' means to declare one's presence openly, without apology and to an extent, to adopt an unambiguous identity (Pausé, 2012; Saguy & Ward, 2011). As Murray (2005) points out, this is difficult, in practice, as it seemingly asks you to "simply *forget* the dominant discourses that shaped my understanding of my body, that I lived out corporeally in every interaction, every gesture" (p. 270, *original emphasis*). Perhaps, then, it is more appropriate to consider the claiming of a 'fat' identity as complex and multifaceted, as Pausé (2012) suggests, with the "occasional questioning, dissonance, or feeling of uncertainty" (p. 43). Indeed, this was the case for the majority of the 'fat' participants I interviewed. For instance, Jane called herself 'fat' but said that she was "trying to get to a place of that just being a neutral descriptor like 'tall'". Jane's use of the word 'trying' above speaks to the contention felt by many participants who still struggle with the complicated relationship the word 'fat' has to ridicule. For instance, Hope indicated that while she used the word fat to describe herself, she also suggested that fat people have a specific 'look'. By this, she was not referring to a specific distribution of fat, but rather seemed to be speaking to a perceived inability to pass for thin. This relies on a common trope of the 'extreme other', wherein fatness or 'obesity' is imagined as a form of undeniable or 'extreme' largeness. For Hope, then, the word 'fat' signals unambiguous fatness and is an almost 'last resort' label and thus something to be reconciled.

A particular struggle in the reconciliation of identity for participants who identified as 'fat' was a lingering sense of shame. The issue of shame was particularly apparent in the in-terview with Sarah. Sarah grew up in South America and was fat from a young age. In our conversation, she told me that she was the only fat person in her family, and as a result, there was little to no understanding or empathy for what it meant to be fat. More often, her body size was something to be feared, and she spent a great deal of her youth in a range of different medical offices and on a variety of diets and exercise regimes. In this context, Sarah's use of the word 'fat' to describe herself both signified an emancipatory distance from the damaging experience she had with the medical establishment over her size as well as a continued sense of shame that she still felt over her body. Shame was similarly present in Shashank's use of fat in the term 'skinny-fat'. For Shashank, identifying in this way was propelled by bullying he experienced from friends and family over his body, who would tease him in Hindi *'mote, mote, mote'* or, in English, 'fatty, fatty, fatty' and tell him to "go out and exercise". He told me that only after he started being 'called out' by his family did he start viewing his body as a problem and start seeing himself as 'fat'. Similarly, Rob told me that "in conversation amongst friends I would say 'fat' but y'know, in any other contexts I would say 'obese'". Here, there is a vulnerability to the word 'fat' that demarcates it as a word to be used among friends, and which separates it from the more sterile term 'obese'. In this sense, Rob's use of 'fat', only in trusted settings, signals that he views it as inappropriate for general public consumption, likely as a form of self-deprecation, and speaks to a perceived degree of social shame associated with the word and identity.

In considering participant responses, I felt the need to reflect on my own reasons for using the word fat. My own fat identity was something I wrote extensively about in my research diary, as despite every effort, my body became intertwined in my research in ways I could not predict and did not choose. Upon honest reflection, my professional desire to help re-evaluate the way in which the relationships between fatness, health, and identity are publicly imagined, paralleled my personal wish to rewrite how I saw my own body, health, and identity. In this respect, the road to using fat confidently and neutrally has been hard and is not over, as I wrote here:

> At that time [early twenties], my use of the word fat was in the painful stages of reclamation, it was uncomfortable and in part I said it to make others feel uncomfortable. It was as freeing as it was ensnaring: I felt agency for the first time in setting an agenda about my body, about making the unsaid said, but the word 'fat' and all its associated meanings still held power over me. I had come to accept my fatness at this point, but I would be lying if I said it wasn't begrudgingly so. I had not experienced fatness like mine as anything other than a negative identity marker, and so acceptance for me was not positive, but neutral. I tolerated my body. I came to accept myself as fat after a long time of trying and failing to wish away my size.

My use of the word 'fat' is not uncomplicated or apolitical. Like Sarah, my use of fat has a long and complex history relating to fat shame, emancipation, and reclamation. In looking back on the above diary entry, written in late 2017, those sentiments seem both a distant memory and yet are bubbling away just below the surface. The lingering presence of shame, in particular, illustrates how sticky the process of reframing a marginalised identity can be. From a Foucauldian perspective, fat as an embodied identity is both a product of, and a response to, dominant obesity discourses (Murray, 2008, p. 90). For instance, as a researcher who critiques and deconstructs obesity discourses, I am in essence critiquing and dismantling the parts of my own identity that still harbour these beliefs. This is clearly visible in the extract above with respect to my understanding of my own fat identity. My use of the words 'begrudgingly', 'not positive, but neutral' and 'tolerated' communicate a persisting underlying hostility towards my own fatness. Yet, I also describe feeling 'agency' and an ability to set an 'agenda' about my self and body through the use of the word 'fat'. Here then, my experience of, as Jane says, 'getting to a place' where fat is neutral and okay involved simultaneously accepting and rejecting my fat identity. A similar struggle was described by Murray (2005, p. 270, *original emphasis*) who surmised "the ways in which I live my fat body are *always* multiple, contradictory and eminently ambiguous". In this sense, to be a 'fat' person is to face, engage with, and negotiate one's identity and its relationship to lingering stigma and shame.

'Overweight'

Similar to the fat participants above, those who were 'overweight' also felt that their word was neutral. The use of the same word 'neutral' is interesting here, as it was used to signify very different things. Where fat participants used the word to mean non-specific, general, or widely applicable, for people who called themselves overweight 'neutral' was used to indicate apolitical, objective, descriptive, and value-free. Take the example of Jessie, who, when contacting me to participate in the study said that her BMI was 'technically' overweight, provided me with her height and weight, and indicated that she had a complex relationship with food. Even though at no point during recruitment was any metric of physical size requested, it is interesting that she offered them all the same. Jessie's use of metrics and the word 'technically' suggest a confirmation of fatness through numbers. In addition, the fact that she told me about her relationship with food doubles down on the coding of her body as problematic through eating behaviours. In this sense, her body is both scientifically or 'technically' problematic as well as socially problematic. In a similar vein, when asked, Nick defined 'overweight' as "weighing more due to excess adipose tissue than would be ideal for my frame, I suppose". The use of 'adipose tissue' – the scientific term for 'fat' – generates meaningful distance between fatness and any kind of embodied experience. It is interesting that, in a study which asked for people to self-identify, arguably, an inherently embodied question, some participants provided such externalised and disembodied answers. To do this, participants relied on the trustworthiness of science in order to support normative beliefs about the body. In this way, fatness is presented as a sterile 'fact'; yet, it is clearly underpinned by moral judgements about an 'ideal' body.

Of note here is the presence of the BMI in the interactions with both participants. Both Nick and Jessie draw upon this ratio of height and weight as a way to talk about their bodies and overweight status. The reliance on the BMI in overweight narratives was stronger than in fat narratives, but its usage was not always as prescribed. For instance, Mira referred to herself as 'overweight', but when speaking of her body in relation to the BMI, she said "I am in the higher end of the normal range but the lower end of the ... um ... *fat* range". By this measure, Mira would be classified as 'normal' bodied; indeed, she is clear to distinguish herself from others who are 'fat'; yet, she does not see herself this way. Her use of this terminology along with the BMI puts her assertion in the 'ballpark' of science, just as Nick affiliated his definition of overweight with science by using 'adipose tissue'. These words are powerful signifiers in their relationship to science, and their usage alone indicates an association with truth or reality even if what is said contradicts official usage. Note that, following this, she said "[overweight] is where I am because if I'm in China, people are more skinnier in general, so if you go buy clothes you can maybe go for like a large size or extra-large". Here, we see the distinction between the social and clinical meaning of words such as 'overweight'.

A common critique from critical scholars and activists is to question 'overweight? Over *what* weight?' (e.g. Burns & Gavey, 2004; Fitzgerald, 1985; Ross, 2005; Wann, 2009) as a way to highlight the issue of ambiguity. As one participant, Maggie critically articulated "[overweight] means you're not the ideal weight, but therefore what *is* the ideal weight?" In this sense, 'overweight' can easily be applied to any*body* and often more accurately communicated how participants saw their own body in relation to the bodies of others. For some participants like Mira, this meant that they felt out of place and excessive, while others such as Kirsten and Hardy Girl communicated to me that to be overweight was to be 'normal' or 'average'.

Being over an 'ideal' was a common thread among 'overweight' participants. For instance, returning to Mira's quote above where she stated that in her home country of China "people are more skinnier in general", it is clear that 'overweight' for her has strong ties to social norms and ideals regarding body size. Here, she indicates that clothing sizes – buying large or extra-large – are significant to her understanding of her overweight identity. The notion of an 'ideal' came up in interviews with other participants, too. While Jane described herself as fat, she indicated that this notion and the concept of 'overweight' was something that she struggled with. In her interview, Jane told me that the prescription medication she took to alleviate chronic fatigue had the side effect of weight gain. So, although she had accepted this change in body size, in part, because altering this prescription was not an option for her, she also felt that her current weight was over a personal ideal. Jane's struggles illustrate how interwoven stories of body size can be with stories of control. For many 'overweight' participants, the notion of 'control' was central to their identity. For instance, consider the way that Abby situated her body in relation to 'obesity' when describing herself "I'm definitely a little bit overweight, but not… that much towards like obesity? I think I'm still like okay-ish, but if I lose control, I might have some problems". For Abby, being 'overweight' is constructed as 'okay-ish', meaning that she feels that she is not wholly 'normal' but that she is closer to 'normal' than she is to 'obese' because she perceives herself as having a level of self-control that 'obese' people do not. Thus, the use of the term 'overweight' served two key functions for my participants. First, the use of the term 'overweight' – in conjunction with the casual usage of the word 'fat' as a shorthand for general malaise about one's body – signalled that their bodies, and bodies like theirs are something to be monitored, manipulated, and dissatisfied with. Finally, it also served as a way for some participants to elevate their relative social position through the continued oppression of others within their community, in that they were 'fat' but not as fat as *'some* people'.

'Obese'

Of all the terms that participants used, 'obese' was the least frequently chosen and the most controversial. Consider how Cheryl differs between 'fat' and 'obese' here when she says

> So it's weird, I don't like the word obese at all. It's not commonly used to be offensive but I just really don't like the term […] I commonly call myself fat in like mixed company, but I would never sit there and be like "So I'm obese" y'know what I mean?

Jane, who also hated the term, hit on a similar note when she reasoned that it was 'really reductive' and suggested that "it's unnecessarily stigmatised. […] I think it would be a harder road to reclaim [obese] than it was to reclaim fat". Another participant, Lisa, also raised the issue of stigma in her discussion of the term 'obese'. Her experience with the word was complex; on the one hand, she noted how 'obese' and 'obesity' was normal for her. It spoke to a lifetime of being fat herself, and growing up and living in a fat community, but at the same time, like many others, it related to a lifetime of having her fat medicalised and problematised. In this way, Lisa's fatness was mundane but also maligned by harmful stigma and stereotyping.

Other participants, like Lisa, associated the term 'obese' with a doctor's office; as a label that was prescribed by practitioners and imbued with stigmatising medical discourses, more so than other medical terms such as 'overweight'. For instance, both Hope and Rob saw it as an "objective medical term" while Abby described it as a 'disease', which sat in contrast to her fairly normal or average 'overweight' body. Similarly, Hardy Girl told me that her doctor had said she was 'clinically obese', but that this did not match her own perception of what it meant to be 'obese'. Here then, 'clinically' assumes a comparable discursive role to Jessie's use of 'technically' in the previous section. The status of Hardy Girl as 'obese' was presented to me as a sterile fact and one that positions medical definitions and medical spaces as separate from an external social world.

Where the inherent vagueness of the term 'overweight' enabled participants to normalise and neutralise the social significance of their fat bodies, 'obese' conveyed an inescapable sense of gravity and severity of one's size. As Ross (2005) points out, the word 'obese' stems from the Latin route word 'obedere' meaning *to devour* which exemplifies much of the symbolism – and often assumed causal reasoning – associated with 'obese' bodies. The word 'devour' communicates a stigmatising sense of grossness – in both the sense of physical size and level of revulsion – which is then mapped onto fat bodies and their behaviour. Interestingly, when used by 'overweight' participants, the label 'obese' was invoked to establish a 'cut-off' point, wherein fatness was no longer perceived as acceptable and instead was excessive, unnatural, or wrong. In these interviews, the word 'obese' was more readily defined by social or visual indications of significant size rather than measurements such as the BMI. For example, when Kirsten defined the term 'obese' in our interview, she said the following:

> I feel like 'obese' is like, like once again a very medical term, and I guess 'overweight' is as well, but like… *'obese'*, when I think of 'obese' I'm like, I think of someone who is… really, *really, really* big, who can't like get around on their own.
>
> *(Kirsten)*

It is clear to Kirsten that 'obese' is a medical term – indeed, it was a key reason why she did not like the word – but the assessment that 'overweight' was also borne of medicine was more of an afterthought when she said 'I guess 'overweight' is as well'. In this sense, 'obese' was perceived to be an undeniably severer term. The use, repetition, and tonal stressing of 'really' is significant here. When combined with the stressing of 'obese' in 'but like… *'obese'*, the word 'really' serves to enforce the distance between herself as 'overweight' from the other. This gap is further widened, and the 'obese' body further othered by the use of a visual narrative of someone whose fatness had presumably made them immobile. The issue of mobility ties into related ableist discourses which perceive differently abled bodies as defective and diseased (Campbell, 2012). By this measure, fatness which is seen to coincide with disability is constituted as wrong and dangerous.

To this end, 'obese' is often presented as neutral or factual; yet, it remains a harmful term. It is so closely aligned with the disease of 'obesity' that it would be almost impossible, as Jane suggests, to conceive of this term outside of dominant obesity discourses. Perhaps, this is the reason that it was so vehemently disliked by participants, as it is both a product and co-producer of oppressive beliefs about fatness and fat people that are *ongoing*. In this respect, how can something that is actively and powerfully being used to marginalise bodies be reclaimed? In using words like 'obese', are we not complicit participants in the marginalisation of fat bodies? And, furthermore as a term, is 'obese' even useful? If we consider Cheryl's statement that 'obese' is not a word that she would use, and Rob's exclusive use of 'fat' among friends, it indicates that the word 'obese' shuts down meaningful dialogue about bodies of size, in which ideas and beliefs about fat people can be challenged and grown.

Concluding remarks

The manner in which we label ourselves and others relies upon a composite network of meaning-making. In particular, the labels of 'fat', 'overweight', and 'obese' took on numerous meanings for participants and were informed by their histories as fat individuals as well as wider discourses relating to health and body ideals. While this chapter has examined the ways in which people 'self-identify' – and indeed perceive other commonly used labels – this is not to suggest that such interpretations should be viewed in isolation. As has been argued above, the meanings associated with these labels are tethered to wider discourses surrounding the body and 'obesity' and as such are collectively defined and agreed upon. This raises important questions regarding which labels are available to 'choose', how this process is impacted by the ascription of, and being ascribed by others and the extent to which these labels are universally applicable. Certainly, while not directly addressed in this chapter, the role of the 'other' – including both friends and family as well as imagined, extreme 'others' – in defining acceptable and unacceptable expressions of fatness was significant. In particular, the 'other' contributed to the meaning of labels and influenced the settings in which participants used them in. These nuances illustrate how complicated and multiple the issue of fat identity formation is and highlighted the need to look deeper into not just language use, but also language *in* use.

References

Anderson, J. (2012). Whose voice counts? A critical examination of discourses surrounding the body mass index. *Fat Studies*, *1*(2), 195–207. https://doi.org/10.1080/21604851.2012.656500

Bacon, L. (2008). *Health at every size: The surprising truth about your weight*. Dallas: BenBella Books, Inc.

Burns, M., & Gavey, N. (2004). 'Healthy weight' at what cost? 'bulimia' and a discourse of weight control. *Journal of Health Psychology*, *9*(4), 549–565. https://doi.org/10.1177/1359105304044039

Campbell, F. K. (2012). Stalking ableism: Using disability to expose "abled" narcissism. In D. Goodley, B. Hughes, & L. Davis (Eds.), *Disability and social theory* (pp. 212–230). Houndmills: Palgrave Macmillan.

Cooper, C. (2010). Fat studies: Mapping the field. *Sociology Compass*, *4*(12), 1020–1034. https://doi.org/10.1111/j.1751-9020.2010.00336.x

Dickins, M., Thomas, S. L., King, B., Lewis, S., & Holland, K. (2011). The role of the fatosphere in fat adults' responses to obesity stigma. *Qualitative Health Research*, *21*(12), 1679–1691. https://doi.org/10.1177/1049732311417728

Fitzgerald, F. T. (1985). Space-age snake oil. *Postgraduate Medicine*, *78*(3), 231–240. https://doi.org/10.1080/00325481.1985.11699127

Moon, M., & Sedgwick, E. K. (2001). Divinity: A dossier, a performance piece, a little-understood emotion. In J. E. Braziel & K. LeBesco (Eds.), *Bodies out of bounds: Fatness and transgression* (pp. 292–328). Berkeley: University of California Press.

Murray, S. (2005). Doing politics or selling out? Living the fat body. *Women's Studies*, *34*(34), 265–277. https://doi.org/10.1080/00497870590964165

Murray, S. (2008). *The "fat" female body*. New York: Palgrave Macmillan.

Pausé, C. (2012). Live to tell: Coming out as fat. *Somatechnics*, *2*(1), 42–56. https://doi.org/10.3366/soma.2012.0038

Rich, E., Monaghan, L. F., & Aphramor, L. (2011). Introduction: Contesting obesity discourse and presenting an alternative. In L. Aphramor, L. F. Monaghan, & E. Rich (Eds.), *Debating obesity: Critical perspectives* (pp. 1–35). Houndmills: Palgrave Macmillan.

Ross, B. (2005). Fat or fiction: Weighing the "obesity epidemic." In M. Gard & J. Wright (Eds.), *The obesity epidemic: Science, morality and ideology* (pp. 86–106). New York: Routledge.

Saguy, A. C., & Ward, A. (2011). Coming out as fat: Rethinking stigma. *Social Psychology Quarterly*, *74*(1), 53–75. https://doi.org/10.1177/0190272511398190

Wann, M. (2009). Forward: Fat studies: An invitation to revolution. In E. Rothblum & S. Solovay (Eds.), *The fat studies reader* (pp. xi–xxvi). New York: New York University Press.

21

SKINNY SELVES IN A FAT-OBSESSED WORLD

Susan Greenhalgh

In the late 1990s and early 2000s, with obesity rates rising to "epidemic" levels, the US Government declared an urgent, nationwide public health campaign enlisting the entire society to get people – especially the young – to eat more healthfully and be more active, in an effort to achieve a "normal" Body Mass Index (BMI; Office of the Surgeon General 2001; Dietz 2015). Taking root in an entrenched culture of thin-worship and fat-loathing, what started as a critical public health call to action quickly grew into a society-wide war on fat[1] that involved every sector of American society – from education to health care to the economy – and left few domains of life untouched (Farrell 2011; Boero 2012; Saguy 2013). Although the use of warlike language has declined in the last five to ten years, both the fight against the nation's high levels of obesity[2] and the cultural oppression of the "wrong-weighted" remain vital parts of the landscape of corporal power in the US.

Growing bodies of work in fat studies and critical obesity studies have illuminated how the war on fat, introduced in a fat-phobic and fat-oppressive society, has worsened the stigma and discrimination against heavy people (Puhl & Heuer 2010; Fikkan & Rothblum 2011). The anti-fat campaign has also given rise to new forms of fat subjectivity, oppressive to perhaps the majority, but celebrated by fat scholars and activists working to regain control of their lives by creating fat-positive identities and more corporally, sexually, and racially inclusive analytic approaches (Rice 2007; Murray 2008; also Rothblum and Solovay 2009; Strings 2019; Pause & Taylor 2021).

Given the celebration of thinness in American society, one might expect the very thin to live charmed lives. As everyone of slight build knows, however, there is a fine line between *pleasingly thin* and *too thin* that, in Southern California ("SoCal" to the locals), where I lived and worked for almost two decades, falls around BMI 16–17 for girls and somewhat higher for boys. Skinny people – the term they themselves use – have long been the butt of jokes, but the medicalized discourse of the war on fat makes their condition something else: a biologically based abnormality ("underweight") which predisposes them to numerous diseases.[3] (Someone 5' 6" tall weighing 114 or less is "underweight.") The discourse that dominates the war on fat created a radically new weight-based identity and a new target of surveillance, discipline, and control.

With all the concern about excess weight, the impact of the war on fat on those deemed "underweight" (but not eating-disordered) has been woefully neglected – in critical weight

DOI: 10.4324/9780429344824-26

studies, in popular culture, and even in medicine.[4] The neglect can be traced not only to the intense focus of the campaign on heavy weights but also to their small numbers, and perhaps to the fact that most are (East and Southeast) Asian-Americans, a group whose voice is underrepresented in critical weight studies. Though small, those numbers are significant. Although only 2 percent of Whites are underweight, 10.9 percent of Japanese- and Vietnamese-Americans and 3.9 and 5.7 percent of Korean- and Chinese-Americans are underweight (Barnes et al. 2008).[5] If obesity is 12–25 times more prevalent than underweight among Whites, Blacks, and Hispanics, among Asians, the categories are reversed: Among Vietnamese, underweight is twice as prevalent as obesity, while among Chinese, Korean, and Japanese, it is 1.3–1.4 times more common (Barnes et al. 2008). Numbers aside, in the Asian-American communities that dot the SoCal landscape, skinniness is a sociologically salient and personally felt problem. The experiences of these Americans are important both because they constitute a form of weight-based discrimination that is poorly understood and because of what they newly reveal about the racialized dynamics and larger consequences of the war on fat.

Fat-talk and the making of weighty subjects: the SoCal project

In 2010, I began anthropological research on how the war on fat is playing out in American society, focusing on southern California. My aim was to systematically study, in one locality, the broader human consequences of this nationwide campaign against all "wrong-weighted" persons. How is the war unfolding on the ground? What are its intended and unintended effects, especially on the young, its main targets? Although body standards and pressures are intense in the region – after all, it's home to Hollywood – Southern Californians share the belief of other Americans that the good body brings the good life, allowing the region to serve in many ways as a microcosm.

In *Fat-talk Nation: The Human Costs of the War on Fat* (2015), I draw on 245 auto-ethnographies of "diet, weight, and the BMI in everyday life" written by my students at the University of California, Irvine, to answer these questions.[6] Although each case is unique, evidence from elsewhere in the country suggests that the dynamics of weight struggles they describe are quite general. Auto-ethnography provides rare insight into selfhood or subjectivity – people's own sense of who they are and what's important in their lives. Extending work in critical obesity studies to the US case, I develop a broad theoretical framework that illuminates how the war works on the ground and produces the effects noted by others as well as a host of consequences not yet brought to light.

The war on fat seeks to achieve a well-ordered (i.e., healthy and productive) society by creating new kinds of weight-based selves, or subjects, based on a biomedical definition of weight, and recruiting them to the effort. The scientific discourse on fat establishes weight-based categories based on the BMI: 18.5–24.9 is "normal," 25–29.9 is "overweight," 30 and higher is "obese," while below 18.5 is "underweight." The BMI discourse, then, is not only *normalizing* – specifying an ideal and urging all to normalize their status – it is also *subjectifying*, setting out weight-based identity categories or labels that people are encouraged to take as their own. These are medical or biological categories; I introduce another set of social identities just below.

In its effort to construct that well-ordered society, the war on fat seeks to turn all Americans into virtuous biocitizens (citizens whose political belonging is connected to their bodily attributes and who have social responsibilities) (Rose & Novas 2005; Halse 2009). What I call *thin, fit biocitizens* have two social responsibilities: first, taking care of their own diet and exercise to achieve a normal-weight, fit body, and second, helping others – family, friends, even perfect strangers – reach normal weight and become good biocitizens (cf. Halse 2009).

The most important tool available to the virtuous biocitizen for persuading "bad," "unhealthy" citizens to become good ones is *fat-talk*, everyday communications about weight – not just fatness – that circulate in popular culture through talk, the media, advertisements, and so forth, often accompanied by concrete practices (e.g. inducements to diet). My research shows how the war on fat produced a veritable explosion of fat-talk and how different kinds of pedagogical and abusive fat-talk work together to turn people in heavier weight classes into *fat subjects* (Evans et al. 2008; Royce 2009). A social category, a fat subject is different from an obese person (someone with a BMI of 30 or higher). A fat subject is someone who, regardless of weight, identifies as fat, organizes his or her life around that fatness, and acquires the attributes of a typical "fat person" (Rice 2007; Greenhalgh 2015).

In *Fat-talk Nation*, I present in-depth accounts of the weight struggles of 45 Californians of different genders, ethnicities, and income levels. In this chapter, I highlight two main findings, or contributions, of this research: the existence of a distinctive skinny subjectivity and the co-constitution of weight-based subjectivities. In SoCal, my research reveals, the duties of the biocitizen to work on the "abnormal" extend to the underweight end of the spectrum. Very thin people are subject to a variant of fat-talk that I call *skinny-talk* – suggestions that they are unhealthily skinny, together with associated material practices. People so teased often start seeing themselves as abnormally "underweight" or, in the colloquial, *skinny persons*, a social label I use for them. By systematically examining the dynamics of weight-based subjectification across the full spectrum of weights in a fairly large sample (for a qualitative, anthropological study), my work reveals that weight-based identities are in important ways *co-constituted*. By that, I mean fatness and skinniness are constituted in the same moment and in relation to one another. Just as, in other norm-setting social classification schemes, one category cannot be understood except in reference to other categories, and especially its supposed opposite, skinniness cannot be fully understood without understanding fatness and vice versa. Attending to skinny selfhood shows the dynamics of war on fat to be more complicated than previously thought.

The problem of skinniness plagues some categories of individuals more than others. If being overweight is especially difficult for women, for whom thinness is essential to femininity, being underweight poses major challenges for men because norms of masculinity make bigness, strength, and muscularity the signs of "real manhood." Thin men must struggle to prove not only their "normality" but also their masculinity. Ethnicity is also important. In the U.S., the idealized (or hegemonic) masculine figure is white (and tall and buff). Nonwhite males who inhabit subordinated masculinities cannot hope to change their skin color or height, but they can try to get closer to the ideal masculine form by bulking up.

As the statistics presented above suggest, within nonwhite groups, some racial-ethnic groups – especially East and Southeast Asians – are more biologically predisposed than others to being underweight and thus face challenges trying to bulk up. Ethnic differences in parent–child relations play a role in the formation of skinny-person identities as well.[7] While virtually, all parents are concerned about their kids' health and well-being, in the East and Southeast Asian families I studied, many parents, believing their kids must be near-perfect to overcome their minority status and gain acceptance in mainstream society, routinely commented on their weight, berating them if they were "too fat" or "too thin."[8] In these groups, it is especially difficult for young people to reject the perception that something is seriously wrong with them.

In this chapter, I present auto-ethnographic material from my study to understand the lives and worlds of the very thin. I explore three questions. First, how do skinny-talk and biocitizenship work at this end of the weight continuum? Second, do those labeled "underweight and defective" internalize that identity; if so, what are the attributes of the "skinny subject"? Finally, what are the larger consequences for the health, well-being, and lives of uber-skinny young people? I begin with excerpts from two auto-ethnographies, those of Jason, a 21-year-old of Chinese descent, and Linh, a 22-year-old Vietnamese-American, then draw together the findings from all the essays on underweight people.

Yellow swan: Jason's life as a skinny male

I am currently 5' 8" and 117 pounds. [BMI 17.8] I'm completely aware that I'm really skinny. Unfortunately, I've been told that I was skinny all my life, and it's really started to piss me off. I've struggled with attaining a normal weight ever since I can remember. I really don't know what's wrong with me. I eat normally – about as much as my friends who are normal weight – so why can't I gain weight? I've never even talked about [this] with my closest friends because, frankly, I'm a "man" and something like this, and the frustrations I would like to share, could make me come off as – pardon my language – a "pussy."

The handball champion gives up his game

Back in elementary school, I was the school's best handball player. I loved playing that game, and I really was known school-wide as the "handball champion." I had one of the deadliest serves around. Some people couldn't believe how far I could hit the ball, to the point where it was almost impossible for my opponent to return it.

I made many friends playing that game. Quite frankly, I also made some enemies. The reason I was able to hit the ball the way I did, according to the bullies, was not because I knew the basic concepts of physics, but because I didn't have any of the fat that normal kids had that could prevent the ball from going as far as it did. It sucked, it really did. My outlet for success and recognition on the school playground was becoming a venue for bullies to make fun of me. I quit handball when I started the fifth grade. I didn't want to be made fun of anymore.

Every time I socialize with other people, I'm always wondering what they think of me. Do they think I'm too skinny? Will they not want to be my friend because I'm too skinny? Some people even give suggestions on how to gain more weight. Now, I completely understand that people just want to help me when they give tips and diets for me to try to gain weight, but it pisses me off because, frankly, do they seriously think I haven't been trying that for the past few years of my life??

Responsible for parental loss of face

Now I'm going to share something that really made me angry. My mom is always telling me that I'm too skinny and that she wants me to get bigger so that I can "save face." Well, my aunt from my father's side recently came to visit from Taiwan. Guess what the first thing this aunt said to me after I gave her a hug and introduced myself. YEP! She said in Mandarin, "Wow! John (my father), why is your son so skinny?" Great first impression, Jason, good going! Right when I heard that, my heart sank, I was so close to just yelling a big F★★★ YOU! right then and there. But I didn't. I wanted to "save" whatever "face" my father had left by not verbally destroying my aunt so that she couldn't bundle up my being skinny and completely rude and use it against my father. My father pulled me off to the side and said "thanks," because he saw my subtle facial expressions and my fists clenching. I teared up a little when my dad thanked me; in fact, I'm a little teary writing this now.

I really am trying to gain weight, though mostly not for myself but for my mom and dad, because I'm tired of having them hear "your son is too skinny" from church friends and family members. One of my most distinct memories is of when my father introduced me to his church friend who is also our insurance agent. I really remember this occasion clearly because it sucked. This male church friend, after my father exchanged introductions, stated, in Mandarin: "John, you have to stop focusing on your business and start feeding your son." This comment doesn't seem too bad, right? Until I tell you that my father is now the owner of a restaurant. So, this church friend told my father that he had paid too much attention to feeding his customers and neglected feeding me.

Humph, I just remembered something. In one class discussion, a female stated that she doesn't like Asian guys because we're too short and skinny. I will probably remember that, for a very long time, because it kind of describes me, ha ha. I haven't seen the movie *Black Swan*, but from what I've heard, it [features a ballet dancer with a] significantly low BMI. I hope my experiences of being a skinny Asian male – a yellow swan, as it were – provide some insight into how brutal society can be toward people who aren't of normal weight.

"A weakling": Linh's struggles to escape the curse

I have a BMI of 17.9 and yes, I do know I am underweight. However, that does not seem to stop people from perpetually drawing that fact to my attention. I am not anorexic and have never been drawn to the "cult of thinness." Contrary to popular belief, I do eat, at least three meals a day to be exact. I do not frequent the gym religiously and do not partake in the diets endorsed so powerfully by celebrities. No matter how many times I tell people that I am healthy (I have the doctor visits to prove that), and that I do not harbor some obsession about my weight, they still assume I live my life around a set of numbers: BMI, weight, and caloric intake. Many times people tend to focus on my weight more than who I am as a person.

"Too frail for the job"

Despite my accomplishments, people still think of me as mentally and physically weak, a quality that my family members assume comes with being thin. Whenever I go to family [functions], there will always be comments made by my relatives about my weight. They always assume that I am on a diet and tell me to eat more. They also advise me to take easier courses [in school so] as to not increase my stress and my chances of being sick. In addition, they also assume I am not physically and mentally strong enough to [handle] the stresses of graduate school and thus should settle for a more passive path, a path more [suited] to my physique and my female status. It is also very bothersome that my mother constantly worries about my health whenever the weather changes slightly.

Even though size discrimination is getting more media attention, people tend to neglect the fact that thin people as well as fat people suffer discrimination. When I applied for a job at a local pharmacy, I was passed over in favor of a young, normal-weight man, not because of my qualifications but because [the manager] felt I was too thin to lift boxes, type and stand at the computer, and talk to customers for a whole work period. My weight has always led people to underestimate my abilities when it has come to finding and performing in jobs.

213

"It's your choice"

The belief that being underweight is [something I have chosen] due to vanity or some sick obsession with anorexia is quite common but utterly untrue. My mom has put me on high-protein, high-calorie diets along with medicine that supposedly increased my appetite. All this was to no avail, not because I chose to be thin, but because there is just some part of me that cannot gain and maintain healthy weight for a long period of time. I do not like being so thin and I despise all the disadvantages that come with it. To this day, I am on a diet plan to increase my weight. The media are obsessed with fad diets linked to the "cult of thinness," but there is little help for people who are thin and want to gain some weight in a healthy manner. I despise the fact that all the clothes that I would like to wear do not fit me. I despise the fact that people still mistake me for a lost child whenever I walk alone by myself. For me, being thin is a curse, not a choice.

Becoming a skinny person

These essays and others I gathered open up an entire world of skinniness that few outside the skinny community even know exists. In some ways, the experience of skinniness paralleled that of fatness. Both identities were biologized, and both categories were subject to nonstop weight-talk. In other ways, though, the difficulties faced by the very thin were products of the treatment of, or actions by, the very fat. For example, the excessive attention to the uber-fat entailed the excessive *in*attention to the uber-thin, with both over- and under-attention producing many, mostly unwanted additional effects. (I provide more examples just below.) Thin and thick were co-constituted in surprising ways.

Skinny-talk and -practices: the world of the uber-thin

Regardless of gender or ethnicity, the young people I worked with reported remarkably similar experiences of being skinny in a fat-obsessed world. All were subject to a constant barrage of unwelcome skinny-talk. Acting as responsible biocitizens who seek to coax – or ridicule – the abnormally thin to become normal, the people in their social worlds felt compelled to remark on their skinniness, as though that were the most important thing about them. Some of the comments were pedagogical (diet tips, disingenuous compliments), but many more were abusive, meant to stigmatize, and shame them to motivate supposedly healthful change. Meantime, the wider culture of media images, clothing offerings, and so on provided constant reminders that those with skinny bodies did not belong to mainstream society.

Underlying the comments and cultural images that emerged in my study was a set of assumptions about ultra-skinny people that appears to be remarkably widespread in these California communities – yet almost wholly untrue. Precisely because fatness is so common in the US, skinny people were presumed to be abnormal, unhealthy, and closet anorexics. Since most fat people are able to lose weight, even if only temporarily, skinniness was assumed to be the result of a deliberate choice to under-eat or remain on a diet and not an uncooperative biology. Since skinny people were not gaining, evidently, they were bad Americans who, through inattention, vanity, or sickness, did not take proper care of their bodies. Thinness was deemed a moral defect through and through. Just as obese people were assumed to have character flaws, some of my thin informants were subject to additional assumptions about their character defects. Linh, in particular, was believed to be physically and mentally weak, incapable, childlike, and unable to take care of herself. Whereas obese people were said to be irresponsible, abnormal, and lacking in self-control, at least they remained part of the human community; others could relate to their putative weaknesses. Skinny people, by contrast, were sometimes placed beyond the pale, labeled "outcasts" or "freaks" because no one could fathom why they would "choose" to remain so unappealingly thin. Many of my informants believed that heavier people called them such dehumanizing names to make their own heaviness seem human and normal; they shamed the skinny to hide their own insecurities about being fat. Thick and thick were connected in complicated and little understood ways.

Skinny-talk was attached to a set of material practices designed to name, address, and fix the "problem." Doctors diagnosed my young informants as underweight and anorexic and began surveilling and managing their eating to correct their "disease." Many of the moms, including Linh's, put their kids on special diets and medicines intended to increase their body weight. Schoolmates placed them on "anorexia watch" in the lunchroom. Worst of all, the anti-obesity campaign has been so focused on helping heavy people lose weight that it has created few diets or medicines with proven ability to help the underweight add pounds and become "normal." (Fitness routines helped a few bulk up.) No wonder these young people felt "left behind" by society and the medical world alike.

Skinny selves: the inner world of skinny personhood

Of all the young people I worked with, the ultra-thin were among the most tormented by weight worries. Living in a world that is constantly telling them they are defective and socially unacceptable, it is not surprising that most took on the identity of the unhealthily skinny subject. In a typical pattern of identity formation, as children, most never cared about or noticed their low weight. Then, as suggested theoretically above, as the weight-talk aimed at them accumulated, they increasingly took on the subjectivity of the skinny person. When friends and family started making fun of them, they became self-conscious about their bodies. Then, as the skinny-abuse and pressure to add pounds persisted year after year, they came to see themselves as abnormal, skinny people who needed to gain weight to become "normal." One even took on the identity of "anorexic" to fit peers' perception of him and to get attention for something. While most took on the skinny identity, there was a continuum, from those who, like Jason and Linh, adopted it as a dominant identity, to others who eventually managed to see beyond or grow out of it.

In the essays I gathered, the young people of Asian background seemed more likely to internalize the shame of "bad weight" than those of Caucasian descent. Many lived in ethnic communities where they and their parents were subject to intense cultural pressures to conform. These pressures around weight reflected both ethnic bodily norms and the fairly widespread conviction that, as minorities, Asians needed to try harder and be more perfect than Caucasians to get ahead in American society. For many Asian young people, demanding families and high-pressure communities were obsessed with their skinniness and constantly badgered them about it, whereas the families and communities of white people expressed less concern about low weight. In the communities Jason and Linh inhabited, the individual was decentered in favor of the group, and individual "voluntary" flaws, like skinniness, were seen as stains on the group. Jason suffered a double dose of shame for bringing dishonor to his parents and disgrace on himself.

The characteristics of the "skinny person" were similar in many ways to those of the better understood fat subject. First, being skinny was considered a despicable condition that

215

was bad in almost every way. Most of these young people hated their skinniness and felt that it made them deviant, flawed, and sickly. Skinniness was profoundly staining, "tantamount to the shame of being fat," as one put it. Being skinny brought a host of negative emotions that ranged from hurt to anger, humiliation, and low self-esteem. What made it so difficult, many stressed, was the absence of a like-weighted community to provide support, a product of their minuscule numbers relative to the "too fat." Finally, most were obsessed with their low weight and engaged in constant struggles to eat more to gain weight. For the majority, exercise was not part of the program because it was seen as dangerously weight-shedding.

Larger consequences of pathologizing and stigmatizing skinniness

Yet, all the skinny-talk of the concerned biocitizens did not work to turn these young people into good biocitizens. Not only did no one gain weight and keep it on, but also some turned to patently unhealthy eating practices in an effort to add pounds. Believing that high-calorie foods make people fat, several stuffed themselves with such foods, becoming bad biocitizens – people who used *un*healthy practices – to achieve normality. Desperate to conform, they prioritized their weight over their health. And with little proven professional weight-gain advice available, they saw no way out.

The essays make clear that, for these young people, skinniness was not a disease but just another way of being in the world. Just as fat-studies scholars have insisted that fat can be healthy, and that body diversity, not BMI between 18.5 and 24.9, should be the norm, my informants insisted that they were skinny and healthy and deserved recognition like everyone else (Bacon 2010). Yet, they were treated as freaks simply because they were "too thin" rather than the more common "too fat." The larger effects on their lives are troubling. Skinny youngsters suffered not only emotional distress from all the stigma and biobullying; as Linh's essay shows, their lives were diminished in many ways. Some of these effects are likely to be long-lasting.

The essays I gathered provide stark evidence that regardless of weight category – underweight, overweight, obese, and even normal – the biocitizenship approach is not only not producing healthy weights but it has also remade individual subjectivity and is doing real damage to America's selves, psyches, families, and especially to its young people. While others have made related points in other, especially non-American, contexts (classic studies include Gard & Wright 2005; Evans et al. 2008), what is new here is the connection of theories of biocitizenship to the real-life experiences of a relatively large number of people and viewing the formation of weight-based subjectivities through the eyes of the subjects themselves. The subjectification narratives of my informants have allowed us to discover new kinds of selves and dynamics not reflected in previous theorizing. Relatively new as well is observing the dynamics of weight politics along a full spectrum of weights (other than the "severely obese"). That wide-angled view makes clear that our theories of weight-based politics need to be broadened to recognize the importance of the skinny end of the continuum and to acknowledge the co-constitution of the selves and lives of people along different parts of the weight spectrum. Finally, through the ethnographies, we have glimpsed the rather different ways the racialized dimensions of fat politics work in Asian-American families and communities. To be truly inclusive, critical weight studies must be broadened to include those of Asian descent. I've suggested some lines along which that work could develop.

Notes

1 This chapter draws material from and expands on arguments in *Fat-Talk Nation: The Human Costs of America's War on Fat.* I call the campaign a war both because some public health advocates used that metaphor and because the word captures the feeling of many of its targets that not just their bodies but also their persons are under ceaseless attack. I use the word fat because many heavy people prefer the term, finding obesity, the official term, objectifying.

2 In 2017–2018, 73.1 percent of US adults aged 20 or over were overweight (30.7) or had obesity (42.4) (age-adjusted figures). Among children and adolescents aged 2–19, 35.4 percent were overweight (16.1) or had obesity (19.3) (Fryar, Carroll, & Afful 2021a,b).

3 A BMI of 17.5 or below is commonly used as a possible indicator of anorexia nervosa. Below that, specialists recognize tiers ranging from mild to extreme probability (under BMI 15). The underweight subjects in my sample did not report anorexic behaviors.

4 Before obesity burst onto the cultural scene, historians, sociologists, and women's studies scholars focused on America's obsession with thinness, documenting cults of dieting, the power of the weight-loss industry, risks of eating disorders, and many other mid- to late 20th-century maladies (Chernin 1981; Schwartz 1986; Fraser 1997; & Hesse-Biber 2007; to name a few).

5 Statistics from 2004 to 2006, the most complete data available.

6 The ethnographies were written in 2010 and 2011. Of the 245 narratives used, 11 were collected orally. Most were about the young people themselves, but some were about friends and relatives. Of the total, 92.7 percent focused on Californians, and 78 percent of the subjects were from Southern California or from SoCal and another area.

7 Key sources on Asian-Americans in SoCal are Choi and Hahm 2017; Kibria 1995; Lee and Zhou 2004; and Zhou 2009.

8 This generalization is based on the 119 ethnographies on East and Southeast Asian subjects.

References

Bacon, L. (2010). *Health at Every Size: The Surprising Truth about Your Weight.* Dallas, TX: Benbella.

Barnes, P. M., Adams, P. F. & Powell-Griner, E. (2008). Health characteristics of the Asian adult population: US, 2004–2006. *Advance Data* no. 394. https://www.cdc.gov/nchs/data/ad/ad394.pdf

Boero, N. (2012). *Killer Fat: Media, Medicine, and Morals in the American "Obesity Epidemic."* New Brunswick, NJ: Rutgers University Press.

Chernin, K. (1981). *The Obsession: Reflections on the Tyranny of Slenderness.* New York: Harper and Row.

Choi, Y., & H. C. Hahm (eds.) (2017). *Asian American Parenting: Family Process and Intervention.* Cham: Springer.

Dietz, W. H. (2015). The response of the US Centers for Disease Control and Prevention to the obesity epidemic. *Annual Review of Public Health,* 36, 575–596. https://doi.org/10.1146/annurev-publhealth-031914-122415

Evans, J., Rich, E., Davies, B. and Allwood, R. (eds.) (2008). *Education, Disordered Eating and Obesity Discourse: Fat Fabrications.* London: Routledge.

Farrell, A. E. (2011). *Fat Shame: Stigma and the Fat Body in American Culture.* New York: New York University Press.

Fikkan, J. L. & Rothblum, E. D. (2011). Is fat a feminist issue: Exploring the gendered nature of weight bias. *Sex Roles: A Journal of Research,* 66(9), 575–592. https://doi.org/10.1007/s11199-011-0022-5

Fraser, L. (1997) *Losing It: False Hopes and Fat Profits in the Diet Industry.* New York: Penguin.

Fryar, C. D., Carroll, M. D. & Afful, J. (2021a). Prevalence of overweight, obesity, and severe obesity among adults aged 20 and over: United States, 1960–1962 through 2017–2018. National Center for Health Statistics, US Centers for Disease Control and Prevention (revised report). https://www.cdc.gov/nchs/data/hestat/obesity-adult-17-18/obesity-adult.htm

Fryar, C. D., Carroll, M. D. & Afful, J. (2021b). Prevalence of overweight, obesity, and severe obesity among children and adolescents aged 2–19 years: United States, 1963–1965 through 2017–2018 (revised report). https://www.cdc.gov/nchs/data/hestat/obesity-child-17-18/obesity-child.htm

Gard, M., & Wright, J. (2005). *The Obesity Epidemic: Science, Morality and Ideology.* London: Routledge.

Greenhalgh, S. (2015). *Fat-talk Nation: The Human Costs of America's War on Fat.* Ithaca, NY: Cornell University Press.

Halse, C. (2009). Bio-citizenship: Virtue discourses and the birth of the bio-citizen. In J. Wright & V. Harwood (Eds.), *Biopolitics and the "Obesity Epidemic"*, pp. 45–49. New York: Routledge.

Hesse-Biber, S. N. (2007). *The Cult of Thinness* (2nd ed). New York: Oxford University Press.

Kibria, N. (1995). *Family Tightrope: The Changing Lives of Vietnamese-Americans*. Princeton, NJ: Princeton University Press.

Lee, J., & Zhou, M. (Eds.) (2004). *Asian American Youth: Culture, Identity, and Ethnicity*. New York: Routledge.

Murray, S. (2008). *The 'Fat' Female Body*. New York: Palgrave Macmillan.

Office of the Surgeon General (2001). *The Surgeon General's Call to Action to Prevent and Decrease Overweight and Obesity*. Rockville, MD: Office of the Surgeon General (US), US Department of Health and Human Services, Public Health Service.

Pause, C. & Taylor, S. R. (eds.) (2021). *The Routledge International Handbook of Fat Studies*. New York: Routledge.

Puhl, R. M., & Heuer, C. A. (2010). Obesity stigma: Important considerations for public health. *American Journal of Public Health,* 100(6), 1019–1028. https://doi: 10.2105/AJPH.2009.159491

Rice, C. (2007). "Becoming 'the fat girl': Acquisition of an unfit identity." *Women's Studies International Forum,* 30(2), 158–174. https://doi.org/10.1016/j.wsif.2007.01.001

Rose, N. & Novas, C. (2005). "Biological citizenship." In A. Ong & S. J. Collier (eds.) *Global Assemblages: Technology, Politics, and Ethics as Anthropological Problems*, pp. 439–463. Malden, MA: Blackwell.

Rothblum, E. and Solovay, S. (Eds.) (2009). *The Fat Studies Reader*. New York: New York University Press.

Royce, T. (2009). The shape of abuse: Fat oppression as a form of violence against women. In E. Rothblum and S. Solovay (Eds.), *The Fat Studies Reader* (pp. 151–157). New York: New York University Press.

Saguy, A. C. (2013). *What's Wrong with Fat?* Oxford: Oxford University Press.

Schwartz, H. (1986). *Never Satisfied: A Cultural History of Diets, Fantasies and Fat*. New York: Doubleday.

Strings, S. (2019). *Fearing the Black Body: The Racial Origins of Fat Phobia*. New York: New York University Press.

Zhou, M. (2009). *Contemporary Chinese America: Immigration, Ethnicity, and Community Transformation*. Philadelphia, PA: Temple University Press.

22

THE UBIQUITY OF THE EXPERIENCE OF BEING "TOO FAT"

Perspectives from young people in Germany

Eva Barlösius

Typifications in the everyday world

The question of how people know they are fat seems trite at first glance. The answers are obvious, as a look in the mirror or at the reading on a set of bathroom scales reveals. But it is not quite that simple. Only by comparing your own body to bodies regarded as fat do you know how your body is perceived – or is to be perceived. The same applies to objective weight. You conclude that you weigh too much only by taking account of what standardized weight charts say. Being fat or thin is not a natural given. These conditions emerge through comparison with other people and are based on benchmarks and evaluations. It is thus a social rather than a personal experience. It is the reactions of others, the comparisons with socially set norms, that let people know they are regarded as being too fat. How, then, is this knowledge conveyed in the reality of everyday life?

To answer this question, I turn to Berger and Luckmann's (1967) theory of the social construction of reality, which makes it possible to examine the reality of daily life and reconstruct common-sense knowledge. According to Berger and Luckmann (1967, p. 15), "the sociology of knowledge must first of all concern itself with what people 'know' as 'reality' in their everyday, non- or pre-theoretical lives." This knowledge determines the reality of everyday life and regulates the behaviour in it. By knowledge, Berger and Luckmann mean the "certainty that phenomena are real and that they possess specific characteristics" (p. 1). "Commonsense knowledge is the knowledge I share with others in the normal, self-evident routines of everyday life" (p. 23). It therefore has a social character.

"The social reality of everyday life is thus apprehended in a continuum of typifications" (Berger & Luckmann, 1967 p. 33). Typifications are an essential part of everyday life because social interaction cannot succeed without them. They make it possible to determine the individual's place in society and set forth corresponding social "treatment" (p. 43). Typifications are ubiquitous in character and thus all but inevitable. They are templates with which everyday life is recognized. They have a reciprocal quality, for they more or less define the framework for acting and reacting.

There are many different kinds of typifications. Some stem from direct social interactions, such as those characteristic of face-to-face encounters, channelling how one looks at,

DOI: 10.4324/9780429344824-27

and is looked at by the interlocutor, how gestures, facial expressions, physical appearance, and movements are perceived. With bodies always being present in face-to-face encounters, many typifications relate to physical phenomena. Other typifications refer to anonymous or formalized social interactions. They often have an abstract quality and take on "objective character." For example, feelings and attitudes are objectified as typical physical expressions. A stooped posture can be seen as an "objectivation" of subservience; a fat body, as an objectivation of unbridled eating and low self-control.

Typifications also serve to separate "unproblematic" from "problematic." Agreement with everyday routines will thus be experienced as unproblematic; deviation from them, as problematic. Accordingly, there are typifications of what is considered "normal" and typifications that identify something as outside the "routines of everyday life" (Berger & Luckmann, 1967, p. 24) and, hence, as deviant. Building on this theoretical framework, the present contribution focuses on two questions: What kinds of typification of being fat can be differentiated? And how is the ubiquity of typifications of fat young people experienced?

Empirical material: group discussions with fat youth

Empirically, this investigation rests on a major project on obesity among young people in Germany.[1] Data were collected in three ways: (a) group discussions with fat young people from socially disadvantaged quarters of Hanover, (b) group discussions with parents of fat children, and (c) a World Café with experts on practices for preventing overweight. This chapter draws only on the group discussions with young people. Group discussion served as the method because it is particularly well suited to documenting collective patterns of orientation and experience, such as legitimation (Bohnsack, 1997; Loos & Schäffer, 2001; Moscovici & Doise, 1992). Thematically, the group discussions began with prompts that stemmed from "society as objective reality" (Berger & Luckmann, 1967, p. 47), such as common typifications of the everyday world and their social legitimation. Subsequent prompts inquired into subjective comments on the legitimations and explored expectations the participants had of their future biographical trajectory.

Eight group discussions with the young people took place, with 60 boys and girls participating. Each group consisted of six to ten persons, and the discussions lasted from 90 minutes to 2 hours. The discussions were segmented by gender, family background (German or Turkish), and age (11–13-year-olds and 14–16-year-olds). The young people had been recruited primarily from city quarters in which social reporting had recorded (a) an above-average percentage of the population to be receiving unemployment benefits or social welfare, (b) overrepresentation of persons with migration background in comparison to other city quarters with high percentages of dwellings under public-housing regulations, and (c) other indices of high socio-spatial disadvantage. This socio-spatial recruitment was intended to ensure that young people from socially disadvantaged families took part in the group discussion. In Germany, as in most European countries, socially disadvantaged groups have an especially high incidence of obesity.

The young people were recruited through a flyer entitled "*Dicke Freunde*" (Fat Friends, or Best Friends). We wanted to benefit from the two meanings of the German word for "dicke": (a) "close" or "best" for characterizing friends who enjoy getting together and (b) "fat" for qualifying bodies that are regarded as "obese." This word play was designed to ensure that mainly fat young people would feel addressed by, and that the flyer would convey, a positive meaning of fat, namely "best friends." Using this approach, we aimed (to the extent possible) to avoid a stigmatizing recruitment process.

In keeping with the project's premise that being fat is, above all, a socially experienced condition, the idea was to involve young people who perceived themselves to be fat. Therefore, no medical criteria were set in the recruitment process. In medical terms, most of the young people who attended the group discussions could be classified as "overweight" and "obese." Only a few could be categorized as "significantly obese." The young people assigned themselves into a German or a Turkish discussion group. In some cases, parents classified their children in one of these groups when registering them for the study. In the following pages, I analyse the segments of group discussions that were intended to elicit the typifications of being regarded as fat. As to be expected with common approaches, those typifications were not differentiated by gender, family background, or age, so the dissimilar constellations of participants in the group discussions are not discussed further.

Typifications of being fat

To have the young people in the group discussions describe the typifications confronting them in everyday reality, a cartoon was projected onto a screen. It depicted comparatively fat and comparatively thin young people standing in front of a snack bar. The cartoon represented a typical face-to-face encounter in young people's everyday life, in which, according to Berger and Luckmann (1967), simple mutual typifications are created and applied. The young people's narrative task was to look at the picture and respond to the question, "What goes through your mind when you see this picture?" This openly formulated item was intended to avoid making the participants feel pressured to talk about their own experiences. The idea was to give them the opportunity to comment, as observers, on the social interaction that appeared in the cartoon.

The analysis of these passages of the group discussions revealed that the three kinds of typifications were used to describe the social situation shown in the cartoon. They differed by their degree of abstraction. The first kind of typification referred directly to the bodies of the persons depicted and had a predominantly descriptive character. It was a relational typification in which fatter bodies are described as opposed to thinner ones. With a few exceptions, the young people spoke simultaneously of the "fatter" and the "thinner" ones, of "getting fatter" or "thinner," "a bit fatter," or "somehow thinner" and "a bit leaner." They used nouns, adjectives, and adverbs in comparative formulations. The typification into "fatter" or "thinner" only denoted different somatic manifestations.

The second kind of typification encompassed characterizations of attitudes and interactions linked to social perception of the body. This typification provided information about how the social interactions between the comparatively fat and comparatively thin young people take place. These participants used forceful, pejorative words for this purpose, but almost exclusively for the heavier adolescents. Examples were "fatties," "fatsos," "the fat people are being ignored," and "the fat people are ashamed." Only at one point in the eight group discussions was there a characterization of the thinner young people, which was meant disparagingly but nevertheless consisted of appreciative words: "the cool, thin ones who can check off all the boxes." Apart from this instance, the typifications of social attitudes and interactions focused only on those involving social interaction with fat people, not thin ones. This kind of typification seemed to be unilateral rather than relational and addressed only the fat young people. The obvious interpretation of the relational counterpart's absence is that the corpulent young people experience the attitudes toward and interactions with the thinner young people as axiomatic social "normality," which needs no specific explanation. By contrast, the typifications applied to the corpulent young people are those that indicate deviation. They classify the attitudes and manners, justifying the pejorative social interactions to which the overweight persons are socially subjected.

The third kind of typification completely consisted of abstract terms that characterized the situation depicted in the cartoon as a general societal phenomenon. They supplied a short title and categorized the overall phenomenon under the prevailing social framework and treatment. The young people turned to abstract technical terms originally used in discourses by therapeutic specialists. "Outsider," "excluded," and "bullying" are examples of this third kind of typification.

These words abstract preconceptions from human physique as well as from attitudes and comportment. The terms shape the social treatment of fat people, who are bullied and excluded and cast as outsiders. This language conveys values because bullying, excluding, or ostracizing people are forms of social interaction not regarded as socially legitimate. It contains the denigration, stigmatization, exclusion, and harassment to be ended.

Employing therapeutic jargon, the fatter young people could count on approval in social interactions. They could also be sure that their views would be seen as self-explanatory. One word such as *outsiders* was enough to determine a corpulent person's social place. Above all, however, recourse to the therapeutic language of experts enabled the fat young people to step back and discuss obesity. In this way, they avoided the necessity of talking about themselves. A typical example is, "Maybe if you're fat, you're excluded by many people who straightaway have the attitude 'fat people aren't cool', so they prefer to keep to themselves" (GD 14–16).[2]

The third typification's inherent abstraction from everyday life – the daily experience of being perceived and treated as too fat – enabled the young people to name events and embed them in an objectified context. The young people thus explained the causes of their obesity with socially legitimatized causes such as bullying and stress.

H[3]: "Stress would have to end in any case because when you're stressed you can't lose weight."
C: "You actually tend to gain weight when you're stressed."
H: "Yes." (GD 11–13)

However, by resorting to jargon, the young people also confirmed what the problems of being fat are and how and in what sequence they should be solved. They perceived these typifications as neutral representations of objective reality, as also shown by the fact that they used the typifications – "outsiders" and "bullying" – to label all that they go through.

Reconstructing the course of the conversation about the cartoon shows that typifications of the third kind were the most prominent ones and were highly spontaneous in most of the group discussions.

"A fatso is an outsider." (BD 11–13)
"So, fatsos are misfits." (GT 11–13)

Thereafter, the participants explained the physicality of the cartoon characters and compared the fat ones to the thinner ones. They then typified the attitudes and interactions and described the social exchanges between the fat and thin characters in the cartoon. Across the eight group discussions, there was a high degree of agreement about the three kinds of typifications. That concurrence and the uniformity of the sequence of conversations are persuasive indications that the typifications have an "objective character" for the young people and are perceived as representations of society's objective reality.

The ubiquity of typifications

"I have several siblings … They're not perfect, meaning they're fatter than I am …, and my brother is even more extreme… When he walks by somewhere, everyone looks at him as if he were, I don't know, as if he had a chicken perched on his head or something" (GD 11–13). The experience of being considered too fat was ubiquitous for the young participants in the group discussions. They explained that this omnipresence arises from fleeting, seemingly unconscious hints and reactions, as well as from conscious staring, provocative remarks, and denigrations. These social interactions shape the relationship between these young people and society and mould their view of the social world (Barlösius, 2017). According to the participants, their practices, behaviours, actions, clothing, what they eat, how they spend their leisure time, and so forth are primarily typified according to whether they are considered thin or fat. From their perspective, all other typifications, such as young or old, poor or rich, female or male, are secondary in drawing and justifying differences. The distinction between fat and thin is something they are incessantly reacting to not only in their perceptions and evaluations but also in their behaviour and actions. These young people acted as though the typifications were operative even in such interactions and situations in which the distinction between fat or thin had no relevance at all in the immediate context.

These fat young people found the typification of fat and thin to be as prevalent and unchallengeable as, say, society's distinction between genders. These participants found it to be just as natural, too; there was no in-between. It was intuitively and universally recognized, mostly at the subconscious level. Almost all movements, clothing, foods, sports, activities, and professions were assigned to one of these two worlds. As with the gendering of the world, the world, to them, was arguably embodied in terms of fat or thin. Whether succeeding or failing in sports, sitting or standing in the subway, eating in public, wearing tight jeans or a wide sweatshirt – the entire experience of the social world among these individuals was related to their bodies. They were unable to escape this pervasiveness unless they withdrew, and even that retreat was interpreted as both a cause and a consequence of their being fat.

The power of typification is measurable only when it is realized that the differentiation between fat and thin is not confined to bodies, associated modes of behaviour and action, and jargon. Directly or indirectly, it also extends to most other things and practices, many rules and regulations, essential obligations, and sanctions. For fat young people, it is not just one typification among many. To them, this typification constitutes the order that dominates all others. In the following paragraphs, this persuasion is illustrated by examples taken from three areas of life: eating, dressing, and sexuality and love.

In terms of eating, one boy described his experiences while having meals in school. "At our school you can eat, and if someone suddenly comes and says: 'Oh, you eat too much', or something like that, you take it as a threat, of course, or, [if] not as a threat, then something very close to it" (BD 14–16). A girl explained what happens to her when she goes to McDonald's: "That's right, when you sit at McDonald's, you get the same line: 'Yeah, you sit here every day'. It's so bad that you don't dare go in there by yourself. It's so stupid" (GD 14–16).

Both quotations convey something about exposure in public. Something similar happens to them at the family table, where they are requested not to put so much on their plate: "Well, then better take only half of it" (GD 14–16), "Oh, you're not full yet" (GT 14–16). Both public and family reprobation included disparagement. These observations, however, do not capture what the omnipresence of typifications means. The constant and undeniable immediacy of typifications for young people become apparent only in situations in which they feel compelled to emphasize their knowledge of, and basic agreement with, a given typification even though there is no danger of being exposed or belittled (Barlösius & Philipps, 2015). Among themselves in the group discussions, the participants felt called upon to distance themselves from social typifications. "I like to eat a lot of fruit, although it doesn't show" (GT 14–16). "I eat one for dinner … without anything and not fried in fat" (BD 11–13). They react to the ubiquity of this typification even when they are part of a conversational situation in which they can be sure that there is no threat of being discredited.

The same applied to shopping for clothes. They experience insults and disparagement, which can be interpreted as contempt. In hip fashion shops, for example, they are told that there is nothing for them there. But the pervasiveness of the typification means more. "I wish … I didn't need extra-large clothes anymore so that I could wear normal clothes again … Same with my underwear so that I could wear normal sizes again" (GD 11–13). "I don't want to be some anorexic right now; I just want to be more comfortable and be able go shopping" (GT 14–16). The young people, especially the girls, differentiated between clothes that are "normal" and "really nice" and those they have to wear but do not look good in. For them, clothing falls into two categories: (a) as apparel designed for people with bodies that are considered normal and (b) as clothes that are made especially for overweight people and that emphasize that condition. From the perspective of the discussants in our groups, every part of a wardrobe expresses either fat or thin. Each time they go shopping, they feel addressed above all as "fat girls," not like other girls, who are regarded as fashion-oriented young people.

Even when it comes to the experiences that fat teenagers have with love and sexuality, understanding the import of ubiquity means more than considering only direct degradations. One boy reported a particularly hurtful direct confrontation: "And they say, 'You have breasts like a woman', and stuff like that" (BD 14–16). The reproach that one looks like a woman is unsettling and problematic for a boy in puberty. Such insults are directly communicated in the social interactions between the fat and thin teenagers. But to these fat young people, its ubiquity went beyond that context. Because they are socially classified as "obese," it was hard for them to imagine that someone could fall in love with them. If it does happen, they tend to withdraw in order to avoid exposing themselves to hurt that they see as inevitable because of their body. For example, one female adolescent stated that, contrary to her feelings, she shunned involvement in a relationship with a boy to escape what she anticipated would be the inevitable, insulting comments about her body:

> [One boy] liked me the way I am and didn't mind that I was fat. But … I felt really shitty because everyone rejected me because of my looks. And then suddenly he comes and acts completely different. And then I was angry at myself for not being able to handle it … I thought: 'Yeah, if we're together' [and] he says: 'Oh, you're fat' or something, I wouldn't be able to handle it, so I just pretended not to be interested in him, though I'd actually been hoping for it for a while.
>
> *(GD 14–16)*

The omnipresence of the distinction between fat and thin, and the clear denigration of everyone and everything associated with being fat, meant that the fat young people were constantly confronted with being judged as too fat no matter where they are. The everyday world signalled to them that their bodies are read as a reification of their deviation from the desirable patterns of behaviour and action in daily reality. Above all, they felt the typification even if it was not present at all in the minds of people who are not fat. This characteristic of typecasting was best illustrated by the fact that the fat young people had no words to describe or even ridicule the attitudes and manners of their thin counterparts as typical of people who are too thin. The fat kids regarded the thin ones as representing the normal, an assessment so self-evident that there was no need to communicate about it at all. The consequence was that the fat young people are certain they would be treated primarily as too fat and that conviction drove their behaviour toward thin persons. They always commented on the typifications and distanced themselves from the associations attached to them. It was difficult for them to express this ubiquity, so they resorted to imagery – "a chicken perched on his head" (GD 11–13) – to convey this experience.

Their everyday reality was coloured by these experiences, and they wished for nothing more than not to be perceived as too fat. They wanted to lose weight, but not in order to become thin, that is, to change their body. Instead, losing weight meant to them the possibility of being seen as normal and no longer as "different": "I'm not somehow different right now just because I'm a bit heavier" (GT 14–16). "Because we want to fit in and not look so different now" (GD 11–13).

In other words, being fat is essentially a social experience for young people and therefore much truer to life than what the scales show. For them, this experience involves being perceived as "abnormal" and being treated as "deviant." Being stereotyped as fat not only addresses the body but it also extends to most areas and dimensions of life and thus conditions the ubiquity of this evaluative distinction. Social objectivation thereby pegs being fat as a deviation, and that perception becomes an all-encompassing social reality.

Notes

1 The study, entitled "Improvement in the Effectiveness of Obesity Prevention for Socially Disadvantaged Children and Youth—Targeted Strategies to Enhance the Health-Related Resources for Encouraging Responsibility for Diet and Exercise" (01E0813), is based on a project funded by the German Federal Ministry of Education and Research. All results are presented in the book *Dicksein. Wenn der Körper das Verhältnis zur Gesellschaft bestimmt [Being fat: When the body determines your relationship to society]* (Barlösius, 2014).
2 The quotations are excerpts from the group discussions. The language in some of the quotations has been revised to improve their comprehensibility, but neither the substance nor the manner of expression has been altered. In the transcripts, B stands for boy; G, for girl; T, for Turkish; and D, for German. The numerals give the age ranges.
3 One girl's first name started with H; the other with C.

References

Barlösius, E. (2014). *Dicksein. Wenn der Körper das Verhältnis zur Gesellschaft bestimmt [Being fat: When the body determines your relationship to society]*. Frankfurt am Main: Campus.

Barlösius, E. (2017). Being Fat – As "objectivation of deviance" from the societal order. In J. Martuschukat & B. Simon (Eds.). *Food, power, and agency* (pp. 147–168). New York: Bloomsbury.

Barlösius, E., & Philipps, A. (2015). Felt stigma and obesity: Introducing the generalized other. *Social Sciences & Medicine, 130*, 9–15. doi: 10.1016/j.socscimed.2015.01.048

Berger, P. L., & Luckmann, T. (1967). *The social construction of reality: A treatise in the sociology of knowledge*. Garden City, NY: Doubleday.

Bohnsack, R. (1997). Gruppendiskussionsverfahren und Milieuforschung [Group discussion procedure and milieu research]. In B. Friebertshäuser & A. Prengel (Eds.), *Handbuch Qualitative Forschungsmethoden in der Erziehungswissenschaft* (pp. 492–502). Weinheim, DE: Jeventa.

Loos, P., & Schäffer, B. (2001). *Das gruppendiskussionsverfahren: Theoretische grundlagen und empirische anwendung [The group discussion procedure: Theoretical principles and empirical application]*. Opladen, DE: Leske und Budrich.

Moscovici, S., & Doise, W. (1992). *Dissensions et consensus. Une théorie générale des décisions collectives [Dissent and consensus: A general theory of collective decision-making]*. Paris: Presses Universitaires de France.

23

A MOTHER OF A PROBLEM

Addressing the gendering of obesity panic

George Parker

Introduction

The war waged on obesity in the Global North since the mid-1990s has more recently been focused on pregnant bodies not only as the latest manifestation of the obesity epidemic but also more disturbingly as its cause. The emerging discourse of "maternal obesity"[1] has problematised fatness during pregnancy as a major reproductive health risk associated with an increase in almost all pregnancy and birth complications as well as initiating a programming effect that leads to future obesity and unwellness in the off-spring of fat mothers (e.g., Poston et al., 2016). Mirroring the drivers of obesity panic more generally, the gendering of obesity panic has occurred at the confluence of expanding medical interest in maternal obesity and the rapid and uncritical uptake of the resulting research in sensationalised news media coverage and reactive health policies. The result has been the problematisation of pregnancy fatness as a major public health crisis with significant consequences for the maternal health care offered to fat pregnant people and the negotiation of fat maternal identity.

This chapter explores the emergence of maternal obesity as a problematising discourse and its effects through a critical feminist intersectional lens. I begin this chapter by charting the rise of maternal obesity as a contemporary health crisis resulting in significant changes to reproductive health care policy and practice, along with contemporary understandings of fat reproductive bodies. Drawing on examples from my own research (Parker, 2019; Parker & Pausé, 2018a, 2018b, 2019; Parker, Pausé, & LeGrice, 2019), I demonstrate the value of critical obesity scholarship that draws on feminist, intersectional, and other critical social theoretical analyses to disrupt the certainty of problem discourses about pregnancy fatness and reveal their harmful discursive and material effects in the lives of fat women and gender diverse people who birth babies. I conclude by emphasising the key role of critical obesity scholarship in attempting to retrieve discourses of reproductive health from the toxic politics of anti-fatness and to argue for a much more complex and socially just view of the relationship between fatness, reproductive health, childbearing, and parenting.

DOI: 10.4324/9780429344824-28

Making pregnancy fatness into a big problem

The problematisation of pregnancy fatness as a significant reproductive health risk and public health challenge is now accepted as something of a contemporary certainty. The physical characteristics of a pregnant person, including both size and age, are commonly named as the driver for most maternity care challenges, including maternity service budget blow-outs and workforce shortages, growing rates of childbirth interventions, and all manner of day-to-day practice issues such as ultrasound availability and demands for equipment (e.g., Bayer, 2015). Body mass index (BMI) is now used to govern access to publicly funded fertility treatment in Aotearoa New Zealand and other Global North countries including Australia, the United Kingdom, and Canada, meaning that those classified as obese cannot access fertility care unless it is self-funded (Farquhar & Gillett, 2006). The medical management of fatness as an obstetric risk factor is now the norm, restricting fat pregnant people's access to low-risk birthing environments and practices such as immersion in water for labour and birth, and leading to increased medical screening and interventions for those classified as "overweight" or "obese" (Royal Australian & New Zealand College of Obstetricians & Gynaecologists, 2013). Fat pregnant people are now routinely targeted with mainstream weight-management discourses and practices such as weight surveillance and advice on diet and exercise management, leading to fear of, and attempts to restrict, weight gain during pregnancy despite its physiological inevitability (e.g., Goodwin, 2011).

It would be easy to understand the weight-centric practices of contemporary maternity care as a "common-sense" approach to improving maternal and child health; however, they are, in fact, a recent and contested development. As a researcher in this field for the past decade, I can still remember my first encounter with the emerging discourse of maternal obesity as a health issue. It came in the form of a chance reading of an online newspaper article in Wellington's[2] daily newspaper, *The Dominion Post*, late in 2010. The relatively brief article, titled "Mum's obesity might have role in baby deaths" (Newton, 2010), was reporting on the release of the Perinatal and Maternal Mortality Review Committee's periodic review of perinatal and maternal deaths in Aotearoa New Zealand. The article detailed a focus on bereaved mothers' body weight as a possible causal factor in the stillbirth or early infant death of their babies. The article (Newton, 2010, para. 1) began as follows: "Nearly half of all newborn babies that die are born to overweight or obese mothers, prompting concerns that increasing obesity rates could spark a rise in the number of baby deaths". I remember being struck at the time by the "heaviness" of this observation and wondered what it might be like for a family experiencing the trauma of the unexpected and often unexplained loss of a baby to be presented with this association with fatness, and the terrible burden of guilt, self-blame, and shame that could ensue as a result. I think it's fair to say that my interest was piqued.

The framing of obesity as a reproductive health complication that might be associated with stillbirth and neonatal infant death was unknown to me until encountering this article, which is not insignificant considering that I had spent most of the previous decade practising as a midwife and was thus intimately acquainted with reproductive health knowledges. In my midwifery education in the early 2000s, we were not taught that pregnancy fatness was an obstetric risk factor, and further, we were actively discouraged from routinely weighing pregnant people on the basis that there was no established relationship between maternal weight and perinatal outcomes. I had carried this knowledge into my early years in practice as a community midwife where fatness during pregnancy was not something considered particularly clinically relevant, was not included in obstetric consultation and referral guidelines,[3] and did not shape the kind of care that was provided in any explicit or intentional way.

In the months following *The Dominion Post* article, a steady stream of increasingly alarmist and definitive national news media articles reported on the risks posed by high maternal body weight across all aspects of reproductive health, with headlines such as "Over-eating while pregnant leads to obese babies" (Associated Press, 2010), "Birth, pregnancy complications worse for obese mums" (Newton, 2011), "Some babies already obese in the womb" (Hope, 2011), and "Big mums risk babies' health" (Grunwell, 2011). The opening sentence of the latter captured the general thread of reporting: "Pregnant women are packing on too many kilograms, risking their health and that of their babies—and costing the health system a fortune" (Grunwell, 2011, para. 1). Digging into the issue further, I discovered that media coverage was referencing, and being driven by, a veritable avalanche of new medical science publications on the phenomenon termed "maternal obesity". This was evident in my review of the articles listed on the Medline database with *maternal obesity* in the title. In the ten-year period from 1999 to 2009, there were under 100 such articles, and in the subsequent ten-year period from 2009 to 2019, this had risen to well over 700. These studies describe growing rates of obesity amongst reproductive-age women and an association between maternal obesity and almost all adverse reproductive health outcomes including infertility, miscarriage, stillbirth, congenital abnormalities, caesarean section, postpartum haemorrhage, infection, failed breastfeeding, and neonatal unit admission (e.g., Denison & Chiswick, 2011; Heslehurst, 2011; Nagle et al., 2011; Poston et al., 2016; Rowlands, Graves, de Jersey, McIntyre, & Callaway, 2010; Stacey, Thompson, Mitchell, Ekeroma, & Zuccollo, 2011).

Further, some of the studies, drawing on the scientific developments in epigenetics, also suggested that fatness before and during pregnancy may have long-term effects on the health of offspring as a result of foetal or in-utero programming (e.g., Low, Gluckman, & Hanson, 2015). These studies associated fatness during pregnancy with the development of childhood and adult obesity and a range of other chronic health conditions in offspring from autism to asthma (e.g., O'Reilly & Reynolds, 2013). Represented as posing both immediate reproductive health harms and long-term effects on offspring, these studies and their recitation in the national news media elevated pregnancy fatness to the status of a major public health crisis presenting, as claimed by one study, "the biggest challenge for maternity services today" (Heslehurst, Bell, & Rankin, 2011, p. 161).

Over the next few years, the so-called "crisis" of maternal obesity was front-page news in Aoteaora New Zealand, triggering a range of reactive government and health service responses. A leading epigenetics scientist, Professor Peter Gluckman, was appointed as the Chief Science Advisor to the Office of the Prime Minister. Obesity was added to the national obstetric consultation and referral guidelines, meaning that it was now regarded as an obstetric risk factor (Ministry of Health, 2012). Measuring and monitoring BMI became a compulsory component of the delivery of maternity care. And a range of government inquiries and action plans on maternal fatness would result in the reallocation of public health funding formerly invested in addressing the obesity epidemic in the general population to the new priority area of maternal obesity. It was clear that the war waged on obesity in Western countries since the mid-1990s (Gard & Wright, 2005) was now being focused on the womb not only as the latest manifestation of the obesity epidemic but also more disturbingly, as its cause.

Carving out critical responses

As the chapters throughout this handbook attest, critical obesity scholarship plays a vital role in responding to the social, political, and biomedical processes implicated in the problematisation and medicalisation of the fat body. Such scholarship draws on a range of critical tools and analytical approaches that call into question the objectivity of medical and scientific knowledge claims about fat bodies and their uptake in heath policy and practice, pointing to the influence of social, political, and indeed economic forces in constituting knowledges that produce the fat body as abject, inferior, and risky. Revealing obesity knowledges as constructs in service to political and other interests, critical obesity scholarship both seeks to intervene in and resist the meanings attached to fat bodies, opening up spaces for other cultural possibilities for fat embodiment and subjectivity.

Responding to the cultural moment in which maternal obesity has emerged as the new frontline in the "war on obesity", a growing body of critical obesity scholarship has adopted feminist, intersectional, and other critical lenses to disturb the problematisation of pregnancy fatness and reveal its harmful effects. Pregnancy has traditionally been regarded by feminist scholars as a time of release from the pressures to uphold the feminine ideal of a slender body and for a more enjoyable and less anxious experience of embodiment (Earle, 2003; Williams & Potter, 1999). However, more recently, the slenderness ideal has encroached on pregnancy (e.g., Harper & Rail, 2012; Johnson, Burrows, & Williamson, 2004; Longhurst, 2005; Nash, 2006, 2011). Scholars attribute this both to the rise of popular cultural representations of "fit", "fat-free", and "sexy" pregnancies (e.g., Longhurst, 2005; Nash, 2012) in tandem with this burgeoning medical scientific concern with the health impacts of maternal obesity (e.g., McPhail, Bombak, Ward, & Allison, 2016). Research exploring the discursive and subjectification effects of this heightened medical and social concern with the size of the pregnant body remains nascent, but is forming an important critical response to maternal obesity discourse (e.g., Bombak, McPhail, & Ward, 2016; Furber & McGowan, 2011; McPhail et al., 2016).

Several such studies have critiqued the medical framing of pregnancy fatness through a textual-based analysis of the medical science studies on maternal obesity, policy documents, clinical guidelines, news media representations, and popular cultural discourse (Davidson & Lewin, 2018; Herndon, 2018; Jette & Rail, 2012; McNaughton, 2011; Sanders, 2017; Strings, 2015; Warin, Moore, Zivkovic, & Davies, 2011). These studies have called into question the objectivity of medical knowledge, media, and health policy claims about pregnancy fatness, pointing to the influence of neoliberal political values of the self-managing citizen and gendered constructs of "good mothering" in constituting fat reproductive bodies as abject, inferior, and risky. A strong theme across this literature is how maternal obesity knowledges extend the pernicious effects of maternal responsibilisation for child health and obesity (e.g., Boero, 2010) to pregnancy or even prior to conception, subjecting pregnant people to increasing surveillance, discipline, and control (McNaughton, 2011). Fewer studies have responded critically to the emergence of maternal obesity discourse by centring the voices and experiences of fat people themselves. Canadian scholars McPhail, Bombak, Ward and Allison (2016) explored the experiences of fat people accessing reproductive health care through a feminist poststructural lens. Their study identified the stigmatising effects on fat pregnant people produced through the discourses and practices associated with maternal obesity and a "new eugenics" (McPhail et al., 2016, p. 110), whereby fat people's reproductive potential is actively restricted through reproductive health policy and practice that limits access to fertility and maternity care.

My own research adds to this nascent scholarship by drawing on fat people's voices and experiences through in-depth, semi-structured face-to-face interviews with 27 self-identified fat and ethnically diverse women[4] who were trying to conceive, were currently pregnant, or who had recently had a baby in Auckland,[5] Aotearoa New Zealand. My overtly political interest in the research was cultural analysis and critique, asking how (and why) maternal obesity knowledges coalesce around and constitute fat pregnant embodiment in seemingly oppressive ways, with the goal of opening up other possibilities for transformation. This means that, while I was interested in fat people's experiences of reproduction, my analytical work with their accounts was not simply descriptive. Rather, I also wanted to know how their experiences were enmeshed in culture, seeking to reveal the discursive forces that shape the conditions of possibility for those experiences (Gavey, 2011).

This approach to research is consistent with Foucault's notion of problematisation as elaborated by Bacchi (2010, 2012, 2016). Foucault (as cited in Bacchi, 2012) was interested in "how and why certain things (behaviour, types of bodies, phenomena, processes) become a problem" (p. 1) and how they are shaped as objects of thought that are taken up in the process of subjectification as truth. Problematisations are constituted in discourse (Bacchi, 2010). Discourse, in the Foucauldian sense, are ways of constituting authoritative knowledge; they are regulated systems of statements, "that systematically form the objects of which they speak" (Foucault, 2002, p. 41). The focus of analysis is to identify and distil those dominant discourses, or authoritative ways of thinking, that produce an object of thought as a taken for-granted truth (Bacchi, 2010). The analyst seeks to "dismantle" knowledge claims as "fixed essences" asking how the fat pregnant body is "questioned, analysed, classified and regulated" at "specific times and under specific circumstances" (Deacon, 2000, p. 127). By rendering apparently fixed objects "fragile" and "mutable", they can then be challenged, dismantled, and reconstituted (Bacchi, 2012, p. 4).

Thinking problematically about fat pregnant people's experiences of their maternity care, I was also conscious of the challenge laid by feminist black, indigenous, and people of colour (BIPOC) to be attentive to the raced, classed, and other kinds of differences in order to avoid making hegemonic generalisations about experience (Price, 2011, p. 55; see also Collins, 1986). Intersectional analysis seeks to ensure attention to the "interlocking effects of identities, oppressions, and privileges to fully understand the range and complexity of women's experiences" (Price, 2011, p. 55; see also Collins, 1986). Examining the research data through an intersectional lens allowed me to identify the ways in which participants' experiences were refracted through the axes of privilege and oppression, most clearly those of race and class. A commitment to intersectionality means that the experience of pregnancy fatness cannot simply be universalised or generalised but rather must be understood for the ways that it intersects with and compounds other axes of oppression. The problematisation of pregnancy fatness should therefore be understood for the ways in which it perpetuates and amplifies the legacy of reproductive injustices endured by minority women, particularly Indigenous women, women of colour, and poor women (Parker et al., 2019).

Vulnerable babies and bad (pregnant) mothers

Thinking problematically (and intersectionally) in relation to my research data, I identified dominant discourses of fat pregnant people as bad mothers who are wilfully harming their babies through their poor self-management and as problem citizens who are adding pressure to the health system and costing the tax payer (Parker, 2019; Parker & Pausé, 2018a, 2018b, 2019; Parker et al., 2019). These dominant discourses were constituted and reproduced in participants' interactions with maternity care providers, in the medicalised processes instigated in response to pregnancy fatness, and in media stories about maternal obesity. Nadine, for example, recalled the midwife's very negative response to her size when she attended her first prenatal appointment, leading her to feel like she was putting her baby at risk: "she [midwife] made it [fat] sound very, very scary, like it was AIDS, you know, like it was a real, real bad thing". Leilani also described a negative reaction from her doctor about her size and the potential impact on her pregnancy leading her to question her suitability as a mother-to-be and to associated feelings of guilt and self-blame: "It was scary to know that, it's depressing to know that these bad things are going to happen because of my choices and my body".

The discourse of fat people as problem citizens adding pressure to the health system was encountered in the ways in which some participants struggled to access maternity care and unkind and inappropriate treatment when they did. Emma, for example, described ringing around a number of midwives only to be turned away once they asked her about her weight. When asked why she thought she was refused care, Emma reflected: "you know I think they thought I was too much trouble, and just that they were worried about the risks to them and their reputation and how much hard work it would be". The discourse of being a problem or burden to health services was also evident in Emma's treatment during her stay in hospital after the birth of her baby by caesarean section:

> They never gave me a shower, I had to get my family to shower me, even though they [staff] knew I couldn't walk, I had to have two people holding me in the shower so I didn't fall over, but yeah they [staff] wouldn't do anything, they [staff] basically just treated me like a big inconvenience and that I was fat and deserved what I got, because what the hell was I doing having a baby in the first place?

Examined through an intersectional lens, these negative discursive effects are compounded for participants already marginalised along racial and other lines. Specifically, Māori and Pacific[6] participants in my study experienced the problematisation of their fatness as racialised. Participants reflected that negative attitudes towards their fatness were yet another expression of the racial discrimination they experienced in health care. Māori and Pacific women described feeling positioned, in highly dismissive ways, as just another number to add to the "problem" of Māori and Pacific obesity, and unwelcome in the maternity care system. As Talia described:

> "you're just a Pacific Island girl who's overweight, typical, and you're going to have a baby, and you're young, get out" that's just how I felt. Yeah I felt that with the midwife and with everything, you know, it was like "oh, you're just another friggin' number to add to the problem…

Participants' exposure to these dominant discourses resulted in a range of oppressive effects, limiting their possibility for being in relation to reproduction and mothering. In particular, fat pregnant people took up subjectivities of failed mothers and citizens, casting a shadow over their pregnancies and driving engagement with a range of self-governing practices such as efforts at restricting weight gain, or even achieving weight loss, during pregnancy as they tried to manage their fat bodies and salvage their maternal identities. Participants in my research described a range of harmful responses including swinging from depriving themselves of food to comfort eating, excessive or significantly reduced physical activity, anxiety, and hypervigilance over their pregnancies and lowered self-esteem leading to social withdrawal and depressive feelings. These practices did not support mental health and wellbeing during pregnancy with participants describing the loss of enjoyment and happiness in pregnancies and the experience of distress. Maia, for example, described her anxiety and hypervigilance over her pregnancy resulting from the problematisation of her fatness: "There was that anxiety that came with it because it was implied that you were very lucky to be pregnant because you were overweight and therefore you needed to do everything you could to manage the risks". Nadine described the stress induced by trying not to gain any weight while pregnant, constantly watching what she ate, and trying to engage in exercise even when she felt unwell: "I didn't realise until after the birth how naturally happy I was with all the endorphins of being pregnant, because during that time I was always stressed, I always watched what I ate". Alice described a vicious cycle in which exposure to maternal obesity risk discourse led to negative feelings resulting in comfort eating which, in turn, compounded her fear for her baby and her own self-loathing:

> Oh, I think it just makes you stressed, and it's a time when you should be relaxed, and happy and taking care of yourself. But if you feel this bad you're not going to, you're going to want that bag of chips, and that chocolate, and then you feel like, oh god I'm destroying my baby, those really extreme negative views come into your head because of what you've been told.

Conclusion

As this discussion has demonstrated, the great irony of the problematisation of pregnancy fatness is that the medical science, popular media, and health policy discourses and practices deployed in the interests of addressing the so-called health crisis of maternal obesity, are actually implicated in a public health crisis. The toll of the oppressive discourses produced in maternal obesity knowledges on fat women's pregnancies, emerging maternal identities, and their physical, mental, and spiritual health was significant and long-lasting. The key role of critical obesity scholarship in disturbing and peeling back the logics of maternal obesity, in order to reveal the harmful and inequitable effects on fat parents and their babies, has been highlighted. By revealing these harmful effects, critical obesity scholars can challenge the prioritisation of maternal obesity as a public health crisis and the centring of weight in the delivery of maternity care.

However, the role of the critical obesity scholar is not simply confined to *critique*. We also have an important role to play in transformation, opening up possibilities for generating counter-knowledge of pregnancy fatness that might begin to transform the conditions in which fat women navigate reproduction (McKenzie-Mohr & Lafrance, 2014; Parker & Pausé, 2018a). A counter-knowledge of pregnancy fatness, for example, could reject the emphasis within dominant maternal obesity discourse on individual gendered (maternal) responsibility for the current challenges facing Western health care systems. It could also de-centre body weight as the determining force of health during pregnancy on the basis that such a focus diminishes, rather than enhances, the health and bodily sovereignty of fat women.

In its place, a counter-knowledge of pregnancy fatness could draw on a much more holistic and arguably non-Western epistemological view of pregnancy health that takes account of the social, political, and cultural context of health, body weight, and mothering (Parker et al., 2019). It could draw on the knowledges afforded by whakapapa[7] and other elements of a mātauranga Māori[8] epistemology of reproduction (Le Grice & Braun, 2016) to emphasise the significance of the social, spiritual, and ecological, alongside the biological, in the life-giving forces of human reproduction.[9] From this perspective, pregnancy health could never be achieved through the derogation of pregnant people, and healthy pregnancy would be understood in the context of a complex web of relationships and factors that include cultural differences in patterns of fertility and reproductive norms, socio-economic disparities, food and housing security, diverse family realities and challenges, access to education and healthcare, safe, and sustainable communities, and love, care, and support.

Notes

1   I use single inverted comments on first usage to denote terms that are contested and in order to avoid reproducing the dominant discursive meanings attached to them.
2   Aotearoa New Zealand's capital city.
3   In Aotearoa New Zealand, the Ministry of Health's (2012) *Guidelines for Consultation with Obstetric and Related Medical Services (referral guidelines)* provide primary maternity care services with a list of conditions and criteria about referring pregnant people for consultations with other clinicians, transferring clinical responsibility for care to specialists, and transferring care in emergencies.
4   All participants in this study identified as cisgender women. However, I acknowledge that not all gestational parents identify as women and that not all women give birth. I have endeavoured to use gender-inclusive language in this chapter where possible, however aknowledge that I have done so imperfectly.
5   Auckland is New Zealand's largest city of approximately 1.6 million inhabitants.
6   Māori are Indigenous (tangata whenua) to Aotearoa New Zealand. Pacific people are Indigenous to further islands of Te Moana Nui a Kiwa (The Great Ocean of Kiwa – The Pacific Ocean).
7   Whakapapa is a fundamental principle in Māori culture that describes human connection and belonging through ancestry, incorporating past influences, and future potential.
8   The knowledges, understandings, and world view of Māori.
9   Acknowledgement and sincere gratitude to Dr Le Grice for her cultural guidance in my research.

References

Associated Press. (2010, August 6). Over-eating while pregnant leads to obese babies. *Stuff*. Retrieved from http://www.stuff.co.nz/life-style/3997417/Overeating-while-pregnant-leads-to-obese-babies

Bacchi, C. (2010). Poststructuralism, discourse and problematisation: Implications for gender mainstreaming. *Kvinder, Køn & Forskning, 4*, 62–72. doi: 10.7146/kkf.v0i4.28005

Bacchi, C. (2012). Why study problematisations? Making politics visible. *Open Journal of Political Science, 2*(01), 1–8. doi: 10.4236/ojps.2012.21001

Bacchi, C. (2016). Problematisations in health policy: Questioning how "problems" are constituted in policies. *Sage Open, 6*(2), 1–16. doi: 10.1177/2158244016653986

Bayer, K. (2015, September 2). Lifestyles burden on midwives' workload. *New Zealand Herald*. Retrieved from https://www.nzherald.co.nz/nz/news/article.cfm?c_id=1&objectid=11506924

Boero, N. (2010). Fat kids, working moms, and the "epidemic of obesity": Race, class, and mother blame. In E. D. Rothblum & S. Solovay (Eds.), *The Fat Studies Reader* (pp. 113–119). New York: New York University Press.

Bombak, A. E., McPhail, D., & Ward, P. (2016). Reproducing stigma: Interpreting "overweight" and "obese" women's experiences of weight-based discrimination in reproductive healthcare. *Social Science & Medicine, 166*, 94–101. doi: 10.1016/j.socscimed.2016.08.015

Collins, P. H. (1986). Learning from the outsider within: The sociological significance of black feminist thought. *Social Problems, 33*(6), S14–S32. doi: 10.2307/800672

Davidson, M., & Lewin, S. (2018). Eating for two: The fear and threat of fatness in pregnancy. In J. Verseghy & S. Abel (Eds.), *Heavy burdens: Stories of motherhood and fatness* (pp. 45–60). Bradford, ON: Demeter.

Deacon, R. (2000). Theory as practice: Foucault's concept of problematization. *Telos, 2000*(118), 127–142.

Denison, F. C., & Chiswick, C. (2011). Improving pregnancy outcome in obese women. *Proceedings of the Nutrition Society, 70*(4), 457–464. doi: 10.1017/S0029665111001637

Earle, S. (2003). "Bumps and boobs": Fatness and women's experiences of pregnancy. *Women's Studies International Forum, 26*(3), 245–252. doi: 10.1016/S0277–5395(03)00054-2

Farquhar, C. M., & Gillett, W. R. (2006). Prioritising for fertility treatments: Should a high BMI exclude treatment? *BJOG an International Journal of Obstetrics and Gynaecology, 113*(10), 1107–1109. doi: 10.1111/j.1471–0528.2006.00994.x

Foucault, M. (2002). *Archaeology of knowledge.* London: Routledge.

Furber, C. M., & McGowan, L. M. E. (2011). A qualitative study of the experiences of women who are obese and pregnant in the UK. *Midwifery, 27*(4), 437–444. doi: 10.1016/j.midw.2010.04.001

Gard, M., & Wright, J. (2005). *The obesity epidemic: Science, morality, and ideology.* New York: Routledge.

Gavey, N. (2011). Feminist poststructuralism and discourse analysis revisited. *Psychology of Women Quarterly, 35*(1), 183–188. doi: 10.1177/0361684310395916

Goodwin, E. (2011, April 16). Call for ministry to lead in checking pregnant women. *Otago Daily Times.* Retrieved from http://www.odt.co.nz/news/ dunedin/156448/call-ministry-lead-checking-pregnant-women

Grunwell, R. (2011, January 30). Big mums risk babies' health. *New Zealand Herald.* Retrieved from http://www.nzherald.co.nz/nz/news/article.cfm?cid=1&objectid=10702999

Harper, E. A., & Rail, G. (2012). 'Gaining the right amount for my baby': Young pregnant women's discursive constructions of health. *Health Sociology Review, 21*(1), 69–81. doi: 10.5172/hesr.2012.21.1.69

Herndon, A. (2018). Overfeeding the floating fetus and future citizen: The "war on obesity" and the expansion of fetal rights. In J. Verseghy & S. Abel (Eds.), *Heavy burdens: Stories of motherhood and fatness* (pp. 45–60). Bradford, ON: Demeter.

Heslehurst, N. (2011). Identifying 'at risk' women and the impact of maternal obesity on National Health Service maternity services. *Proceedings of the Nutrition Society, 70*(4), 439–449. doi: 10.1017/S0029665111001625

Heslehurst, N., Bell, R., & Rankin, J. (2011). Tackling maternal obesity: The challenge for public health. *Perspectives in Public Health, 131*(4), 161–162. doi: 10.1177/1757913911412477

Hope, J. (2011, September 26). Some babies already obese in the womb. *New Zealand Herald.* Retrieved from http://www.nzherald.co.nz/lifestyle/news/article.cfm?c_id=6&objectid=10754502

Jette, S., & Rail, G. (2012). Ills from the womb? A critical examination of clinical guidelines for obesity in pregnancy. *Health, 17*(4), 407–421. doi: 10.1177/1363459312460702

Johnson, S., Burrows, A., & Williamson, I. (2004). 'Does my bump look big in this?' The meaning of bodily changes for first-time mothers-to-be. *Journal of Health Psychology, 9*(3), 361–374. doi: 10.1177/1359105304042346

Le Grice, J. S., & Braun, V. (2016). Mātauranga Māori and reproduction: Inscribing connections between the natural environment, kin and the body. *Alternative: An International Journal of Indigenous Peoples, 12*(2), 151–164. doi: 10.20507/AlterNative.2016.12.2.4

Longhurst, R. (2005). (Ad)dressing pregnant bodies in New Zealand: Clothing, fashion, subjectivities and spatialities. *Gender, Place & Culture, 12*(4), 433–446. doi: 10.1080/09663690500356842

Low, F. M., Gluckman, P. D., & Hanson, M. A. (2015). Evolutionary and developmental origins of chronic disease. In M. P. Muehlenbein (Ed.), *Basics in Human Evolution* (pp. 369–381). London: Academic Press.

McKenzie-Mohr, S., & Lafrance, M. N. (Eds.). (2014). *Women voicing resistance: Discursive and narrative explorations.* London: Routledge.

McNaughton, D. (2011). From the womb to the tomb: Obesity and maternal responsibility. *Critical Public Health, 21*(2), 179–190. doi: 10.1080/09581596.2010.523680

McPhail, D., Bombak, A., Ward, P., & Allison, J. (2016). Wombs at risk, wombs as risk: Fat women's experiences of reproductive care. *Fat Studies, 5*(2), 98–115. doi: 10.1080/21604851.2016.1143754

Ministry of Health. (2012). *Guidelines for consultation with obstetric and related medical services (referral guidelines).* Wellington: Ministry of Health.

Nagle, C., Skouteris, H., Hotchin, A., Bruce, L., Patterson, D., & Teale, G. (2011). Continuity of midwifery care and gestational weight gain in obese women: A randomised controlled trial. *BMC Public Health, 11*(1), 174–179. doi: 10.1186/1471-2458-11-174

Nash, M. (2006). Oh baby, baby: (Un)veiling Britney Spears' pregnant body. *Michigan Feminist Studies, 19,* 27–50.

Nash, M. (2011). "You don't train for a marathon sitting on the couch": Performances of pregnancy 'fitness' and 'good' motherhood in Melbourne, Australia. *Women's Studies International Forum, 34*(1), 50–65. doi: 10.1016/j.wsif.2010.10.004

Nash, M. (2012). Weighty matters: Negotiating 'fatness' and 'in-betweenness' in early pregnancy. *Feminism & Psychology, 22*(3), 307–323. doi: 10.1177/0959353512445361

Newton, K. (2010, October 10). Mums' obesity may have role in baby deaths. *The Dominion Post.* Retrieved from http://www.stuff.co.nz/national/health/4239829/mums-obesity-

O'Reilly, J. R., & Reynolds, R. M. (2013). The risk of maternal obesity to the long-term health of the offspring. *Clinical Endocrinology, 78*(1), 9–16. doi: 10.1111/cen.12055

Parker, G. C. (2019). Mothers at large: Governing fat pregnant embodiment (Doctoral dissertation). University of Auckland, Auckland.

Parker, G., & Pausé, C. (2018a). "I'm just a woman having a baby": Negotiating and resisting the problematization of pregnancy fatness. *Frontiers in Sociology, 3,* 5. doi: 10.3389/fsoc.2018.00005

Parker, G., & Pausé, C. (2018b). Pregnant with possibility: Negotiating fat maternal subjectivity in the "War on obesity". *Fat Studies, 7*(2), 124–134. doi: 10.1080/21604851.2017.1372990

Parker, G., & Pausé, C. (2019). Productive but not constructive: The work of shame in the affective governance of fat Pregnancy. *Feminism & Psychology, 29*(2), 250–268. doi: 10.1177/0959353519834053

Parker, G., Pausé, C., & LeGrice, J. (2019). "You're just another friggin' number to add to the problem": Constructing the raciliased (m)other in contemporary discourses of pregnancy fatness. In M. Friedman, C. Rice, & J. Rinaldi (Eds.), *Thickening fat: Fat bodies, intersectionality and social justice* (pp. 97–105). New York: Routledge.

Poston, L., Caleyachetty, R., Cnattingius, S., Corvalán, C., Uauy, R., Herring, S., & Gillman, M. W. (2016). Preconceptional and maternal obesity: Epidemiology and health consequences. *The Lancet Diabetes & Endocrinology, 4*(12), 1025–1036.

Price, K. (2011). It's not just about abortion: Incorporating intersectionality in research about women of color and reproduction. *Women's Health Issues, 21*(3, Supplement), S55–S57. doi: 10.1016/j.whi.2011.02.003

Rowlands, I., Graves, N., de Jersey, S., McIntyre, H. D., & Callaway, L. (2010). Obesity in pregnancy: Outcomes and economics. *Seminars in Fetal and Neonatal Medicine, 15*(5), 94–99. doi: 10.1016/j.siny.2009.09.003

Royal Australian and New Zealand College of Obstetricians and Gynaecologists. (2013). *Management of obesity in pregnancy.* Retrieved from http://www.ranzcog.edu.au/college-statements-guidelines.html

Sanders, R. (2017). The color of fat: Racializing obesity, recuperating whiteness, and reproducing injustice. *Politics, Groups, and Identities, 7*(2), 1–18. doi: 10.1080/21565503.2017.1354039

Stacey, T., Thompson, J. M. D., Mitchell, E. A., Ekeroma, A. J., & Zuccollo, J. M. (2011). Relationship between obesity, ethnicity and risk of late stillbirth: A case control study. *BMC Pregnancy and Childbirth, 11*(3), 1–7. doi: 10.1186/1471-2393-11-3

Strings, S. (2015). Obese black women as "social dead weight": Reinventing the "diseased black woman." *Signs: Journal of Women in Culture and Society, 41*(1), 107–130.

Warin, M., Moore, V., Zivkovic, T., & Davies, M. (2011). Telescoping the origins of obesity to women's bodies: How gender inequalities are being squeezed out of Barker's hypothesis. *Annals of Human Biology, 38*(4), 453–460. doi: 10.3109/03014460.2011.591829

Williams, L., & Potter, J. (1999). 'It's like they want you to get fat': Social reconstruction of women's bodies during pregnancy. In J. Germov & L. Williams (Eds.), *A sociology of food and nutrition: The social appetite* (pp. 228–241). Melbourne: Oxford University Press.

24

FIGHTING FAT IN FAMILIES?

Lisette Burrows

Introduction

In 2017, a preschool teacher in New Zealand was accused of removing food from children's lunch boxes at the early childhood centre she worked at: "The teacher said she removed children's food because of research around childhood obesity rates. She said it had always been part of her career in early childhood to help children make healthy choices" (Franks, 2019, para. 8). At first blush, one could read this incident as a lone example of an educator over-stepping her role – a random, albeit regrettable, act by an over-zealous teacher with the best interests of children in her care at heart. On the other hand, this incident gestures towards a contemporary climate where it is entirely conceivable that an educator may override family food preferences for the "good" of a child, premised on their understanding about obesity.

There is certainly no shortage of evidence that families are indeed being drawn into fat-fighting practices via governmental strategies enacted by health professionals, school-based resources and teachers themselves (Burrows, 2009, 2016; Fullagar, 2009; Pike and Leahy, 2016; Rich, 2011). In New Zealand, programs like "Healthy Families New Zealand" (Ministry of Health, 2014) provide abundant resources designed to shape and, in some cases, reset family dispositions and everyday practices on route to achievement of a healthier (often read as slimmer) state and parents are squarely in the line of sight (Maher, Fraser, & Wright, 2010; Warin, Turner, Moore, & Davies, 2008).

Positioned variably as allies or as hindrances, in volumes of on and off-line resources, the culpability of parents for fat that accumulates on their children's bodies is barely concealed (Boero, 2010; McCormack, 2012). Parents, particularly mothers (Maher, Fraser, & Lindsay, 2010), are advised to limit screen-time, facilitate "play", restrict "junk" food, bake sugar-free treats, cook nutrient-rich meals and, as signalled in the opening exemplar, carefully reflect on the constituents of their children's lunchboxes. Indeed, as Parker and Pause (2018) have compellingly shown, even parents who are not yet parents (e.g., pregnant mums) are falling under the watchful health promotor's eye, with fatphobia producing discomforting levels of mental, emotional and social distress during the antenatal care experience.

Relatively, recently, however, this targeting of parents and/or children has given way to an ostensibly more open, holistic understanding that genuine change requires not simply

DOI: 10.4324/9780429344824-29

pedagogised parents but also a collective effort involving the "whole family". Healthy Families New Zealand, for example, endorses an approach that makes a difference where people "live, learn, work and play" (Ministry of Health, 2014). Their desire to move services "close to home" comes with a dawning acknowledgement that Western approaches to family health change don't necessarily suit families whose cultural practices and dispositions toward food differ wildly from the norms espoused. While the latter can be regarded as a "good" thing, even community-based initiatives ostensibly framed by indigenous knowledge, tend to embrace neo-liberal, individualistic health ideals where "choosing wisely" remains the pedagogy of choice (Burrows, 2016).

As is often the case, schools, as places where volumes of children reside, have waded in to obesity prevention initiatives (Gard & Pluim, 2014). School-based resources often contain veiled or explicit messages about healthy family life. New Zealand's "Healthy Homework" programme, for example, is designed to maximise family engagement in nutrition and physical activities through asking children to complete weekly tasks in their home. These include activities like "organising family walks, walking to and from school, limiting screen time, testing the fitness of the family, eating 5+ fruit and vegetables each day, comparing food labels at the supermarket, helping with dinner, preparing a healthy lunch box" (Auckland University of Technology (AUT), 2019, paragraph 6). Researchers claim that "the findings support the integration of compulsory home-focused strategies for improving healthy behaviour into the primary education curriculum" (AUT, 2019, paragraph 5).

Pike and Leahy's (2016) examination of three "eating well" teaching resources used by primary Health and Physical Education teachers in Australia provides compelling analysis of the "pedagogical force" fuelling these kinds of initiatives. As they put it, this force "consists of a constellation of discourses about food, health, risk, morality and changing family structures and in turn invokes particular approaches to learning about how families should (and should not) eat" (Pike & Leahy, 2016, p. 88). The resources invite assessment of family eating practices against normative notions of what families should eat and how they should eat. They potentially foster family relationships imbibed with surveillant and judgemental tendencies (e.g., monitoring each-others' dietary choice and patterns of consumption). They also work to position children (and sometimes very young children) as change agents for family eating practices. In other words, it is presumed that children can, should and will be able to shift the way family meals are done once armed with knowledge about how to do so (Pike & Leahy, 2016).

While the nuances of family-focussed interventions and resources differ across geographic and cultural context and not all will share the characteristics referred to above, most initiatives do appear to share a commitment to both a monolithic notion of what constitutes family and a moral purview that casts particular kinds of families as good and others as not so. The ways class (and other markers) shapes family food practices are well documented (e.g., Wills, Backett-Milburn, Roberts, & Lawton, 2011); yet, these distinctions rarely register in normative prescriptions for what a healthy life entails. What also underpins many of these initiatives is an uncomplicated claim to the veracity of obesity science and its use as a guide in shaping family-focused change. Simplistic equations that posit obesity prevention as a matter of diet and exercise have been roundly troubled by scholars (e.g., Aphramor, 2005; Campos, Saguy, Ernsberger, Oliver, & Gaesser, 2006; Evans, Rich, Allwood, & Davies, 2004; Gard & Wright, 2005; Guthman, 2009; Lupton, 2013); yet, obesity findings are repeatedly drawn on to bolster support for or, at times, mandate healthy food initiatives in schools, early childhood centres and within families.

There is little doubt that a pedagogisation of families in the service of obesity reduction is well underway. What is less clear is how families themselves are making sense of the health imperatives and pedagogical suggestions conveyed to children in schools. It is this reach of school-based health pedagogies into the intimate environs of the family home that is the focus of this chapter.

Methodology

Drawing on data derived from a 20 family New Zealand research project entitled "Children as change agents for family health", in descriptive fashion, I trace the ways school-based health messages reach (or not) into family homes and with what effect for family dynamics for relationships between family members and for practices families undertake in their daily lives. The broader project involved a discourse analysis of the kinds of health initiatives, policies and practices schools are engaging with to provide some context for the next stage which saw children between ages of 5 and 12 being loaned i-Pad Minis to take pictures and videos of food and/or physical activity moments, events and things that matter to them. These were used as prompts for interviews with the children and provided a rich source of visual information about what is important to children about their food and physical activity environments. We interviewed parents as well. We were particularly interested in their response to information imparted in school contexts. All of the field work took place in family homes, often around dinner time, which yielded multiple opportunities to understand family dispositions and everyday practices "in situ".

None of the families had high levels of disposable income, although most could be described as fairly "comfortable" in the context of careful budgeting. Two sole-parented families were the exception; yet, for one of these, financial hardships were ameliorated by high levels of familial support, and for the other, an impending return to work was set to alleviate the current economic hardship. Two families were of Māori[1] ethnicity, while the rest were Pākehā.[2]

Carrying out the research in family homes and the visual portrayals of family food events provided by children in each of the families yielded opportunities to glean nuanced understandings of what mattered to individual family groupings and how this intersected with the socio-cultural contexts of their lives. I begin by discussing parents' perspectives on information transfer across school and home boundaries and follow this with analysis of the key threads of children's testimony. Occasionally, I draw on video and photographic material that children produced, as the latter often powerfully conveys affect in ways that words may not. Given the broader imperatives around obesity prevention, briefly sketched above, I was particularly keen to see whether and how fat-fighting discourse may have shaped their experiences.

What travels home?

There is no shortage of resources and initiatives available to schools in New Zealand and elsewhere currently to assist with teaching children about what comprises healthy food. Government-sponsored programs like Project Energize (Waikato District Health Board), research initiatives like Healthy Homework and corporate-funded initiatives like "Fruit in Schools", "Life Education" and "Garden to Table" share the school space with health education resources created by teachers themselves. A recent survey of New Zealand primary school principals identified 163 different external providers for year 4 classes and 176 for year

8 classes (Ministry of Education, 2018). Many of these providers are particularly focused on pedagogies related to food (Petrie, Penney, & Fellows, 2014; Powell & Fitzpatrick, 2015). Given this scenario, we assumed that parents would have plenty to say about what goes on at school for their children. We were mistaken.

In a nutshell, our interviews with parents across seven different school districts yielded little evidence of information transfer across school and home boundaries. Few could recall their children talking about specific school-based programs or resources, and those they did mention were perceived by parents as having relatively little impact on home life. As one parent declared:

> The most obvious one lately would be when they had Harold[3]...this year it was about food and eating a variety...Mary came home with this message, it was a song about eating variety of food... "this is good because we're eating variety" she'd say for about two weeks.
>
> I feel like maybe because healthy food and exercise is such a normal part of our life, they don't come home and talk about it...because we give the everyday messages at home, the kids talk about other things, like a dog visiting the school...

Most parents expressed a level of comfort with the food-based school rules and routines their children were exposed to (e.g., water only, no cling wrap, and no sweets), and if not, they were confident enough in their own family practices to refute or ignore them. As long as food rules did not shame their child nor encroach too rigorously on food values and habits prioritised in the home, parents managed to accept "over the top" policies that did not necessarily connect with the realities of their daily lives. For example, a "no pies rule" at one school rendered an $8 pita pocket as the cheapest available lunch to buy – an unaffordable one for the parent(s) with three school-aged children. While the Dad thought that this rule was "stupid" because of both the cost and the demonisation of pies it implied, it was not an issue worth railing against. One mum thought a school rule that children eat their sandwiches before their fruit was "daft" and a parent of a nine-year-old girl observed that "Brain food" schemes (i.e., a requirement to revitalise the brain through eating healthy snacks during class time) meant that their "children were expected to eat too much food in the day". Still others referred to increasing pressures to provide nude food (i.e., food devoid of wrapping) as unrealistic – "no way – six kids – imagine washing them (the lunch-boxes) every night! As soon as you put anything sticky in there like cheese or sauce... imagine!"

The aforementioned school-based practices were irritants rather than deal breakers though. As suggested earlier, it was only when any hint of shame or blame around food policies was detected, that parents expressed any resistance. For example, one mum withdrew her child from the "brain food" initiative in her school after teachers rejected her carefully selected dried banana pieces as "improper" brain food. The same mum expressed anger over another incident where sports ambassadors branded her child's favourite weekend family ritual food, pancakes, as "bad". Almost all parents described some school practices as hypocritical and inconsistent, citing instances where sweets, chips and fizzy drinks were banned in the school setting yet present in abundance at school events, in school fundraisers and gifted as rewards for student achievement. These incidents aside, parents generally described school rules, philosophes and messages about food as closely aligned or as one put it, "close enough" to not be bothersome. Parents were certainly interested in providing their children with food and engaging them in some of the practices linked to it. They were keen to ensure that their children had enough to eat, and a "balanced" diet that enabled them to do the things they enjoyed rather than overly worried about whether or not food met approved "health guidelines".

Parents held particular philosophical positions and attitudes about food, largely developed prior to and/or outside of their child's current school setting. Amongst our cohort were health teachers, a nurse, families who had engaged in other health-related research and parents who drew insight from friends' and extended family's experiences. Parents had read widely, listened to what "experts" had to say and woven these sources together with their own knowledge about their children's likes, dislikes, allergies and needs. Their food knowledge and practices were drawn from heterogeneous and fragmented sources (e.g., Plunket, parent groups, community organisations, corporations, media, family and friends) and assembled in ways that made sense for each family's life. Affordability of food, availability of food and the practicalities of managing busy lives were pivotal regulators in family food choices, and alongside, these were broader philosophical positions contoured by family relationships, politics, rituals and traditions together with religious and cultural beliefs. Whether it be the nightly dinner time ritual of a prayer, Dad making pancakes on Sunday mornings, the allure of Auntie's fudge, a sister's caramel square, a Friday takeaway night or the pizza after swimming, food was deeply embedded with ritual, with history, with relationships and with commitments to living and being a certain way "as a family". Commitments to sustainability were expressed in parental practices around growing food, rubbish disposal, sharing food and, in one case, a device-free household. Food, its gathering, its function and its form, was a utilitarian matter *and* an expression of family norms and culture.

Children and food

Children's recall of school messages about health in general and food in particular was minimal. Harold, the giraffe from Life Education, did feature in their recollections, as did the food pyramid, a lesson on learning how to make sandwiches, messages about drinking water and the odd worksheet where children coloured in different kinds of fruit and vegetables. Children's narratives together with the photos and videos they prepared painted a picture of co-learning about food in the context of daily conversations and the routines and rituals of family life rather than in schools. There are two tropes that stand out across their testimony and visual expressions of food in their family life. The first is their level of engagement in food production and presentation. The second is the extent of children's pleasure in relation to food in their family contexts.

Children, across each of the 20 families, were thoroughly involved in most aspects of food preparation, collection and presentation. They peeled and chopped vegetables, rolled sushi, baked, collected vegetables from the garden, cooked meals, set and cleared tables, did dishes and, in some cases, assembled their own lunchbox each day. Some took out the compost and/or took responsibility for recycling while others assisted in the garden. Some clearly regarded supermarket shopping as an opportunity for a family "outing". While the extent and nature of children's engagement differed across families and in relation to factors such as age, child motivation, parental philosophies, and time constraints, the involvement of children in family food practices and their knowledge of the properties of different foods were unexpected.

Sometimes portrayed as passive consumers of food chosen and prepared by adults (Benton, 2004; Birch, Savage, & Ventura, 2007; Dietz, 2001), these children were intimately engaged with their food in collaborative and agentic ways that challenge developmental assumptions of what children can, should and will do at particular ages and stages. Some children were particularly adept at mimicking Master Chef[a] celebrities, creating long videos demonstrating each moment of a meal's presentation. These children understood food as not simply fuel, but also as an expression of aesthetic style. They were able to perform food in ways that impressively mirrored those exhibited by television chefs. Indeed, for several families viewing Master Chef together was a family ritual, one that wrought togetherness and a sense of culinary delight which was repeatedly expressed in the children's visual representations of family food events.

Pleasure and delight in food permeated children's narrative and visual creations. They relished food in all its different forms. Bananas, frozen peas, roast kumara, pancakes, Grandma's soup, home-baked scones and lamb chops were just some of the foods ascribed the status of "yummy" by the children. The children who adored Grandma's soup were not that fond of the lentils it contained; yet, it was Grandma's, so they "love it". A photo of an odd-looking biscuit placed alone on a wooden floor was described as a favourite food, as "my biscuit", made by the child and thereby imbued with a special quality. Infused in the children's choices about what to photograph and their narratives about their pictures, were relationships with friends and with family, memories of celebrations and pivotal moments in their lives. A picture of five children eating ice creams while resting their bikes in the sun was a favourite for one child, not because they were eating something "yummy" or because their cycling was a "good" thing to do. Rather, "being with my cousins" was what the picture represented to her. Home-baked scones may have been tasty or not. It was the visit to Nana's place and the association of scones with Nana that made the difference for another. For one young child, what she liked most about her dinner was the fact her Mum had "made it with love". Children also roamed beyond food in their photography. A picture of an empty sky signalled "fresh air" for one, "which of course, is good for your health". Another photographed her sister lying on the couch, explaining how rest is important for a person's well-being. Another declared that laughing was crucial for health. As he put it, "It's good for you to laugh, it keeps you alive longer, it keeps you fit and healthy and keeps you very very happy – and, you need love too, it makes you laugh".

Discussion

This necessarily brief traverse of findings from the family project affords some counterpoint to the oft-times gloomy predictions I, and others, have made about the impact fat-fighting imperatives in schools may yield in family homes. First, is the spectacular amnesia both parents and children expressed regarding what gets taught about food in schools. While extraordinary financial and personnel resources have been invested in school-based programs designed to educate children around healthy eating, parents' and children's recall of school food knowledge is modest, to say the least. There was minimal indication that anything beyond the odd school rule, the food pyramid and an animal puppet (i.e., Harold) remained front of mind for any of our cohort. As Gard and Pluim (2014) have repeatedly asked, why do governments and health professionals persist with the notion that information transmitted in schools will effect significant change in children's thought patterns and behaviour, when there is little evidence to suggest that this happens?

Second, while one might have assumed that the saturation of schools with resources designed to not only change children's habits but those of their families (e.g., Healthy Homework) might yield some impact in the home, our admittedly small study would suggest otherwise. Families in our study already had their routines and rituals associated with the production and consumption of food. While peripherally aware of some of the school practices and policies, these yielded little impact on family life. If schools are pursuing fat busting practices, then families would seem to be providing considerable insulation against most of their pernicious affects. That is, the school–home boundaries appear, at least in the case of these families, relatively impermeable. What goes on in school stays there, and families get on with feeding their children and educating their children about food in ways that make functional and cultural sense in the context of their busy daily lives.

Third, qualitative research that has sought to understand children's perspectives on health has repeatedly suggested that children hold narrow, individualistic and certain conceptual-isations of "good" and "bad" food (Beausoleil, 2009; Burrows, 2010; Burrows & Wright, 2007; Rail, 2009). It has also suggested that many children and young people link food and obesity in causal relation, tying food consumption in intimate relation to "health" and "slimness" (Beausoleil, 2009; Evans, Rich, Davies, & Allwood, 2008; Sykes and McPhail, 2008). Further, school-based resources and pedagogies steeped in ideologies of healthism (Crawford, 1980) and individualism are often apportioned at least some culpability for the aforementioned state of affairs (Burrows & Wright, 2007; Evans et al., 2008; Leahy, 2014). The children in this cohort never mentioned the word "fat" or "obesity" and rarely linked their food preferences explicitly to health. Their representations of what mattered to them about food were rather filled with descriptions of joy, of connection and of the way food, in a vast array of shapes, sizes and types, made them feel. Similarly, the "worried well" that some commentators speak of – that is, people who have enough to eat yet worry excessively about the health status of the food and practices they engage in – were nowhere to be found in our study. The worries expressed by these parents were centred around ensuring that their children had enough to eat and that other children (not their own) had sufficient food. Any concerns they raised about school-based food policies and practices were motivated by a sense of fairness, social justice and issues around time, cost and the mundane challenge of filling children's lunch boxes.

These insights will, of course, not necessarily reflect the situation for all New Zealand families. Families with low incomes, families who are already regarded as "problematic" in health discourse, and those with fat children, may air very different reflections. Re-cently released figures from New Zealand's Ministry of Health point to significant house-hold food insecurity among children in New Zealand. As they suggest, one in five children in 2015/2016 lived in food-insecure environments, with most of these housed in rented accommodation in the most deprived neighbourhoods (Ministry of Health, 2019). There is no doubt that families in our cohort do not fit this demographic; yet, some would argue that this is precisely the point. A re-distribution of resource that is allocated to school-based healthy eating programs towards alleviating the food poverty many experience may make better sense.

Returning to the title of this chapter, "fighting fat in families", there is little to suggest that any of the families in our cohort were fighting fat. Parents were confident in their fam-ily food knowledge, and there appeared no linear or predictable mode of transmission of food messages from school to home. Family narratives yielded a tangible absence of anxiety, guilt or shame about food. Rather, the joy and mundaneness of sharing and preparing food in ways that work for particular families would seem to trump any public or school-based efforts to incite change.

Notes

1 Māori refers to indigenous people of New Zealand.
2 Pākēha refers to non-Māori New Zealanders.

3 Harold is a puppet – the front animal for the Life Education Trust – an organisation that runs health programs across New Zealand and claims to teach over 250,000 children every year (Life Education, 2019).

4 Master Chef is a reality television cooking show that pits aspiring chefs against each other. It is aired in New Zealand and based on an original show created in the United Kingdom.

References

Aphramor, L. (2005). Is a weight-centred health framework salutogenic? Some thoughts on un-hinging certain dietary ideologies. *Social Theory & Health, 3*(4), 315–340. doi:10.1057/palgrave. sth.8700059

Auckland University of Technology (2019*). Healthy homework gets results: Study.* Wellington: Scoop Independent News, Education [on-line]. Retrieved from http://www.scoop.co.nz/stories/ED1909/ S00045/healthy-homework-gets-results-study.htm (September 16, 2019).

Beausoleil, N. (2009). An impossible task? Preventing disordered eating in the context of the current obesity panic. In J. Wright & V. Harwood (Eds.), *Biopolitics and the obesity epidemic: Governing bodies* (pp. 93–107). London: Routledge.

Benton D. (2004). Role of parents in the determination of the food preferences of children and the development of obesity. *International Journal of Obesity 28*(7), 858–869. doi: 10.1038/sj.ijo.0802532

Birch, L., Savage, J.S., & Ventura, A. (2007). Influences on the development of children's eating behaviours: From infancy to adolescence. *Canadian Journal of Dietetic Practice and Research, 68*(1), s1–s56.

Boero, N. C. (2010). Fat kids, working moms, and the "epidemic of obesity": Race, class, and mother blame. In E. D. Rothblum & S. Solovay (Eds.), *The fat studies reader* (pp. 113–119). New York: New York University Press.

Burrows, L. (2009). Pedagogizing families through obesity discourse. In J. Wright & V. Harwood (Eds.), *Biopolitics and the Obesity Epidemic: Governing Bodies* (pp. 127–140). London: Routledge.

Burrows, L. (2010). Kiwi kids are Weet-Bix™ kids: Body matters in childhood. *Sport, Education and Society, 15*(2), 235–251. doi: 10.1080/13573321003683919

Burrows, L. (2016). Close to home: What kind of family should we become? In S. Dagkas and L. Burrows (Eds.), *Families, young people, physical activity and health: Critical perspectives* (pp. 57–68). London: Routledge.

Burrows, L. & Wright, J. (2007). Prescribing practices: Shaping healthy children in schools. *International Journal of Children's Rights, 15*(1), 83–98. doi: 10.1163/092755607X181685

Campos, P., Saguy, A., Ernsberger, P., Oliver, E., & Gaesser, G. (2006). The epidemiology of over-weight and obesity: Public health crisis or moral panic? *International Journal of Epidemiology, 35*(1), 55–60. doi: 10.1093/ije/dyi254

Crawford, R. (1980). Healthism and the medicalization of everyday life. *International Journal of Health Services, 10*(3), 365–388. doi: 10.2190/3H2H-3XJN-3KAY-G9NY

Dietz, W. (2001). The obesity epidemic in young children. *British Medical Journal, 322*, 313–314. doi: 10.1136/bmj.322.7282.313

Evans, J., Rich, E., Allwood, R., & Davies, B. (2004). Fat fabrications. *British Journal of Teaching Physical Education, 36*(4), 18–21.

Evans, J., Rich, E., Davies, B., & Allwood, R. (2008). *Education, disordered eating and obesity discourse: Fat fabrications.* London & New York: Routledge.

Franks, J. (2019). Pre-school teacher accused of grabbing children, taking 'unhealthy' food off them. *Stuff* [online]. Retrieved from https://www.stuff.co.nz/national/education/114947768/preschool-teacher-accused-of-grabbing-children-taking-unhealthy-food-off-them (September 18, 2019).

Fullagar, S. (2009). Governing healthy family lifestyles through discourses of risk and responsibility. In J. Wright & V. Harwood (Eds.), *Biopolitics and the obesity epidemic: Governing bodies* (pp. 108–126). London: Routledge.

Gard, M., & Pluim, C. (2014). *Schools and public health: Past, present and future.* Lanham, MD: Lexington.

Gard, M., & Wright, J. (2005). *The obesity epidemic: Science, morality and ideology.* London: Routledge.

Guthman, J. (2009). Teaching the politics of obesity: Insights into neoliberal embodiment and con-temporary biopolitics. *Antipode, 4*(5), 1110–1133. doi: 10.1111/j.1467-8330.2009.00707.x

Leahy, D. (2014). Assembling a health[y] subject: Risky and shameful pedagogies in health education. *Critical Public Health, 24*(2), 171–181. doi: 10.1080/09581596.2013.871504

Life Education. (2019). *Welcome!* Retrieved from https://www.lifeeducation.org.nz/

Lupton, D. (2013). *Fat.* New York: Routledge.

McCormack, J. (2012). *Obesity, parents and me.* (PhD dissertation, University of Otago, Dunedin, NZ).

Maher, J., Fraser, S., & Lindsay, J. (2010). Between provisioning and consuming? Children, mothers and 'childhood obesity'. *Health Sociology Review, 19*(3). 304–316. doi: 10.5172/hesr.2010.19.3.304

Maher J. M., Fraser, S., & Wright, J. (2010). Framing the mother: Childhood obesity, maternal responsibility and care. *Journal of Gender Studies, 19*(3), 233–247. doi: 10.1080/09589231003696037

Ministry of Education. (2018). National monitoring study of student achievement Report 16: *Health and Physical Education: 2017 – Key Findings.* Educational Assessment Research Unit, University of Otago, Dunedin and New Zealand Council for Educational Research.

Ministry of Health. (2014). *Healthy Families NZ.* Retrieved from http://www.health.govt.nz/our-work/preventative-health-wellness/healthy-families-nz (July 12, 2019).

Ministry of Health. (2019). *Household food insecurity among children: New Zealand health survey: Summary of findings.* Wellington: Ministry of Health.

Parker, G., & Pause, C. (2018). The elephant in the room: Naming fatphobia in maternity care. In J. Verseghy & S. Abel (Eds.), *Heavy Burdens: Stories of motherhood and fatness* (pp. 19–31). Bradford, ON: Demeter Press.

Petrie, P., Penney, D., & Fellows, S. (2014). Health and physical education in Aotearoa New Zealand: An open market and open doors? *Asia-Pacific Journal of Health, Sport and Physical Education, 5*(1), 19–38. doi: 10.1080/18377122.2014.867791

Pike, E., & Leahy, D. (2016). "The family that eats together stays together": Governing families, governing health, governing pedagogies. In S. Dagkas & L. Burrows (Eds.), *Families, young people, physical activity and health: Critical perspectives* (pp. 84–95). London: Routledge.

Powell, D., & Fitzpatrick, K. (2015). "Getting fit basically just means, like, non fat": Children's lessons in fitness and fatness. *Sport, Education and Society, 20*(4), 463–484. doi: 10.1080/13573322.2013.777661

Rail, G. (2009). Canadian youth's discursive constructions of health in the context of obesity discourse. In J. Wright & V. Harwood (Eds.), *Biopolitics and the obesity epidemic: Governing bodies* (pp. 141–156). London: Routledge.

Rich, E. (2011). 'I see her being obesed!': Public pedagogy, reality media and the obesity crisis. *Health, 15*(1) 3–21. doi: 10.1177/1363459309358127

Sykes, J., & McPhail, D. (2008). Unbearable lessons: Contesting fat phobia in physical education. *Sociology of Sport, 25*(1), 66–96.

Warin, M., Turner, K., Moore, V., & Davies, M. (2008). Bodies, mothers and identities: Rethinking obesity and the BMI. *Sociology of Health and Illness, 30*(1), 97–111. doi: 10.1111/j.1467-9566.2007.01029.x

Wills, W. J., Backett-Milburn, K., Roberts, E. M., & Lawton, J. (2011). The framing of social class distinctions through family food and eating practices. *The Sociological Review, 59*(4), 725–740. doi: 10.1111/j.1467-954X.2011.02035.x

25

GOLDILOCKS DAYS

Optimal activity mixes in Australian children

Tim Olds, Dorothea Dumuid, and Melissa Wake

The foundation principle of time-use epidemiology is that the way we use our time affects our health. Use of time includes physical activity (PA), sitting, and sleep, while health outcomes can range from depression to diabetes from anxiety to eczema. One outcome of interest, because it is associated with health, is fatness. An important question is how children can best use their time to optimise fatness, and whether that optimal mix is also optimal for other important outcomes such as mental health and academic achievement. In this analysis, we used compositional data analysis (CoDA) to examine the relationship between time use and fatness in 938 11–12-year-old Australian children from a nationally representative sample. Time use was measured using 8-day 24-hour wrist accelerometry. Fatness was operationalised as percent body fat, percent truncal fat, and percent non-truncal fat measured by bio-electrical impedance analysis, body mass index z-score (zBMI), and waist:height ratio. Analyses were adjusted for age, sex, pubertal stage, and socio-economic status (SES). Heat maps were used to plot the modelled distribution of fatness variables across the activity footprint (the mix of sleep, sedentary time, and physical activity which characterised this sample). The lowest levels of fatness occurred when children slept between 9.25 and 11.5 hours a day were physically active (including light PA) between five and seven hours a day and were sedentary for less than 8eight hours a day. However, the optimal activity mix for low fatness was different from that for other outcomes such as quality of life. Ultimately, choices about the best way children can use their time depend on value decisions around the relative importance of outcomes. "One-size-fits-all" recommendations from various governments and the World Health Organization – and the body of research which informs them – implicitly privilege certain outcomes (such as obesity) above others (such as well-being and academic achievement).

Background

The way children and adults use their time has a profound impact on their physical and mental health, relationships, economic fortunes, educational outcomes, cultural flourishing and spiritual well-being. Sleep duration (Chaput et al., 2016), sedentary time (Carson et al., 2016), and physical activity (PA) (Janssen & LeBlanc, 2010) have all been found to be

DOI: 10.4324/9780429344824-30

associated with a wide range of health-related outcomes in children. One important outcome which has both mental and physical health implications is fatness.

Cross-sectional and longitudinal studies find strong associations between fatness and a wide range of health outcomes (Hruby et al., 2016), albeit less strongly marked in children (https://www.cdc.gov/obesity/childhood/causes.html). However, intervention studies are often confounded by the methods used to lose weight, so it is difficult to know whether benefits accrue from fat loss or from the exercise and dietary changes used to achieve fat loss.

As a result, various national governments and the World Health Organization (WHO; https://apps.who.int/iris/rest/bitstreams/1213838/retrieve) have issued recommendations around how children should use their time – physical activity, screen time, sleep – for optimal health, with obesity being one of the principal outcomes targeted. Traditional analyses looking at the relationship between time use and health assume that activity domains (such as sleep, sitting, and PA) are independent. They are not: they are co-dependent, mutually exclusive, and exhaustive and limited by the 24 hours in the day. If we want to increase the amount of time we spend in PA, for example, we must decrease the total amount of time we spend across the other two domains (sleep and sitting) by exactly that amount. The overall health impact depends on the mix of activities, the *activity composition*. In fact, it makes no sense to talk about the relationship between sleep and fatness or PA and fatness or sitting and fatness – we can only talk about different activity compositions which have different mixes of sleep, PA, and sitting.

Some recent studies have included multiple time-use variables in their analyses (Saunders et al., 2016). Unfortunately, it is impossible to use traditional statistical approaches to model the whole day because time-use domains collectively are perfectly multi-collinear. Recently, a new mathematical approach, *compositional data analysis* (CoDA), has been used to address this issue (Pedišić, 2014; Chastin et al., Palarea-Albaladejo, Dontje, & Skelton, 2015). CoDA can tell us whether the activity composition as a whole is related to health outcomes and can quantify the effects of re-allocating time from one domain to another (telling us, e.g., that re-allocating × minutes of time from sitting to PA will reduce body fat by *y*%). CoDA is based on the appreciation that all the relative information contained in a compositional dataset can be expressed as a set of isometric log ratios which are coordinates in real Euclidean space (Dumuid et al., 2017). Log ratios express the time spent in one or more parts of the composition relative to another amount of time spent in one or more other parts, for example, the ratio of time spent in PA to time spent in sitting and sleep. The set of log ratios can be used to represent the composition in standard statistical models (such as regression models) without violating the principles of compositional data analysis.

The concept of the optimal activity composition, the "best day", is novel in public health. In Australia, NZ and Canada, there has been a recent move towards framing public health guidelines in terms of the 24-hour day. So far, guidelines have been developed for pre-school in Canada (Tremblay et al., 2017) and Australia (http://www.health.gov.au/internet/main/publishing.nsf/content/npra-0-5yrs-brochure) and for school-aged children in Canada (http://www.csep.ca/view.asp?x=696), Australia (https://www1.health.gov.au/internet/main/publishing.nsf/Content/health-24-hours-phys-act-guidelines) and New Zealand (https://www.health.govt.nz/system/files/documents/pages/physical-activity-guidelines-for-children-and-young-people-may17.pdf). However, these guidelines are so far just combinations of existing guidelines covering sleep, screen time, and moderate-vigorous PA. They set lower and/or upper limits, but don't identify an "ideal day" covering the whole 24 hours.

In this chapter, we will use data from a large population-derived sample of Australian 11–12-year-olds to explore the associations between the activity composition and fatness. Our basic research question was whether there is a "Goldilocks Day", an optimal mix of physical activity, sitting and sleep, associated with the body composition characteristics which characterise good heath – that is, lower overall percentage body fat and regional fat, smaller relative waist circumference, and lower BMI.

Methods

Study design and participants

Participants were aged 11–12 years, drawn from the cross-sectional Child Health Check-Point study, nested between Waves 6 and 7 of the Longitudinal Study of Australian Children (LSAC). LSAC commenced in 2004 with a nationally representative B (birth) cohort of 5107 infants recruited through a two-stage random sampling design. The initial recruitment rate was 57 percent. In 2014, during LSAC wave 6 (*n* = 3764, 74% retention), 3513 families consented to provide their contact details to the Child Health CheckPoint team. In 2015, these families were mailed an information pack, followed by a recruitment phone call. Data for the Child Health CheckPoint were collected from 1874 child participants between February 2015 and March 2016. Ethical approval was granted by The Royal Children's Hospital (Melbourne) Human Research Ethics Committee (HREC33225) and the Australian Institute of Family Studies Ethics Committee (AIFS14-26). A parent/guardian provided written informed consent. Details regarding the CheckPoint study design and methods are available elsewhere (Clifford et al., 2019).

Measurements

Participants were measured either at the CheckPoint Assessment Centres in one of Australia's seven major cities, at one of the Mini Centres set up in eight regional cities, or during a one-hour home visit (Clifford et al., 2019). Demographics, pubertal status, and body composition were collected during these visits; at the end of the visit, a research assistant fitted the participant with a GENEActiv accelerometer (Activinsights Ltd., UK) on their non–dominant wrist. They were also given an activity log to record when they went to bed, woke up, and the time and reasons for device removal.

Exposure: activity composition

The daily activity behaviour composition was derived from accelerometry. Participants were asked to wear a GENEActiv accelerometer for eight days, 24 hours a day. Accelerometry data were downloaded at 50 Hz using GENEActiv PC Software, Activinsights, UK, and converted to 60-s epoch files. These files were then analysed in MATLAB using a customised software program, *Cobra* (Fraysse, Grobler, Muller, Wake, & Olds, 2019), to determine sleep and non-wear time (visual interpretation of daily data for each participant combined with self-reported sleep and time and reason for device removal from activity logs). If the reason for device removal was "sport", the associated period of non-wear was replaced with PA.

The 60-s epochs were classified into energy expenditure bands using cutpoints defined in Phillips, Parfitt, and Rowlands (2014) – the only validated cutpoints available for the GENEActiv in this age group. These cutpoints were linearly adjusted to account for the

50 Hz sampling frequency, so that the cutpoints were 244 and 878 g min for sedentary time and physical activity (including light, moderate, and vigorous), respectively. Accelerometer days were considered invalid if waking wear time was ≤10 h or if daily average sleep duration was ≤200 min or sedentary time ≥1000 min. Participants with <4 valid days were excluded.

Outcome: fatness

Body composition was measured with bioelectrical impedance analysis using the InBody230 four-limb segmental body composition scale (Biospace, Seoul, Korea; Clifford et al., 2018). Bio-electric impedance analysis has been shown to be valid (r = 0.69–0.79 vs. underwater weighing) and reliable (CV_{intra} = 3%) for estimating body fat in school-aged children (Jensky-Squires et al., 2008). We distinguished between truncal fat and non-truncal fat, both expressed as a percentage of body mass, as these body compartments have been differentially associated with health outcomes (Ali et al., 2014; Staiano et al., 2014). Height and weight were also measured, from which we derived BMI, which we expressed as an age- and sex-specific z-score using WHO criteria (http://www.who.int/growthref/who2007_bmi_for_age/en/). Waist circumference was measured with a Lufkin W606PM steel girth tape at the midpoint between the bottom of the 10th rib and the top of the iliac crest in the mid-axillary line according to the protocols of the International Society for the Advancement of Kinanthropometry (Marfell-Jones, Olds, Stewart, & Carter, 2012). Waist circumference was expressed relative to height. There were therefore five outcome measures: overall percentage body fat, percentage truncal fat, percentage non-truncal fat, BMI z-score, and waist:height ratio.

Covariates: sex, age, socio-economic status, and pubertal status

Sex and age were obtained from the LSAC dataset. Children completed an iPad question-naire to report pubertal signs using the Pubertal Development Scale (Bond et al., 2006). From this, they were categorised as either pre-pubertal, early pubertal, mid-pubertal, late pubertal, or post-pubertal. A previously constructed composite z-score for LSAC wave 6 (at child age ten), based on occupation, household income, and education, was used to indicate the family-level socio-economic position (Blakemore, Strazdins, & Gibbings, 2009).

Data treatment and analysis

Average minutes spent in each intensity band (sleep, sedentary time, total PA including light, moderate, and vigorous) were weighted at 5:2 for weekday and weekend days. The times were linearly adjusted to collectively sum to 24 hours creating an "average" three-part activity composition per participant. The composition was expressed as a set of isometric log-ratio *(ilr)* coordinates (Mateu-Figueras, Pawlowsky-Glahn, & Egozcue, 2011). The *ilrs* contain all the relative information regarding the 24-h composition, but they are not per-fectly multi-collinear meaning that they can be used in regression models unlike raw activity behaviour values (min/day).

Analyses were conducted in R (R Development Core Team, 2016) using the packages *compositions* (van den Boogaart & Tolosana-Delgado, 2008), *zCompositions* (Palarea-Albaladejo & Martín-Fernández, 2015), and *robCompositions* (Templ, Hron, & Filzmoser, 2011). Descrip-tive analysis of the compositions included their central tendency (the geometric means of each component, adjusted to sum to 1440 min for interpretation in min/day) and dispersion (matrices of variances of all possible log-ratios among parts).

To explore whether the activity composition was associated with fatness indicators, multiple linear regression models were used with activity composition *ilr* coordinates as the explanatory variables and fatness (overall % body fat, % truncal fat, % non-truncal fat, BMI z-score, and waist:height ratio) as the dependent variables. Models were adjusted for sex, age, pubertal status, and socio-economic position.

To create heat-map response surfaces, the multiple linear regression models were used to estimate fatness for 1000 randomly selected activity compositions within the empirical activity footprint of the study population. The randomly selected activity compositions were plotted on ternary diagrams and colour-coded according to their estimated fatness, where an increasing red gradient indicated higher fatness and an increasing blue gradient indicated lower fatness. The space between the plotted points was interpolated using linear models with the MATLAB *alchemyst/ternplot* package (https://www.mathworks.com/matlabcentral/fileexchange/2299-alchemyst-ternplot) to create a continuous heat-map response surface.

Results

Children with complete data (*n* = 938) were included in the analyses. Descriptive characteristics of the sample are shown in Table 25.1.

Table 25.1 Descriptive characteristics

Characteristic	
Sex (males); *n* (%)	471 (50)
Age (y); mean (SD)	11.9 (0.4)
Socio-economic position z-score; mean (SD)	0.3 (1.0)
Pubertal status; *n* (%)	
Prepubertal	101 (11)
Early pubertal	241 (26)
Midpubertal	480 (51)
Late pubertal	113 (12)
Postpubertal	3 (0)
Activity composition (min/d)★	
Sleep	572
Sedentary time	680
Physical activity	188
BMI z-score; mean (SD)	0.26 (0.97)
%Body fat	21.6 (8.3)
%Truncal fat	9.1 (5.3)
%Non-truncal fat	12.5 (3.2)
Waist:height ratio	0.43 (0.05)

★ Activity composition is described using compositional means (geometric mean of components, adjusted so that all components sum to 1,440 minutes). To describe the spread of compositional data, multivariate variation matrices are used instead of standard deviations, which are univariate measures.

Multiple linear regression models

The activity composition was associated with all of the fatness indicators (p < 0.0005 for all outcomes). The relationships remained significant after sequential Bonferroni correction. Figure 25.1 shows the heatmaps for the five fatness outcomes (overall % body fat, % truncal fat, % non-truncal fat, BMI z-score, and waist:height ratio). The shaded area represents the *activity footprint*, the range of activity mixes actually achieved by the children. While there

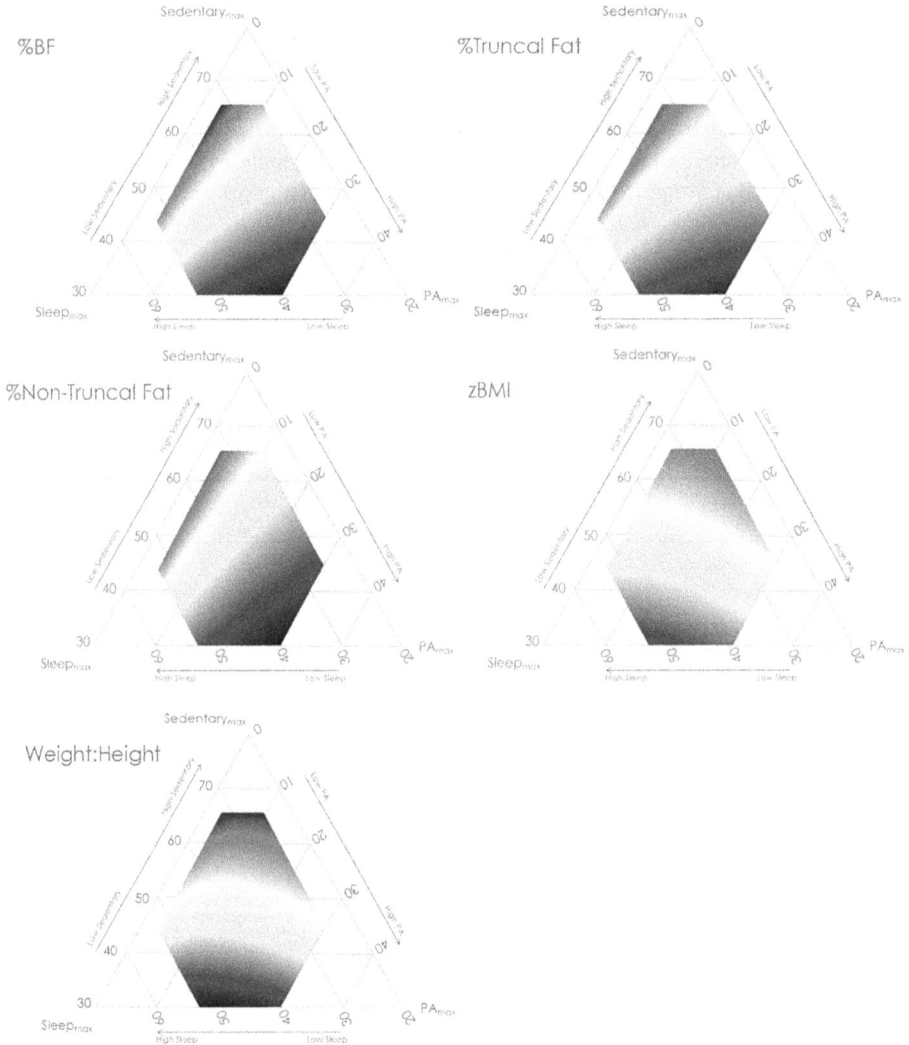

Figure 25.1 Ternary plots showing the relationship between the three-part activity composition and fatness indicators (%body fat, %truncal fat, % non–truncal fat, BMI z–score, and waist:height ratio).

Note: On each plot, the apex represents high sedentary, but low PA and sleep; the bottom left-hand vertex represents high sleep, but low PA and sedentary; and the bottom right-hand vertex represents high PA, but low sleep and sedentary. Red areas indicate unfavourable (high) values, while blue areas indicate favourable (low) values. For example, the highest (most red) value for %body fat occurs at approximately 66% (16 h) sedentary, 2% (0.5 h) PA, and 32% (7.5 h) sleep.

are small differences in the exact location of the optimal activity mix for each outcome, they cluster in the same general area of the footprint. The general pattern is clear: the activity mix associated with the lowest levels of fatness is characterised by low sitting time, high physical activity, and moderate amounts of sleep; the activity mix associated with the highest levels of fatness is characterised by high sitting time, low physical activity, and low amounts of sleep.

Comparison with other outcomes

The optimal activity composition for leanness (sleep = 10.5 h/day; sitting = 8 h/day; PA = 5.5 h/day) can be compared with the optimal compositions for other outcomes using the same dataset. Using a similar methodology, we found that the best time-use composition for a range of other outcomes (unpublished data; Table 25.2). There are substantial differences in the optima: they vary by up to 3 h/day for sleep, 6.5 h/day for sitting, and 4.5 h/day for PA.
    PA = physical activity

Discussion

There is a distinct activity composition, or activity composition *zone*, associated with low levels of fatness in Australian children. It is characterised by amounts of sleep close to the range recommended by the National Sleep Foundation (NSF) (https://www.sleepfounda-tion.org/press-release/national-sleep-foundation-recommends-new-sleep-times). We found optimal sleep to be between 9.25 and 11.5 hours per night compared to the NSF recom-mendation of 9–11 hours. In the optimal activity composition, sedentary time was less than eight hours a day, towards the edge of the activity footprint, which is at the lower limit of that typically achieved by children of this age. Total physical activity made up the rest of the composition – about four to seven hours per day.

While it seems likely that the activity composition causally impacts on fatness, the data here are cross-sectional so cannot confirm the causality or the directionality between the activity composition and fatness. It is quite possible that fatness causally affects the activity composition either directly or through stigmatisation. Fatter children may be less likely to participate in sport and exercise (perhaps because they are less adept or because they feel sub-ject to ridicule) and have poorer quality and longer duration sleep. It is equally possible that a third factor causally affects both the activity composition and fatness, that is, unmeasured confounding. Although we have adjusted our analyses for SES, puberty, and sex, factors

Table 25.2 Optimal activity mixes (h/day, rounded to nearest 0.5 h) for a range of outcomes.

Outcome	Sleep	Sitting	PA
Cardiovascular[a]	11.5	8.0	4.5
Health-related quality of life	11.0	7.5	5.5
Fatness	10.5	8.0	5.5
Numeracy	10.0	13.0	1.0
Metabolic[b]	9.0	11.5	3.5
Literacy	8.5	14.5	1.0

a   Pulse wave velocity, blood pressure
b   Cholesterol:HDL ratio, triglycerides
PA = *Physical activity*

such as diet and parenting style may play a role. Furthermore, this analysis refers only to a very limited age range (11–12 years) of an Australian sample which, although derived from a population-representative survey, had, through self-selection and attrition, come to represent a narrower and slightly higher socio-economic band (IRSD = 1020 ± 64).

Nonetheless, the optimal activity composition found in this study is consonant with results from non-compositional longitudinal and intervention studies, which have consistently found lower fatness to be associated with higher levels of physical activity (Janssen & LeBlanc, 2010), optimal sleep (Chaput et al., 2016), and low amounts of sedentary time (Carson et al., 2016). Furthermore, there are plausible mechanistic links between this activity pattern and lower adiposity. The optimal activity composition zone is characterised by relatively high levels of overall energy expenditure (PAL = 1.60–1.85 METs).

The activity composition zone associated with lower fatness, however, is quite different from that associated with other outcomes, such as academic performance. In a previous compositional study (Dumuid et al., 2017), we found that better academic performance was characterised by much higher sedentary time and very low levels of light PA. The "Goldilocks Days" for fitness, academic performance, and quality of life also differ from the optimal activity composition for fatness. This is consistent with other (non-compositional) studies. Fuligni and colleagues (2018), for example, found that, in 15-year-old US boys, the optimal sleep duration for mental health was 8.75 hours, while the optimal duration for academic performance (GPA) was 7.75 hours, less than the minimum recommended by the NSF.

Guidelines around optimal sleep, sitting, and physical activity (collectively known as "movement behaviours") seek to regulate everyday activities through standardising practices in institutions such as schools and childcare centres, promoting "movement hygiene" practices to parents and encouraging children to self-regulate. The current recommendations for children have largely been framed around concern over the "obesity pandemic" with less attention to other outcomes. For example, a recent systematic review of the literature designed to inform the development of the 24-hour Australian movement guidelines (https://www1.health.gov.au/internet/main/publishing.nsf/Content/4FA4D308272BD065CA2583D000282813/$File/Australian%2024%20Hour%20Guideline%20Development%20Report%20for%20Children%20and%20Young%20people.pdf) identified almost 150 studies looking at the relationship between physical activity and adiposity, but only one related to self-esteem, six related to well-being and four related to prosocial behaviour. The review identified over 300 associations between sedentary behaviour and fatness, 40 relating to antisocial behaviour, and 8 to distress. More than 80 studies report on the association between sleep and fatness, but fewer than ten on the relationship between sleep and well-being.

Governmental guidelines therefore privilege certain types of outcomes above others. It is arguable that this represents an unjustified focus on fatness, given the potential risks and counter-productive effects of stigmatisation (Tomiyama et al., 2018), the recent plateauing of the prevalence of overweight and obesity in children in the developed world (Olds et al., 2011), and consistent findings that overweight (although not obesity) in adults is associated with *lower* all-cause mortality (Flegal, Kit, Orpana, & Graubard, 2013).

A compositional approach could help to redress this imbalance by identifying optimal activity compositions for a range of outcomes. Outcomes could be weighted using objective criteria such as contribution to burden of disease or by subjective decisions on the part of children and their parents. For example, an app could be used to model the likely effects of different activity mixes on a range of outcomes, informing children, parents, and caregivers of different options – a pathway towards the democratisation of health decision-making.

References

Ali, O., Cerjak, D., Kent, Jr J., James, R., Blangero, J., & Zhang, Y. (2014). Obesity, central adiposity and cardiometabolic risk factors in children and adolescents: A family-based study. *Pediatric Obesity, 9*, e58–e62. doi: 10.1111/j.2047–6310.2014.218.x

Blakemore, T., Strazdins, L., & Gibbings, J. (2009). Measuring family socioeconomic position. *Australian Social Policy, 8*, 121–168.

Bond, L., Clements, J., Bertalli, N., Evans-Whipp, T., McMorris, B. J., Patton, G. C., Toumbourou, J. W., & Catalano, R. F. (2006). A comparison of self-reported puberty using the Pubertal Development Scale and the Sexual Maturation Scale in a school-based epidemiologic survey. *Journal of Adolescence, 29*(5), 709–720. doi: 10.1016/j.adolescence.2005.10.001

Carson, V., Hunter, S., Kuzik, N., Gray, C. E., Poitras, V. J., Chaput, J.-P., ... Tremblay, M. (2016). Systematic review of sedentary behaviour and health indicators in school-aged children and youth: an update. *Applied Physiology, Nutrition, and Metabolism, 41*, S240–S65. doi:10.1139/apnm-2015–0630

Chaput, J.-P., Poitras, V., Carson, V., Gruber, R., Olds, T., Weiss, S., ... & Tremblay. M. (2016). Systematic review of the relationships between sleep duration and health indicators in school-aged children and youth. *Applied Physiology, Nutrition, and Metabolism, 41*, S266-S82. doi: 10.1139/apnm-2015–0627

Chastin, S.F., Palarea-Albaladejo, J., Dontje, M.L., & Skelton, D.A. (2015). Combined effects of time spent in physical activity, sedentary behaviors and sleep on obesity and cardio-metabolic health markers: A novel compositional data analysis approach. *PLoS ONE, 10*, e0139984.

Clifford, S. A, Davies, S, & Wake, M. for the Child Health CheckPoint Team (2019). Child Health CheckPoint: Cohort summary and methodology of a physical health and biospecimen module for the Longitudinal Study of Australian Children. *BMJ Open; 9*. doi: 10.1136/bmjopen-2017–020261

Dumuid, D., Olds, T., Martin-Fernandez, J. A., Lewis, L. K., Cassidy, L., & Maher, C. (2017). Academic performance and lifestyle behaviours in Australian school children: A cluster analysis. *Health Education & Behavior, 44*(6), 918–927. doi: 10.1177/1090198117699508

Dumuid, D., Stanford, T. E., Olds, T., Lewis, L. K., Martin-Fernandez, J. A., Pedisic, Z., ... Maher, C. (2017). Compositional data analysis for physical activity, sedentary time and sleep research. *Statistical Methods in Medical Research, 27*(12), 3726–3738. doi: 10.1177/0962280217710835

Flegal, K. M., Kit, B. K., Orpana, H., & Graubard, B. I. (2013). Association of all-cause mortality with overweight and obesity using standard Body Mass Index categories: A systematic review and meta-analysis. *JAMA, 309*(1),71–82. doi:10.1001/jama.2012.113905

Fraysse, F., Grobler, A., Muller, J., Wake, M., & Olds, T. (2019). Physical activity and sedentary activity: Population epidemiology and concordance in 11–12 year old Australians and their parents. *BMJ Open, 9*. doi: 10.1136/bmjopen-2018–023194

Fuligni, A. J., Arruda, E. H., Krull, J. L., & Gonzales, N. A. (2018). Adolescent sleep duration, variability, and peak levels of achievement and mental health. *Child Development, 89*(2), e18–e28. doi: 10.1111/cdev.12729

Hruby, A., Manson, J. E., Qi, L., Malik, V. S., Rimm, E. B., Sun, Q., Willett, W.C., & Hu, F. B. (2016). Determinants and consequences of obesity. *American Journal of Public Health, 106*(9), 1656–1662. doi:10.2105/AJPH.2016.303326

Janssen, I., & LeBlanc, A. (2010). Systematic review of the health benefits of physical activity and fitness in school-aged children and youth. *International Journal of Behavioral Nutrition and Physical Activity, 7*, 40 et ss. doi: 10.1186/1479–5868-7–40

Jensky-Squires, N.E., Dieli-Conwright, C.M., Rossuello, A., Erceg, D.N., McCauley, S., & Schroeder, E.T. (2008). Validity and reliability of body composition analysers in children and adults. *British Journal of Nuitrition, 100*(4), 859–865. doi: 10.1017/S0007114508925460

Marfell-Jones, M., Olds, T., Stewart, A., & Carter, J.E.L. (2012). *International standards for Anthropometric Assessment.* International Society for the Advancement of Kinanthropometry.

Mateu-Figueras, G., Pawlowsky-Glahn, V., & Egozcue, J. (2011). The principle of working on coordinates. In V. Pawlowsky-Glahn & A. Buccianti (Eds.). *Compositional data analysis: Theory and applications* (pp. 29–42). Chichester, UK: John Wiley & Sons.

Olds, T., Maher, C., Aeberli, I., Bellisle, F., Castebon, K., de Wilde, J., ... Zimmermann, M. (2011). Evidence that the prevalence of childhood overweight is plateauing: data from nine countries. *International Journal of Pediatric Obesity, 6*(5–6), 342–360. doi: 10.3109/17477166.2011.605895

Palarea-Albaladejo, J., & Martín-Fernández, J. A. (2015). zCompositions—R package for multivariate imputation of left-censored data under a compositional approach. *Chemometrics and Intelligent Laboratory Systems, 143,* 85–96. doi: 10.1016/j.chemolab.2015.02.019

Pedišić, Ž. (2014). Measurement issues and poor adjustments for physical activity and sleep undermine sedentary behaviour research—the focus should shift to the balance between sleep, sedentary behaviour, standing and activity. *Kinesiology, 46*(1), 135–146.

Phillips, L. R., Parfitt, G., & Rowlands, A. V. (2013). Calibration of the GENEA accelerometer for assessment of physical activity intensity in children. *Journal of Science and Medicine in Sport, 16*(2), 124–128. doi: 10.1016/j.jsams.2012.05.013

R Development Core Team. R: A language and environment for statistical computing. In. Vienna, Austria: R Foundation for Statistical Computing. Retrieved from http://www.R-project.org, 2016.

Saunders, T. J., Gray, C. E., Poitras, V., Chaput, J.-P., Janssen, I., Katzmarzyk, P. T., … Carson, V. (2016). Combinations of physical activity, sedentary behaviour and sleep: Relationships with health indicators in school-aged children and youth. *Applied Physiology, Nutrition, and Metabolism, 41,* S283–S293. doi: 10.1139/apnm-2015–0626

Staiano, A.E., Gupta, A.K., & Katzmarzyk, P.T. (2014). Cardiometabolic risk factors and fat distribution in children and adolescents. *Journal of Pediatrics, 164*(3), 560–565. doi: 10.1016/j.jpeds.2013.10.064

Templ, M., Hron, K., & Filzmoser, P. (2011). robCompositions: an R-package for robust statistical analysis of compositional data. In V. Pawlowsky-Glahn & A. Buccianti (Eds.), *Compositional data analysis: Theory and applications.* (pp 341–355). Chichester: John Wiley & Sons.

Tomiyama, A., Carr, D., Granberg, E., Major, B., Robinson, E., Sutin, A. R., & Brewis, A. (2018). How and why weight stigma drives the obesity 'epidemic' and harms health. *BMC Medicine, 16,* 123 (2018). doi: 10.1186/s12916-018-1116-5

Tremblay, M.S., Chaput, J., Adamo, K.B., Aubert, S., Barnes, J. D., Choquette, L. … Carson, V. (2017). Canadian 24-hour movement guidelines for the early years (0–4 years): An integration of physical activity, sedentary behaviour, and sleep. *BMC Public Health, 17,* 874 et ss. doi:10.1186/s12889-017-4859-6

van den Boogaart, K.G., & Tolosana-Delgado, R. (2008). "Compositions": A unified R package to analyze compositional data. *Computational Geoscience, 34*(4), 320–338. doi: 10.1016/j.cageo.2006.11.017

26

FAT ACTIVISM AND PHYSICAL ACTIVITY

Jenny Ellison

Now a movement over 40 years old, fat activism shifts depending on the time and place where it emerges. The basic idea that it is okay to be fat has been taken up in different ways across many western nations, including the United States, Canada, Australia, England and the Netherlands. For this reason, activists have never had a uniform approach to physical activity. Among fat activists, whether and how to engage with stereotypes about "fitness" has been the subject of debate. Some activists claim to be fit and fat or promote "health at every size." Others see physical fitness promotion negatively, as way to discipline and contain unruly fat bodies. This debate echoes a perceived division in the movement between radicalism and assimilation, that is, those who seek to fundamentally transform social structures and those who seek acceptance of fat bodies. In practice, fat activism doesn't necessarily fall easily along these theoretical lines. Fat activist approaches to physical activity illuminate how other social movements like feminism and disability rights use movement to articulate their critiques of embodied oppression.

To understand the hybridity of the movement, this essay considers aerobics classes organized by Vancouver, B.C. activist group Large as Life (LAL) from 1981 to 1985. Formed in 1981, LAL's motto was "stop postponing your life until you lose weight and start living now!" (*The Bolster* (Vancouver) October 1981, p. 1). Like fat activists of earlier decades, their newsletters feature critiques of looksism, the fashion industry, doctors, dieting and weight loss surgery. Departing from American predecessors like the Fat Underground and their Canadian contemporaries *Lesbiennes Grosses Cinq* (*LG5* [five fat lesbians]), however, LAL embraced opportunities to participate in feminine fashion and beauty culture of the 1980s. Alongside work critiquing medical professionals' approaches to weight, weight-loss surgeries and sexism, LAL organized fashion shows, clothing swaps, personal style seminars, dance classes and a physical fitness program (Ellison, 2016). Their approach blurred the boundaries between feminine and feminist, radical and assimilationist.

LAL aerobics classes reflect foundational feminist approaches to women's health: creating programs by-woman-for-woman, emphasizing safety and privacy, and challenging mainstream assumptions about women's physical ability (Feldberg, Ladd-Taylor, McPherson, & Li, 2001; Murphy, 2004). At the same time, members of the group traded information in their newsletter about finding fitness clothing. LAL's aerobics program shows that the participation in aerobics is not the same thing as complicity with negative cultural scripts about

DOI: 10.4324/9780429344824-31

fatness and femininity. It is the opposite. LAL's work is evidence of a creative and critical engagement with popular culture, physical activity and fat activism. While LAL reflects limitations of activism of their era – such as a lack of critical reflection on race and gender – their approach is an important example of the unexpected ways that people can take up fat activism and apply it critically to problems they encounter in their everyday lives.

Aerobics for fat women only

In September 1981, LAL hired a fitness instructor from the YWCA, a "skinny little person," who taught eight women at a local community centre (Partridge, 2005). Classes lasted for one hour and were offered two mornings or evenings a week (*The Bolster* (August 1981), 4). While enrolment was sufficient to run the course, LAL founder Kate Partridge believed that more women would attend if the instructor were fat. She and another member, Joan Dal Santo, enrolled in the local YWCA fitness leadership course. They saw themselves as outsiders among the "30 fitness Nazis with hard bodies" they encountered every week in the course (Dal Santo, 2005). Partridge was nervous going into the course, so much so that she scribbled to herself on the cover of her course notes: "Get Binder; Nametag; Be Enthusiastic" (YWCA, 1981; Partridge, 2005). The women may have had some reason to feel nervous. Among the five "S's" of physical fitness, the YWCA espoused on day 1 of the course was "STAMINA – STRENGTH – SUPPLENESS – SLENDERNESS and SPIRIT" (YWCA, 1981). Dal Santo and Partridge completed the course successfully despite the negative assumptions about weight that underpinned their training.

Partridge's hunch was correct. Enrolment multiplied after fat women began teaching LAL classes. Within five months, LAL's program expanded to three more community centres (*The Bolster* (July 1982), 10). Two years later, their classes were offered in ten Vancouver, Canada community centres. Expansion was possible as more and more LAL members took the YWCA course. Each instructor adapted the YWCA program for their audience. Documentary sources describe the approach:

> The class begins with a long warm-up, slow-paced and lots of fun. This is designed to slowly warm the body and prepare the muscles for more action… Now we are ready for a little up-paced movement. Don't panic – we are all in this together, and we won't be doing any Jigs!…We slow the pace and stretch out our leg muscles, we continue to stretch other parts of the body until we have cooled down … then we work on strengthening our major muscle groups …We also spend time on exercises for the care of the back… Finally, after our bodies are just about to groan, we relax and stretch to very soft music until we are cool and happy to leave, feeling great.
>
> *(Bell, May 1982, p. 14)*

Suzanne Bell, who became LAL's fitness coordinator in 1982, believed that adapting the classes to larger bodies was key (Bell, 2005). She also changed the way she talked to students about fitness. Using the YWCA principles of physical fitness she learned in her leadership training course, she taught LAL participants the *four* major principles of physical fitness: "strength, stamina, stature, and suppleness" (Bell, September 1982, pp. 7–8). Contrary to the "feel-the-burn" and "no-pain-no-gain" image of aerobics classes from this period, LAL classes were intended to be supportive environments. Bell eliminated "slenderness" from the discourse of the class because it was not the goal (Bell, 2005). In a 1981 interview, LAL president, Kate Partridge, described the classes as a way "to get healthy, to start feeling better about your body, to start understanding it, to move around more" (Partridge, 2005).

Like women's health activists of the 1970s and 1980s, Bell drew on her personal experience in the way she talked to members and wrote about aerobics in LAL's newsletter. One of her primary messages was that fat people could be fit. In an article titled *LAL Fitness Program Needs YOU!* Bell called on readers to become "role models" for fellow members; "if you are a large woman, active in sports and in good physical condition you may be interested." Addressing herself to doubtful readers, Bell continued, "don't assume you are not 'fit enough' – speak to us first" (Bell, 1982b, p. 8). Her message resonated, and at least seven women went on to train as LAL instructors in Vancouver (Laue, 1982, p. 8). Historical sources also show that Bell's experiential approach resonated with participants. Responding to a questionnaire about the program, a respondent described Bell in the following way:

> To see a "mirror image" when looking at the instructor, to have a role model, would seem to me to be the greatest motivator. Suzanne (very trendy in peach tights, black leotards, and colour-coordinated head-band) can coax marvelous things out of everybody... she is completely in control, encouraging, cheerfully vocal, changing from one routine to another in a very fluent fashion, all of them expertly synchronized and executed without apparent effort.
>
> *(Thomson, 1983, p. 16)*

In interviews, LAL aerobics' participants returned frequently to the topic of the body size of the instructor. They were emblems for the potential of other women to participate in physical activity. In this respect, the appeal of classes for fat women may not have been so different from the appeal of Jane Fonda for other women. Hilary Radner argues that Fonda was an example to her students rather than an unattainable idea. Her popularity was rooted in her ability to claim, "membership within the group to whom she speaks" (Radner, 1997, p. 116). Fonda was honest (seemingly) about her desire to stay fit, and her books underlined her normalcy rather than her expertise (Radner, 1997). Normalcy is relative in Fonda's case, but it speaks to the connections between fat activism and other cultural phenomena of the 1980s.

Unlike popular culture *representations* of aerobics as a site of competition among women, documentary sources and oral history interviews reveal that women negotiated and expanded the boundaries of physical activity in conversation with each other. LAL members wrote stories and published editorial cartoons in their newsletter, *The Bolster*, celebrating their physical fitness. In April 1982, member Sal Thompson described her "astonishment and delight" at exercising with "a group of my contemporaries – large women – who were starting from square one like me" (Bell, April 1982, p. 11). Another woman reported, "I weigh 255lbs … and I am a borderline diabetic. But I challenge anyone, slim or not, to keep up with me for even one day!" (Berry, 1982, p. 11). *The Bolster* editor, Ingrid Laue, chastised Canadian public health program ParticipACTION for their "Fat is NOT where it's at!" ad campaign, Laue charged: "fitness has little to do with body size, although it may take more effort, initially, to move 200lbs around the Stanley Park seawall than it takes to move 125lbs … your slim friend who does not believe in exercising the body beautiful may have trouble keeping up with you" (Laue, 1982, p. 1). In interviews conducted between 2005 and 2008, LAL members continued to be enthusiastic about their former classes. Janet Walker of LAL recalled a sense of security in their classes, "it felt wonderful to know you had a place you could go and people weren't going to be laughing at you" (Walker, 2005).

By claiming aerobics as an activity for fat women, participants were taking control of the structural and social exclusions they had experienced in the past. Documentary sources and oral history interviews conducted 25 years after their participation show how people can "endure as well as react against discursive practices on multiple bodily, emotional, and intellectual levels" (Shari Stone-Mediatore as cited in Davis, 2007, p. 133). In other words, participants didn't necessarily think of themselves in singular terms as fat activists, or as women, or any other category. Their participation was driven by personal experiences rather than a singular ideology. Seen through the lens of contemporary understandings of gender identity and race, however, LAL programs had their limitations. LAL practice presumed common experiences of being fat – pressure to lose weight, snide comments from friends and family, difficulty finding clothing, negative experiences with medical professionals, and a sense of un-belonging in the fitness world. These experiences were specific to members of the group and not shared by all fat women. LAL was primarily a white women's organization, with working and middle-class members, the majority of whom were heterosexual. These demographics reflect (what is known about) the overall demographics of fat activism.

Charlotte Cooper argues that fat activism appeals mostly to white women because of its focus on consumption and challenging the obesity epidemic. To grow, she suggests, fat activism must align itself with other marginalized groups to regain its true momentum (Cooper, 2016). While the whiteness of fat activism is problematic, my research suggests a different path forward. LAL's aerobics classes, and other Canadian and American groups, reflect a tendency within individual fat activist groups to universalize the category "fat woman." "Fat women" needed to radicalize and/or challenge hetero-social norms and/or find more stylish clothes and/or exercise together and/or reform representations of women on TV and/or work with fat men. Narrow and singular approaches limit the impact of the movement because they silence and erase some voices. Time, place, and situation mean that embodied experiences of fatness vary, and there is no one right way to be a fat (or a fat activist). Negative messages about fatness are deeply ingrained in western culture, and people have different levels of ability to participate in acts of cultural resistance. Rather than privileging some forms of activism over others, LAL's aerobics classes are suggestive of the potential for playful forms of activism deployed in response to the needs of particular groups.

Commercialization

Tie-ins like clothing have also been interpreted as evidence of the negative impact of aerobics. I argue that services developed by fat women for fat women challenge straightforward readings of commercialization. In *The Bolster*, we can see how finding clothing became politicized for fat women, who compared notes about where to find sizes. LAL members reviewed local retailers and brands, published lists of what sizes/styles were available in Vancouver, and also shared stories about crossing the border to Washington State, where a greater variety of clothing options were available. Once they found what they were looking for, participants remembered "getting into" leotards "in a big way." Joan Dal Santo explained: "I started getting leotards that were coloured instead of getting leotards that were all black. I'd start getting coloured leotards with black tights, and I'd get some coloured tights with other coloured leotards. And, it was fun, it got to be fun" (Dal Santo, 2005). Janet Walker kept her treasured hot pink leotard set. Sharing it with me in a 2005 interview, she remembered, "I had gotten to a stage where I was exploring my body and being more bold. I loved to wear it under a black coat…It was fun to begin to play" (Walker, 2005). Fitness facilitated other pleasures and forms of self-expression for participants. Aesthetics were central to, rather than separate from, LAL's understanding of physical fitness.

While experimenting with aerobics clothing was new for members like Walker and Dal Santo, LAL fitness coordinator Suzanne Bell loved to dress up. In a 2006 interview, she laughed out loud remembering her favourite ensemble, "I had a purple leotard that I bought in the States and this wild top that had cut through with silver or something. I mean, I was just a sight" (Bell, 2005). Within about a year of starting to teach fitness, Bell hit upon the idea of manufacturing fitness clothing for large women. Having done the research on finding leotards in Vancouver, she saw a space to begin her own business. She approached a company that agreed to manufacture a fitness line for larger women called the Suzanne Bell Collection. Initially, Bell sold the clothes "from the trunk of her car" and later held home parties (Bell, 2005). Photographs for this era show women wearing coordinated leotards and tights. There was a wide range of styles in colourful fabrics. Janet Walker's treasured pink leotard was from an early Suzanne Bell collection. Bell's leotards were colourful, trendy, and showed off the wearer's body. If one were to imagine a politicized and woman-centred fashion brand, this might not initially be what comes to mind. But Bell's decision to manufacture clothing was a targeted and critical response to the erasure and marginalization of fat bodies by the fashion industry. She maintained the line until the early 1990s, after which she opened a plus-size woman's clothing store.

Recess for adults

After LAL disbanded in 1985, Suzanne Bell used the model to set up her own exercise business. She expanded into more community centres and eventually opened an exercise studio, all for fat women only (Bell, 2005). During this period, another one-time LAL instructor, Jody Sandler, released a best-selling fitness video, "In Grand Form" in 1986 and "In 2 Grand Form" in 1998, and began to offer her own group fitness classes at local recreation centres (Sandler, 2005). Outside Vancouver, in the 1980s and early 1990s, aerobics classes by-and-for-fat-women could be found across the United States. *Radiance: A Publication for Large Women* (1984–2000) was the most significant single resource for publicizing aerobics for large women in the US. A 1985 "Celebrate Your Body" special issue featured profiles of women in the San Francisco Bay area offering fitness classes for large women. Subsequent issues of *Radiance* featured classified ads announcing the arrival of "low impact aerobics for BBWS with BBW instructors" in Illinois, New York, Texas, and Virginia (*Radiance*, Summer/Fall 1986, p. 30; *Radiance*, Spring 1988, p. 48; *Radiance*, Summer 1991, p. 48). The concept of fat and fit also gained momentum with the publication of *Great Shape: The First Exercise Guide for Large Women* in 1988. The book was co-authored by Pat Lyons and Debby Burgard, two women who connected through *Radiance*. In addition to guidance on starting a fitness program, the book included an extensive appendix listing other aerobics programs for large women, sources of fitness clothing, and exercise videos. According to Lyons and Burgard, there were at least 27 fitness programs for fat women operating in 10 different states in 1988 (Lyons & Burgard, 1988).

The affirmative focus of aerobics classes and emphasis on pleasure were important fat activist strategies. Remembering her experience teaching in a 2019 radio interview, Debby Burgard described her dance-based aerobics program "We Dance" as "recess for adults." Her course was based on the "idea of play as opposed to the idea of punishment" (Ayers, Balogh, Freeman, & Connolly, 2019). Embedded in Burgard's commentary is a critique of the ways that government, commercial, and cultural forces have positioned physical activity as an antidote to obesity (Rice, 2007; Monaghan, 2008; Zanker & Gard, 2008; Beausoleil &

Ward, 2010; Saguy, 2013). Discipline, rather than pleasure, has become the discursive focus of public health programs and physical education (Sykes & McPhail, 2008). In these decades, "physical fitness" has replaced "physical activity" as a framework for describing exercise, recreation and leisure. Fitness is a seemingly measurable and objective goal, whereas activity is a descriptive term. In the early 1980s, activist Elly Janesdaughter described this phenomenon as "healthism... setting an arbitrary standard for determining whether a person is healthy and persecuting anyone who does not conform to this definition" (Scott-Jones, 1983, n.p.). Fat Underground member Karen-Scott Jones warned fat activists not to use it against each other. Instead, she encouraged activists to "assert our right to decide for ourselves whether, how, and how much we should exercise... without guilt, fear of censure or ostracism, or pressure from society or OUR OWN MOVEMENT" (Scott-Jones, 1983, n.p.).

In spite of these early fat-positive engagements with aerobics, much feminist scholarship has been sceptical about the liberatory potential of physical activity. Aerobics have been interpreted through the lens of healthism, as evidence of the amplified individualism of late-capitalist America (Burr, 2011). Scholars have also compared aerobics classes to panopticon, describing them as places where women went to observe and be observed (Lloyd, 1996). Studies also described women's aerobics classes as spaces that were "geared toward the reproduction" of "cultural standards of beauty" (Radner, 1997, p. 130). Collectively, these studies conclude that women participated in aerobics in order to keep "their bodies in line with dominant messages about femininity" (Maguire & Mansfield, 1998, p. 125). Later, studies have made more room for agency and choice and subjectivity (Haravon-Collins, 2002). Rather than a panopticon, aerobics are framed in relation to Foucault's notion of a "technology of the self." Pirkko Markula argues that fitness activities focusing on an ethic of self-care can become a "feminist alternative politics under two conditions: they have to involve an active critical attitude and an act of self-stylization" (Markula, 2003; Markula & Pringle, 2006).

Building on this rich debate about the meaning of aerobics, I argue that feminization is not a meaningful measure of the level of critical engagement with physical activity. Rather, part of the truth about aerobics lies in the meaning that participants take away from their classes. Like other forms of fat activism, LAL aerobics classes were created because members did not see their concerns reflected in either the women's movement or the broader culture. What LAL's program allows us to see is the way that women drew from both feminist discourses of liberation and contemporary popular culture to create activities tailored to their needs, interests, bodies and schedules.

LAL's critical approach to physical activity nonetheless reflects broader silences within the movement, specifically the limited engagement of activist groups with questions of gender, race, and ability. In spite of their hybrid approaches to activism, individual activist groups have tended to universalize fat experiences. LAL and most activist groups operate on the assumption that women experience being fat in similar ways or that the solution lies in addressing particular aspects of fat oppression. Activists did not consider the complex ways being fat could intersect with other experiences (Ellison, 2020). Rather than being an ideal example of fat activism, LAL is suggestive of the potential for pluralism within fat activism. Rather than drawing a narrow boundary around "types" of activism, LAL met women where they were and developed an approach that responded to participants' needs.

Conclusions

In this chapter, I have argued that aerobics for fat women reflect a fluid approach to fat activism, which focused on pleasure, was driven by personal experience, and drew on feminist and feminine popular culture of the 1980s. For LAL members, the value of these activities was not determined by the extent to which they promoted health or femininity, but rather their affective impact on being fat. It is unlikely that aerobics participants had singular motivations that could easily be divided into good/bad or pro-woman/hegemonic reasons for exercising. Participants enjoyed the music and the camaraderie, and many also had fun finding aerobics clothing to wear to class. In aerobics classes, participants were literally embodying the ideas about fat and health that had been circulating among groups of fat women for the previous ten years. In this respect, aerobics departed from *and* added to the knowledge and knowledge practices built up by activists in Canada and the United States. Women experienced their bodies anew in aerobics classes and, in turn, shared physical activity fuelled LAL's response to fat oppression.

References

Ayers, E., Balogh, B., Freeman, J., & Connolly, N. (7 June 2019). Mind, body and spirit. *Backstory* [Audio Podcast], Retrieved from https://www.backstoryradio.org/shows/mind-body-and-spirit/

Beausoleil, N., & Ward, P. (2010). Fat panic in Canadian public health policy: Obesity as different and unhealthy. *Radical Psychology, 8*(1), http://www.radicalpsychology.org/vol8-1/fatpanic.html

Bell, S. (April, 1982). Feeling Great. Fitness Anyone? *The Bolster*, 11. Canadian Women's Movement Archives, University of Ottawa, Canada, HQ 1459 B7 B64.

Bell, S. (May, 1982). Fitness anyone? *The Bolster*, 14. Canadian Women's Movement Archives, University of Ottawa, Canada, HQ 1459 B7 B64.

Bell, S. (September, 1982). Before and after. *The Bolster*, 7–8. Canadian Women's Movement Archives, University of Ottawa, Canada. HQ 1459 B7 B64.

Bell, S. (October 4, 2005). *Oral History Interview with Jenny Ellison*. New Westminster, British Columbia.

Berry, B. (January, 1982). Naturally the choice is up to you. *The Bolster*, 11.

The Bolster (newsletter). (1981–1985). Canadian Women's Movement Archives, University of Ottawa, HQ 1459 B7 B64.

Burr, C. (2011). "The closest thing to perfect": Celebrity and the body politics of Jamie Lee Curtis. In C. Krasnick-Warsh (Ed.), *Gender, health, and popular culture: Historical perspectives* (pp. 215–236). Waterloo: Wilfred Laurier University Press.

Cooper, C. (2016). *Fat activism: A radical social movement*. Bristol: HammerOn Press.

Dal Santo, J. (October 7, 2005). *Oral history interview with Jenny Ellison*. Sechelt, British Columbia.

Davis, K. (2007). *How feminism travels across borders: The making of our bodies, ourselves*. Durham, NC: Duke University Press.

Ellison, J. (2016). From "F.U." to be yourself: Fat activisms in Canada. In J. Ellison, D. McPhail, & W. Mitchinson (Eds.), *Obesity in Canada: Historical and critical perspectives* (pp. 293–319). Toronto, ON: University of Toronto Press.

Ellison, J. (2020). *Being fat: Women, weight and feminist activism in Canada*. Toronto, ON: University of Toronto Press.

Feldberg, G., Ladd-Taylor, M., McPherson, K., & Li, A. (2001). Comparative perspectives on Canadian and American women's health care since 1945. In G. Feldberg, M. Ladd-Taylor, & K. McPherson (Eds.), *Women, health, and nation: Canada and the U.S. since 1945*. Montréal & Kingston: McGill-Queen's University Press.

Haravon-Collins, L. (2002). Working out the contradictions: Feminism and aerobics. *Journal of Sport and Social Issues, 26*(1), 85–109. doi: 10.1177/0193723502261006

Interview of Kate Partridge and Joan Dal Santo by Stan Peters and Ann Mitchell, *CBC Radio Noon* (September 15, 1981). Tape recording, Personal Collection of Kate Partridge.

Laue, I. (December, 1982). Fitness Circuit. *The Bolster, 2*, 7–8. Canadian Women's Movement Archives, University of Ottawa, Canada, HQ 1459 B7 B64.

Lloyd, M. (1996). Feminism, aerobics and the politics of the body. *Body & Society, 2*(2), 79–98. doi: 10.1177/1357034X96002002005

Lyons, P., & Burgard, D. (1988). *Great shape: The first exercise guide for large women*. New York: Arbor House–William Morrow.

Markula, P. (2003). Technologies of the self: Sport, feminism, and Foucault. *Sociology of Sport Journal, 20*, 87–107. doi: 10.1123/ssj.20.2.87

Markula, P., & Pringle, R. (2006). *Foucault, sport and exercise: Power, knowledge and transforming the self.* New York: Routledge.

Maguire, J., & Mansfield, L. (1998). "No-body's perfect": Women, aerobics, and the body beautiful. *Sociology of Sport Journal, 15* 109–137. doi: doi.org/10.1123/ssj.15.2.109

Monaghan, L. (2008). Men, physical activity, and the obesity discourse: Critical understandings from a qualitative study. *Sociology of Sport Journal, 25*, 97–129. doi: 10.1123/ssj.25.1.97

Murphy, M. (2004). Immodest witnessing: The epistemology of vaginal self-examination in the U.S. feminist self-help movement. *Feminist Studies, 30*(1), 115–147.

Partridge, K. (September 20, 2005). *Oral history interview with Jenny Ellison.* Crediton, ON.

Radner, H. (1997). Producing the body: Jane Fonda and the new public feminine. In H. Radner, P. Sulkunen, J. Holmwood & G. Schulze (Eds.), *Constructing the new consumer society* (pp. 108–133). New York: St. Martin's Press.

Rice, C. (2007). Becoming the fat girl: Emergence of an unfit identity. *Women's Studies International Forum, 30*(2), 158–172. doi: 10.1016/j.wsif.2007.01.001

Saguy, A. (2013). *What's wrong with fat: The war on obesity and its collateral damage.* New York: Oxford University Press.

Sandler, J. (October 5, 2005). *Interview by author, digital recording.* North Vancouver, BC.

Scott-Jones, K. (October, 1983). Fat, fitness and exercise – health or health*ism*? *Ample Apple.* Retrieved from https://web.archive.org/web/20050410202305/http://largesse.net/Archives/healthism.html

Sykes, H., & McPhail, D. (2008). Unbearable lessons: Contesting fat phobia in physical education. *Sociology of Sport Journal, 25*, 66–95.

Thomson, S. (March, 1983). Fitness circuit. *The Bolster, 3,* 15–16. Canadian Women's Movement Archives, University of Ottawa, Canada, HQ 1459 B7 B64.

Walker, J. (6 October, 2005). *Oral history interview with Jenny Ellison.* White Rock, BC.

YWCA Canada. (1981). *Fitness leadership course manual.* Personal Collection of Kate Partridge, London, ON, Canada.

Zanker, C., & Gard, M. (2008). Fatness, fitness and the moral universe of sport and physical activity. *Sociology of Sport Journal, 25*, 48–65. doi: 10.1123/ssj.25.1.48

27

WAYFINDING OBESITY WITHIN THE VA' OF CRITICAL BEAUTY

Fetaui Iosefo

'The Sisterhood of the underpants' is a family group of six Samoan women. They all sat eating in a cafe discussing why we don't publicly talk about 'obesity'. One woman responded "why would we bother? That's what white people do plus we already, are, the poster girls for it". In this chapter, the aim is to be 'bothered' by speaking back, using critical autoethnography and the Va' (Samoan Indigenous Reference for the spaces in-between) to the aversion of the word 'obesity'.

Introduction

Wayfinding obesity within the Va' and Critical Beauty begins with wayfinding the Samoan Indigenous Reference (SIR) (His Highness Tui Atua, 2008) and how Va' is synonymous with Samoans. Wayfinding is a term used by indigenous voyages within Pacific Ocean (Barclay-Kerr, 2016). It is intentional in making claim to our ancestral ways of navigating without Western elements. Hence this piece is grounded in the SIR, namely the Va'. Following the discussion of Critical Autoethnography (CAE) and its intermediary with Critical Beauty, we introduce examples of Critical Autoethnography and Critical Beauty through story and poetry. Our first narrative is the 'skinny white man'. We then move to the ambiguity of the 'O' word and time travel into the relational space of Critical Beauty with the poetics of the interpretation of the dusky maiden. Following the poetics of the dusky maiden, we wayfind into our present time with the Critical Autoethnographic poetics as a means of activism and Critical Beauty. Finally, we close with ten helpful tips to consider for all future critical researchers.

Samoan indigenous reference and the Va'

Samoan philosopher His Highness Tui Atua Tupua Tamasese (2008) is the primary scholar/philosopher who writes about the SIR. It is a collection of who we were, who we are, and who we maybe in the future. It enables Samoans within Samoa and the diaspora to wayfind/navigate through life-academia through our sacred ancestral lenses. One way that we wayfind/navigate is with our Va', described by Wendt (1999) as the relational space in-between. Within the SIR, there are 37 Va' 'spacial relations' (Tuagalu, 2008). Many Samoan academics have since used the Va' to create meaning for their aiga/whanu-families within education (Iosefo, 2014, 2016, 2019; Iosefo et al., 2018, 2020), anthropology (LilomaiaVa'-Doktor,

DOI: 10.4324/9780429344824-32

2009, Anae, 2010), and sociology (Suaalii-Sauni, 2017). Every year, the number of Samoan academics who immerse the Va' into their praxis is rapidly growing. This is reflective of the gravitas of the Va' for Samoans.

For Samoans, the Va' space is pivotal in wayfinding/navigating identity. Faulkner and Ruby (2015) discuss the importance of the discourse that takes place within relationships of past, present, and the future. This is also in alignment with the Va' as the impact of what is said between people, place, and space shapes personal identities. Within the SIR, the personal is not one person, but rather, it is the aiga (family). The personal is regarded as the collective.

Critical autoethnography and critical beauty

Within critical autoethnography (CAE), Holman-Jones (2016) emphasises that the frame work of CAE is critical theory; therefore, CAE is never static. It engages with theory and the personhood via poetry and story-sharing as a means of critical analysis. Spry (2009; 2016a; 2016b) argues that the qualitative research, namely autoethnography, is effective/affective in the crafting of the personal and political. She suggests that both the personal and the political resides within our bodies and uses autoethnography as a praxis for articulation. Boylorn (2016) uses critical autoethnography to explore what she calls 'blackgirl autoethnography' and deconstructs racism, classism, and misogynistic cultures. Furthermore, she situates research that begins and/or ends at home. Boylorn, Spry, Faulkner and Holman-Jones embody critical autoethnography as a means of activism.

In May 2017, I attended the International Congress of Qualitative Inquiry (ICQI) in Urbana-Champaign, Illinois, USA. At this conference, I attended 'Doing Justice' (Wyatt & Diversi, 2019). This session was based on 'acts of activism' inspired by Professor Soyini Madison (2010). Global scholars had been invited to share examples of their acts of activism. Although each scholar was amazing, the person who I most resonated with was Professor Soyini Madison. She shared her experience of 'Doing Justice'. She showed us pictures of herself and woman of different colours, shapes, and sizes protesting against the Trump administration. These pictures moved me. What I saw was a beautiful, black, powerful woman protesting, challenging white supremacy, and systemic racism. What I saw was a plethora of marginalised bodies speaking back to power. What I saw was the creation hope and courage for all marginalised bodies. What I heard, what I saw, was/is 'Critical Beauty'. For this chapter, we continue to embody Madison's (2010) activism as Critical Beauty.

'Skinny white man'

In 2016, I was invited to attend the 'obesity-café' event by a skinny white guy. First, let's take a moment to pause and review the conundrum of the word of 'obesity' and skinny white guy. The skinny white guy in this narrative is my dear friend/colleague. When I first met skinny white guy, it was at a critical ethnography reading group. During the first session, I observed that he leaned in to listen to whoever was speaking and gently affirmed them with either a nod and or a smile. My experiences with white men up to this point hadn't been positive, so to see this skinny white man pay genuine attention to everyone around the table was quite intriguing for me. Then he did the unfathomable and spoke on the issue of fat activism as an ally. In my mind, I was like 'are you freaking kidding me', and then he did the inconcei-Va'ble, unspeakable; he owned his white male privilege! Part of me wanted to jump up and celebrate with a Yes and Amen! The rest of me was totally still yet in my head I had freaked me out. I sat like a stunned group of mullet weighing in at 130 kilograms.

In all the years of being in academia, that was the first time I had ever heard a white man own his privilege. Not only own his white privilege, but purposefully use it to speak up for fat activists. When we finished that session, I rung my sister Fadi (who is part of the Sisterhood of the underpants) and shared with her about this totally weird and random experience and how it left me dumbfounded. During our conversation, Fadi asked about his family. I told her how he shared about his wife and two children. She said 'Fetaui, he sounds like good people'. 'Hmmm…. maybe' I replied.

Over the next few months, every interaction with the skinny white man was positive. One particular time, we both sat in a planning meeting with other faculty members. The landscape of colour was heavy-laden in white, and so my chocolate brown skin felt like it didn't belong. However, throughout this meeting, I knew that the skinny white guy would speak up for the marginalised and he did.

As our tradition, I rung my sister Fadi to debrief and told her what had happened with skinny white guy and how at that meeting I finally agreed with her that he is good people. She laughed and said for me to invite him and his wife to the launch of *Oceanus* (a waka hourua-double-hulled canoe which wayfinders used to traverse the Pacific Ocean) at the Auckland waterfront. I did, and they came. Skinny white guy and his beautiful wife met all our aiga (family), my parents, siblings, the sisterhood of the underpants, my hot husband and representatives of our next two generations. All in all skinny white guy and his beautiful wife met four generations of our aiga. That moment is forever imprinted in our family. White people accepted our invitation and turned up, they sat with us, ate with us, laughed, and cried with us.

So, when skinny white guy invited me to the 'obesity café' event (despite me cringing over being the poster girl of obesity), I knew that regardless I would be safe. The conclusion of the skinny white guy narrative is at the end of this chapter.

'Ambiguity of the O word'

'Do we have a word in Samoa that is the equiVa'lent to the word "O"?', asks Fetaui. 'Shhhh Fetaui, we are not allowed to talk about the O word in public or in priVa'te', whispers Luse to her sister Fetaui. 'O word? What are you talking about? What is the 'O word?', Luse replies in a hushed tone. 'You know', she nudges Fetaui in the ribs and raises her eyebrows. 'Oh…that O WORD!! Um yeah, I suppose it's not kosher to mention it', Fetaui sighs. Luse continues, 'yes Fetaui we best be Obedient and not Obnoxious because the O word spoken in public can be quite Obscene and not Ok'.

Fetaui sits pondering this thought and then says out loud, 'Does anyone Object to me using the O word in public?' She scans the café. The looks from other patrons are amusement and shock. A couple of people nod signalling that they did Object to the O word being used in public. Luse slaps Fetaui and says, 'OMG shut up I told you that you aren't allowed to use that word!' Fetaui is saddened. She looks at Luse and says 'I just don't get it! The O word is so rich and full we should all be speaking about it Out loud and proud!', Luse interrupted Fetaui: 'Shush, shut up the O word is gross for some people and they have anxiety over this word, so we do not talk about it'. Fetaui is Oblivious to Luse's frustration and replies: 'I don't get it…we live in a climax era of knowledge and discussing the O word shouldn't give people anxiety that is so…anti-climax'. Luse is now at her wits' end with Fetaui and semi yells at her, 'Well for some people the weight of it can be Overbearing and Overwhelming so it's best not to speak about it, so just SHUT UP!!' Fetaui replies Optimistically, 'Huh??... Overbearing? Are you serious? Yes, I agree with Overwhelming but Overbearing?... how about Overawed Or Overjoyed!'

Luse's face begins to contort, and her eyebrows are raised so high that they are not part of her forehead. Her jaw drops, and she howls with laughter and turns to Fetaui and says, 'Wait, wait, what O word are you talking about?' Fetaui says proudly, 'Ah hello... Orgasm'. Luse, still laughing, adds snorting to the laughter and responds 'that's not the O word I'm talking about!!!'. Fetaui is miffed. Luse continues, 'the O word I was talking about', she leans into Fetaui and whispers, 'the O word you idiot is 'Obesity'.

A point to consider, Darder (2009), a critical theorist, asserts the need to decolonize ideologies on/of the body. Therefore, the question is why the 'O' word within this context is something that is spoken about in hushed tones with Samoans? Within the Samoan language, we do not have a word that translates the O word of Obesity. We have/use 'puta', which means fat; 'lapoa', which means large; but there is no Samoan word for 'obesity'. This word has no direct connections to who we were/are as a people. Furthermore, the words puta and lapoa, when spoken, are used in context of endearment or with humour.

When hearing the 'O' word, as a Samoan within Aotearoa, it reminds us of how we are viewed as problematic and the end of the tail of underachievement in this nation. 'Obesity' leaves a slight distaste when we hear it. As discussed with 'the sisterhood of the underpants', we don't talk about obesity because who wants to be reminded that we are the poster girls for obesity. Unfortunately, with the 'well meaning' health promotion/awareness for obesity you will see us, Pasifika, with the highest statistics for adult and children obesity within Aotearoa. Once again, we are advertised as being problematic. Over the years, we had heard the deficit, we have seen the deficit, we have felt the deficit, we have lived the deficit, so why would we want to continue this rhetoric of deficit? For us, the Samoan words of puta and lapoa don't bring with it the derogatory reminder that we are being exposed as a collective of people who have failed in their health. The 'O' word – obesity – when spoken or displayed is dehumanising, which causes the Va'-relationship of those being labelled 'obese' and those who inflict this label to be at opposite ends of the spectrums of power. Darder (2009) asserts that we must continue to decolonize western assertions placed on our bodies because our bodies are reflexive of our history. Pasifika bodies have lived within Aotearoa as obese and problematic. We have been dehumanised in believing we are the deficit. As a result, our bodies have felt the pain and shame of this stigma.

Wayfinding I/eye and we with critical beauty

Dusky maiden time

During the mid-18th century, European seafarers and the Pacific wayfinders relationship began to emerge. This is demonstrated with the visual historical imagery of Indigenous Pacific woman (Tamaira, 2010). According to Cocker[1], there were two Victorian fetish archetypes that had become the dominant perspective of the Pacific woman: the dusky maiden and the noble saVa'ge. These two Victorian fetish archetypes collectively became the poster-images of that era. The imagery portrayed the dusky maidens as naked sexual beings, inviting those lusting after them to come hither and freely deflower them by having their ways with them (Jones, Herda & Sua'ali'i-Sauni, 2000). This was and is the power of art, and today, there is no difference. The power of posters subjugates those that are on display. They are an open invitation to continue stereotyping and dehumanising (Farrell, 2011).

Below is a dual poem created by JOFI[2] that depicts a European seafarer and the dusky maiden and their journey of thoughts. For the seafarer, it begins from seeing the dusky maiden painting/poster in the United Kingdom 1800s–1900s to seeing her on her Island.

His thoughts	Her response
The visual painting of the dusky maiden a world away:	*The visual painting of the dusky maiden a world away:*
A dusky maiden beckon me	Really, he saw a picture of me and decided that
A dusky maiden awaits me	him and I, would be, we?
A dusky maiden wants me	From the picture/poster surely that cannot be.
A dusky maiden entices me	How un-nobly of he.
A dusky maiden	*The dusky maiden now in the flesh:*
The dusky maiden now in the flesh:	O dear another white man, has come to ogle us
Her dark brown eyes are alerted to my presence	O dear another white man thinks we can't see his
Her long alluring black hair shimmering and shiny	thoughts
cascades down her back	When clearly his face is gleaming in shades of red
Her chocolate brown skin glistens from the sun	O dear I can feel his breathe from here
Her slender neck an open invitation to touch	His panting is so very near
Her breasts are titillating and longing to be caressed	And his inability to see clear
Her shapely shoulders and arms signally her need and	Awakens my fear
desire for me	There is nowhere near for me to disappear
Her hips are curVa'ceous	He saw the poster/painting of me and desired to
A sense of ownership overwhelms my throbbing third	be near and now he is here
member	With a smirk and a leer
This dusky maiden is mine	Whilst I am still in fear
I will take pleasure in dominating her	As I watch him near,
My dusky maiden has saVa'ge markings on her toned	His burgeoning third eye has lengthened to its
thighs and past her knees	fullest size
Her honeypot is covered.	Protruding out the top of his pants
This cannot be	His stance is not one of romance
As her master I will unmask her honey pot	Rather
And make her part of me.	Of cognizance and dominance
JOFI	

Although the dusky maiden reflects our history, there are remnants of that historical trauma that are concurrent with our present:

What you see determines who we will be
What you see determines who we will be
What you see is not me
What you see determines who will get the money
What you see is what you want to see of me
You see my Body Mass Index as my ID
You see my colour
You see the circumference of my waist
You see the monetary gain
You see you use your cultural capital
You see you use me this present time
For money

What you see should not determine who/how we will be
What you see should determine how to free WE~
JOFI

You say	Eye say	We say
You are fat	Eye am cureVa'lcious	Alofa mai
You are poor	Eye see richness	Alofa mai
Your skin colour is offensive	Eye see chocolate brown	Alofa mai
Your culture is offensive	Eye see humanity	Alofa mai
Your choice of sexuality is unacceptable	Eye see sadness	Alofa mai
Your body offends me	Eye sense judgement	Alofa mai
You chose to be fat	Eye see hatred	Alofa mai
JOFI		

Conclusion

In the beginning of this chapter, the skinny white guy narrative connected with Fadi; this was an intentional ploy to conclude with them both. Fadi, at that time, was a Traditional Sailing Master/Captain of the waka hauroa. She worked with young indigenous and non-indigenous people, educating them in the art of our ancestors in wayfinding. Fadi was mentored by the late Matua Hector Busby and served alongside her waka hauroa brothers, Hoturoa Barclay Kerr, James/Hemi, Stan, Jacko, and Piripi in reclaiming and restoring wayfinding. Fadi was accepted into this space because of her solemnity in and with the Va'.

The gravitas of the Va' and relational space not only connects you in the moment but also, if done right, connects you for a lifetime. The skinny white guy exuded the sacred qualities of the Va', and he didn't even know it. Fadi passed away in 2019, but before she did, she had her final sail. For this sail, she/family chose specific people to be part of this ceremony. The aiga invited the skinny white guy, and he came and brought his son. They were on the waka with the aiga. Fadi, for her final time, was our Traditional Sailing Master/Captain for that waka. Skinny white guy and his son were on the waka that day. They again stayed and ate and laughed and cried with us.

When thinking about the 'obesity café' event, I was the only full Pasifika Samoan woman at that gathering. I went because of the skinny white guy. Imagine if every person at that event had done what the skinny white guy had done. I imagine that there would be less of us on posters and more of us in that room actively contributing to the obesity research; not as participants or data, but as informed, educated scholars.

In closing, we offer ten possible ideas for all critical researchers to consider:

1 Be the skinny white guy.
2 Do not tell me your qualifications (seriously zzzz).
3 Introduce yourself as a person not a researcher.
4 Take time to get to know us (all of us our aiga/whanau).
5 Show that you care for us beyond the research.
6 Introduce your family to us (not just pics on your phone).
7 In the flesh allow your kids to play with ours.
8 Don't try and change us – we don't need another white saviour.

9 When you are doing research that involves us, instead of writing on us as data, invite us to write with you.

10 Stay connected for life.

Notes

1 There is no year attached to this reference; however, it is included as Cocker in the reference list. I spoke with the author, and she said that it was in 2013, however, until the date changes online I cannot insert the year within this chapter.

2 JOFI is the poet. This is a joint pseudonym to represent the three people who collaboratively write these poems: an 'annoying narrator', an 'annoying academic analyser', and the 'trashy/erotica/ happy ending identity'.

References

Anae, M. (2010). Teu le Va': Toward a native anthropology. *Pacific Studies, 33,* 19–19.

Barclay- Kerr, H. (2016). From myth and legend to reality: Voyages of rediscovery and knowledge. In E. Emerald, R. E. Rinehart & A. Garcia (Eds.), *Global South ethnographies: Minding the senses* (pp. 87–91). Sense.

Boylorn, R. M. (2016). On being at home with myself: Blackgirl autoethnography as research praxis. *International Review of Qualitative Research, 9*(1), 44–58. https://doi.org/10.1525/irqr.2016.9.1.44

Cocker, C. (2016). *Fa'a Fafine; In the manner of a woman: Shigeyuki Kihara.* artsonline.tki.org.nz.

Darder, A. (2009). Decolonizing the flesh: The body, pedagogy, and inequality. *Counterpoints, 369,* 217–232. https://www.jstor.org/stable/42980390

Farrell, A. E. (2011). *Fat shame: Stigma and the fat body in American culture.* NYU Press.

Faulkner, S. L., & Ruby, P. D. (2015). Feminist identity in romantic relationships: A relational dialectics analysis of e-mail discourse as collaborative found poetry. *Women's Studies in Communication, 38*(2), 206–226. https://doi.org/10.1080/07491409.2015.1025460

His Highness Tui Atua T., T., T., E. (2008). The Samoan indigenous reference: Intimations of a romantic sensibility. In T. Suaalii-Sauni, I. Tuagalu, T. Kirifi-Alai & N. Fuamatu (Eds.), *Su'esu'e manogi: Tui Atua Tupa Tamasese Ta'isi and the Samoan indigenous reference* (pp. 288–314). The Centre of Samoan Studies.

Holman-Jones, S. (2016). Living bodies of thought: The "critical" in critical autoethnography. *Qualitative Inquiry, 22*(4), 228–237. https://doi.org/10.1177%2F1077800415622509

Iosefo, J. (2014). *Moonwalking with the Pasifika Girl in the Mirror: An autoethnography on spaces in higher education* (Masters dissertation, ResearchSpace@ Auckland).

Iosefo, F. (2016). Third spaces: Sites of resistance in higher education? *Higher Education Research & Development, 35*(1), 189–192. https://doi.org/10.1080/07294360.2016.1133273

Iosefo, F. (2019). Settling the soul through Va'(relational) ethics: An ekphrastic review of Hinekura Smith's "Whatuora": theorizing 'new' Indigenous methodology from 'old' Indigenous weaving practice. *Art/Research International: A Transdisciplinary Journal, 4*(1), 420–424. https://doi.org/10.18432/ari29453

Iosefo, F., Jones, S. H., & Harris, A. (Eds.). (2020). *Wayfinding and Critical Autoethnography.* Routledge.

Iosefo, F., Siope, L. E. T. F. V., Siope, F., & Iosefo, J. (2018). Way finding faasinomaga (identity-i/eye) in higher education. *Departures in Critical Qualitative Research, 7*(4), 97–105. https://doi.org/10.1525/dcqr.2018.7.4.97

Jones, A., Herda, P., & Sua'ali'i-Sauni, Tamasailau. (2000). *Bitter sweet: Indigenous women in the Pacific.* University of Otago Press.

LilomaiaVa'-Doktor, S. I. (2009). Beyond "migration": Samoan population movement (malaga) and the geography of social space (vā). *The Contemporary Pacific,* 1–32.

Madison, D. S. (2010). *Acts of activism: Human rights as radical performance.* Cambridge University Press.

Spry, T. (2009). Bodies of/as evidence in autoethnography. *International Review of Qualitative Research, 1*(4), 603–610. https://doi.org/10.1525%2Firqr.2009.1.4.603

Spry, T. (2016a). *Autoethnography and the other: Unsettling power through utopian performatives.* Routledge.

Spry, T. (2016b). *Body, paper, stage: Writing and performing autoethnography.* Routledge.

Suaalii-Sauni, T. (2017). The Va' and kaupapa Māori. In T. K. Hoskins & A. Jones (Eds.), *Critical conversations in Kaupapa Māori* (pp. 132–44). Huia Publishers.

Tamaira, A. M. (2010). From full dusk to full tusk: Reimagining the "Dusky Maiden" through the visual arts. *The Contemporary Pacific, 22*(1), 1–35.

Tuagalu, I. U. (2008). Heuristics of the Vā. *AlterNative: An International Journal of Indigenous Peoples, 4*(1), 107–126. https://doi.org/10.1177/117718010800400110

Wendt, A. (1999). Afterword: Tatauing the post-colonial body. In P. Grace, D. Hanlon, D. S. Long, E. Hau'ofa, S. T. Marsh, R. Nicole & A. Wendt (Eds.), *Inside out: Literature, cultural politics, and identity in the new Pacific* (pp. 399–412). Rowman & Littlefield.

Wyatt, J., & Diversi, M. (2019). Doing justice: Introduction to the special issue. *International Review of Qualitative Research, 12*(1), 1–4. https://doi.org/10.1525/irqr.2019.12.1.1

PART F

Media

The media has been central in the construction of the so-called obesity epidemic. In the last two decades, thousands of newspapers articles have translated, sometimes mistranslated, scientific knowledge about body weight and its negative relation to health for the general public. Newspapers around the world have also constantly reported the economic costs that obesity represents for the population and for the health, financial, and pensions systems in different countries. Reality television shows where people with large bodies are made objects of discipline through exercise and diets have popularized globally. With almost identical designs, these reality shows exalt that lifestyle change – which in their view is fundamental for transforming an ill, fat body into a lean, vigorous one – is achievable through will power and the correct use of freedom to choose.

As some of the chapters in the history section of this handbook show, the communication of ideas around body weight and its relation to health has been present in the printed media since the early-20th century. From her historical analysis of newspapers and magazines in Sao Paulo between the 1900s and the early 1980s, Denisse Bernuzzi de Sant'Anna, for example, describes how large bodies were depicted as sign of vigour in newspapers, and how this perception started to change by the 1960s due to the circulation of new, 'modern' diet regimes through middle-class lifestyle magazines. Sant'Anna also shows that, more recently, social media has potentiated the reimagination of body sizes, shapes, and colors in Brazil. History, then, tells us that different forms of media have conceptualized body weight in particular ways under particular circumstances.

This section includes four chapters that, in a different but complementary way, critically discuss how obesity has been communicated in different media outlets, reality television shows and social media. Abigail C. Saguy explains how the concept of framing can be used in the analysis of what is said and unsaid about obesity in news media and discusses how particular issues around obesity have been emphasized while others have been obscured in the debate. Through a narrative that carefully interweaves a series of theoretical, methodological and personal reflections, Saguy explains her interest in theorizing and researching the forms in which obesity is communicated as 'frames' and how she has used this approach to show that the 'fat frame' has position large bodies as a medical problem requiring intervention and created stigma against them. Saguy's critical research on fat frames in the news media also

DOI: 10.4324/9780429344824-33

shows us that embracing a scholarship that questions taken-for-granted ideas in the obesity debate implies risk.

The media is central to our understandings of things and to the position we take towards particular issues. The media also shapes cultures. An example of this is seen in the extent to which television programs from the United States (US) have shaped the content of local television in other countries. US-based 'make-over' shows where 'fat bodies' are the protagonist, for example, have widely influenced the creation of alike shows across Latin America. In their chapter, Valeria Radrigán and Tania Orellana examine the similarities and differences between a US and a Chilean anti-obesity make-over shows to explore how the discourses in these programs become frames of reference of a set of beliefs about bodies, health, and morality. The authors show that, similar to its US counterpart – *The Biggest Looser*, the Chilean make-over show – *Sueño XL: La Transformación de tu Vida* [*XL Dream: Transforming your Life*] – has generated discrimination against fat people, depicting obesity as a personal failure resulting from the lack of will power. The chapter also makes an important contribution mapping out how critical obesity studies and fat studies have been debated and adapted in the growing Latin American scholarship in these areas.

While these two chapters explicitly deal with media-related issues about obesity, the next two chapters in this section, as the reader will notice even from their titles, are not particularly focused on this area. For example, Travis' and Poudrier's rich discussion on why and how the idea that an all-meat diet can shape an ideal body has become quite appealing for white, usually, right-wing men could have also fit either in the food or bodies sections of this volume. However, we decided to situate the chapter in this media section to highlight how social media is working to spread ideas and shape practices about the relation between food, body weight, health, and even, politics. Travis and Poudrier's chapter do not have the interrogation of obesity as its main focus either. Instead, the authors argue that social media forums such as YouTube, Instagram, and Facebook have enabled the emergence of a dietary movement and the development of a bodily politics among white, right-wing men in Canada and the US that is 'downright dangerous,' among other things, for their intensely fatphobia.

In the last chapter of this section, Jessica Lee's and Ben Williams discuss how diverse knowledges were put together in the process of designing an anti-obesity campaign, *Healthier. Happier.*, in Australia. Drawing on interviews conducted with six key informants who were involved in the development of the campaign and on the analysis of its online materials, the authors show that *Healthier. Happier.* is an heterogenous construction out of epidemiological, market research and political knowledge, which is also hybrid to the extent that it is composed of both traditional and online media. While it could have been included in the policy section, we decided to bring this chapter into dialogue with the others in this section because it shows how the Internet and mobile technologies are transforming, and enriching the reach of, government actions to promote ideal body weights, and sizes.

28

NEWS REPORTING ON THE "OBESITY EPIDEMIC" AND HOW IT WORSENS WEIGHT-BASED STIGMA

Abigail C. Saguy

I came to the topic of body size and health in 2001, as a Robert Wood Johnson Foundation (RWJF) health policy research scholar at Yale University – a postdoctoral fellowship for economists, political scientists, and sociologists within four years of earning their PhD. I was a sociologist straight out of graduate school. My dissertation research was a socio-legal study of how and why sexual harassment had been defined differently in the United States and France. I had a long-term interest in social mobilization and the power of framing, or how we present issues in particular ways that emphasize some aspects of reality while obscuring others (Snow, Rochford, Worden, & Benford, 1986).

Some of the other RWJF scholars – political scientists including Eric Oliver, Taekun Lee, and Rogan Kersh – were asking in our weekly meetings why "obesity" was not on the public agenda given that it was, or so we thought, catching up with smoking as the leading cause of "preventable death." For shorthand, these political scientists asked, "why isn't obesity political?" They meant: why had politicians not taken up the issue? But, as a sociologist with an interest in personal politics, I began exploring the extent to which body size was politicized for ordinary people. I quickly stumbled upon the fat acceptance activists, including those – such as Lynn McAfee – who had spent years becoming a self-made expert on the science of body size. I read published works including Glenn Gaesser's *Big Fat Lies* (G. A. Gaesser, 1996) that convincingly questioned the very premise that being heavier caused bad health. I learned that the fat acceptance movement rejects the terms *overweight* and *obese* as pathologizing and reclaims the term *fat*. Fat acceptance activists taught me, drawing on their own experiences, that stigma against fat people is intense and suggested that the increased talk about the so-called obesity epidemic may be worsening that stigma. I subsequently spent two decades of my life studying those questions.

Fat frames

I did not call what I was doing "critical obesity studies." Indeed, I was coming to question the initial framing of bigger bodies as "obese" – a term that implies medical pathology. Reading work by sociologist Jeffrey Sobal, I learned that doctors had coined the term "obese" in the middle of the 20th century as part of an effort to gain control and authority over the issue of body weight (Sobal, 1999). I began to conceptualize obesity as a specific kind of *fat frame*,

DOI: 10.4324/9780429344824-34

one that implied that larger bodies were a medical problem requiring weight-loss diets, drugs, and/or surgery under medical supervision. I began to realize that every time people uncritically used terms such as *overweight* or *obese*, they were buying into and reinforcing this medical frame.

I also began to see that a shift was occurring at the time I was first thinking and starting to write about this – the late 20th century and early 21st century. People were beginning to talk about "obesity" not just as a medical problem but also as a public health crisis and as an epidemic. A 2001 Surgeon General's report declared that "overweight and obesity have reached nationwide epidemic proportions" and the World Health Organization (WHO, 2000) labelled obesity "a global epidemic." Following their lead and that of obesity re-searchers, the news media was also sounding the alarm. Originally referring to the rapid and episodic onset of infectious diseases, the term *epidemic* elicits fear and compels swift action (Rosenberg, 1992). It glosses over the fact that body weight is *not* an infectious disease and that the relationship between weight and health is crude as best (Campos, Saguy, Ernsberger, Oliver, & Gaesser, 2006).

I saw the medical and public health crisis frames as distinct, in that the former portrayed "obesity" as a clinical problem to be handled at the individual level under medical supervi-sion, while the latter framed it as a population-level crisis that warranted government inter-vention. Yet, these two frames reinforced each other and heightened the stakes. Now, the reasoning went, the individual person who had put on 50 pounds was not just putting their own health at risk but was also threatening the future solvency of Medicare and the readiness of our troops. I also started to see how the medical and public health crisis frames reinforced – rather than replaced – earlier understandings of fatness as a sign of moral failing, that is, of sloth and gluttony, attitudes that historian Peter Stearns traces back to the beginning of the 20th century (Stearns, 1997). News media reports conjured up images of lazy people stuffing their faces with junk food while watching television on the couch, harming their own health and the health and economy of the nation.

Meanwhile, I learned of the fat acceptance movement's efforts to push back against the medical and public health crisis frames. In the summer 2001, I attended the annual conven-tion of the National Association to Advance Fat Acceptance (NAAFA), where the keynote speaker was Glenn Gaesser, author of *Big Fat Lies* (G. Gaesser, 2002). At that conference, I spoke to veteran fat activist and member of the 1970s radical feminist group Fat Under-ground (FU) Lynn McAfee who explained:

> I recognized very early on that if we are ever to succeed, we have to get a foothold in the medical world and make them understand. And that's what I've tried to do because, when it comes down to it, the last argument is, "oh but it's so unhealthy for you…." Peo-ple get to discriminate against us because they're just trying to help us with our health.

McAfee's advocacy reminded me of what sociologist Steven Epstein (1996) had shown in the case of AIDS – how laypeople with a personal stake in the disease had converted them-selves into experts and engaged in "credibility struggles" with scientists, blurring the line between layperson and expert and shifting public understandings of the science of AIDS. Similarly, here were people like McAfee whom doctors and researchers would categorize as "morbidly obese" who were becoming self-made obesity experts and contesting taken-for-granted understandings about the relationship between body size and health. These laypeople were joined by clinicians and researchers who were also questioning the notion that higher weight is itself a disease or causes illness. Over time, this position would come to be known as "Health at Every Size" (HAES) – the idea that higher weight is not in and of itself a health problem or public health crisis and that people can be healthy at every size (Bacon, 2010; Campos, 2004; Campos et al., 2006; Flegal, Graubard, Williamson, & Gail, 2005).

At the same time, some fat acceptance activists started to see that debating the health risks of obesity was a trap. As long as the questions being asked focused on health risk, credentialed researchers would enjoy more credibility than self-made lay experts. Moreover, as long as the question was about diabetes, epidemiology, and heart disease, it was difficult to talk about stigma and discrimination. That required a different framing of bigger bodies not in terms of health but in terms of rights and dignity. Charlotte Cooper, Marilyn Wann, Katie LeBesco, and others argued that fat people should not have to prove that they are healthy or engaged in healthy behavior to deserve to be treated like human beings (Cooper, 1998, 2008; LeBesco, 2001; Wann, 1999). They emphasized that the stigma and discrimination that fat people face is wrong regardless of how a person became fat. I have called this the "fat rights frame" (Saguy 2013).

I wrote about these competing frames – including three that frame fatness negatively as a medical, public health or moral problem and three that framed the issue in more positive terms as beautiful, healthy, or a basis for rights claims – in a 2005 piece with Kevin Riley and in my 2013 book, *What's Wrong with Fat?* (Saguy, 2013; Saguy & Riley, 2005). In these pieces, I examined how the material and symbolic resources of those pushing the medical and public health crisis frames dwarf those of the people and groups advocating for health at every size and recognition of fat stigma. I argued that this inequality went far in explaining why the medical and public health crisis frames are so taken for granted, and why fat rights activists and health at every size researchers and clinicians are disadvantaged in credibility struggles with obesity researchers.

Something that I have never before shared in print was that I found myself caught in the very politics about which I was writing circa 2006, as a young assistant professor at UCLA. The UCLA Sociology Department had recommended me for promotion to Associate Professor with tenure, and my case had gone to the University-wide committee on academic personnel. I learned in a private meeting with the then-acting vice chancellor of academic personnel that my 2006 co-authored piece in the *International Journal of Epidemiology* titled, "The Epidemiology of Overweight and Obesity: Public Health Crisis or Moral Panic?" (Campos et al., 2006), had hit a nerve with one or more members of the committee who had appointments in the medical school. At their urging, the committee had unanimously voted to deny my promotion. The vice chancellor gave me the option to withdraw my candidacy and come up again three years later – at the end of my extended academic clock, which included two extra years for the birth of my two children – when most of the current members of the committee would have rotated off. In the meantime, I was advised to "tone down" my claims about the science of obesity.

While painful, this experience revealed another mechanism by which the production of certain kinds of knowledge is discouraged and penalized. In interviews, other researchers told me how they have sometimes reframed their research to make it more palatable to peer reviewers who take for granted the idea that "obesity" represents an urgent health crisis and are skeptical of any research that questions this view (Saguy & Riley, 2005). Psychologists call this tendency to believe information that is consistent with a preexisting worldview and to be skeptical of evidence that challenges it, confirmation bias (Nikerson, 1998).

News media reporting on body weight

I suspected that peer reviewers were not the only ones vulnerable to confirmation bias and that journalists were also affected by it. I wondered what would happen if two articles were published – by equally reputable researchers in equally prestigious journals – that came to different conclusions about the health risks associated with obesity. Would the news media report subject them to similar levels of scrutiny or would confirmation bias lead journalists to scrutinize more the study that questioned taken-for-granted understandings of the urgency of the obesity crisis than the study that reinforced the received wisdom?

These musings remained hypothetical until 2005, when senior researchers at the Centers for Disease Control and Prevention (CDC) published an article in the *Journal of the American Medical Association* (*JAMA*) that contradicted a study published the previous year – also in the *JAMA* and authored by a different team of senior CDC researchers – about the number of "excess deaths" associated with overweight and obesity in the year 2000 (Flegal et al., 2005; Mokdad, Marks, Stroup, & Gerberding, 2004). The 2004 study, which I have nicknamed the "Eating-to-Death" study (Saguy, 2013), estimated that there were 400,000 "obese" or "overweight" people who died in the year 2000 who would not have died if they had been of "normal" weight. "Obesity," "overweight," and "normal" weight were based on body mass index (BMI) – calculated by dividing one's weight in kilos by one's height in meters squared. Normal weight is defined as having a BMI equal or greater than 18.5 and less than 25. Overweight is defined as having a BMI equal or greater than 25 but less than 30, and obesity is defined as having a BMI equal or greater than 30. The estimate of 400,000 excess deaths was close to the number of excess deaths associated with tobacco use that year (435,000), leading the authors to predict that overweight and obesity "may soon overtake tobacco as the leading cause of death," a claim echoed in news media reporting on the study (Mokdad et al., 2004, p. 1238).

There were serious flaws, however, in the data analysis, which began to come to light following the publication. The following year, the authors published a correction, in which they updated their estimate to 365,000 (Mokdad, Marks, Stroup, & Gerberding, 2005). Concerns about the calculations persisted, however, and later, in 2005, a separate team of CDC researchers published an article, which I have called the Fat-OK study (Saguy, 2013) that estimated that having a BMI over 30 was associated with only 111,909 excess deaths and that having a BMI at or above 25 but less than 30, was associated with 86,094 *fewer* deaths, bringing the total excess deaths associated with "obesity" and "overweight" to fewer than 26,000 (Flegal et al., 2005).

Ultimately, the CDC recognized the Fat-OK study as providing the more accurate estimate (Saguy, 2013). Yet, you would never have guessed that if you were reading the news. As I showed in *What's Wrong with Fat?*, the news media cast doubt on the Fat-OK study, whereas the previous year they had presented the findings in the Eating-to-Death study as self-evident.

Specifically, over 75 percent of news reports on the Eating-to-Death study suggested that the findings confirmed what was already known, compared to less than 10 percent of the news reports on the Fat-OK study. In contrast, more than one-third of the news reports on the Fat-OK study, but less than 3 percent of the Eating-to-Death study, framed its findings as surprising. Moreover, over 30 percent of news reports on the Fat-OK study quoted researchers who questioned the study's validity, something that happened in *none* of the news reports I found on the Eating-to-Death study. Thus, news media reporting has reinforced public understandings that obesity is a public health crisis while resisting evidence that higher body weight may not be such an urgent public health problem after all.

Another mechanism through which the news media end up reinforcing the idea that obesity is a major public health crisis is by reporting disproportionately more on the most alarmist of studies. I demonstrated how this works in a 2008 paper with Rene Almeling (Saguy & Almeling, 2008). For this paper, we tracked news media coverage of 20 scientific articles appearing in one of two special issues of *JAMA* on obesity published in 1999 and 2003, respectively. By looking at articles published within the same issue of the same journal, we were able to control for both prestige of journal and timing in the news cycle, both of which are expected to affect news reporting. The scientific articles varied in the extent to which they portrayed obesity as a public health crisis, offered a more nuanced perspective, or were more technical. We expected that the news media would be more likely to cover the more alarmist scientific articles, while being more likely to ignore the more nuanced or technical ones.

Our analyses lent support to these expectations, showing the role the news media have played in heightening concerns about the so-called obesity epidemic. Specifically, the news media were almost 250 percent more likely in 1999 and 50 percent more likely in 2003 to portray obesity as an epidemic. Part of the reason for this is that the news media dramatized more than the studies on which they were reporting. Another part is that the news media focused proportionately more attention on scientific studies that used such alarmist language to begin with. We also found that the news media were more likely than the original scientific study to highlight individual blame for weight and were more likely to report on scientific studies that emphasized individual blame (Saguy & Almeling, 2008).

I began to wonder if the patterns I was seeing for news media reporting on "obesity" were specific to this issue or were part of a general pattern of how the news media report on medical issues generally. I wondered how news media reporting on anorexia – a medical problem associated with thinness instead of fatness – might differ. I also wondered whether there was something specific about how the issue of weight was covered in the United States compared to elsewhere. I and others (Lawrence, 2004) had noticed that the US news media tended to heap blame on individual people for their weight. Would this be different, I wondered, in countries – like France – with a greater tradition of social solidarity and social structural critique (Lamont & Thévenot, 2000)?

To answer these questions, my students and I created a database of news media articles on obesity and anorexia in France and the United States between 1995 and 2005, ultimately publishing two separate papers from the analyses of these data. The first paper showed that the news media reports in our sample typically discussed how a host of complex factors beyond individual control contribute to anorexia and bulimia, focusing on sufferers who are young white women or girls, thereby reinforcing cultural images of young white female victims (Saguy & Gruys, 2010). In contrast, the news media reports on overweight and obesity predominantly attributed these conditions to bad individual choices, while focusing on overweight and obesity among the poor and ethnic minority groups, thereby reinforcing social stereotypes of fat people, ethnic minorities, and the poor as out of control and lazy. This paper further showed that while appreciation for bigger female bodies among African Americans was hailed as protecting against thinness-oriented eating disorders, this same cultural preference was partially blamed for overweight and obesity among African-American women and girls. In other words, while some of the patterns on reporting on overweight and obesity could be attributed to media routines that favor dramatization, there was also something specific about how the issue of obesity was being racialized and moralized.

A second paper focused on the extent to which the United States was exceptional in its approach to obesity, contrasting news reporting on overweight and obesity in the United

States with news reporting on this topic in France (Saguy, Gruys, & Gong, 2010). This paper showed that French news reports were significantly more likely to discuss social structural contributors to overweight and obesity policy solutions, whereas US news reports were significantly more likely to discuss individual-level solutions. However, more recent work that I have published with French collaborators suggests that – despite the French news media's greater emphasis on social-structural causes of obesity – French policies have focused on individual level solutions (Bergeron, Castel, & Saguy, 2019).

How news media reporting worsens anti-fat bias

In my 2001 interview with Lynn McAfee, McAfee argued not only that many of the scientific claims about the dangers of obesity were wrong but also that by constantly talking about the health risks associated with obesity, researchers and journalists were worsening weight-based prejudice. McAfee explained:

> They continue to write epidemiology, scare epidemiology, and all these horrible associations. There's nothing practical and useful that comes out of that except more funding from the NIH [National Institutes of Health] for this disease, and that is 100 percent the purpose of that. But what they don't understand is that there are social repercussions. Who's going to hire me if they think it's so expensive to have me on their health plan?... They're supposed to be advocating for fat people, [but] they simply don't understand that a direct result of that is an increase in the discrimination that we suffer and people saying all the time, "it's just too expensive to hire fat people, you're going to cost me too much money."

In subsequent years, this argument stuck with me and I wondered if I could test it. In 2008, I began a series of experiments with psychologist David Frederick to find out.

Our findings supported McAfee's fears (Frederick, Saguy, & Gruys, 2016; Frederick, Saguy, Sandhu, & Mann, 2016; Saguy, Frederick, & Gruys, 2014). Across our experiments, some people – either college students or a broader sample of adults – read a real or constructed news report that discussed the dangers of obesity. A consistent finding across 12 experiments in three peer-reviewed articles is that, compared to people who had not read this kind of article, those who read an obesity-is-a-big-problem article reported not only greater concern over the medical risks of obesity but were also more likely to endorse anti-fat sentiments or agree that it was acceptable to discriminate against heavy people (Frederick, Saguy, & Gruys, 2016; Frederick et al., 2016; Saguy et al., 2014). We also found some evidence that reading articles that condemned weight-based discrimination led people to be less likely to endorse such views (Frederick, Saguy, & Gruys, 2016). Given research showing that weight-based stigma and discrimination worsen health (Incollingo-Rodriguez, Heldreth, & Tomiyama, 2016; Tomiyama, 2014), we should all be concerned about current discourse about "obesity" as a public health crisis.

Conclusion

What began for me as a postdoctoral research project in 2001 turned into almost two decades of multi-methods research about how and why we talk about body weight in the ways we do and the social consequences of such talk. Like many others, I was inspired by the courageous work of fat acceptance activists who have a personal stake in this issue. While the field has progressed since I began, there remains much more work to be done. I hope this chapter and the larger volume will inspire others to join us.

References

Bacon, L. (2010). *Health at every size: The surprising truth about your weight.* Dallas, TX: BenBella Books.

Bergeron, H., Castel, P., & Saguy, A. C. (2019). A French paradox? Toward an explanation of inconsistencies between framing and policies. *French Politics, Culture & Society, 37*(2), 110–130.

Campos, P. (2004). *The obesity myth: Why America's obsession with weight is hazardous to your health.* New York: Gotham Books.

Campos, P., Saguy, A. C., Ernsberger, P., Oliver, E., & Gaesser, G. (2006). The epidemiology of overweight and obesity: Public health crisis or moral panic? *International Journal of Epidemiology, 35*(1), 55–60. https://doi.org/10.1093/ije/dyi254

Cooper, C. (1998). *Fat and proud: The politics of size.* London: Women's Press.

Cooper, C. (2008). *The bizarro world of the obesity stakeholder.* Retrieved from http://www.charlottecooper.net/docs/fat/obesity_stakeholder.htm

Epstein, S. (1996). *Impure science: AIDS, activism, and the politics of knowledge.* Berkeley: University of California Press.

Flegal, K. M., Graubard, B. I., Williamson, D. F., & Gail, M. H. (2005). Excess deaths associated with underweight, overweight, and obesity. *Journal of the American Medical Association, 293*(15), 1861–1867. https://doi.org/10.1001/jama.2009.2014

Frederick, D. A., Saguy, A. C., & Gruys, K. (2016). Culture, health, and bigotry: How exposure to cultural accounts of fatness shape attitudes about health risk, health policies, and weightbased prejudice. *Social Science & Medicine, 165*, 271–279.

Frederick, D. A., Saguy, A. C., Sandhu, G., & Mann, T. (2016). Effects of competing news media frames of weight on antifat stigma, beliefs about weight, and support for obesity-related policies. *International Journal of Obesity, 40*, 543–549.

Gaesser, G. A. (1996). *Big fat lies: The truth about your weight and your health.* New York: Fawcett Columbine.

Gaesser, G. A. (2002). *Big fat lies: The truth about your weight and your health.* Carlsbad, CA: Gurze Books.

Incollingo-Rodriguez, A. C., Heldreth, C. M., & Tomiyama, A. J. (2016). Putting on weight stigma: A randomized study of the effects of wearing a fat suit on eating, well-being, and cortisol. *Obesity, 24*, 1892–1898. https://doi.org/10.1002/oby.21575

Lamont, M., & Thévenot, L. (2000). *Rethinking comparative cultural sociology: Repertoires of evaluation in France and the U.S.* Cambridge/Paris: Cambridge University Press and the Presses de la Maison des Sciences de l'Homme.

Lawrence, R. G. (2004). Framing obesity: The evolution of news discourse on a public health issue. *Press/Politics, 9*(3), 56–75.

LeBesco, K. (2001). Queering fat bodies/politics. In J. E. Braziel & K. LeBesco (Eds.), *Bodies out of bounds: Fatness and transgression* (pp. 74–87). Berkeley: University of California Press.

Mokdad, A. H., Marks, J. S., Stroup, D. F., & Gerberding, J. L. (2004). Actual causes of death in the United States, 2000. *Journal of the American Medical Association, 291*(10), 1238–1245.

Mokdad, A. H., Marks, J. S., Stroup, D. F., & Gerberding, J. L. (2005). Correction: Actual causes of death in the United States, 2000. *JAMA, 293*, 293–294.

Nikerson, R. S. (1998). Confirmation bias: A ubiquitous phenomenon in many guises. *Review of General Psychology, 2*(2), 175–220. https://doi.org/10.1037/1089-2680.2.2.175

Rosenberg, C. (1992). *Explaining epidemics and other studies in the history of medicine.* Cambridge: Cambridge University Press.

Saguy, A. C. (2013). *What's wrong with Fat?* New York: Oxford University Press.

Saguy, A. C., & Almeling, R. (2008). Fat in the fire? Science, the news media, and the 'obesity epidemic'. *Sociological Forum, 23*(1), 53–83.

Saguy, A. C., Frederick, D., & Gruys, K. (2014). Reporting risk, producing prejudice: How news reporting on obesity shapes attitudes about health risk, policy, and prejudice. *Social Science & Medicine, 111*, 125–133.

Saguy, A. C., & Gruys, K. (2010). Morality and health: News media constructions of overweight and eating disorders. *Social Problems, 57*(2), 231–250. https://doi.org/10.1525/sp.2010.57.2.231

Saguy, A. C., Gruys, K., & Gong, S. (2010). Social problem construction and national context: News reporting on 'overweight' and 'obesity' in the U.S. and France. *Social Problems, 57*(4), 586–610.

Saguy, A. C., & Riley, K. W. (2005). Weighing both sides: Morality, mortality and framing contests over obesity. *Journal of Health Politics, Policy, and Law, 30*(5), 869–921. https://doi.org/10.1215/03616878-30-5-869

Snow, D. A., Rochford, E. B., Jr., Worden, S. K., & Benford, R. D. (1986). Frame alignment processes, microbilization, and movement participation. *American Sociological Review, 51*(4), 464–481.

Sobal, J. (1999). The size acceptance movement and the construction of body weight. In J. Sobal & D. Maurer (Eds.), *Interpreting weight: The social management of fatness and thinness* (pp. 231–249). New York, NY: Aldine de Gruyter.

Stearns, P. N. (1997). *Fat history: Bodies and beauty in the modern West.* New York and London: New York University Press.

Tomiyama, A. J. (2014). Weight stigma is stressful. A review of evidence for the cyclic obesity/weight-based stigma model. *Appetite, 82*, 8–15.

Wann, M. (1999). *FAT!SO? Because you don't have to apologize for your size.* Berkeley, CA: Ten Speed Press.

World Health Organization (2000). Obesity: Preventing and managing the global epidemic. *Technical Report Series* No. 894. http://libdoc.who.int/trs/WHO_TRS_894.pdf.

29

THE SPECTACLE OF OBESITY IN REALITY MAKEOVER SHOWS IN CHILE[1]

Valeria Radrigán and Tania Orellana

Introduction

Reality television shows have had a relevant presence in TV schedules during the last three decades in Chile, occupying prime time slots with a large audience. The generation of a 'reality effect' has involved changes in the ways of being a viewer and of being related to the 'television device' (Eco, 2012; Orellana, 2016a). This format has thematically addressed several dimensions of life, establishing a close model and a normative relationship with areas such as education, health, the organization of the domestic space, the affective bonds with others and the relationship with one's body. In regards to the last point, reality makeover shows about body transformation (specially through plastic surgery) have proliferated in Chilean TV. The first show of this kind, *Quiero un Cambio* [I Want to Change], was released in 2011.

In this kind of TV shows, the body is subjected to scrutiny and correction, and certain corporeal forms are negatively signified based on the excess of fat. These judgments rely on indicators taken from the medical field and from criteria that respond to a highly mediated notion of health, integrating referents from the beauty, fashion and fitness industries. Prototypes, values and habits are promoted and assumed as an indispensable condition to achieve health or a satisfactory state of well-being. In this way, the fat body is constructed as ill, deformed, unbalanced and without beauty. At the same time, in makeover shows, fatness is exposed as the lack of will, good habits and harmony, which justifies the medical gaze/intervention in the form of a discourse and of a specific anatomical aesthetic technique.

In this chapter, we analyse two reality shows: *Sueño XL: La Transformación de tu Vida* [XL Dream: The Transformation of your Life] (Sepúlveda, 2013; we will use the shorter title, *Sueño XL*, in this chapter) and *The Biggest Loser* (Gaha, 2004; We will use the shorter title, *TBL*, in this chapter) to show how the medical gaze and the associated techno-scientific discourses in these programs are raised as frames of reference and foundations of a set of beliefs. We have opted to compare one Chilean and one American reality show to describe how the 'obese' body is made a spectacle in mass media through social spaces across different countries. At the end of the chapter, we describe how some Latin American scholars and activists have started to challenge the spectacle of fatness in mass media from a critical approach to obesity.

DOI: 10.4324/9780429344824-35

Sueño XL: medical discourses and the normalisation of bodies in TV

Sueño XL is a make-over show focused on people medically classified as 'morbidly obese'. On a weekly basis, these 'participants' are exposed to a routine of exercises, diet and a general re-education of their way of living in order to reduce weight and transform their being. Submitting themselves to this TV monitoring and control plan, the participants have the chance to win a body 'transformation' that includes beauty treatments and surgeries, notably, a gastric bypass surgery. The decision about who deserves such prizes depends on a panel, headed by a bariatric surgeon. A relevant point of the program is the differentiation that is constructed between the participants—unable to control the problems associated with their body appearance—and the panel of experts that decides and/or performs the interventions (health professionals, fashion specialists, physical trainers). Thus, the body of the participants is presented as a defective, unmanageable for the subject itself. Consequently, *Sueño XL* proposes a transformation that emerges from the dissatisfaction of the participants regarding their body and a negative evaluation of themselves. The experts, in particular, the doctors and surgeons, are depicted as having the technical knowledge to intervene into the bodies, judge these habits and decide the relevance of participant's body transformation.

In *Sueño XL*, the testimony of each of the participants is exposed, showing their daily life and their family relationships, highlighting the issues associated with their morbidity. Through technical and discursive strategies, the cases are exposed in a personal, intimate and dramatic perspective—incarnated by the participants, which contrasts with the erudite view of the panel of medical experts. Besides the dramatization, the program incorporates touches of humour and the mockery of attitudes of the participants, mainly related to their eating habits and to the constraints caused by the physical training to which they are subjected.

This makeover show also uses elements of medical documentary, inserting explanatory sequences from surgical interventions, including images of the procedures. However, most of the program is constituted by the exhibition of the daily life of the participants, their difficulties in correcting habits and routines and the moments of weighing. The latter are carried out in the studio in front of a live audience and the hosts of the show, who watch the participants wearing minimal clothing that allows to appreciate their obesity and to exacerbate certain parts of their bodies. The exhibition of the nakedness of the body in specific sections reinforces the vulnerability of the participants in front of the scrutiny of the public in the studio, of the viewers and of the specialists. In this case, undressing is a symbol of scarcity.

Another figure of authority is the personal trainer, for whom the participants also have a position of submission. For example, in episode 14, Samantha, a participant, addresses the personal trainer: 'I absolutely trust you, so I totally surrender, I will be a good student' (Sepúlveda, 2013). In these similar scenes, the personal trainer fulfils the role of unveiling the physical deficiencies of obese people, the problems of will of the participants, as well as their difficulties to carry out the program of weight loss. This is achieved through hard training but also via dramatization, in scenes where obesity equals ineptitude and suffering.

In general terms, the show reinforces the idea that medical action and physical discipline are necessary interventions for deviant and passive subjects. These strategies, applied in their daily life and family structure, manage to correct what they are not able to solve by themselves, since they cannot develop a controlled relationship with food. At the same time, it is claimed that being thinner not only implies a benefit for health but it is also shown as a widely accepted social condition, validating a reductionist and unambiguous relationship between thinness and beauty. This is clearly depicted in Episode 7 of *Sueño XL*, where Karina, a participant, is introduced to the show. Karina is presented as a beautiful woman, but it also emphasised that the large size of her body undermines her beauty and her personality, which impedes her to have a 'normal' life. Karina is presented to be addicted to food, which frustrates her possibilities of being happy. Nevertheless, when she realised that her large size was a 'problem', Karina became motivated to join *Sueño XL*. Her perseverance paid off, and she managed to join the show (Sepúlveda, 2013, Episode 7).

In this case, the participant represents a prototype of western beauty: white skin, blue eyes and fine features. Also, she has a body structure that preserves, on a larger scale, the hierarchy of the 'hourglass' figure. However, there is an association between fatness, shame, disgust and ugliness. To the same extent, and despite 'having a partner', fatness is related with the inability to 'be' a woman and to experience her sexuality. Finally, her behaviour towards food is doubly sanctioned: she is accused of involving her son in her bad habits, and at the same time, she lies hiding what she eats, reinforcing the moral condemnation towards obese people.

Sueño XL and the biggest loser: comparative aspects of relevance

The Biggest Loser (TBL) is a US reality show also aimed at people with obesity. This program, as an international prototype, has been subject to several criticisms regarding its procedures and results. Probably, the most watched reality about obesity at a worldwide level (Callahan, 2015), and attending to its originality, we believe that its influence over the cultural construction of fatness is a relevant factor not only in the US but also in our Chilean context. Economic deregulation and liberalism have contributed to the consolidation and importation of American cultural models to Chile (Ossandón & Santa Cruz, 2005; Rinke, 2013). In the words of the *Consejo Nacional de Televisión de Chile* (CNTV) [National Television Council of Chile] (2013, p. 11), the audio-visual environment in Chile is dominated by a 'standardized fictional programming of strong North American influence, even in the local models'. In this sense, we have not only copied programs but also adopted a series of 'models' about success, family, love and beauty. Even more, the assumption of a certain kind of humour has been incorporated and culturally consolidated in this country.

TBL focuses on a group of obese people who fight, in teams and individually, for a cash prize (about US$250,000), obtainable by losing the largest amount of weight. In this case, authority figures are also presented, including the host, physical trainers and medical doctors. The latter play a supplementary role in the eyes of the audience. Although in the first episodes an evaluation of the 'health' of each participant is shown, and at the end of each program it is highlighted that the program is supervised by doctors, the medical role does not evolve in the following episodes. The attitude of the doctors is categorical and unquestionable. Facing these prescriptions, the participant is unable to make judgments. The obese must comply. This is extreme in cases where the participant attempts to express his or her opinion, being taken to physical collapse with close-ups, quick questions and with an emphasis in emotional aspects.

In terms of resources, each episode closes with a weighing-in scene. Like in *Sueño XL*, in TBL, participants are presented wearing minimal, fitness clothing: shorts for men and crop tops with tights for women, with the purpose of highlighting body fat. In contrast, the presenters and personal trainers usually wear sportswear or casual outfits. As the participants lose weight, and especially during the final phases of the program, the clothing increases. For instance, in both genders wearing loose and longer shirts is allowed, which can be understood as a form of 'dignifying' their condition of thin individuals. Finalists and winners are presented with 'posh' or fashionable apparel and also are benefited with hairdressing and makeup sessions.

The scales are monumental, 'industrial' type. In some way, this resource takes away obese persons from humankind, placing them as livestock similes, products or objects. The weight is shown in a large and luminous display (an element shared with *Sueño XL*). Both elements refer to a scene of public judgment that we could relate with human zoos or freak shows from the 19th century. As an 'exhibition of the monstrous', those scenes confront the spectator with body normativity at its hardest core (Vigarello, 2011). Then, this reality show contributes to strengthen the social structures and all the stereotypes previously mentioned and associated with obesity (Álvarez, 1995).

Following Álvarez (1995, p. 238), we suggest that *Sueño XL* and TBL present the fat body as 'the unusual side of a spectrum without limits', a tragedy that is expressed in the deformation 'of the flesh that fell to the floor, of improbable creatures, of disproportioned bellies'. In TBL, these aspects are treated through strategies of humiliation. It can be said that a hallmark of the program is that the participants are always shown in extreme situations, usually presented while having a physical or psychological breakdown. This is emphasized during the training sessions, characterized by high physical and psychological demands. The trainers shout at the protagonists: 'You are fat! You have failed in life!', looking at them with disgust and reprove. Sometimes, during intense exercises and at the climax of fatigue, personal information (emotional and biographical) of the participants is alluded: deaths of relatives due to a history of obesity, affective failures, etc. At this point, doctors reappear as an emergency team, whose role is to take charge of those who collapsed during the process.

In both shows, habits are moralized and behaviours that are considered harmful are sanctioned, contributing to the solidification of stereotypes culturally associated with obesity (sedentary lifestyle, laziness, lack of control). This validates the interpretation of reality makeover shows as a device that reaffirms social modalities and, in this case, acts with a double function: morbidity represents a disease and a deformity, in both corporal and anatomical way and, at the same time, obesity is associated with wrong practices that must be corrected (Orellana, 2016b). However, there are some relevant differences between the two shows that we would like to highlight.

Homogenization vs. particularity. In TBL, we see an apparent standardization in the diet, the exercises and the competitions. As we suggested before, the focus is on the massive loss of weight. On the other side, *Sueño XL* highlights the uniqueness of each character's drama: his/her history (usually of failures) and, associated with it, the struggle and the spirit of overcoming. This focus on drama and emotional particularity arises from the aim to generate compassion and/or identification of the viewers with the participants. This aspect is supported by a research led by the CNTV (2016, n/p), where it is mentioned that the exposure of privacy in reality shows 'is the main component to attract the audience to consume the format'.

Competition. While *Sueño XL* is not properly a competition program, we can state that the competitive factor is transferred to the subjectivity of the participants. They compete *against themselves*, and they compete *against obesity*. In this sense, the victory overweight is seen as the result of both a personal and a collective effort (the medical team, personal trainers, family, etc.), an aspect that is shared with TBL. However, in TBL, the winner results from the failure of the other participants. From a social point of view, this turn towards the subject reflects the individualism of our neoliberal society. Individualism is at the core of multiple anti-obesity treatments, which are centred on the re-education of individual behaviours. In a reductionist and moralizing vision, fatness is equivalent to a personal failure in multiple dimensions. Whether there is a distortion of one's own food intake and/or an inability to exercise effectively, this focus of attention disregards the cultural, social, economic, political or even commercial conditions that foster what is nowadays considered an 'unhealthy lifestyle' (Radrigán & Orellana, 2016). Given this, it is the sick, defective, maladjusted individual, who must manage its own weaknesses to construct a coherent image with a productive and aesthetically functional subject.

Discrimination and ridicule. In both shows, the fat people constitute a spectacle of bodies presented as sick, grotesque and in overflow. Their correction is, therefore, a moral exemplification against the supposed signs of personal, affective and productive failure. However, we think that, in TBL, this is taken to an extreme, which is revealed by the audio-visual strategies used and by the way in which the protagonists are treated by the authority figures. The fascination encouraged by the denigration entails a duality. On one hand, it promotes high ratings worldwide and gives a sort of identity label to the US reality format. On the other hand, it has generated a series of criticisms and denunciations in the local and global context. In Chile, although neither complaints nor major accusations have been made public regarding *Sueño XL*, the CNTV (2016) has pointed out that TV shows must adhere to social responsibility norms, which entails 'not losing sight of respect for the dignity and privacy of people'. *Sueño XL* does not adhere to these recommendations. Instead, the participants are constantly disqualified by the authority figures who constantly associate their body weight as a tragedy and social failure, which are obvious promoters of discrimination and fatphobia. Those elements put us at the centre of an ethical debate that concerns, on one hand, the media and its strategies, and on the other, the professionals (doctors, trainers, communicators, etc.) who validate this violence and who, given their position of power, influence a naturalization and social internalization of these discourses.

The doctor. The doctor does not have the same function in the shows analysed here. In TBL, doctors are practically absent, except for some episodes and specific moments. On the contrary, in *Sueño XL*, they are a main element. We watch them as an authority figure that personalizes and executes a behavioural normalizing/rectifying discourse, occupying spaces outside the set according to its role (medical consultations or surgical pavilions). This emphasizes the social position that these professionals fill in our context, validating their expertise as owners of a knowledge about the body that participants do not have, highlighting the passive nature of the participant as a patient. This figure legitimizes the status of medical institutions in general, an aspect that is also related to a moralization of the obese body: disobeying the authorized voice equals to a failure in the subjection of the individual to certain prescriptions based on corporality (Foucault, 2004). The medical discourse hegemonically positions views and opinions regarding health that, as truths, transcend the scope of the medical-scientific field, impacting on the cultural and social construction of fatness, assuming the notion of the scientific field as a space of symbolic production, and the inherence of scientific paradigms into the social (Bourdieu, 2008).

The social class domain. This is a crucial aspect in the Chilean case, with no great preponderance in TBL. *Sueño XL* focuses on people who cannot afford medical treatments, so the participation in the program is represented as a 'reward' in itself. In a context of privatization of health and the absence of comprehensive anti-obesity public programs in Chile, TV offers a sort of economic and social response in exchange for the exhibition of intimacy and the dramatization of the relationship with the body. The Chilean Ministry of Health (MINSAL, 2019) has created programs focused on the promotion of 'healthy habits' and on the ideal of a 'healthy life', being nutrition a key foundation. However, these perspectives ignore the complexity of the phenomenon of food from the perspective of its social constitution as well as the consideration of inequity in the access to quality food. Therefore, the 'responses' to obesity in Chile are illusory: what has been constructed as healthy food is more expensive and, often, more difficult to get than food rich in carbohydrates, saturated fats and additives. Diets are not consistent with the needs and daily lives of people from the lower socioeconomic classes, so the maintenance of an 'ideal' weight becomes a chimera (Braghetto *et al.*, 2006).

To report, to reveal

The aforementioned makeover shows have been subjected to multiple criticisms, being TBL an emblematic example. Well known is the case of Kai Hibbard, who after her participation in TBL in 2006, became an activist, sharing her negative experiences in the program (Poretsky, 2010). Hibbard's critiques, along with that from other former members of the show, are focused on revealing the dangers—training against medical orders, injuries to participants, harassment outside the set by the production team—of the strategies used for extreme weight loss. Furthermore, the recovery or increase of the original weight after the end of the show is a common sign among the participants, an aspect made visible by reports, declarations of the participants and a series of scientific studies of relevance (Fothergill *et al.*, 2016). In the same vein, movements such as Health at Every Size (see Bacon, 2008), have challenged the stereotyped views of obesity and reaffirmed the need to understand it not as a failure of willpower, placing the problem in a complex that includes different variables. We believe that these denounces contribute to a required change in the health paradigm (understood in the broad field of the social), beauty standards and weight stigma, recognizing the right to inhabit a more widely and diverse range of bodies.

In the Chilean context, beyond isolated comments on social media and concerns from the CNTV (2016) about the general reality shows phenomena, we have not been aware of more articulated criticism towards *Sueño XL* (or to other makeover shows). The visibility of fat-phobia as well as the discrimination against fat people has not seemed to be a topic of great concern in our national context, a reason that motivated our pioneering book published in 2016. However, in the frame of globalization, the notions of borders and countries have become diffuse, generating a hybrid cultural panorama (Canclini, 2001). Thus, issues such as big sizes in fashion (with the gradual and new association between fatness and beauty); the widespread growth of cyber-cultural movements such as *bodypositive* and the absorption of world trends such as #fattitude, #stopbodyshame, #allbodiesaregoodbodies and #stophatenotweight through social media; and the promotion of blog activism and independent magazines have been incorporated in Chile and other Latin American countries to challenge reductionist perspectives between body and weight.

Some examples of critical approaches to obesity in Latin America are proposals such as *Orgullo Gordo* (n.d.) in Venezuela; AnyBody Argentina (n.d.); and the work of activists Lucrecia Masson (2014) and Constanza Álvarez-Castillo (2012, 2014). In a general sense, these approaches are marked by decolonial and dissident postures to mainstream circles in fashion, advertising and mass media and to the traditional knowledge institutions such as universities. This condition, as well as the reiteration of the oppressive/oppressed logic, has kept several of these proposals into a marginal zone, detaching themselves from the academic discourse and from more massive movements of popular culture. However, their wide presence on social media has expanded their messages in unprecedented ways and with unsuspected reaches, which are inevitably infected with other types of strategies, being re-appropriated in hybrid forms by web users.

From Latin America, we believe that spaces of denunciation and report of fatphobia, as well as the reflections about the cultural and political construction of obesity, occur precisely in these integrated spaces, inside and out of the institutional and academic framework, coming from dissident activists and the popular culture, mixed with network strategies of interactivity and the exposure of disobedient bodies. However, any kind of subversive action over the dominant body stereotypes is, in our context, still complex to analyse in its political effectiveness. We need to consider that although other bodies are created and transmitted in cyber-culture, at the same time, a paradigm of dominance over the 'bodies in excess' continues to be reaffirmed and intensified through several platforms. In this regard, the discourses of rejection of fatness that are transversally established, from the field of health and the beauty industry, to the mass media (including TV and reality shows), reinforce a reductionist vision of the fat bodies and have a strong interference in how, every day, we relate to our corporality. One of the main challenges is to dismantle these narratives and the symbolic order in which fatness is relegated to a marginal zone and disconnected apparently from all social responsibility.

Note

1 This chapter is part of a broader research published in our book *Extremos del volumen. Poderes y medialidades en torno a la obesidad y la anorexia* [*Extremes of body mass. Power and media discourses around obesity and anorexia*] (Radrigán & Orellana, 2016). This is the first publication of the text in English. (Translation by Rodrigo Arenas-Carter and Valeria Radrigán).

References

Álvarez, R. (1995). La era americana del reality show. Un territorio intermedio entre información y entretenimiento [The American era of reality show. An intermediate territory between information and entertainment]. *Telos, Cuadernos de comunicación, tecnología y sociedad, 43*, 63–70.

Álvarez-Castillo, C. (2012, November 19). *Manifiestx Gordx* [Fat Manifesto]. Retrieved from http://missogina.perrogordo.cl/manifiesto-gordx/

Álvarez-Castillo, C. (2014). *La Cerda Punk. Ensayos desde un Feminismo Gordo, Lésbiko, Antikapitalista & Antiespecista* [The Punk Pig. Essays from a Fat, Lesbian, Anti-Capitalist & Anti-Speciesist Feminism]. Valparaíso, Chile: Trío Editorial.

AnyBody Argentina. (n.d.). Timeline [Facebook page]. Retrieved March 10, 2019, from https://www.facebook.com/anybodyargentina/

Bacon, L. (2008). *Health at every size*. Dallas, TX: BenBella Books.

Bourdieu, P. (2008). *Los usos sociales de la ciencia* [The social uses of science]. Buenos Aires: Ediciones Nueva Visión.

Braghetto, I., Ibarra, O., Rojas, J., Korn, O., & Valladares, H. (2006). Reoperaciones por fracaso tardío de la cirugía bariátrica. Reporte de 5 casos clínicos [Reoperations due to late failure of bariatric surgery. Report of 5 clinical cases]. *Revista Chilena de Cirugía, 58*(6), 456–463. http://dx.doi.org/10.4067/S0718-40262006000600011

Callahan, M. (2015, January 18). The brutal secrets of the biggest loser. *New York Post*.

Canclini, N. (2001). *Culturas híbridas. Estrategias para entrar y salir de la modernidad* [Hybrid cultures. Strategies for entering and leaving modernity]. Barcelona: Paidós.

CNTV. (2013). *Experiencias de televisión local en Latinoamérica. Estudio de revisión bibliográfica* [Experiences of local television in Latin America. A bibliographic review].

CNTV. (2016). *Reality shows y la relación con las audiencias* [Reality shows and the relationship with the audience].

Eco, U. (2012). *La Estrategia de la Ilusión* [The Strategy of Illusion]. Barcelona: Ed. De Bolsillo.

Fothergill, E., Guo, J., Howard, L., Kerns, J. C., Knuth, N. D., Brychta, R., Chen, K. Y., Skarulis, M. C., Walter, M., Walter, P. J. & Hall, K. D. (2016). Persistent metabolic adaptation 6 years after "The Biggest Loser" competition, *Obesity, 24*(18), 1612–1619. DOI: 10.1002/oby.21538.

Foucault, M. (2004). *Historia de la Sexualidad 3. La Inquietud de Sí* [The History of Sexuality III. The Care of the Self]. Buenos Aires: Siglo XXI.

Gaha, E. (2004) *The Biggest Loser* [Television series]. Los Angeles, CA: NBC.

Masson, L. (2014). *El cuerpo como espacio de disidencia* [The body as a space of dissent]. Retrieved from https://hysteria.mx/el-cuerpo-como-espacio-de-disidencia/

MINSAL. (2019). *Obesidad* [Obesity]. Retrieved from https://www.minsal.cl/?s=obesidad

Orellana, T. (2016a). Cirugía plástica y telerealidad: Antecedentes y articulaciones a partir de la incursión del makeover show en Chile [Plastic surgery and reality TV: Background and articulations from the entrance of makeover shows in Chile]. In M. Correa, A. Kottow & S. Vetö (Eds.), *Ciencias en escena. Saberes científicos y espectáculo en América Latina, siglos XIX y XX* (pp. 323–356). Santiago de Chile: Ocho Libros.

Orellana, T. (2016b). Estereotipos femeninos de salud y belleza en Chile a través del género magazine: Revista Familia (1910–1928) [Female stereotypes of health and beauty in Chile through the magazine genre: Revista Familia (1910–1928)]. In L. Araya, C. Leyton, M. López & M. Sánchez (Eds.), *República de la salud. Fundación y ruinas de un país sanitario. Chile siglos XIX y XX* (pp. 203–224). Santiago de Chile: Ocho Libros Editores.

Orgullo Gordo. (n.d.). Timeline [Facebook page]. Retrieved March 10, 2019, from https://www.facebook.com/OrgulloGordo/

Ossandón, C. & Santa Cruz, E. (2005). *El estallido de las formas. Chile en los albores de la cultura de masas* [Outbreak of the forms. Chile at the dawn of mass culture]. Santiago de Chile: LOM.

Poretsky, G. (2010). A dose of reality: My exclusive interview with biggest loser finalist, Kai Hibbard (Part 2 of 3). Retrieved from http://www.bodylovewellness.com/2010/06/16/kai-hibbard-biggest-loser-finalist-part-2-of-3/

Radrigán, V. & Orellana, T. (2016). *Extremos del volumen. Poderes y medialidades en torno a la obesidad y la anorexia* [Extremes of body mass. Power and media discourses around obesity and anorexia]. Santiago de Chile: Cuarto Propio.

Rinke, S. (2013). *Encuentros con el Yanqui: Norteamericanización y Cambio Social en Chile 1898–1990* [Encounters with the Yankee: Americanization and Social Change in Chile 1898–1990]. Santiago de Chile: DIBAM.

Sepúlveda, J. (2013). *Sueño XL La Transformación de tu Vida* [XL Dream The Transformation of your Life] Television series. Santiago de Chile: Canal 13.

Vigarello, G. (2011). *Historia de la Obesidad. Metamorfosis de la Gordura* [History of Obesity. Metamorphosis of Fatness]. Buenos Aires: Ed. Nueva Visión.

30

THE RISE OF THE CARNIVORE DIET AND THE FETISHIZING OF INDIGENOUS FOODWAYS

Travis Hay and Jennifer Poudrier

Introducing "man the hunter"

In this chapter, the authors confront the rise of dietary trends premised upon primal, paleolithic, and so-called carnivore approaches to health and wellness. Our analysis has been provoked by the recent surge in popularity of the "all-meat diet" and the increasingly extreme influence that white male celebrity podcasters are having on their listeners. For example, in January 2020, internet podcast celebrity and mixed martial arts commentator Joe Rogan announced to his Instagram followers that he was beginning a two-month "strict carnivore diet" that consisted nothing save "meat and eggs" (Rogan, 2020). Rogan explained that a group of his friends were "pretty disgusted with how fat [they] were" and averred to support one another in a collective eight-week weight loss exercise (Rogan, 2020). Rogan stopped the all-meat diet after 30 days, citing digestive difficulties (read: diarrhoea); however, he also claimed that he lost 12 pounds, that his energy levels were higher, and that it had a tonic effect on an autoimmune disorder from which he suffers (vitiligo) (Munson, 2020). In pursuing this diet, Rogan was following the example of another online white male celebrity with legions of dedicated followers: Dr Jordan Peterson. Peterson, who originally curried the favour of the alt-right following his critique of and refusal to use gender-neutral pronouns, became a best-selling author in the self-help sector when he published *12 Rules for Life: An Antidote to Chaos* (2018). In the past two years, Peterson and his daughter Mikhaila have both made headlines and garnered significant attention following their claims that an all-meat diet consisting of salt, beef, water, and the occasional bourbon is as a cure-all to a long list of autoimmune disorders, dermatological problems, and even mental illnesses (Hamblin, 2018). More broadly, podcasters across multiple platforms are extolling the virtues of intermittent fasting, ketogenic diets, and other dietary strategies that are designed to shed body fat by acute changes to one's caloric intake or macronutrient profiles. For example, another Los Angeles podcaster and martial arts figure – former heavyweight fighter Brendan Schaub – capitalized on the popularity of ketogenic diets and sold a T-shirt associated with his podcast that read: "Keto Kid – Get Yo Slim On".

On the surface, an all-meat or protein-exclusive diet appears to be metabolically dangerous or at any rate unsustainable. Indeed, in 2010, professional wrestler and mixed martial artist Brock Lesnar underwent multiple surgeries following serious damage to his digestive

DOI: 10.4324/9780429344824-36

system pursuant to a "carnivore" diet lacking in vegetables. When asked about his inadvisable dietary practices, Lesnar responded:

> I'm a carnivore. I'm not a big fan of PETA. I'm a member of the NRA, and whatever I kill, I eat. Basically, I was just for years surviving on meat and potatoes. When the greens came by, I just kept passing them.
>
> *(UFC Champ Brock Lesnar Slams Canadian Healthcare, 2010)*

As Lesnar's words suggest, the decision to eat meat and avoid vegetables is not only a dietary decision but a political act in which multiple identities are performed and values enacted. In this chapter, we discuss this particular trajectory of dietary extremism as an outgrowth of the larger "paleo" movement (Chang, 2016). Though we place due focus on the politics of gender as well as what Carol J. Adams termed "the sexual politics of meat," we are also heavily preoccupied with the operation of colonial mythologies within the registers of the emergent paleo, primal pattern, caveman, and carnivore dietary trends (Adams, 1990). We recall and reference here what Brenda Parlee and Kristine Wray called "man the hunter" – that oversimplified and profoundly gendered figure often used as a lens through which knowledges about food, health, and environment are produced (Parlee & Wray, 2016). In what follows, we locate the figure of "man the hunter" within emergent dietary discourses and critique the extent to which these coded constructions of Indigenous foodways continue to inform non-Indigenous understandings of health, wellness, meat, and land in both past and present.

The legacy of the thrifty gene

Buried beneath most popular discourses that relate men's health to protein consumption, hunting, and body fat rests the legacy of the ill-fated thrifty gene hypothesis. Both authors of this chapter have spilled considerable ink on this particular hypothesis in our respective disciplines. Invented in 1962 by the American geneticist James V. Neel, the hypothesis held that Indigenous peoples were predisposed to diabetes, obesity, and other metabolic syndromes because their bodies remained programmed for a pre-agricultural environment or "hunter-gatherer" lifestyle wherein food was not plentiful. Neel's claim was "that during the first 99 per cent or more of man's life on earth, while he existed as a hunter and gatherer, it was often feast or famine" (Neel, 1962, p. 354). These assumed chronic food shortages were cited by Neel as a significant selection pressure presumedly absent in agricultural civilizations who (he believed) had more reliable food production strategies. In this frame, Indigenous peoples were biologically unfit for civilization due to their inability to metabolize steady food supplies without the generation of significant adipose tissue, or fat. Put more directly, "Neel imagined Indigenous peoples as camel-like beasts with an inherited ability to over-eat during times of plenty" (Ferreira & Lang, 2006, p. 11). After he spent much of the 1960s hunting (always unsuccessfully) for thrifty genes in the blood of Indigenous communities in Brazil and Venezuela, Neel rejected his own hypothesis. In 1989, he wrote that "the data on which that (rather soft) hypothesis was based has now largely collapsed" as he could discover "no evidence of a predisposition to diabetes in… unacculturated Indians" (Neel, 1989, p. 817). And yet, the thrifty gene lived on.

In the mid-1990s, a team of Canadian researchers signed an unprecedented DNA deal with a remote northern Indigenous community that was grappling with very high rates of type-II diabetes. Sandy Lake First Nation, located near the northwest border of the province of Ontario, thus became the location of a genetic study funded to the tune of $750,000 CAD by the provincial government. In March 1999, this research team – led by the geneticist Dr Robert Hegele – made headlines the world over and put Canadian genomic science on the map when they made the incredible announcement that they had discovered the long-lost thrifty gene. For example, The *Canadian Medical Association Journal* ran an article with the title "Gene Defect Driving Diabetes Epidemic on Ontario Reserve" (Basky, 1999). The *British Medical Journal* reported that:

> a study conducted in a reservation in northern Ontario has identified a genetic mutation that seems to have allowed the Indians there to survive famines in the past but to have triggered diabetes when food became plentiful and their lives became sedentary.
>
> *(Stergeon, 1999, p. 828)*

A Chinese news agency also found the study newsworthy, reporting in March of that year: "Canadian researchers have found that a 'thrifty' gene, or genes, may account for the world's third highest rate of diabetes in the Ojibway-Cree native reserve at Sandy Lake in Northern Ontario province of Canada" (Canadian Researchers Uncover Genetic Link for Diabetes, 1999). By March 2000, *Health Canada* had already started to produce literature on "Aboriginal Diabetes" as if all Indigenous bodies (not merely those in Sandy Lake) were victims of thrifty genes, deleterious alleles, and metabolic maladaptation. The hypothesis had not only been revived in the laboratories of southern Ontario and reanimated in the headlines of newspapers worldwide, but it had also become institutionalized within the Canadian state apparatus and healthcare system.

Jennifer Poudrier was the first to contest this geneticization of "Aboriginal Diabetes" in a 2003 publication. In 2006, the thrifty gene hypothesis was devastated empirically by biological anthropologists who drew attention to the myth of pre-contact Indigenous food insecurity and the false claim that peoples who rely on land-based food procurement strategies are unable to produce food surpluses (Benyshek & Watson, 2006; Fee, 2006). In this same year, British biologist John Speakman introduced the provocative analytic gesture of underscoring that European agricultural societies were not less likely to experience famines than other civilizations with "undernourishment rampant in the Greco-Roman empire and Europe both before and during the Industrial Revolution" (p. 10). In 2007, Dr Poudrier published an article that deployed Indigenous critical theory and philosophy to articulate the thrifty gene hypothesis as a "trickster". Though we unpack this concept in more detail in the conclusion to this chapter, it will suffice here to define it as a narratological device that helps describe wild oscillations, ironic inversions, or unexpected reversals within the context of Indigenous critical theory, in general, and Anishinaabe philosophy, in particular. For those unfamiliar with the term "Anishinaabe", it refers to the Cree, Ojibway, and Ojicree peoples whose traditional territory covers much of central Canada. Though sharing similarities to many Indigenous peoples of Turtle Island (or North America), Anishinaabe philosophy is heavily exercised with dualities of meaning, the deconstruction of seemingly solid binaries as well as the pedagogical impact of humour, unexpectedness, and inversion.

Like Neel before him, the main geneticist associated with the thrifty gene discovery (Dr Robert Hegele) soon rolled back his findings. In 2011, Hegele told the *Globe and Mail* that "newer genetic data suggest it's incorrect to pin the blame for type 2 diabetes on a single gene in any population" and that "the whole thrifty-gene idea seems to me not to capture the subtlety and complexity... of type 2 diabetes in First Nations communities" (quoted in Abraham, 2011). Significantly, in 2012, the Tri-Council Policy Statement on Ethical Conduct for Research Involving Humans cited "genetic research on diabetes in a First Nations community" as an example of a scientific study that is "unlikely to benefit the community in the short term" (Canadian Institute of Health Research, 2012). Finally, in 2013, Hegele wrote that while

> the 'thrifty gene' hypothesis might have seemed like a good idea many years ago…current research suggests that in most cases a single mutation in a single gene is unlikely to predispose an entire group of people to a complex outcome like type 2 diabetes.
>
> *(quoted in Kuhnlein, 2013, p. 14)*

However, as Hay showed in a 2018 article, Hegele et al.'s study continued to be cited in public health literature, clinical guidelines, and a long list of publications from the Canadian Diabetes Association, the Canadian Pediatric Society, and Health Canada. And though the thrifty gene hypothesis continues to lose credibility in the official registers of Canadian healthcare, the figure of the meat-eating, often-starving, pre-agricultural North American biosubject (read: "man the hunter") is more popular and influential than ever.

The increasing popularity of "going paleo"

Strictly speaking, dietary fads and fitness regimens that fetishize the primitive, paleolithic, or caveman approach to health and wellness first emerged as scholarly bioanthropological discourses in the same era of scientific thought as the thrifty gene. In 1985, for example, an article in the *New England Journal of Medicine* titled "Paleolithic Nutrition" underscored the extent to which paleolithic and pre-agricultural humans did not ingest any dairy foods and "consumed cereal grains rarely" (Eaton & Konner, 1985, p. 283). Notably, this article compared "Neanderthals and Cro-Magnons" to "technologically primitive societies" studied by contemporary anthropologists; further, it explained that "Eskimos" were able to obtain sufficient sources of calcium from the consumption of meat (Eaton & Konner, 1985, pp. 284–285). This original study thus made the same kind of racist ontological bait-and-switch accomplished by the Neel, the inventor of the thrifty gene hypothesis: mainly, it viewed contemporary Indigenous peoples and their foodways as a reflection of an earlier stage in human civilizational development prior to the practice of agriculture. Three years later, this article became the basis of a popular book titled *The Paleolithic Prescription: A Program of Diet and Exercise and a Design for Living* (Keaton, Konner, & Shostak, 1988). A spear figured prominently on the cover of this book, which was to become a treasured symbol of the movement-to-come. As Nowell Chang noted in their study of the paleo movement, the authors of these publications

> used data on six diverse modern hunter-gatherer diets drawn from the literature, ranging from the!Kung San to the Greenland Inuit to Australian Aborigines…these data were effectively merged to produce a single reconstruction of the "average" Paleolithic diet, which [the authors] considered to be comparable to what they referred to as the 'average' North American diet.
>
> *(Chang, 2016 p. 229)*

Indigenous peoples of Turtle Island (or North America) were therefore a primary reference point of the paleo diet as originally conceived. Of course, what was advised within the paleo diet was not an accurate representation of Indigenous foodways so much as it was a reflection of non-Indigenous investments in the figure of "man the hunter".

In 1999, the same year as the claimed thrifty discovery, *Men's Health* magazine included an extended series on "Caveman Fitness" that seems to suggest the opening stages of a more popular paleolithic movement that exists in non-peer-reviewed venues (Ballard, 1999). Discussing the alleged ancestors of its male readership, the author extolled their fit, lean, and muscular bodies

> They pumped rocks and chucked spears, conquered tribes, toted women, and ambushed giant wildlife. They spent every day in God's gym, and the results showed. Scientists will tell you that no matter how much you can bench-press, no matter how far you can run, the average tundra-trekker who lived and worked out thousands of years ago was in much better shape than you, for one simple reason: You're not using your body to do what it was meant to do!
>
> *(p. 108)*

This "mismatch hypothesis," which compared the contemporary human body to its primitive and much fitter form, was reproductive of the thrifty gene hypothesis and increasingly common to see covered in popular literature. For example, in 2001, the American scientist Loren Cordain published *The Paleo Diet: Lose Weight and Get Healthy by Eating the Food You Were Designed to Eat*, which arguably eclipsed *The Paleolithic Prescription* (Keaton et al., 1988) as the official reference point for what was fast becoming the paleo movement. Though it is ultimately impossible to extract this particular paleo movement from the CrossFit movement that was emergent at the same time, the analytic gesture of doing so is not necessary here beyond signalling the fact that the two movements were mutually supportive of one another and doubly so in the emerging online space. Other scholars have also cited this period (1996–2006) as exhibiting a marked explosion in popular interest in the ketogenic diet (Freeman, Kossof & Hartman 2007).

In 2007, Israeli health and fitness guru Ori Hofmekler (whose qualifications are dubious) published *The Anti-Estrogenic Diet: How Estrogenic Foods and Chemicals Are Making You Fat and Sick*. The effect of this text has been far reaching as it was arguably the nucleus of what has since become known as the "soy boy conspiracy", wherein men on the internet promote a widespread fear that the ingestion of soy or the release of female hormones into water and food supplies will cause men significant hormonal challenges, make them less "manly", cause them to grow breasts (gynostemia), promote erectile dysfunction, or cause other gendered or sexual impacts on their health (Henderson, 2018). The publication and popularity of this book and its central idea marks a point of departure in the online men's health and fitness movement to the extent that it began to divorce itself from scientificity and began to embrace a more conspiratorial culture cultivated almost exclusively in the online space. In the coming years, a long list of publications picked up on many of the themes, ideologies, and mythologies embedded in the paleo and other movements. The following is a representative list of some best-selling books with provocative and telling titles: *The Primal Blueprint* (Sisson, 2009), *Cavewomen Don't Get Fat* (Blum, 2013), *The Paleo Manifesto* (Durant & Malice, 2014), *The Ancestral Table* (Crandall, 2014), *Paleo Perfected* (America's Test Kitchen, 2015), *The Paleo Intermittent Fasting Program* (Parry, 2016), and *The Paleo Solution: The Original Human Diet* (Wolf, 2017). And while these are all monographs or print publications, it is important to note, as others have, that the "modern Paleo movement lives primarily on the Internet, where it is disseminated via dozens of websites, online discussion boards, Facebook groups, and other social networking tools" (Chang, 2016, p. 228). As noted at the start of this chapter, the recent rise of the all-meat diet as advocated by the likes of Joe Rogan and Jordan

Peterson has emerged as the most recent development in this curious history of increasingly extreme and limited diets. Though the paleo movement was to some degree problematic, the all-meat diet appears to be downright dangerous and warrants serious consideration for several reasons.

First and foremost, the movement is intensely fatphobic and treats thinness and leanness as synonymous with health and wellness (notably, at the expense of digestive health). Second, the movement is gynophobic in that its advocates commonly state hostility towards the influence of feminist politics or fear and anxiety over the prospect of the circulation of female hormones. Further, the fact that the paleo and carnivore community is increasingly and exclusively online raises red flags to many feminists, as the radicalization of isolated and disaffected white male teens who find online communities of support from similarly situated men is the form taken by several regressive movements currently undercutting democracy and posing a public safety threat across the world. We are thinking here not only of white supremacist organizing but also of the emergent "Incel" movement – that is, young men who identify as "involuntarily celibate" and who blame women, feminism, or non-celibate men for their own perceived place near the bottom of a social sexual hierarchy. Indeed, we would go so far as to suggest that there is a direct parallel between refusing to wear a mask in the middle of a global pandemic and making the decision to eat only meat and eggs when western nations struggle with staggering rates of heart disease and cancer. Within this framing, the Romantic construction of "man the hunter" is being cross-pollinated with libertarian fundamentalism given that the powerful image of man in his natural state is being increasingly employed as a coded celebration of freedom from government regulation (and doubly so in the middle of the COVID-19 pandemic). This trajectory of analysis was vindicated during the writing of this contribution, which took place within and around the January 2021 protests on Capitol Hill in the United States. In the aftermath of this protest, a particular fur-clad figure seen sporting a buffalo head and other ancestral imagery became broadly discussed in the media following his arrest. This individual – Jake Angeli – refused to eat the food served to him until Phoenix Judge Deborah Fine made a special ruling allowing him to continue his "organic" diet while under arrest (Falcon, 2021). While this alignment between libertarianism and the paleo movement offers a partial and speculative explanation for the sudden rise of the all-meat diet, in the past several years, we conclude by drawing ironic attention to the competing fetishes and pathologies that have been attached to Indigenous foodways within popular dietary trends between the 1980s and today.

Conclusion: the thrifty gene as trickster

The "trickster" is an Indigenous narratological device often associated with Anishinaabe philosophy, literary studies, and critical theory. It helps describe wild oscillations, ironic inversions, or unexpected reversals within a given story, history, or narrative. In the field of Indigenous Studies, the figure of the "trickster" is strongly associated with the literary theory and works of fiction of Anishnabe scholar Gerald Vizenor, whose *Trickster Discourse* (1998) helped to unpack the ways in which Indigenous scholars and storytellers employ this device to animate or theorize stories in which "hierarchies are leveled, distinctions are dissolved, and roles reversed" (Fox, 2009, p. 72). Importantly, for our purposes, the figure of the "trickster" helps to navigate, denaturalize, or deconstruct binary structures of thought by avoiding totalized narratives and finished knowledges.

In 2007, near the beginning of the paleo movement's rise to online popularity, Dr Poudrier had the foresight to publish an article that, in Dr Hay's reading, neatly predicted the wild inversion in discourses related to Indigenous foodways and fitness by "envisioning the thrifty gene story as a trickster tale" (Poudrier, 2007, p. 239). Poudrier argued that

> the story of the thrifty gene is a powerful example of the complex interplay between genes, race and society, and a provocative reason why it is essential to look back at seemingly finished knowledge, to challenge it, and to produce emancipatory and valid knowledge for the future, indeed, for the purposes of looking back on the future.
>
> *(Poudrier, 2007, p. 240)*

As we have shown in the above, the thrifty gene hypothesis and the enduring figure of "man the hunter" has played a curious role in the creation of both scientific and popular discourses of health and wellness. The thrifty gene has, as predicted, acted as a trickster – whereas the hypothesis originally constructed the foodways of Indigenous peoples as a potential public health crisis of "Aboriginal Diabetes", the discourse has oscillated wildly to the extent that eating like an Indigenous person of Turtle Island is now seen by many as the very best way to deal with excess adipose tissue and develop a lean, muscular, and fit body. Ironically, the on-going erosion in the trust of public health authorities has facilitated these dietary movements in their most extreme and carnivorous variants. Ultimately, then, the "trickster" helps us to makes sense of the all-meat diet as an inversion of the thrifty gene and as the ironic return of the primitive origins of modern science.

References

Abraham, C. (2011, February 26). The life and death of a seductive theory. *The Globe and Mail*, F1.

Adams, C. J. (1990). *The sexual politics of meat : A feminist-vegetarian critical theory*. London: Continuum.

America's Test Kitchen (Ed.) (2015). *Paleo perfected: A revolution in eating well with 150 kitchen-tested recipes*. Brookline, MA: America's Test Kitchen.

Ballard, C. (1999, September 1). Caveman fitness. *Men's Health*, pp. 108–110.

Basky, G. (1999). Gene defect driving diabetes epidemic on Ontario reserve. *The Canadian Medical Association Journal*, 160(12), 692.

Benyshek, D. B., & Watson, J. T. (2006). Exploring the thrifty genotype's food-shortage assumptions: A cross-cultural comparison of ethnographic accounts of food security among foraging and agricultural societies. *The American Journal of Physical Anthropology*, 131, 120–126. https://doi.org/10.1002/ajpa.20334

Blum, E. (2013). *Cavewomen don't get fat: The paleo chic diet for rapid results*. New York: Gallery Books.

Canadian Institute of Health Research. (2012, December). *Tri Council Policy Statement: Ethical conduct for research involving humans*. Retrieved from https://ethics.gc.ca/eng/tcps2-eptc2_2018_chapter9-chapitre9.html?wbdisable=true

Canadian researchers uncover genetic link for diabetes. (1999, March 9). *Xinhua News Agency*.

Chang, N. (2016). How to make stone soup: Is the 'paleo diet' a missed opportunity for anthropologists? *Evolutionary Anthropology*, 25(5), 228–231. https://doi.org/10.1002/evan.21504

Cordain, L. (2001). *The paleo diet: Lose weight and get healthy by eating the food you were designed to eat*. New Jersey: Wiley and Sons.

Crandall, R. (2014). *The ancestral table: Traditional recipes for a paleo lifestyle*. New York: Victory Belt Publishing.

Durant, J., & Malice, M. (2014). *The paleo manifesto: Ancient wisdom for lifelong health*. New York: Harmony Books.

Eaton, S., & Konner, M. (1985). Paleolithic nutrition: A consideration of its nature and current implications. *The New England Journal of Medicine*, 213(5), 283–289. https://doi.org/10.1056/NEJM198501313120505

Falcon, R. (2021, January 12). 'QAnon Shaman' Jake Angeli will be fed organic diet while he's in custody for Capitol riot. *KXAN News*. Retrieved from https://www.kxan.com/news/national-news/qanon-shaman-jake-angeli-will-be-fed-organic-diet-while-hes-in-custody-for-capitol-riot/

Fee, M. (2006). Racializing narratives: Obesity, diabetes and the 'aboriginal' thrifty genotype. *Social Science & Medicine, 62*(12), 2988–2997. https://doi.org/10.1016/j.socscimed.2005.11.062

Ferreira, M. L., & Lang, G.C. (2006). Introduction: Deconstructing diabetes. In P. Stewart & A. Strathern (Eds.), *Indigenous peoples and diabetes: Community empowerment and wellness* (pp. 1–18). Durham, NC: Carolina Academic Press.

Fox, T. (2009). Realizing fantastic trickster liberations in Gerald Vizenor's 'Griever: An American Monkey King in China'. *Journal of the Fantastic in the Arts, 20*(1), 70–90.

Freeman, J. M., Kossoff, E. H., & Hartman, A. L. (2007). The ketogenic diet: One decade later. *Pediatrics 119*(3), 535–543. https://doi.org/10.1542/peds.2006-2447

Hamblin, J. (2018, August 18). The Jordan Peterson all-meat diet. *The Atlantic.* Retrieved from https://www.theatlantic.com/health/archive/2018/08/the-peterson-family-meat-cleanse/567613/

Hay, T. (2018). The invention of Aboriginal diabetes: The role of the thrifty gene hypothesis in Canadian health care provision. *Ethnicity & Disease, 28*(1), 247–252. https://doi.org/10.18865/ed.28.S1.247

Health Canada (2000, March 10). *Diabetes among Aboriginal (First Nations, Inuit, and Métis) peoples in Canada: The evidence.*

Henderson, A. (2018, November 15). Inside the 'soy boy' conspiracy theory: It combines misogyny and the warped world of pseudoscience. *Salon.* Retrieved from https://www.salon.com/2018/11/14/the-soy-boy-conspiracy-theory-alt-right-thinks-left-wing-has-it-out-for-them-with-soybeans_partner/

Hofmekler, O. (2007). *The anti-estrogenic diet: How estrogenic foods and chemicals are making you fat and sick.* Berkeley, CA: North Atlantic Books.

Keaton, S., Konner, M., & Shostak, M. (1988). *The paleolithic prescription: A program of diet and exercise and a design for living.* New York: Harper & Row.

Kuhnlein, H. V. (2013). *Indigenous peoples' food systems and well-being: Interventions and policies for healthy communities.* Rome, Italy: Food and Agriculture Organization of the United Nations.

Munson, M. (2020, February 7). *What happened to Joe Rogan's body after 30 days of the carnivore diet?* Retrieved from https://www.menshealth.com/health/a30813388/joe-rogan-carnivore-diet-review-youtube/

Neel, J. V. (1962). Diabetes mellitus: A "thrifty" genotype rendered detrimental by "progress"? *American Journal of Human Genetics, 14*(4), 353–362.

Neel, J. V. (1989). Update to "The study of natural selection in primitive and civilized human populations." *Human Biology, 61,* 811–823.

Parlee, B., & Wray, K. (2016). Gender and the social dimensions of changing Caribou populations in the Western Arctic. In N. Kermoal & I. Altamirano-Jiménez (Eds.). *Living on the Land: Indigenous Women's Understanding of Place* (pp. 161–190). Edmonton: Athabasca University Press.

Parry, B. (2016). *The paleo intermittent fasting program.* Scotts Valley, CA: CreateSpace Publishing.

Peterson, J. (2018). *12 rules for life: An antidote to chaos.* Toronto, ON: Random House.

Poudrier, J. (2003). Racial categories and health risks: Epidemiological surveillance among Canadian First Nations. In D. Lyon (Ed.), *Surveillance as social sorting: Privacy, risk, and digital discrimination* (pp. 125–148). New York: Routledge Publishing.

Poudrier, J. (2007). The geneticization of Aboriginal diabetes: Adding another scene to the story of the thrifty gene. *The Canadian Review of Sociology and Anthropology, 44*(4), 237–261. https://doi.org/10.1111/j.1755-618X.2007.tb01136.x

Rogan, J. (2020, January 3) *Instagram* post. Retrieved from https://www.instagram.com/p/B64KT3GFfdx/?utm_source=ig_embed

Sisson, M. (2009). *The primal blueprint: Reprogram your genes for effortless weight loss, vibrant health, and boundless energy.* London: Vermillion Publishing.

Stergeon, D. (1999). 'Thrifty gene' identified in Manitoba Indians. *British Medical Journal, 318*(7187), 828.

UFC champ Brock Lesnar slams Canadian health care. (2010, January 20). *CTV News.* Retrieved from https://www.ctvnews.ca/ufc-champ-brock-lesnar-slams-canadian-health-care-1.475750

Wolf, R. (2017). *The paleo solution: The original human diet.* New York: Victory Belt Publishing.

31

A STUDY OF AN *ANTI*-OBESITY, ANTI-*OBESITY* CAMPAIGN

Jessica Lee and Benjamin Williams

Introduction

Since the declaration of the "war on obesity," there have been many attempts to curb the so-called "obesity epidemic." Indeed, anti-obesity campaigns communicating a "fat-as-fatal" message have become a regular and accepted public health strategy in most economically developed countries (Bombak, Monaghan, & Rich, 2018). Despite their ubiquity, a growing number of researchers have critiqued the ways these campaigns frame obesity as a health issue and promote problematic weight-loss methods (Monaghan, Bombak, & Rich, 2017). Nevertheless, such critiques have had little impact on the most highly funded, government-sanctioned interventions on people's bodies (Monaghan et al., 2017). In this chapter, we consider why critical perspectives on obesity have not been more influential in public health practice. To this end, we focus on the Australian anti-obesity campaign, *Healthier. Happier.* – which sought to deliver positive, supportive, health promotion messages about body weight – and ask how, if at all, this campaign was different from its "fat-as-fatal" predecessors. We begin this task by reviewing existing critiques of mainstream anti-obesity campaigns.

Critical research on anti-obesity campaigns

Two characteristics are particularly common among the plethora of recent anti-obesity campaigns. The first of these characteristics is the centrality of body mass index (BMI), and the second is the use of stigma as a motivator for behaviour change. As the critical research literature illustrates, these characteristics have made a significant contribution to the production and perpetuation of stigma and inequality for people classified as overweight or obese. As the criterion most popularly used by individuals and health professionals to judge both weight status and health status, BMI has played a central role in shaping what has come to be the problem of the so-called obesity epidemic. Not only have BMI ranges come to define the health status of bodies, critical health scholars (e.g., Gutin, 2018) have proposed that BMI is often the *only* measure of health reported in epidemiological research therefore becoming not just a proxy for health, but also a replacement for "the definition of health itself" (Gutin, 2018, p. 261). Given the moral imperatives attached to health, those who are understood to be unhealthy are exposed to marginalisation and stigma (Gutin, 2018).

DOI: 10.4324/9780429344824-37

The power of stigma is regularly utilised by commercial advertisers and developers of public health campaigns (Lupton, 2015) despite being identified as playing a role in creating health inequalities (O'Hara & Gregg, 2006, 2012). Campaigns based on stigma generate fear of ill health, failure, and unattractiveness underpinned by the logic that body discontent motivates "beneficial" lifestyle changes that will lead to weight loss (Bacon & Aphramor, 2011). In this way, fat stigma is overtly (re)produced through government policies and resulting anti-obesity campaigns (O'Reilly & Sixsmith, 2012; Pausé, 2017).

It has been demonstrated, however, that adults who face weight stigmatisation and discrimination are less likely to engage with public health messages about fatness (Pausé, 2017) and, furthermore, report increased food consumption, exercise avoidance, and the postponement or avoidance of medical care (Bacon & Aphramor, 2011). It is clear within the literature summarised here that from the perspective of efficacy, as well as ethics, body weight is a poor target for public health intervention. There is considerable evidence to recommend a paradigm shift away from conventional weight management to a focus on health regardless of body weight (Bacon & Aphramor, 2011; O'Hara & Taylor, 2018). In sum, weight-focused approaches to health promotion have not gone unchallenged. Within the academic literature, concerns have been raised over the continued use of BMI, disgust, and stigma in anti-obesity health promotion campaigns across much of the Western world. Chief among these concerns is that such campaigns have shown little success in changing health behaviours or reducing obesity rates. To the contrary, there is ample evidence to suggest that they actually increase health inequalities by contributing to fat stigma. It is in the context of this complexity and contestation that the *Healthier. Happier.* campaign emerged.

Healthier. Happier.: the *anti*-obesity, anti-*obesity* campaign

Healthier. Happier. is a Queensland Government social marketing campaign launched in 2013 (continuing at the time of publication) to reduce the population levels of overweight and obesity. The campaign has consisted of two m-health initiatives supported by television, online, outdoor, and print advertising. A campaign website (Queensland Government, 2019a) containing tools, information, and resources (such as "how-to" videos) has also been a central feature.

The campaign began with advertisements posing the question, "What's your health and fitness age?," directing consumers to the campaign website to complete the Health and Fitness Age Calculator (Queensland Government, 2019b). The calculator uses an algorithm to convert user-entered data about height, weight, physical activity levels, food consumption patterns, and smoking and alcohol behaviours into a personal Health and Fitness Age (see Lee, Williams & Sebar, 2018).

The Health and Fitness Age Calculator was incorporated into the campaign's second major tool: the Health and Fitness Age Challenge app (now discontinued). This piece of smartphone software allowed users to take a four-week challenge to change selected behaviours that would reduce their Health and Fitness Age. Throughout the challenge, users received regular alerts and tips from a virtual personal trainer as well as prompt to record their progress.

In this chapter, we draw on data generated through semi-structured interviews with six key informants who were involved in the development of the *Healthier. Happier.* campaign. These individuals came from the state health department and their collaborating agencies. We also analyse a sample of campaign materials that we collected during our study from sources such as the official campaign website (Queensland Government, 2019a), open letters about the campaign to stakeholders from the state Chief Health Officer (CHO), as well as campaign television advertisements and billboards/posters.

Presence, absence, and heterogeneity in design

Throughout our investigation of *Healthier. Happier.*, a recurring feature was the alternating role of obesity within the campaign. To this end, we have found Law's (1987, 2002) work on heterogeneity and heterogeneous engineering useful in understanding how *Healthier. Happier.* came together as a campaign and the function of obesity within that process.

Law (1987) argues that technological entities (such as *Healthier. Happier.*, with its online and mobile presence) are composed of disparate elements of varying malleability that have been shaped into a relatively stable network within a more or less hostile or indifferent environment (for an explanation of how a public health campaign can be conceptualised as a technological entity, see Williams & Lee, 2020). He terms this network-building process, *heterogeneous engineering* (Law, 1987), and demonstrates how the distribution of relations of difference is central to the process of design (Law, 2002). Law's argument is founded upon the idea of semiotic relationality, that is, that entities owe their existence, their meaning, and their properties to their relations with other entities (see Law, 2009). Some of these relations are those that are or can be captured and presented in some way (i.e., relations of presence), while others are relations that are not or cannot (i.e., relations of absence). From this perspective, the design process can be understood as embodying and expressing, "a set of tensions between what is present and what is absent but also present" (Law, 2002, p. 112). Law uses the term *heterogeneity* to refer to this oscillation between absence and presence.

Through his work, Law (2002) illustrates several forms of heterogeneity. The form to which we primarily attend here is *heterogeneity/Otherness* or "the *heterogeneity of tellable Otherness*" (Law, 2002, p. 102, original emphasis). The logic of this form is underpinned by a positioning of the Other as a danger that is simultaneously excluded (because of the threat it poses to the self) and included (because its incorporation is part of the constitution of the self). In this way, "the forbidden, the abhorrent, sometimes even the unspeakable, is both present in and absent from whatever is being done, designed, or said" (Law, 2002, p. 102). Put differently, the concept of heterogeneity/Otherness is a kind of ambivalence, an element of a design that is "both integrated into a network and antagonistic towards it" (Michael, 2017, p. 154; see also Singleton & Michael, 1993). The analysis we present below focuses on the heterogeneity/Otherness oscillations that were evident in the campaign's design and the heterogeneous engineering performed by the campaign workers to manage these oscillations.

Heterogeneity/otherness in *Healthier. Happier.*

Obesity was a central constituent of *Healthier. Happier.* From the outset, the primary aim of the campaign was to address levels of obesity in the Queensland population. This aim was clear in data sources such as:

- CHO communications to stakeholders – "The Healthier. Happier. campaign was developed as part of a suite of activities to address the issue of obesity in Queensland" (Queensland Government, 2014b);
- Key informant interviews – "... basically we get a brief in saying that we've got an issue with obesity. So that's coming from the epi[demiology] stats" (Kate);
- The campaign website's landing page for phase one (see Figure 31.1).

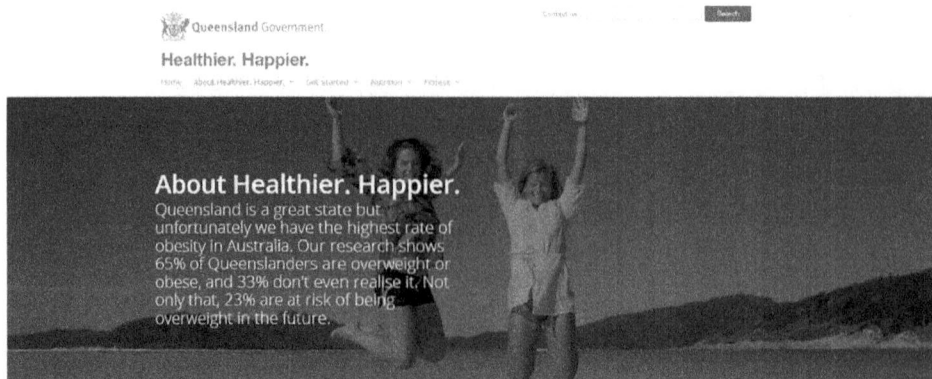

Figure 31.1   *Healthier. Happier.* Phase One website landing page (Queensland Government, 2014a).

An ancillary aim of the campaign was to make obesity a priority within the Health Department. As one informant explained:

> I mean, it [the campaign] was an opportunity... not just in, um, getting messages out to the public, but within the Department and within Government to say, "Yes, obesity is one of our biggest challenges and we need to be investing more." So, the campaign helps to raise the issue of obesity within the Department, except to not wanting to present it as an obesity campaign to the public, we didn't want to do that. It's, it's enabled us to get – I think it's, um, enabled us to get obesity on the agenda within the department.
>
> *(Kathy)*

In addition to highlighting obesity's constitutive role in the campaign, the preceding excerpt foreshadows the simultaneous threat obesity posed to the campaign's success and ongoing existence. Key campaign staff recognised early in the development of the campaign that obesity was an emotive topic that many people were reluctant to acknowledge or discuss. As another informant observed:

> It's something that I don't think has been particularly palatable to do, like talking about overweight and obesity, it's a hard subject to talk about to people... and then I think that's um where the whole *LiveLighter* campaign [a campaign from another Australian state] in concept testing we could really see that the – some of the language, even the words so even yeah the idea of the toxic fats and it's all very negative... I think there's a very emotive side of overweight and obesity which people are really sensitive about.
>
> *(Kate)*

Obesity posed a further threat to the appeal of the campaign in that, during market research conducted to inform the campaign's design, people who did not consider themselves to have a "weight problem" ignored or failed to heed the campaign's messages. This finding was acknowledged by key informants we interviewed and in official campaign communications:

> ... as soon as you say something like obesity or weight loss or fat or kilograms, a thing happens. Straight away you alienate anyone who doesn't consider themselves to have a health issue or a weight problem, they switch off automatically.
>
> *(Kenny)*

... if people generally perceive themselves as being relatively healthy, they are switching off to the messages around nutrition and physical activity because they don't think it applies to them.

(Queensland Government, 2013)

Given the threat of obesity to the campaign, two methods were used to overcome these challenges. First, a "positive, supportive" approach was adopted that emphasised small changes to eating and exercising behaviours rather than body weight:

The creative for the second phase of the *Healthier. Happier.* campaign has the core message 'small changes can make a difference', with a focus on health and fitness rather than weight loss.

(Queensland Government, 2014b)

Second, the Health and Fitness Age concept was developed and implemented, which became a central feature of the "positive, supportive, empowering" approach.

... there's no point talking about weight. So they don't actually talk about weight in the campaign because people don't want to have a conversation about that... Whereas – so that's the whole focus on sort of health and fitness age to try to engage them in a conversation and even put it on their radar.

(Susan)

So, we chose the mass messages to be about this thing called Health and Fitness Age, and then we could have more specific conversations with people as and when they needed.

(Kenny)

Despite threatening the campaign in these ways, obesity was integral to the Health and Fitness Age message. The effect of this positioning was to render obesity both absent and present. The campaign then became anti-obesity, twice over: first, by not wanting people to be obese; and second, by not wanting the concept of obesity to feature in campaign messages.

While the campaign staff spoke of being careful not to include messages around obesity, several examples highlighting obesity as a health issue were conspicuous in the Health and Fitness Age advertisements. There was no verbal reference to obesity in the voiceovers; yet, the message, "being fat is bad for your health," was clear in the imagery when "overweight" people were associated with a higher Health and Fitness Age (see Figure 31.2). In this way, the Health and Fitness Age concept resulted in the oscillation between obesity being absent and present, thus positioning *Healthier. Happier.* as an *anti*-obesity, anti-*obesity* campaign.

A related and overlapping version of obesity's heterogeneity/Otherness is BMI's oscillation between presence and absence. First, within the design of the campaign, obesity was typically defined using BMI classifications. Furthermore, the epidemiological data used to justify the campaign was predominantly based on measures of BMI. The campaign staff and materials attest to BMI as also fundamental to *Healthier. Happier*:

There are so many behaviours but ultimately what they were trying to impress [sic] was BMIs. And so that's why we went back to that, yeah. Because that's what they [i.e., the Department] want to measure over time.

(Susan)

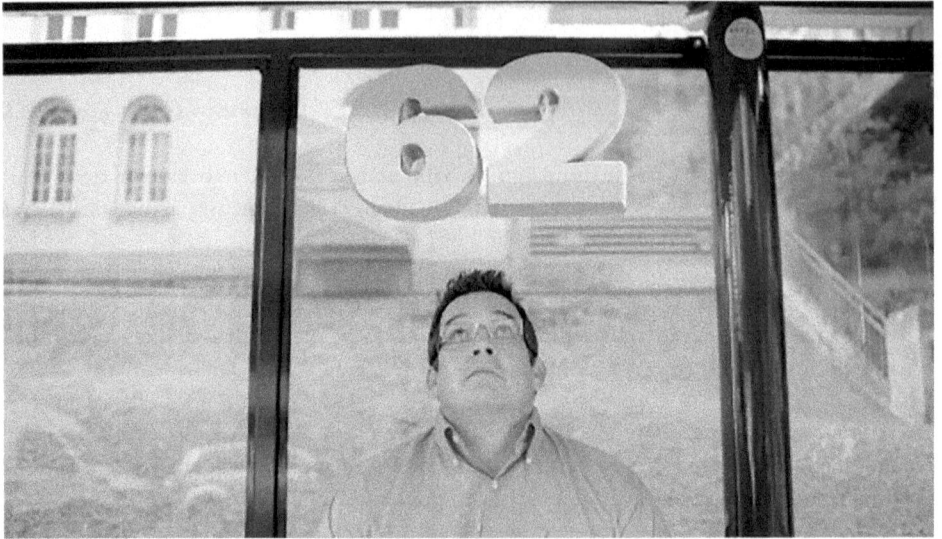

Figure 31.2 "Overweight" people are presented as having a higher Health and Fitness Age (still image from *Healthier. Happier.* television advertisement, 2013).

BMI, however, was also seen as a threat to the campaign as early market research showed that the target audience were sceptical of, or confused about, BMI as a measure. They were therefore unreceptive to messages related to it:

> And one of the actually other big things that came out of the [market] research was no one believes BMI… everyone will discount from this conversation given the opportunity. So, um particularly if you read all those news articles and thinking about overweight and obesity and you read the comments. [People will say] 'Oh BMI, you know Olympic athletes are obese on the BMI scale. It's not accurate.' … anything that they can use to [say] 'I'm not part of it', and people are very much like 'oh, overweight and obesity is a massive problem.' But it's a problem for somebody else.
>
> *(Kate)*

> Perceptions of body shapes have shifted, with overweight body shapes now considered normal. Obesity is considered a problem for 'them' but not for 'me' as my weight and shape is 'normal'. Friends/family/society are being used as a reference point rather than a quantifiable measure such as Body Mass Index (BMI). This is due to the considerable cynicism and confusion over BMI and waist measurement as an indication of healthy weight range.
>
> *(Queensland Government, 2013)*

To overcome BMI as a threat to the campaign, Health and Fitness Age was used as a substitute metric that served as a proxy for BMI:

> So the whole idea about the first phase, is getting people to identify that they – it's kind of something that they should take on board, not necessarily obesity as such, but everyone can make healthier changes and that's what the whole premise of the calculator was,

to take them through that. And sitting behind it is an algorithm, which is largely based on BMI, like 80 percent.

(Kate)

This hidden weighting of BMI in the Calculator algorithm seemed to compromise the ped-agogical intent of the Health and Fitness Age concept. For example, if a respondent has an overweight or obese BMI, their Health and Fitness Age will always be higher than their chrono-logical age, regardless of the other health behaviours they report when using the Calculator. Whilst problematic even at face value, it is demonstrated in the following quote that this factor severely limits the Calculator's intended use in the campaign as a behaviour change motivator:

…there has been a lot of directing back, do your Health and Fitness Age and recheck it [after doing the Challenge]. For most people it's not going to change that much because basically the formula is based on BMI… and changes in the BMI are only going to be very small over time.

(Kathy)

When first completing the Calculator, there are no obvious indicators that the algorithm so heavily relies on BMI. However, when analysing feedback on the Health and Fitness Age Challenge in the App stores, it was clear that users had detected the priority given to BMI and became offended and disinterested. The quote below is from a user who posted feedback (one star) on the Google Play store in 2014:

I put in that I am overweight but eat healthy, dont [sic] drink and exercise 4–5 times a week and got a health age of 49 (I am 27). So I redid it and put in that I was skinny, drink alcohol every day, eat no fruit or vegies [sic] and never exercise. Voila, age of 27. Being overweight doesn't mean I have an unhealthy lifestyle and being thin doesn't mean you're the picture of health. App is pointless and inaccurate.

Our analysis has revealed that, while BMI was intended to be absent from the public-facing component of the campaign, it was indeed present due to the hidden, heavily weighted con-tribution of BMI to the Health and Fitness Age. As such, the stigma associated with obesity and BMI is reproduced and perceived negatively by consumers of campaign messages and m-health tools.

Campaign-as-chimera and the heterogeneities of obesity

The process of designing an anti-obesity campaign is complex, and the constituents out of which it is assembled are heterogeneous (Williams & Lee, 2020). In this chapter, we have magnified one dimension of the *Healthier. Happier.* campaign and examined some of the diverse entities and relations that brought it into being and were intended to maintain its existence. Reflecting on the processes through which *Healthier. Happier.* was assembled, the entities out of which it was composed and the absence/presence oscillations this entailed, we find the figure of the chimera instructive for two reasons both of which correspond to everyday meanings of the word.

The first relevant meaning concerns the use of chimera to refer to a mythical animal formed from parts of various animals (Stevenson, 2010). This use of the word derives from

Greek mythology, where a chimera was a fire-breathing female monster with a lion's head, a goat's body, and a serpent's tail (Stevenson, 2010). *Healthier. Happier.* was chimeric in this fashion as it was constructed out of heterogeneous parts including epidemiological knowledge about obesity, market research knowledge about communicating to target audiences, and political knowledge about being seen to address threats to the population. The campaign was also hybrid to the extent that it was composed of both traditional and new, online forms of advertising. In this way, *Healthier. Happier.* was an amalgam of public education approaches to health promotion and social marketing approaches to behaviour change. However, *Healthier. Happier.* was not only chimeric in the sense that it was formed from multiple presences such as preventive health expertise or market research knowledge. As we sought to demonstrate, the campaign was also a hybrid from the perspective of heterogeneity understood as *"an oscillation between absence and presence"* where "whatever is *not* there is *also* there" and "that which *is* there is also not there" (Law, 2002, p. 96, original emphasis). As a consequence of its *anti*-obesity, anti-*obesity* orientation, obesity was persistently "there" but "not there." To this extent, we suggest that, in the pursuit of an *anti*-obesity, anti-*obesity* campaign, complexity must be managed by concealing some of the parts from view.

The second way in which the image of the chimera is relevant to this study concerns its use to denote something hoped for, yet illusory or impossible to achieve (see Skrabenek's [1994, p. 11] description of the "individual pursuit of the chimera of health"). As demonstrated, it was certainly hoped that *Healthier. Happier.* would be what we term an *anti*-obesity, anti-*obesity* campaign. However, we argue that the campaign's appearance of having a stable, coherent *anti*-obesity, anti-*obesity* orientation is superficial and deceptive. Our analysis shows that what makes a stable, coherent, *anti*-obesity, anti-*obesity* campaign impossible to achieve is the necessity of denying or effacing a fundamental, constitutive element of the campaign, namely, obesity. The reason obesity had to be denied or effaced was because it threatened the campaign's rationale and its likely efficacy. In other words, the epidemiological and political logic of obesity-as-constitutive element interfered and was in tension with the market research and communications logic of obesity-as-threat-to-the-campaign. Since this interference could not be eliminated, the arising instability and precariousness had to be continually managed. In the case of *Healthier. Happier.*, the responsibility for managing obesity's presence/absence oscillations and the resulting instabilities fell on the campaign team. Evident throughout our analysis is a kind of heterogeneous engineering attempted by members of the campaign team as they juggled the heterogeneity of obesity as tellable otherness, of obesity as both rationale for, and risk to, the campaign.

Heterogeneous engineering is a means of dealing with heterogeneity; it is a mode of ordering. From this perspective, the campaign workers can be understood as "trying to order heterogeneity in order to produce healthy bodies" (Niewöhner, et al., 2011, p. 740). For instance, the use of the Health and Fitness Age concept was an attempt to "flatten" (Niewöhner, et al., 2011, p. 728) or tame the heterogeneity associated with BMI. Indeed, the very idea of an *anti*-obesity, anti-*obesity* campaign is an attempt to flatten, tame, or, better still, homogenise the heterogeneities of obesity. The *Healthier. Happier.* campaign workers' efforts at heterogenous engineering entailed deciding from moment-to-moment, task-to-task, audience-to-audience, whether the campaign would be *anti*-obesity or anti-*obesity*. It could not be both at the same time because each formulation (i.e., *anti*-obesity or anti-*obesity*) "othered" core elements of its counterpart. Our research, then, also illustrates the chimeric nature (in this case, at least) of an *anti*-obesity, anti-*obesity* campaign that is perfectly centred, controlled, coherent, and consistent. At the heart of the *anti*-obesity, anti-*obesity* design concept was an oscillating ambivalence or heterogeneity of obesity as tellable otherness. The campaign workers' attempts to engineer or order this source of heterogeneity enacted both complementary and conflicting practices and views.

Following Law's (2004) suggestion that "programmes such as these *always* harbour and enact conflicting practices and views" and "that it is such oscillatory ambivalence that makes them possible and more or less successful in the first place" (2004, p. 92, original emphasis), we argue that the heterogeneous engineering of obesity as tellable otherness was essential to the design phase of *Heathier. Happier.* To this end, we conjecture that, during its design, the campaign was held together as much, if not more, by the non-coherence (Law, 2002) of the *anti*-obesity, anti-*obesity* concept than by the coherence of this element. Yet, during the implementation phase of the campaign, the homogenisations that had been performed (i.e., the flattening/taming presented above) encountered the heterogeneities of people's everyday lives (see similar findings relating to cardiovascular disease interventions in Niewöhner, et al., 2011). At these points, as evident in the app store feedback, the contradictions of the campaign became visible, and so too did the designers' attempts to tame these contradictions.

It is noteworthy that, in their attempts to design an *anti*-obesity, anti-*obesity* campaign, the *Healthier. Happier.* campaign team ultimately replicated the very same neo-liberal discourses and behavioural solutions as its anti-obesity predecessors. A similar pattern is evident in the United Kingdom's *Change4Life* campaign (see Piggin & Lee, 2011). The persistence of neoliberal discourses and behavioural solutions is perhaps due to their familiarity and dominance as a mode of ordering in public health efforts to address obesity. When faced with complex heterogeneities of the kind highlighted here, it is perhaps unsurprising that campaign designers revert to or rely upon the modes of ordering or forms of heterogeneous engineering they know best, or those they have access to, given contextual constraints, even if they are likely to produce the problem designers were attempting to solve in the first place.

The conclusion we draw from our analysis of *Healthier. Happier.* is that the concept of an *anti*-obesity, anti-*obesity* campaign is chimeric and subject to the same threats to its integrity as its simpler anti-obesity campaigns. While *Healthier. Happier.* was an attempt at a different kind of anti-obesity campaign, its designers could not escape the tensions produced by the concept of obesity. We have argued that an *anti*-obesity, anti-*obesity* campaign will always have to contend with the oscillatory ambivalence of obesity's presence/absence. The problem with the *anti*-obesity, anti-*obesity* design concept is indeed obesity itself. It is tempting to think that, if obesity as the enemy or "other" was simply removed, the tension would subside. The result would be perhaps just a campaign where obesity was neither rationale nor target outcome to be reduced – a campaign that focuses on promoting wellness regardless of body shape or size. There are good grounds to believe, however, that such a campaign would merely create a new set of tensions related to how to bring the issue of health promotion onto the agenda of politicians. Within the current health priorities of state and federal governments in Australia, if obesity is not constitutive of the campaign, it is unlikely to receive funding. Therefore, in this case, the tension cannot be escaped – no obesity, no campaign – a central feature of the design architecture (Law, 2002) of these campaigns.

References

Bacon, L., & Aphramor, L. (2011). Weight science: Evaluating the evidence for a paradigm shift. *Nutrition Journal, 10* (9). https://doi.org/10.1186/1475-2891-10-9

Bombak, A., Monaghan, L. F., & Rich, E. (2018). Dietary approaches to weight-loss, Health At Every Size® and beyond: Rethinking the war on obesity. *Social Theory & Health, 17* (1), 89–108. doi: https://doi.org/10.1057/s41285-018-0070-9

Gutin, I. (2018). In BMI we trust: reframing the body mass index as a measure of health. *Social Theory & Health, 16* (3), 256–271. https://doi.org/10.1057/s41285-017-0055-0

Law, J. (2009). Actor network theory and material semiotics. In B. Turner (Ed.), *The new Blackwell companion to social theory* (pp. 141–158). Malden, MA: Wiley-Blackwell.

Law, J. (2004). *After method: Mess in social science research.* London: Routledge.

Law, J. (2002). *Aircraft stories: Decentering the object in technoscience.* Durham, NC: Duke University Press.

Law, J. (1987). Technology and Heterogeneous Engineering: The Case of the Portuguese Expansion. In W. E. Bijker, T. P. Hughes & T. Pinch (Eds), *The social construction of technical systems: New directions in the sociology and history of technology* (pp. 111–34). Cambridge, MA: MIT Press.

Lee, J., Williams, B., & Sebar, B. (2018). Tracing translations: The journey from evidence to policy to physical activity promotion campaigns. In J. Piggin, L. Mansfield & M. Weed (Eds.), *Routledge handbook of physical activity policy and practice* (pp. 139–152). Abingdon: Routledge.

Lupton, D. (2015). The pedagogy of disgust: The ethical, moral and political implications of using disgust in public health campaigns. *Critical Public Health, 25* (1), 4–14. https://doi.org/10.1080/09581596.2014.885115

Michael, M. (2017). *Actor-network theory: Trials, trails and translations.* London: Sage.

Monaghan, L. F., Bombak, A. E., & Rich, E. (2017). Obesity, neoliberalism and epidemic psychology: Critical commentary and alternative approaches to public health. *Critical Public Health, 28* (5), 498–508. https://doi.org/10.1080/09581596.2017.1371278

Niewöhner, J., Döring, M., Kontopodis, M., Madarász, J., & Heintze, C. (2011). Cardiovascular disease and obesity prevention in Germany: An investigation into a heterogeneous engineering project. *Science, Technology, & Human Values, 36*(5), 723–751. https://doi.org/10.1177/0162243910392797

O'Hara, L., & Gregg, J. (2012). Human rights casualties from the "war on obesity": Why focusing on body weight is inconsistent with a human rights approach to health. *Fat Studies, 1* (1), 32–46. https://doi.org/10.1080/21604851.2012.627790

O'Hara, L., & Gregg, J. (2006). The war on obesity: A social determinant of health. *Health Promotion Journal of Australia, 17* (3), 260–263. https://doi.org/10.1071/HE06260

O'Hara, L., & Taylor, J. (2018). What's wrong with the 'war on obesity?' A narrative review of the weight-centered health paradigm and development of the 3C framework to build critical competency for a paradigm shift. *SAGE Open, 8* (2). https://doi.org/10.1177/2158244018772888

O'Reilly, C., & Sixsmith, J. (2012). From theory to policy: Reducing harms associated with the weight-centered health paradigm. *Fat Studies, 1* (1), 97–113. https://doi.org/10.1080/21604851.2012.627792

Pausé, C. (2017). Borderline: The ethics of fat stigma in public health. *The Journal of Law, Medicine & Ethics, 45* (4), 510–517. https://doi.org/10.1177/1073110517750585

Piggin, J., & Lee, J. (2011). 'Don't mention obesity': Contradictions and tensions in the UK Change4Life health promotion campaign. *Journal of Health Psychology, 16* (8), 1151–1164. https://doi.org/10.1177/1359105311401771

Queensland Government (2019a). *Healthier. Happier.* Retrieved from https://www.healthier.qld.gov.au/

Queensland Government (2019b). *Calculate your health and fitness age.* Retrieved from https://www.healthier.qld.gov.au/tools/calculator/#/tools/calculator

Queensland Government (2014a). *Healthier. Happier.* Retrieved from https://www.healthier.qld.gov.au/

Queensland Government (2014b). *Healthier. Happier.* [stakeholder letter]. Brisbane: Queensland Government.

Queensland Government (2013). *Healthier. Happier.* [stakeholder letter]. Brisbane: Queensland Government.

Singleton, V., & Michael, M. (1993). Actor-networks and ambivalence: General practitioners in the UK cervical screening programme. *Social Studies of Science, 23*(2), 227–264.

Skrabenek, P. (1994). *The death of humane medicine and the rise of coercive healthism.* Bury St Edmunds: Crowley Esmonde.

Stevenson, A. (Ed.) (2010). *Oxford dictionary of English* (3rd ed.). New York: Oxford University Press.

Williams, B., & Lee, J. (2020). Public health pedagogy and technology as a mode of existence. In D. Leahy, K. Fitzpatrick & J. Wright (Eds.), *Social theory and health education: Forging new insights in research* (pp. 241–252). Abingdon: Routledge.

PART G

Policies

The set of actions proposed by governing bodies to be taken against obesity, or what is called obesity policies, are complex and common object of debate. Governments, international organisations, non-government organisations (NGOs) of all forms and sizes, and corporations from various sectors have all come together in 'search' for what are praised are 'solutions'. With this multiplicity of actors, of course, come myriad competing interests that need to be negotiated in the construction of solutions. Their scope, design, or rationale can please some groups, but can infuriate others with particular economic interests and a significant lobbying capacity.

Underpinned by the bio-medical premise that situates it as a problem resulting from an unbalance between energy consumption and energy expenditure, the solutions to obesity have focused on regulating what people eat and encouraging them to be physically active. The chapters in this section address the, sometimes unspoken, political, economic, cultural, and ethical dimensions of policies aimed at changing behaviours, many times deemed as 'unhealthy' lifestyles, to reduce obesity. Together, the five chapters implicitly challenge the one-size-fits-all model that, although denied, governing organisations around the world have adopted in their responses to obesity.

In more specific ways, four out of the five chapters offer a contextually situated analysis of the ways in which obesity policy has been done and acted upon in Denmark, Australia, Spain, and Canada. Writing from and about the Danish context, Signild Vallgårda explores how the idea of evidence-based policymaking – which has been widely emphasised in the obesity policy domains – has framed obesity policies in Denmark. Through a critical analysis of the *2019 Recommendations to Municipalities on Lifestyle Intervention Addressing Severe Overweight* published by the Danish Health Authority (DHA), Vallgårda argues that the institutional setting under which evidence is produced significantly shapes policy and that the evidence informing obesity policies is neither neutral nor always the best. Similar to what happens in other countries, the making of obesity policies in Denmark follows a "highly selective" use of the evidence available, which, as Vallgårda concludes assertively, "seems to a larger extent to legitimise the ideas already held by [them], rather than informing them".

Signild Vallgårda's chapter shows that obesity policymaking is, even when tried to be masked behind bio-medical "evidence", a political process. With a different aim of analysis but also highlighting the political dimension of policy, in the next chapter of this section,

DOI: 10.4324/9780429344824-38

Megan Warin discusses her ethnographic work on public health interventions around food, eating and bodies conducted in South Australia since 2002 to argue that these interventions lack, or purposefully avoid, the recognition of a socio-cultural dimension of the 'problem' they are addressing.

Through a discussion of the cultural politics within Australia, Warin shows that obesity policies and interventions in this country are "embedded in medicalised and middle-class cultures" and fail to "address the cultural contexts of the communities they target". As a political process embedded in culture, the decision of which terminology should be used, or avoided, reveals the particular knowledges, beliefs, and ideologies that are prioritised in Australian obesity policymaking. Words such as "social class", "disadvantage", or even "fat", as Warin problematises, can be unpalatable to government staff who prefer a more technical language that links to the "individualising discourses of obesity prevention". This chapter also provides powerful examples of how critical obesity research is in constant tension with the ideas and ideals of policymakers and government staff and also invites the reader to question why "culture and cultural practices" are "remarkably absent in policy and interventions" if they are key to understanding obesity.

The prevailing evidence-based, de-cultured, technical approach to obesity policymaking has produced almost uniform responses to the problem around the world. In the next chapter of this section, Mabel Gracia-Arnaiz shows the problematics of adopting standardised policy measures that do not consider the local context of implementation. Through a critical analysis of the *2005 Spanish Strategy for Nutrition, Physical Activity and the Prevention of Obesity* (*2005 NAOS Strategy*), Gracia-Arnaiz argues that this policy blames individuals for their alleged inadequate eating and exercise behaviours without paying attention to the structural macroeconomic factors that shape these behaviours. Showing how the economic crisis of the late 2000s changed the diet and physical activity patterns in Spain, Gracia-Arnaiz claims that Spanish policymakers should first consider the role of "economic policies in the increase of poverty and social inequality", if obesity policies are to be effective.

One of the main components of the *2005 NAOS Strategy* is the promotion of 'healthy lifestyles' in schools through nutrition and physical activity programs, an anti-obesity policy trend that is widely popular and celebrated as 'effective' around the world (for works challenging this idea, see Burrows', Land's, Leahy's and colleagues', and Tenorio's chapters in this volume). Considered as 'ideal' anti-obesity spaces, schools have been the object of myriad interventions of multiple kinds since the beginning of the so-called obesity epidemic. The strategies to 'fight' obesity from within schools have been implemented both as part of the official curriculum or as separate programs that operate independently from or parallelly to it.

In terms of the former, governments around the world have modified their study plans to match policymakers' and public health experts' desires of addressing obesity through the curriculum. Physical education has, of course, been positioned as the natural space to prevent obesity. In the next chapter of this section, Leanne Petherick and Moss Norman discuss the ways in which two Physical and Health Education (PHE) curriculum documents in British Columbia have changed to accommodate anti-obesity work in this subject area. Through the critical analysis of the two documents, Petherick and Norman discuss the shifting ways in which the obesity discourse "continuous to be a force in influencing public health, even in its apparent absence". Theoretically, the authors draw on the Foucauldian scholarship associated with the study of health as a technology of government. Thus, Petherick and Norman propose to approach the curriculum not an isolated document but a social construction that is "rendered intelligible in relation to broader discursive and affective public pedagogies". From this perspective, the authors claim that the shift in language use between the 2006 and

the 2016 syllabi reflects the integration of the obesity discourse with, let's say, a more encompassing healthy lifestyles discourse rather than the vanishing of the latter.

Similar to the generalised enthusiasm for school-based policies as highly effective
anti-obesity measures, in the last five years, countries around the world have imposed, in
slightly different ways, a tax on sugar as an attempt to disincentivise people from consuming
processed foods and drinks with added sugar, which, some policymakers and public health
experts think, will curb obesity. Given the potential negative economic effects that this fiscal
measure supposes for some actors, the sugar tax has become a widely contested obesity policy
globally. While there have been recent efforts to explore this measure beyond its 'efficacy',
critical discussions about the ethical implications of taxing as an anti-obesity measure are
mostly absent.

In the final chapter in this section, T. M. Wilkinson addresses this gap by questioning
the "fairness", the "welfare", and the "social justice" arguments that are commonly raised in
the discussions to justify the pertinency of sugar tax. For analytical purposes, as he clarifies,
T. M. Wilkinson builds his discussion of the arguments in favour for tax and government
intervention proceeding as "if obesity were bad for health". Imbued by the complexity of
a topic that touches on personal freedom, political systems, and economic interests, T. M.
Wilkinson argues that, while these arguments "could genuinely justify reducing choices",
thinking that obesity can be reduced by "raising the costs of the decisions that cause it" is
not an entirely ethically justified idea. Instead, as the author concludes, the arguments in
favour of taxing sugar for the sake of health rest upon stigmatising assumptions such as "that
the obese do impose substantial costs on others or that badly off people would benefit from
having fewer options".

32

EVIDENCE AS A FIG LEAF

Obesity policies and institutional filters in Denmark

Signild Vallgårda

The increase in the proportion of people with obesity, or severe overweight, as it is called in Danish policy papers, has caused great concern among many people including politicians. In 2017, of the adult population in Denmark, 19 percent reported a BMI above 30 (Sundheds-styrelsen, 2020). This was the case for only 5.5 percent in 1987 (Kjøller & Rasmussen, 2002). Over the years, the Danish Health Authority (DHA) [*Sundhedsstyrelsen*] has published several recommendations regarding treatment and prevention of severe and moderate overweight aimed at municipalities and general practitioners (Dansk Selskab for Almen Medicin, Sund-hedsstyrelsen, 2006, 2009; Sundhedsstyrelsen, 2014, 2018). These publications had their focus on tracing individuals with severe overweight and on behavioural changes. The most recent publication concerns "lifestyle interventions addressing severe overweight" (Sund-hedsstyrelsen, 2019). Politicians in Denmark tend to consider the term severe overweight as having fewer negative connotations than "fedme" (obesity or fatness). Here, I use severe overweight and obesity synonymously.

During the recent decades, the idea of evidence-based policy has become popular in Denmark as well as in other countries (Nutley, Morton, Jung, & Boaz, 2010). Politicians and civil servants commission research more often and they more often use references to evidence in policy documents and debates (Vallgårda, 2003). This suggests a belief in the ability of research to provide answers to policy questions or a need to legitimise policies with references to research or both.

In this chapter, I aim to answer four questions: What is the content of the obesity recommendations? Can one find an explanation for the chosen focus? What role does the institutional setting play for the recommendations given? What is the role of research and evidence in the recommendations?

The text I studied to answer these questions is a draft of the 2019 Recommendations to Municipalities on Lifestyle Intervention Addressing Severe Overweight (Recommendations) published by the DHA (see Sundhedsstyrelsen, 2019). Thus, as the name of the document reveals, from the very beginning, it was restricted in its focus; it should address people's behaviours and intervene among individuals. The recommendations were aimed at professionals in the municipalities, at hospitals, and in general practice who work with people with severe overweight. The Recommendations were preceded by a report commissioned by the DHA on the evidence for the effects of lifestyle interventions and were

DOI: 10.4324/9780429344824-39

written by a group of researchers from the University of Copenhagen (Sundhedsstyrelsen & Københavns Universitet, 2018). The DHA did not wish other interventions to be considered such as surgery and medical treatments. Structural interventions were not mentioned – they were seemingly not considered.

Evidence and policymaking

The role of research in policymaking has been the topic of a wide range of research and theoretical considerations (Weiss, 1979; Davies, Nutley, & Smith, 2000; Sanderson, 2002; Greenhalgh & Russel, 2009; Frey & Ledermann, 2010; Stevens, 2007; Greenhalgh & Wieringa, 2011). Tony Blair's UK Labour government, among others, launched the idea of evidence-based policy, which has since gained ground. The mantra was: "What matters is what works", and research could tell politicians what works (Davies et al., 2000). With the idea of evidence-based policymaking, politicians and civil servants often seem to assume that there can be a linear and direct relation between research evidence and policies. They also seem to assume that a process, with the selection, synthesising, and critical evaluation of the best research evidence, will lead to the obvious answer to a policy problem (Greenhalgh & Russel, 2009). Researchers' faith in the ability of evidence to guide policymaking is a little less strong (Davies et al., 2000). Those who advocate evidence-based policymaking often see research evidence as context neutral and therefore consider that research from one country or population group can easily be translated to another country or population group. Researchers also often consider quantitative research to be superior to qualitative research (Greenhalgh & Russel, 2009).

However, evidence is always produced and used in specific contexts. Using a discursive institutionalist approach (Schmidt, 2010), British health policy researcher Katherine Smith (2013) shows how institutional filters tend to influence which ideas appear, and which ideas survive, in the policymaking setting. Using policies against social inequalities in health as examples, Smith (2013, p. 81) describes how institutions tend to filter, block, or reshape ideas that do not fit with "existing institutional ideas" and encourage or even exaggerate those that do. One might also describe these processes as formed by the "mental maps" of the civil servants and politicians (Pierson, 2000). They, as does everybody else, tend to see what fits into their mental maps and ignore what does not. Another factor forming the policies, which Smith mentions, is the organisation of the administration. Health policies are developed in ministries of health and are therefore usually limited to their field of responsibility – health services and health promotion activities. Moreover, the individual civil servants, Smith writes with reference to Max Weber, are even more limited in their focus by their area of responsibility and their specialisation, and one could add, educational or disciplinary background. These factors make initiatives and interventions in the areas of other ministries less obvious and if considered, difficult to implement. Smith also points out the short memory that policymaking institutions seemingly have. When civil servants change positions, their knowledge and experience are often lost, and their successors do not always learn from initiatives developed prior to their arrival in the organisation.

The institutional setting

Smith (2013, p. 82) states that "ideas are shaped by institutions". In the DHA, medical doctors play a central role, and doctors dominate the DHA's numerous advisory committees. It is situated in the central state administration as a part of the Ministry of Health. Medical doctors usually understand health issues in a biological paradigm rather than psychological or sociological paradigms. The advice the DHA sought when preparing the Recommendations was exclusively from people with a medical or natural science background. Of the five researchers in the group writing the evidence report, one was a biochemist, one was a nutritional scientist, and three were medical doctors. Despite the topic being interventions aimed at making people change their behaviour, no psychologists, sociologists, or health promotion/disease prevention researchers were involved. The working group supporting the DHA in preparing the Recommendations showed the same pattern: four medical doctors, a nurse, a representative from the patient association for people with severe overweight – who was also a postdoc in nutritional science – and the two scientists from the aforementioned group of researchers. From the DHA itself, a nutritional scientist participated as chair with the support of a staff member with a Masters in Public Health. Thus, the domination of biomedically focused experts was almost total among those preparing both the evidence base and the Recommendations supposed to result in behavioural changes of people with obesity.

In the following section, I analyse how evidence is used as defined by the DHA and the researchers. I do not discuss their definition of evidence.

Governing people's lives, changing their behaviours

The DHA suggests interventions aimed at changing people's habits when it comes not only to eating and physical activity but also to sleep, sedentary behaviour, stress, smoking, alcohol, and psychosocial issues. It mentions information, dialogue, counselling, support, and techniques aiming at behavioural changes, but it is not specific when it comes to the interventions.

One premise for the Recommendations is that weight loss will lead to better health. However, the DHA does not refer to a publication from the "Knowledge Council on Prevention", under the Danish Medical Association (Sørensen, Pedersen, Sandbæk, & Overvad, 2015), that concludes that there is no clear evidence that weight loss will lead to better health. That report concludes that a stable weight seems to be the healthiest state of being.

The DHA explains the prevalence of severe overweight as energy imbalance – a higher intake of energy than expenditure of energy. This explanation fits well with the laws of physics and is supported by many medical doctors. The doctors and scientists preparing the Recommendations subscribed to this idea. Other obesity researchers assume that the biological processes are more complex (Bray & Champagne, 2005; Guyenet & Schwartz, 2012). The disciplinary background of the people involved in the process of producing the Recommendations may have influenced their choice of explanation. The point here is not to discuss which theory is correct, but to identify which theory was chosen.

As already mentioned, the Recommendations focus on interventions among individuals with severe overweight. It is not about preventing people from becoming overweight. The suggested interventions will take place in health-care settings. People are to be traced and identified as having obesity and be persuaded to change their behaviours in a healthier direction through different approaches. In the Recommendations, one chapter is dedicated to tracing overweight people and another chapter to the lifestyle interventions.

The DHA states that the interventions are about improving quality of life, and it seems clear that weight loss is viewed as the most important means to achieving that. The authors of the Recommendations state that severe overweight reduces the quality of life for those affected. For adults, whether this reduced quality of life stems from their weight or from the way people with obesity are treated is not discussed. For children with obesity, the issue of bullying is mentioned as an issue to be dealt with.

The strong focus on weight reduction can be illustrated with word counts. Weight loss is mentioned 77 times on 40 pages. Quality of life is mentioned only 13 times. Lifestyle is mentioned 157 times, leaving no doubt that behaviours are the focus of the Recommendations. People with severe overweight shall obtain "healthier habits" (Sundhedsstyrelsen, 2019, p. 5). The suggested lifestyle interventions should not merely be an offer of support to weight reduction activity already desired by the person, but, as the Recommendations state: "If the citizen is not immediately motivated to accept the offer, one should aim at creating such motivation" (Sundhedsstyrelsen, 2019, p. 19). The health professionals should have the abilities to create trust and motivate the citizen, first to actively participate in the weight-loss programmes and then to be helped to maintain the achieved behavioural changes.

In line with the previous recommendations, tracking down and identifying people with severe overweight is envisioned to take place in health facilities, schools, and in other public institutions. When detected, people shall subsequently be offered help with weight reduction. Tracking down people with severe overweight is an activity that should be undertaken not only by health professionals but also by employees in the municipalities – those at job centres and drop-in centres and those offering special housing support [*botilbud*] – and at activities and gatherings organised by the municipality. The tracking-down activities can be described both as an expression of solicitude and as an infringement of people's integrity, and they constitute an activity that may be stigmatising.

The Recommendations note that there is pronounced social inequality in the prevalence of obesity; yet, no explicit interventions to address social inequalities are suggested. However, more individuals with low incomes have severe overweight, making them more likely than others to be offered interventions. Some of the areas where the DHA suggests that tracking should occur, for instance, job centres and drop-in centres, are more often visited by people living in poverty. Thus, poor people are more likely to become objects of these activities. Nevertheless, the detection is not mentioned as a means of reducing health inequalities.

The DHA mentions numerous causes of severe overweight, including individual, societal, genetic, environmental, and psychosocial factors (Sundhedsstyrelsen, 2019, pp. 11–12). But it does not seem to consider other factors apart from behaviour when addressing weight reduction. According to the evidence report, behavioural changes can be achieved not only by finding and contacting people but also by changing their environment – as suggested by the slogan "make the healthy choices the easy choices". The reason why the environment does not play any role in the DHA's Recommendations could be what Smith (2013, p. 90) has described as "institutional filters". These filters prevent activities being considered that are outside the realm of the Ministry of Health.

The Recommendations also illustrate the short memory of institutions. A little more than a decade ago, the DHA published two small books, one on stigma (Sundhedsstyrelsen, 2008) and another on public health ethics (Sundhedsstyrelsen, 2009). The DHA also addressed ethics in a short paragraph in a publication on prevention of overweight from 2018 (Sundhedsstyrelsen, 2018), to which the Recommendations refer. In that publication, the DHA states that it is important to situate obesity as a broad social problem rather than as a matter of exclusive personal responsibility. It also emphasises the risk of stigmatising people with overweight. However, none of these concerns is addressed in the Recommendations; neither stigma nor ethics is mentioned.

The appropriateness of the interventions from perspectives other than weight loss is not considered. Greenhalgh and Russel (2009) argue that the focus on what works in evidence-based policy "eclipses equally important questions about desirable ends and appropriate means" (p. 310). The question about "appropriate means" was what politicians from the two left-wing parties and the right-wing populist Danish People's Party addressed when they expressed concerns that the recommended interventions, especially the tracing, would increase stigmatisation of people with severe overweight (Overgaard, 2020). They asked for a discussion of more aspects of appropriateness than merely the effects on weight and weight maintenance.

The evidence base

The request for evidence-based policies has led Danish authorities to commission overviews of research in their work on policies. Following this pattern, the DHA commissioned researchers from the Department of Nutrition, Exercise and Sports at the University of Copenhagen to provide "evidence for health effects of lifestyle interventions aimed at achieving weight loss or weight maintenance among children, young people, adults and older people with severe overweight" (Sundhedsstyrelsen & Københavns Universitet, 2018, p. 6). Thus, the DHA collection of evidence was limited to the field of behavioural interventions among individuals. The researchers were asked to evaluate and present the evidence from this field. The purpose was to support the DHA in its work with Recommendations about lifestyle interventions. To better cover the field, the researchers carried out the task primarily by using systematic reviews of research.

The researchers used the Grading of Recommendations Assessment, Development and Evaluation (GRADE) approach (Balshem et al., 2011) to evaluate the included systematic reviews. Of the 23 reviews graded, only three had a high grade, implying that the authors were very certain that the true effects were close to the estimated effects. In five reviews, they were moderately certain, meaning that the effect could be as the estimated effect, but it could also be substantially different. In 15 of the reviews, the authors had low or very low trust in the estimated effect. This indicates that the evidence base was relatively poor because much of the research was of poor quality (Sundhedsstyrelsen & Københavns Universitet, 2018). The DHA stated that it would take its starting point from the best possible evidence (Sundhedsstyrelsen, 2019). However, nothing was said about the limited evidence and its poor quality.

Furthermore, very few of the reviews studied could conclude that there were significant effects of the lifestyle interventions. The researchers state in the report that there was "moderate" evidence of a weight reduction of on average 1.5–3.5 kilos, which, for most people with obesity, is less than a 5 percent weight loss. The researchers considered a 5 percent weight loss as clinically relevant, thus having a health effect. They also pointed to the risk of selection bias because participants who achieved an effect of an intervention would be more inclined to continue. They found no reliable evidence of weight loss and weight-loss maintenance in Danish interventions. Accordingly, they had no relevant knowledge from the Danish context. The researchers did not seem to consider the importance of the context in which these studies were conducted or whether the results could easily be translated to a Danish context. This view could be explained by a view of humans as isolated individuals rather than as parts of social contexts, which seems to dominate the research selected for the report.

With their exclusive focus on obesity, the researchers did not include in the report other literature about lifestyle interventions in Denmark not specifically addressing obesity. Notably, a large intervention study with more than 50,000 participants, of whom more than

11,000 were included in the intervention group (Jørgensen et al, 2014), was not included in the systematic review. The intervention included smoking cessation, diet, and physical activity. After ten years' follow-up, no significant effect could be detected on ischaemic heart disease, stroke, or total mortality.

Few studies have investigated differences in lifestyle interventions between subgroups of the population. Thus, there was no knowledge about whether groups differed in their response to the interventions. Accordingly, the DHA recommends the interventions be organised in similar ways across subgroups. The logic was obviously that, since they did not know whether there were differences in the effect across subgroups, municipalities and health professional were encouraged not to differentiate. The recommendation was made based on the lack of evidence.

All in all, the researchers' report documented that the evidence for lifestyle interventions was of poor quality and showed minor effects. Nonetheless, in the Recommendations, the DHA refers repeatedly to evidence, often with reference to the researchers' report. The word evidence is used 44 times. Sometimes, the evidence does not even pertain to what the DHA writes about. One example is when the DHA writes that "new epidemiological studies and randomized controlled studies have shown that a positive health effect can be achieved if overweight is reduced" (Sundhedsstyrelsen, 2019, p.18). The studies referred to did not deal with intended weight loss but with weight loss from childhood to adulthood and the risk of diabetes and colon cancer in adulthood (Bjerregaard, Jensen, Sørensen, & Baker, 2018; Jensen et al., 2018). The studies included neither conclusions about a causal relation between weight loss and health nor about general health effects. A similarly lenient attitude to documentation of evidence can also be found in policy papers from other institutions such as the WHO and the EU (Vallgårda, 2018). This suggests that authorities sometimes use evidence more as legitimation of its standpoints than as something informing them.

An example of how the DHA moulded evidence to fit the positions held is the following statement:

> The evidence did not reveal any difference with regard to adult weight loss depending on whether the session was face-to-face or online. There are, however, indications that face-to-face interventions have a greater effect. Therefore, it is recommended that guidance of adults take place face-to-face.
>
> *(Sundhedsstyrelsen, 2019, p. 29)*

In this case, the DHA recommends the more time-consuming intervention without any evidence base.

The DHA did not mention the limitations of the evidence – there was no mention of the quality of the research or the lack of documented substantial significant effects of the interventions.

There might be different explanations for the DHA's reluctance to use the commissioned research and, instead, use their misinterpretations of the research as "evidence". One reason could be the fact that the DHA had invested much of their own time and prestige as well as that of the researchers, and therefore, they were not prepared to change direction and recognise that lifestyle interventions were perhaps not the best means to achieve weight loss. Another reason could be that the DHA was not interested in the research in the first place and that it commissioned it only to legitimise the intervention it had already decided to encourage. A third possibility is that the focus on lifestyle or behaviour interventions targeting individuals is so strong in Danish public health policies (Vallgårda, 2011) that the mental maps of the employees and the advisors at the DHA had prepared them to see only what confirmed their already-held assumptions. The weaknesses of the evidence were filtered out despite the reactions from general practitioners. The Danish College of General Practitioners withdrew its representative from the expert group advising the DHA that they did not consider the evidence base for the interventions satisfactory. The representative from the College stated that "it is unethical to track people down if you do not have an effective treatment to offer them" (Overgaard, 2020). The representative further criticised the Recommendations for not looking at possible negative effects of detection and of offering weight-loss interventions as well as for not having psychological and other expertise in the evidence group or working group (Olsen, 2020). This illustrates that not all medical doctors subscribe to the same ideas.

Danish obesity policies have similarities with those from other European countries when it comes to the focus on behavioural changes (Vallgårda, 2015). What stands out is their emphasis on tracking down or detecting. They are more individualising. Health professionals and others shall single out people with severe overweight and address them in person and not only through collective measures.

Compared with another country launching an obesity strategy, namely the UK (Department of Health and Social Care, 2020), the Danish strategy is more limited in its approach regarding the means suggested. Focus on behavioural changes is the same in the UK plan, but it does not target individuals to the same extent and in no way suggests tracking down and identifying people with obesity. In the UK plan, it is stated, "Tackling obesity is not just about an individual's effort, it is also about the environment we live in, the information we are given to make choices; the choices we are offered; and the influences that shape those choices" (Department of Health and Social Care, 2020). The UK government wishes to use legislation on advertising and on calorie information on food and drink including those that consumed in cafes and restaurants. It also suggests restrictions on reduced prices on large quantities and organising shops to avoid tempting people to buy foods high in fat, sugar, and salt. In Denmark, some stakeholders suggest a broader approach. Cancer Denmark suggests in a campaign launched in August 2020 that access to food and beverages, portion sizes, and prices are important factors in increasing the obesity prevalence (Rohweder, 2020). It has not yet suggested legislation.

Conclusion

In its Recommendations for dealing with severe overweight, the DHA has focused exclusively on behavioural interventions among individuals concerning nutrition and physical activity. It has stated that it will rely on evidence-based activities, but it does not seem to register or care about the poor quality of much of the evidence or the lack of effect it shows. Moreover, it uses the evidence in a highly selective, even misleading, manner. The DHA addresses severe overweight, a high BMI, as a health issue, without much discussion of whether it is a relevant measure.

The content of the Recommendations about lifestyle interventions seems to be shaped by the institution where they were developed, with medical dominance, institutional boundaries of the DHA, and the long-term focus on individual behaviours dominating Danish public health policies. Institutional filters alone cannot explain the content, but they can contribute to explaining why the DHA chose one specific path out of many possible paths.

When it comes to the evidence base, the problem is not that the DHA has considerations other than those for which it can use evidence. Science cannot answer all questions, and there are values that must also guide the decisions. But it could be seen as a problem if it uses evidence in a misleading way. The DHA cannot use evidence to decide whether intervening among people with severe overweight should be prioritised, but it can use it to inform decision-makers about whether it is plausible to use, as in this case, lifestyle interventions.

One reason why the DHA continued working with Recommendations on lifestyle interventions regarding severe overweight is probably because the work had been going on for so long. The researchers had been asked to provide evidence for such interventions. When this evidence turned out to be relatively weak and often of poor quality, it was seemingly not feasible for the DHA to change direction and look for other ways to address the prevalence of overweight; other ways that might have included using sociological theories and looking at the social contexts.

The idea behind evidence-based policymaking was certainly that it could improve the results, making it possible to better achieve the politically defined goals. The way evidence is used in this case, as in several others, seems to a larger extent to legitimise the ideas already held by the policymakers rather than informing them.

References

Balshem, H., Heland, M., Schünemann, H. J., Oxman, A. D., Kunz, R., Brozek, J., ... Guyatt GH. (2011). GRADE guidelines: 3. Rating the quality of evidence. *Journal of Clinical Epidemiology, 64*, 401–406. doi: 10.1016/j.jclinepi.2010.07.015

Bjerregaard, L. G., Jensen, B. W., Sørensen, T. I. A., & Baker, J. L. (2018). Change in overweight from childhood to early adulthood and risk of type 2 diabetes. *New England Journal of Medicine, 378*, 1302–1312. doi: 10.1056/NEJMoa1713231

Bray, G. A., & Champagne, C. M. (2005). Beyond energy balance: There is more to obesity than kilocalories. *Journal of the American Dietetic Association, 105*(5), suppl., 17–23. doi: 10.1016/j.jada.2005.02.018

Dansk Selskab for Almen Medicin, Sundhedsstyrelsen. (2006). *Opsporing og behandling af overvægt hos førskolebørn.* [Tracing and treatment of overweight among preschool children.] Copenhagen: Sundhedsstyrelsen.

Dansk Selskab for Almen Medicin, Sundhedsstyrelsen. (2009). *Opsporing og behandling af overvægt hos voksne.* [Tracing and treatment of overweight among adults.] Copenhagen: Sundhedsstyrelsen.

Davies, H. T. O., Nutley, S., & Smith, P. (2000). *What works? Evidence-based policy and practice in public services.* Bristol: The Policy Press.

Department of Health and Social Care. (2020). *Tackling obesity: Empowering adults and children to healthier lives.* London: Department of Health and Social Care. Retrieved from https://www.gov.uk/government/publications/tackling-obesity-government-strategy/tackling-obesity-empowering-adults-and-children-to-live-healthier-lives

Frey, K., & Ledermann, S. (2010). Introduction: Evidence-based policy: A concept in geographical and substantive expansion. *German Policy Studies, 6*(2), 1–15.

Greenhalgh, T., & Russel, J. (2009). Evidence-based policymaking: A critique. *Perspectives in Biology and Medicine, 52*(2), 304–318. doi: 10.1353/pbm.0.0085

Greenhalgh, T., & Wieringa, S. (2011). Is it time to drop the metaphor of 'knowledge translation'? A critical literature review. *Journal of the Royal Society of Medicine, 104*(12), 501–509. doi: 10.1258/jrsm.2011.110285

Guyenet, S. J., Schwartz, M. W. (2012). Regulation of food intake, energy balance, and body fat mass: Implications for the pathogenesis and treatment of obesity. *The Journal of Clinical Endocrinology & Metabolism, 97*(3), 745–755. doi: 10.1210/jc.2011-2525

Jensen, B. W., Bjerrregaard, L. G., Ängquist, L., Gögenur, I., Renehan, A. G., Osler, M.,... Baker, J. L. (2018). Change in weight status from childhood to early adulthood and late adulthood risk of colon cancer in men: A population-based cohort study. *International Journal of Obesity, 42*, 1797–1803. doi: 10.1038/s41366-018-0109-y

Jørgensen, T., Jacobsen, R. K., Toft, U., Aadahl, M., Glümer, C., & Pisinger, C. (2014). Effect of screening and lifestyle counselling on incidence of ischaemic heart disease in general population: Inter 99 randomised trial. *BMJ, 348*, g3617. doi: 10.1136/bmj.g3617

Kjøller, M., Rasmussen, N. K. (2002). *Sundhed og sygelighed i Danmark 2000 og udviklingen siden 1987.* [Health and disease in Denmark 2000 and the development since 1987.] Copenhagen: Statens Institut for Folkesundhed.

Nutley, S., Morton, S., Jung, T., & Boaz, A. 2010. Evidence and policy in six European countries: Diverse approaches and common challenge. *Evidence & Policy, 6*(2), 131–144. doi: 10.1332/174426410X502275

Olsen, T. L. (2020). Læger smækker med døren: Nye råd mod fedme er oldnordiske. [Doctors slam the door: New advice against obesity are antediluvian.] Retrieved from http://www.dr.dk

Overgaard, M. (2020). Politikere raser over udskældte anbefalinger: Det stigmatiserer svært overvægtige. [Politicians are furious about severely criticised recommendations: They stigmatise people with severe overweight.] Retrieved from http://www.AvisenDanmark.dk

Pierson, P. (2000). Increasing returns, path dependence, and the study of politics. *American Political Science Review, 94*(2), 251–267. doi: 10.2307/2586011

Rohweder, M. (2020). Kræftens Bekæmpelse lancerer kampagne om overvægt: Vi kobler to tabuer. [Cancer Denmark launches a campaign about overweight: We combine two taboos.] *Sundhedspolitisk Tidsskrift,* 31 August 2020.

Sanderson, I. (2002). Evaluation, policy learning and evidence-based policy making. *Public Administration Review, 80*(1), 1–22. doi: 10.1111/1467-9299.00292

Schmidt, V. (2010). Taking ideas and discourses seriously: Explaining change through discursive institutionalism as the fourth 'new institutionalism'. *European Political Science Review, 2*(1), 1–25. doi: 10.1017/S175577390999021X

Smith, K. (2013). Institutional filters: The translation and re-circulation of ideas about health inequalities within policy. *Policy & Politics, 41*(1), 81–100. doi: 10.1332/030557312X655413

Sørensen TIA, Pedersen BK, Sandbæk A, Overvad K. (2015). *Skal overvægtige tabe sig?* (Shall people with overweight lose weight?) Copenhagen: Vidensråd for forebyggelse.

Stevens A. (2007). Survival of the ideas that fit: An evolutionary analogy for the use of evidence in policy. *Social policy and society, 6*(1), 25–35. https://doi.org/10.1017/S1474746406003319

Sundhedsstyrelsen. (2008). *Stigmatisering – debatoplæg om et dilemma i forebyggelsen.* [Stigma – discussion paper about a dilemma in disease prevention.] Copenhagen: Sundhedsstyrelsen.

Sundhedsstyrelsen. (2009). *Etik i forebyggelse og sundhedsfremme.* [Ethics in disease prevention and health promotion.] Copenhagen: Sundhedsstyrelsen.

Sundhedsstyrelsen. (2014). *Opsporing af overvægt og tidlig indsats for børn og unge i skolealderen.* [Tracing of overweight and early intervention towards children and young people in school age.] Copenhagen: Sundhedsstyrelsen.

Sundhedsstyrelsen. (2018). *Forebyggelsespakke – overvægt.* [Prevention package – overweight]. Copenhagen: Sundhedsstyrelsen.

Sundhedsstyrelsen. (2019). *Livsstilsintervention ved svær overvægt. Anbefalinger for kommunale tilbud til børn og voksne. Høringsudkast.* [Recommendations to municipalities about lifestyle intervention addressing severe overweight. Consultation draft.] Copenhagen: Sundhedsstyrelsen.

Sundhedsstyrelsen. (2020). *Social ulighed i sundhed og sygdom. Udviklingen i Danmark i perioden 2010–2017.* [Social inequalities in health and disease. Development in Denmark 2010–2017]. Copenhagen: Sundhedsstyrelsen/SDU.

Sundhedsstyrelsen, Københavns Universitet. (2018). *Evidens for livsstilsinterventioner til børn og voksne med svær overvægt.* [Evidence for lifestyle interventions towards children and adults with obesity.] Copenhagen: Sundhedsstyrelsen.

Vallgårda, S. (2003). *Folkesundhed som politik. Danmark og Sverige fra 1930 til i dag.* [Public health as policy. Denmark and Sweden from 1930 until today.] Aarhus: Aarhus Universitetsforlag.

Vallgårda, S. (2011). Addressing individual behaviours and living conditions: Four Nordic public health policies. *Scandinavian Journal of Public Health, 39*(6), suppl, 6–10. doi: 10.1177/1403494810378922

Vallgårda, S. (2015). Governing obesity. Policies from England, France, Germany and Scotland. *Social Science & Medicine, 147*, 317–323. doi: 10.1016/j.socscimed.2015.11.006

Vallgårda, S. (2018). Childhood obesity policies – mighty concerns, meek reactions. *Obesity Reviews, 19*(3), 295–301. doi: 10.1111/obr.12639

Weiss, C. (1979). The many meanings of research utilization. *Public Administration Review, 39*(5), 426–431. doi: 10.2307/3109916

33

THE METABOLIC RIFT BETWEEN CULTURE AND LIBERALISM IN OBESITY INTERVENTIONS AND POLICY

Megan Warin

Introduction

Despite over two decades of acknowledging overweight and obesity as a national priority, and admission that "rates of overweight and obesity have risen dramatically in recent decades in all age groups" (Commonwealth of Australia, 2018, p. xv), Australia has no national strategy to tackle obesity. There have been many government reports on obesity since 1997 (e.g. *Acting on Australia's Weight: A Strategic Plan for the Prevention of Overweight and Obesity* [National Health & Medical Research Council, 1997] and *Weighing It Up: Obesity in Australia* [Parliament of Australia, 2009]) as well as the establishment of the National Preventative Health Taskforce in 2007 and the Australian National Preventive Health Agency (ANPHA) (established in 2011 and defunded in 2014). There have been numerous attempts to change people's behaviours (e.g. social marketing and mass media campaigns, school-based and work-place interventions, some community interventions, food labelling attempts, and restriction of advertising to children), but these have been ad hoc, and there is very little research evidence of the effectiveness of interventions (Warin & Zivkovic, 2019).

It is well documented that obesity prevention and intervention programs have limited immediate success, and benefits are rarely sustained (Baum & Fisher, 2014; Roberto et al., 2015; Baker, Gill, Friel, Carey, & Kay, 2017; Wake, 2018). Models of obesity prevention are limited by an emphasis on individualistic, behaviour change strategies (e.g. Cohn, 2014; Prentice, 2015); a lack of theoretical foundations (e.g. Delormier, Frohlich, & Potvin, 2009); a lack of recognition of how the social context shapes behaviour and how social change occurs (Warin, Turner, Moore, & Davies, 2008; Aphramor, Brady, & Gingras, 2013; Warin, 2018); and an inability to address the social gradient of obesity (Olsen, Dixon, Banwell, & Baker, 2009; Broom & Warin, 2011; Farrell, Warin, Moore, & Street, 2016a).

Most health promotion programs and policies aimed at tackling obesity position the individual as a "sovereign consumer" conforming to a model of rational behaviour (Warde & Southerton, 2012) who, once informed about risks, will change their beliefs and their behaviours. Even community-based interventions which use socio-ecological theory as explanatory models, drift back in practice to what Furedi (2006) calls the "politics of behaviour"; lifestyle interventions and social marketing strategies that attempt to change individual behaviours (Baker et al., 2017).

DOI: 10.4324/9780429344824-40

In light of the inability to address this problem, in 2018, the Australian government called an inquiry into the "obesity epidemic" (The Senate Select Committee into the Obesity Epidemic in Australia). The terms of reference sought to examine (broadly) the prevalence and causes of overweight and obesity, the health and economic costs, and the effectiveness of existing policies and programs introduced by Australian governments to improve diets and prevent childhood obesity. Many submissions to the inquiry noted the lack of government investment in supporting children, families, and communities to change eating practices and the need for the government to legislate and regulate to achieve systemic changes within the food system. In his submission, the Chief Executive Officer of the Public Health Association of Australia summed up the lack of government investment in stating that the lack of high-profile education and prevention programs at a national level raises the question of government's commitment and investment in public health: "There seems to be … little appetite to boost investment in public health or prevention, even though we've got an enormous body of evidence that suggests this is one of the best buys we can make in health" (Commonwealth of Australia, 2018, p. 16).

As a social anthropologist, I position cultural knowledges and practices as central to understanding food, eating, bodies, and obesity. In our co-authored Senate submission (Warin et al., 2018), we focused on the cultural contexts of obesity, presenting classed and gendered factors that impact on health inequalities, and people's ability to eat, and to eat well. In putting forward a case for the relationships between disadvantage and obesity, we argued that factors such as economic resources, gender, education, employment, housing, discrimination, and social class fundamentally shape the unequal social patterning of obesity. In foregrounding taste as culturally informed, we drew on Bourdieu's concept of *habitus* to position food and eating as much more than a simple process of bodily nourishment (Bourdieu, 1979/1984, 1977). *Habitus* refers to the ways in which we embody cultural practices in relation to classed consumption, for example, a preference for certain types of foods that signal one's gender, identity, and cultural capital (from a desire for smashed avocado to meat pies). We argued that public health interventions around food, eating, and bodies are symbolic of an idealised middle-class healthy lifestyle, embodying knowledge and bodily regulation to routinely structure daily life (Warin et al., 2008, 2017).

Culture and cultural practices are key to understanding obesity yet remains remarkably absent in policy and interventions.[1] Culture in health relates to the shared meanings and values on which well-being is based. As indicated above, food practices are part of one's *habitus*, and food acts as a medium of gendered caring, social relationships, enacting health, pleasure, conflict, and connectivity. Yet, in Australian obesity debates, food has become decontextualised as nutrition (Scrinis, 2013), and fatness has been historically and culturally constructed as a medical problem called "obesity." In her comparative study of two obesity intervention franchises in France and Australia (EPODE and OPAL), Hartwick notes that OPAL was not linked to any Australian food cultures, and there was no emphasis on taste, conviviality, or food appreciation. In fact, Australia "deliberately discarded the cultural principles of food and eating that were at the foundation of EPODE in France" (Hartwick, 2014, p. 305). The emphasis was on a science-based approach to health, nutrition, and physical activity in which food was narrowly characterised as either "good" or "bad."

The stripping of cultural practices from understanding food and obesity (and the concomitant interventions and policy making) is problematic. In my ethnographic work in an Australian community that has high levels of socio-economic disadvantage and has been targeted for one of Australia's largest obesity programs, our research team has been asked by staff from local and state governments to withdraw words that point to cultural contexts that are intimately related to the social organisation and provision of food – words like "social class" and "disadvantage." We noted how project officers and dieticians who came armed with the ubiquitous *Australian Guide to Healthy Eating* did not make space for different cultural food practices or reflect on their own classed assumptions about food. During cooking demonstrations, one community worker couldn't understand why local people wanted to add salt and sugar to the recipe. She revealed how taken-for-granted her taste preferences were:

> I just don't see the need to add salt. In my house, where I grew up, salt was never added to the food my parents cooked, so I just don't have the taste for it. I like the vegetable frittatas just the way they are.

This project worker understood how her own tastes were shaped by her *habitus* but in setting her experiences as the standard failed to see that others may have a different *habitus*. Community members, for example, would not make or eat polenta that was offered up to them in a "healthy recipe," as this was considered an unfamiliar, high-brow food, and not part of their everyday *habitus* (Warin & Zivkovic, 2019).

The key question that I am continually confronted with is why do socio-cultural contexts of obesities, food, and eating have no traction in health interventions or policy? Why does the mantra of "eat less and exercise more" continue to dominate, even in light of the now widespread acknowledgement that focusing on individuals through education campaigns have failed? Is this a failure of anthropologists and sociologists to make a case for wider socio-cultural factors? Is this an effect of "problem closure" (Guthman, 2013) and policy processes (Warin & Moore, 2020)? Some say that the complexity of obesity renders it impossible to fully know, and it is thus reduced to simpler energy models (think of the UK Foresight map [Ulijaszek, 2015; Sanabria, 2016]), and others say that it's the dominance of neoliberalism, and both have value. Rather than present a classic Foucauldian argument of governmentality that critiques biopower or governmentality as it has unfolded in the obesity debate (already well-covered by a number of scholars, including but not limited to, Gard & Wright, 2005; Coveney, 2006; Wright & Harwood, 2009; Mayes, 2016; Powell, 2020), I want to lay bare the political landscape that makes it difficult for the contexts of culture to reach or influence the contexts of policy and government.

There are three main interconnected parts to my argument. Using Povinelli's (2008, 2011) work, I argue that lack of attention to obesity enacts a form of symbolic violence (or as Nixon [2011] suggests "slow violence"), an ordinary violence that works through the depoliticisation of culture. I then extend this framing to a broader tension that political theorist Brown (2006, 2015) examines between liberal principles and culture. I make the claim that this slow violence is depoliticised by contemporary governments, as liberal values elide political and socio-cultural phenomenon. In Australian obesity debates (and perhaps elsewhere), culture and liberalism are positioned as mutually antagonistic, and this is why there is a rift between the contextual evidence anthropologists provide and the political play of liberalism. In conclusion, I suggest that acknowledging this impasse is important to understanding inaction on obesity as more than political ignorance.

Rejecting cultural work

Since 2002, colleagues and I have been conducting ethnographic fieldwork in suburbs north of the city of Adelaide, the capital of South Australia. Overweight and obesity has been identified by the State and Federal Australian governments as a significant health issue in some of these suburbs, and the State's largest childhood obesity prevention program – Obesity Prevention and Lifestyle program (OPAL) attempted to address this through a community-wide intervention between 2009 and 2017.[2] Our findings identified participants' resistance to the program – all of which were based on cultural understandings of everyday practices of food, relationality, and eating – on *habitus*. We wrote on how local workers in the food banks rejected the middle-class imperatives of healthy eating, the dislike of being told what to eat, when to eat, and the focus on healthy food rather than the more important immediacy of pleasures, taste, or cost (Warin & Zivkovic 2019). There were complaints about OPAL recipes that were unfamiliar, expensive to make, and tasteless. Sweetness, we argued, was not simply about "empty calories", but an important form of exchange and marker of relatedness and care within families and households (Zivkovic, Warin, Moore, Ward, & Jones, 2015). Moreover, small pleasures of sweetness acted as "a form of ballast against wearing out" (Berlant, 2011, p. 116).

Not everyone thought that eating breakfast (let alone cereal) was important, with some participants unable to attend to the temporal ordering of meal times, opting for "a morning fag" [cigarette] or a cup of coffee instead (Warin et al., 2017). South Asian families didn't eat cereal for breakfast, preferring noodles or rice porridge, and African families commented on the undue attention to things like "fibre" and "regularity" since coming to Australia – described as a strange attention to modes of bodily discipline and peristaltic governance. We wrote about how fatness was not always perceived as a problem for local people, and for some, it was a buffer against austerity, as a little extra fat on the bones meant you could last until the next welfare payment, or protect yourself from sexual violence. For many, being thin was not a sign of good health, but of illicit drug use, cancer, or ill-health (Zivkovic, Warin, Moore, & Ward, 2018). We wrote of the humour that some participants used to describe their bodies and interact with each other, and how joking about fatness was a strategy of destigmatising (Peacock, Bissell, & Owen, 2014) the moral weight and shame of being labelled as obese and living in an obesogenic environment. These were all shared cultural understandings concerning the relationality of food and bodies (and creative strategies to resist the stigmatising effects of obesity) that were embodied and practiced in a gendered and class-based *habitus*.

When we talked to the OPAL staff about these cultural understandings of fatness and eating, they were shocked that we would use the vernacular of "fat" rather than the more clinical terms of "overweight and obesity"; that we were critical of the paternalistic moral overtones of healthism (Crawford, 2006); and that our research found positive experiences of eating high-fat, sugary foods, and being fat. While our project was explicitly about social class, health inequalities, and obesity, we discovered that our state and local government partners found the term "class" unpalatable. Rather than viewing class as a powerful structure in society that reproduces disadvantage and inequalities, class was seen as a distasteful category and not relevant to the individualising discourses of obesity prevention (Warin & Zivkovic, 2019; Warin & Moore, 2020).

The soft death of pastoral care

Invested in singular frames that understand obesity as a result of lack of education and the wrong choices, a main platform of many obesity prevention programs is to care for people by educating them about "proper" nutrition and changing their food choices. Care, however, is fraught political terrain. Martin, Myers, and Viseu (2015) state that "practices of care are always shot through with asymmetrical power relations … care organizes, classifies, and disciplines bodies. Colonial regimes show us precisely how care can become a means of governance" (p. 3). Deeply invested in care of the community, public health programs that seek to educate about "the right food choices" can be caught in what Povinelli calls "the soft death of pastoral care" (2011, p. 167).

This soft death of care is a form of ordinary or slow violence. In her work on poverty and government neglect in remote Australian Indigenous communities, anthropologist Povinelli says that slow violence differs from momentous and memorable events like hurricanes or the global financial crisis, as it insidiously creeps into everyday life, as she writes, "distributing misery" (Povinelli, 2008, p. 162) and wearing people down. Povinelli suggests that slow violence is a "quasi-event" as it operates through ordinariness, it remains under the radar, or (as she says), "cruddy", in a way that allows an absence of ethical response.

Obesity is a form of slow violence, as it is not spectacular or instantaneous. Notwithstanding the rhetoric of "epidemic," "crisis," and "time bomb," obesity does not demand immediate attention, and its speed allows all manner of "papering over" and political abandonments to take place. In this abandonment, time is purposefully stretched out, and as Ahmann (2018) suggests, time becomes a process of delay, deferral, attrition, and accumulation. When people are unable to grasp healthy lifestyles (more often due to the unequal distribution of life chances) then they are abandoned and less likely to elicit empathy and to be blamed for their misery. Empathy slides away.

In the so-called fight against obesity in Australia, symbolic or slow violence is manifest in what Mayes (2015) calls "the continual political rejection of research demonstrating the social determinants of health" (p. 66). Because the causes of obesity are seen to be individual, there is no inspiration for genuine political action, and this approach, like in climate-change action, sabotages long-range thinking. Federal funding for the OPAL program was severely cut by a newly elected Liberal government in 2014, and after an evaluation found that there was no significant increase in the proportion of children in a healthy weight range by the end of the intervention (OPAL Evaluation, 2016), all funding ceased in 2017.

The final Senate report into the "obesity epidemic" (Commonwealth of Australia, 2018) similarly abandoned the opportunity to address health inequities: "the case for government intervention is extremely weak and there is no need for government to intervene or legislate". In the report, neither the Australian Liberal nor Labour government supported a tax on sugar-sweetened beverages or unhealthy foods as this "implies that people cannot be trusted to make healthier food choices by themselves" (p. 88), no regulation of the food industry, as this involves "regressive taxes that stigmatise and patronise individuals, harm businesses and risk jobs" (p. 88), and no legislation to restrict discretionary food and drink advertising on free-to-air television. This stance of individual freedoms and liberties was supported by all factions of government. A National Obesity Taskforce (yet another roundtable of the usual experts) was recommended as was the recommendation to add obesity to the list of chronic diseases. The strong emphasis was on more of the same – a universal one-size fits all focus on educating people (including school children) about diets and physical activity.

There was only one minor mention about addressing social determinants of health which came from a submission and not the Committee (p. 64). Nothing on disadvantage, health inequities, or poverty. Nothing on food systems. Culture was only mentioned in relation to "culturally appropriate prevention and intervention programs for Aboriginal and Torres Strait Islander communities" (p. 82). Culture was limited to a taken-for-granted assumption of national, racial, ethnic, or religious affiliation – something that Others have – rather than the embodiment of *habitus*.

Obesity prevention initiatives in Australia are embedded in medicalised and middle-class cultures, and failing to address the cultural contexts of the communities they target is a major oversight. The Senate inquiry similarly marginalised culture, ignoring the existence of different migrant, class, gender, and social relations, ruling out any systemic questions of attention to the social determinants that underpin obesity. Such derision works to depoliticise the issue. Again, I ask why do cultural contexts of obesity have no traction in policy debates, when cultural practices are key?

Depoliticisation

Political theorist Brown states that "depoliticization involves removing a political phenomenon from comprehension of its historical emergence and from a recognition of the powers that produce and contour it" (Brown, 2006, p. 15). When power and history are elided, she states that "an ontological naturalness or essentialism almost inevitably takes up residence in our understandings and explanations" (Brown, 2006, p. 15). Brown places the political ideology of liberalism at the centre of depoliticisation, and it is the convergence of liberalism that erodes the role of culture in obesity.

As a politics, liberalism is a broad church that has a history of multiple factions and constant reinvention (Frew, 2012; Bell, 2014) and has a complicated relationship with neoliberalism. Foucault (2008) states that neoliberalism is a "new programming of liberal governmentality" (p. 94) – a "reprogramming of liberalism" (Brown, 2015 p. 59) that rests on the universality of its basic principles: secularism, the rule of law, equal rights, moral autonomy, and individual liberty. There are positive aspects of liberalism (such as individual freedoms), but there also darker ones, and it is rife with paradox, irony, and double gestures. It is important to note that liberalism is a feature of both major political parties in Australia – on the right, we have arguments for a globalised economic system, and on the left, we have arguments for a more moralised economy. A lot of what transpires in the name of liberalism is considered natural or personal (in any event independent of power and political life) – which is a profound achievement of depoliticisation. We are led to believe that we are liberated, free individuals.

In the case of the "war on obesity," the nutritionist approach appeals to individuals as rational beings engaged in free and autonomous decision-making processes, unconstrained by cultural factors. This is what Yates-Doerr (2012) and others refers to as the "black boxing" of nutrition. Obesity education relies on individuals taking up information and applying this new knowledge to their behaviours (independently of context) (Warin, 2018). If healthy foods cost less than unhealthy foods, then anyone can do it. If there are footpaths to walk on, then anyone can exercise. With a bit of willpower, anyone can eat less and exercise more. If people are obese, bariatric surgery can fix them, and the free market should be open to competition to enable this. This argument was offered by the surgeons at the Senate Committee and in the government recommendations – transforming democracy – equality – into a lucrative market of surgical and tertiary intervention.

If liberalism's concerns are universal, then they are not matters of culture, as culture in this frame is identified with the particular and local. Ethnography and its attention to cultural practices are thus viewed as outside of liberal parameters. Liberalism's unit of analysis is the individual, and its primary project is maximising individual freedom, which together stand antithetically to culture's provision of the coherence and continuity of groups. If individual freedom is upheld, then this explains the distaste for government intervention (the Nanny State – Farrell, Warin, Moore, & Street, 2016b). In rejecting the imposition of a sugary drinks tax and calls to remove marketing of unhealthy food and drink from all children's settings, the Senate Report demonstrated the rule of markets. Markets involve competition, and this means inequalities (again, anathema to principles of health equity).

Liberalism, Brown (2015) argues, thus distinguishes itself from culture and sees itself as above culture, even anti-culture. Liberal principles and culture are mutual antagonists – there is a rift between them. Liberalism presumes to convert culture's collectively binding powers, its shared and public qualities, into individual and privately lived choices. In this ideology, culture (other than essentialised Others) does not get a look in. Despite having its own (unrecognised) culture, liberalism flattens culture – it flattens structures like class and social practices that reproduce cultures and enable them to flourish. As liberalism essentialises culture to ethnically marked religious beliefs, fat positivity in Pacific and Melanesian cultures (c.f. Hardin, 2015) is understood as a cultural difference – but to present findings of the value of fat in Australian contexts (as material and corporeal difference) is unacceptable. Fat – paradoxically itself a result of unbridled liberalism – is negative, bad, and has to be excised from bodies. And when people fail to act according to liberal ideals, abandonment occurs.

Similarly, liberalism helped to explain how all sides of politics in the Senate inquiry came to meet in the central road of liberalist ideals. Often, we think of our political parties being at odds in terms of the individual and the collective, with one side being much more heavily invested in a particular brand of neoliberalism. But, ironically, it was not just the right promoting liberalism, but the left also, both meeting in the middle ground of the liberated, individual self. No party attended to the need to understand cultural practices of food and eating, the social determinants of health, or supported the recommendation for regulation and legislation, as liberalism upholds the freedom to be ourselves and a supposed (yet misrecognised) aversion to government intervention.

Conclusion

If fundamental aspects of culture such as social class, disadvantage, or poverty are viewed in liberalism as unpalatable (despite the growth of inequality in Australian society [Davidson, Bradbury, Wong, & Hill, 2020]), how do we elevate our research to a policy level? How can we make culture matter?

In 2017, the World Health Organisation released a report entitled: "Culture Matters: Using a cultural contexts of health approach to enhance policy-making" (Napier et al., 2017). This is part of an international aim to promote a "culturally grounded approach to enrich policies related to health and well-being ... re-evaluating assumptions about what constitutes evidence and supporting strategies that integrate the complexities of lived experiences into an expanded evidence base" (2017, p. iv). This comes off the back of the 2014 Lancet Commission on *Culture and Health* which argued that "the systematic neglect of culture in health and health care is the single biggest barrier to the advancement of the highest standard of health worldwide" (Napier et al., 2014, p. 1610). But how can we do this when liberalism is at odds with culture?

Brown argues that liberalism and neoliberalism has led to a hollowing-out of contemporary liberal democracy (2015, p. 18), a slow destruction from within and "undoing of demos" as her book title (2015) attests. Like Povinelli's slow violence, this effect she says is "more termitelike than lionlike" (Brown, 2015, p. 35). I have used this framing of liberalism to provide a deeper understanding of the process of depoliticisation of the many cultural practices that are fundamental to food, eating, bodies, and obesity. I have focused on liberalism – rather than neoliberalism – as I have honed in on the values of liberty and freedom that all political parties use, as these undergrid the more recent attention to market rationality that is at the core of neoliberalism. Liberalism enables slow violence to occur and for abandonment of people who cannot make the perceived right choices. Under liberalism, class inequalities are rescripted to appear as a consequence of individual choices, and poverty is "deserved" or "no excuse". Positive values of freedom and liberty have, in this context, been mobilised to disengage people from shared collectives, flattening cultures, universalising cultures, and positioning liberalism as anti-culture. And it is precisely this acultural positioning of liberalism that makes it possible to remove recognition of the power that produces the metabolic rift between food systems, public health, and equity priorities.

Acknowledgements

This work was supported by an Australian Research Council Future Fellowship (Project ID: FT140100825) and the Channel 7 Children's Research Foundation (19/10683447). A version of this paper was delivered as a keynote to the sixth British Sociology Association (BSA) Sociology of Food Study Group Conference in Prato, Italy (2019). Thanks to the BSA, Monash University, Julie Parsons, Deana Leahy, JaneMaree Maher, Sian Supski, Peter Beilharz, John Coveney, and all the participants who provided thought provoking questions and feedback. I am especially grateful to my colleagues Tanya Zivkovic and Vivienne Moore.

Notes

1 Ulijaszek (2015) makes the same observations about the UK project Foresight Obesities, concluding that "key experts to the project showed a bias against critical social science approaches to obesity" (p. 218, c.f. 2017, p. 177).
2 The program ran from 2009 to 2017 and targeted 20 regions (across four timed phases) across the State of South Australia where disadvantage was greatest. The program impacted one quarter of the State's population.

References

Ahmann, C. (2018). "It's exhausting to create an event out of nothing": Slow violence and the manipulation of time. *Cultural Anthropology, 33*(1), 142–171.
Aphramor L., Brady J., & Gingras J. (2013). Advancing critical dietetics: Theorising health at every size. In: E. Abbotts and A. Lavis (Eds.), *Why we eat, how we eat: Contemporary encounters between foods and bodies* (pp. 85–102). Farnham: Ashgate.
Baker, P., Gill, T., Friel, S., Carey, G., & Kay, A. (2017). Generating political priority for regulatory interventions targeting obesity prevention: An Australian case study. *Social Science and Medicine, 177,* 141–149.
Baum, F., & Fisher, M. (2014). Why behavioral health promotion endures despite its failure to reduce health inequities. *Sociology of Health and Illness, 36*(2), 213–225.
Bell, D. (2014). What is liberalism? *Political Theory, 42*(6), 682–715.
Berlant, L. (2011). *Cruel optimism.* London: Duke University Press.
Bourdieu, P. (1977). *Outline of a theory of practice.* R. Nice (trans.). Cambridge: Cambridge University Press.
Bourdieu, P. (1979/1984). *Distinction: A social critique of the judgement of taste.* R. Nice (trans.). London: Routledge and Kegan Paul.
Broom, D. H., & Warin, M. (2011). Gendered and class relations of obesity: Confusing findings, deficient explanations. *Australian Feminist Studies, 26*(70), 453–467.
Brown, W. (2006). *Regulating aversion: Tolerance in the age of identity and Empire.* Princeton, NJ: Princeton University Press.
Brown, W. (2015). *Undoing the demos: Neoliberalism's stealth revolution.* London: MIT Press.

Cohn, S. (2014) From health behaviors to health practices: An introduction. *Sociology of Health and Illness, 36*(2), 157–162.

Commonwealth of Australia. (2018). *Senate select committee into the obesity epidemic in Australia*. Canberra: Senate Printing Unit, Parliament House. https://www.aph.gov.au/Parliamentary_Business/Committees/Senate/Obesity_epidemic_in_Australia/Obesity/Final_Report

Coveney, J. (2006). *Food, morals and meaning: The pleasure and anxiety of eating*. 2nd ed. London: Routledge.

Crawford, R. (2006). Health as a meaningful social practice. *Health: An Interdisciplinary Journal for the Social Study of Health, Illness and Medicine, 10*(4), 401–420.

Davidson, P., Bradbury, B., Wong, M., & Hill, T. (2020). *Poverty in Australia 2020*. Australian Council of Social Service, University of New South Wales.

Delormier, T., Frohlich, K. L., & Potvin, L. (2009). Food and eating as social practice–understanding eating patterns as social phenomena and implications for public health. *Sociology of Health & Illness, 31*(2), 215–228.

Farrell, L., Warin, M., Moore, V., & Street, J. (2016a). Socio-economic divergence in public opinions about preventive obesity regulations: Is the purpose to 'make some things cheaper, more affordable' or to 'help them get over their own ignorance'? *Social Science & Medicine, 154*, 1–8.

Farrell, L., Warin, M., Moore, V., & Street, J. (2016b). Emotion in obesity discourse: Understanding public attitudes towards regulations for obesity prevention. *Sociology of Health & Illness, 38*(4), 543–558.

Foucault, M. (2008). *The birth of biopolitics: Lectures at the College de France, 1978–1979*. M. Seneallart (Ed.). London: Palgrave Macmillan.

Frew, T. (2012). Michel Foucault's *The Birth of Biopolitics* and contemporary neo-liberalism debates. *Thesis Eleven, 108*(1), 44–65.

Furedi, F. (2006). Save us from the politics of behaviour. Spiked. Retrieved from https://www.spiked-online.com/2006/09/11/save-us-from-the-politics-of-behaviour/.

Gard, M., & Wright, J. (2005). *The obesity epidemic: Science, morality and ideology*. London: Routledge.

Guthman, J. (2013). Too much food and too little sidewalk? Problematizing the obesogenic environment thesis. *Environment and Planning A, 45*(1), 142–158.

Hardin, J. (2015). Christianity, fat talk, and Samoan pastors: Rethinking the fat-positive-fat-stigma framework. *Fat Studies, 4*(2), 178–196.

Hartwick, C. (2014). *Transferring an innovation in food and lifestyle education: Development of a French childhood obesity prevention program in Australia. A cultural comparison of childhood obesity prevention in France and Australia* (Unpublished PhD thesis). Université Paris Descartes Ecole doctorale SHS (ED180) CERLIS / Education et Formation and Flinders University School of Public Health, Adelaide.

Martin, A., Myers, N., & Viseu, A. (2015). The politics of care in technoscience. *Social Studies of Science, 45*(5), 625–641.

Mayes, C. (2016). *The biopolitics of lifestyle: Foucualt, ethics and healthy choices*. New York: Routledge.

Napier, A. D., Ancarno, C., Butler, B., Calabrese, J., Chater, A., Chatterjee, H., ... Woolf, K. (2014). Culture and health. *The Lancet, 384*(9954), 1607–1639.

Napier, D., Depledge, M. H., Knipper, M., Lovell, R., Ponarin, E., Sanabria, E., & Thomas, F. (2017). *Culture matters: using a cultural contexts of health approach to enhance policy-making*. World Health Organization Regional Office for Europe.

National Health and Medical Research Council (Australia). (1997). *Acting on Australia's weight : A strategic plan for the prevention of overweight and obesity*. National Health and Medical Research Council, [Working Party on the Prevention of Overweight and Obesity] Canberra: Australian Govt. Pub. Service.

Nixon, R. (2011). *Slow violence and the environmentalism of the poor*. Cambridge, MA: Harvard University Press.

Olsen, A., Dixon, J., Banwell, C., & Baker, P. (2009). Weighing it up: The missing social inequalities dimension in Australian obesity policy discourse. *Health Promotion Journal of Australia, 20*(3), 167–171.

OPAL Evaluation (2016). *OPAL evaluation project final report*. Flinders University OPAL Evaluation Project Team. https://www.sahealth.sa.gov.au/wps/wcm/connect/73c1d1804f54bcf2b396ffdd8959a390/FLINDERSOPALFINALREPORT.PDF?MOD=AJPERES

Parliament of Australia. (2009). *Weighing it Up: Obesity in Australia.* Canberra: Printing and Publishing House of Representatives. http://www.aph.gov.au/house/committee/haa/obesity/report/front. pdf

Peacock, M., Bissell, P., & Owen, J. (2014). Shaming encounters: Reflections on contemporary understandings of social inequality and health. *Sociology, 48*(2), 387–402.

Povinelli, E. A. (2008). The child in the broom closet: States of killing and letting die. *South Atlantic Quarterly, 107*(3), 509–530.

Povinelli, E. A. (2011). *Economies of abandonment: Social belonging and endurance in late liberalism.* Durham, NC: Duke University Press.

Powell, D. (2020). *Schools, corporations, and the war on childhood obesity: How corporate philanthropy shapes public health and education.* London: Routledge.

Prentice, D. (2015). Targeting ignorance to change behavior. In M. Gross & L. McGoey (Eds), *Routledge international handbook of ignorance studies* (pp. 266–273). London: Routledge.

Roberto, C. A., Swinburn, B., Hawkes, C., Huang, T. T., Costa, S.A., Ashe, M., Zwicker, L., Cawley, J. H., & Brownell, K.D. (2015). Patchy progress on obesity prevention: Emerging examples, entrenched barriers, and new thinking. *The Lancet, 385*(9985), 2400–2409.

Sanabria, E. (2016). Circulating ignorance: Complexity and agnogenesis in the obesity 'epidemic', *Cultural Anthropology, 31*(1), 131–158.

Scrinis, G. (2013). *Nutritionism: The science and politics of dietary advice.* New York: Columbia University Press.

Ulijaszek, S. (2015). With the benefit of foresight: Reframing the obesity problem as a complex system. *BioSocieties, 10*(2), 213–228.

Wake, M. (2018). The failure of anti-obesity programmes in schools. *British Medical Journal, 360,* k507. doi: https://doi.org/10.1136/bmj.k507

Warde, A., & Southerton, D. (Eds.) (2012). Introduction. In: *COLLeGIUM: Studies across disciplines in the humanities and social sciences: The habits of consumption,* Vol. 12. Helsinki: Helsinki Collegium for Advanced Studies, pp. 1–25. http://www.helsinki.fi/collegium/journal/volumes/volume_12/index.htm

Warin, M. (2018). Information is not knowledge: Cooking and eating as skilled practice in Australian obesity education. *Australian Journal of Anthropology, 29*(1), 108–124.

Warin, M., Farrell, L., Davis, T., Moore, V., Ulijaszek, S., Coveney, J., … Mayes, C. (2018). Submission 52. https://www.aph.gov.au/Parliamentary_Business/Committees/Senate/Obesity_epidemic_in_Australia/Obesity/Submissions

Warin, M., & Moore, V. (2020). Epistemic conflicts and Achilles' heels: Constraints of a university and public sector partnership to research obesity in Australia. *Critical Public Health.* https://doi.org/10.1080/09581596.2020.1761944

Warin, M., Turner, K., Moore, V., & Davies, M. (2008). Bodies, mothers and identities: Rethinking obesity and the BMI. *Sociology of Health & Illness, 30*(1), 97–111.

Warin, M., & Zivkovic, T. (2019) *Fatness, obesity and disadvantage in the Australian suburbs: Unpalatable politics.* Cham: Palgrave Macmillan.

Warin, M., Zivkovic, T., Moore, V., & Ward, P. (2017). Moral fibre: Breakfast as a symbol of a 'good start' in an Australian obesity intervention. *Medical Anthropology: Cross-Cultural Studies in Health and Illness, 36*(3), 217–30.

Wright, J., & Harwood, V. (2009). *Biopolitics and the 'obesity epidemic': Governing bodies.* New York: Routledge.

Yates-Doerr, E. (2012). The opacity of reduction: Nutritional black-boxing and the meanings of nourishment. *Food, Culture & Society, 15*(2), 293–313.

Zivkovic, T., Warin, M., Moore, V., & Ward, P. (2018) Fat as productive: Enactments of fat in an Australian suburb. *Medical Anthropology: Cross-Cultural Studies in Health and Illness.* 37(5), 373–386.

Zivkovic, T., Warin, M., Moore, V., Ward, P., & Jones, M. (2015). The sweetness of care: Biographies, bodies and place. In E. Abbotts, A. Lavis & L. Attala, (Eds.), *Careful eating: Bodies, food and care* (pp. 109–112). Farnham: Ashgate.

34

A MATTER OF WEIGHT?
ANTI-OBESITY STRATEGIES
IN SPAIN

Mabel Gracia-Arnaiz

Introduction

While there are numerous competing opinions about the rapid development of obesity (Lang & Rayner, 2007, p. 166), there is a broad consensus in the biomedical literature on classifying it as a non-transmissible disease and considering it a product of biological, behavioural, and cultural factors. Given the difficulties associated with the treatment and cure of obesity (Bray & Tartaglia, 2000) and its increasing worldwide prevalence (Dinsa, 2012; Ng et al., 2014), environmental factors have acquired a greater explanatory power, leading some epidemiologists to describe contemporary societies as 'obesogenic' or environmentally 'toxic' (Swinburn, Egger, & Razer, 1999; Brownell & Horgen, 2003). The obesity epidemic discourse dominates public health discussion (Gard & Wright, 2005). Seen as the direct result of high-calorie diets and insufficient energy expenditure (Shelley, 2012), excessive weight gain is understood as a global phenomenon caused by the rapid technological and socioeconomic transformation that has taken place in many countries, including low-income ones (Popkin & Gordon-Larsen, 2004). The phenomena identified as chiefly responsible include urbanization, the mechanization of work and transport, processed food, a reduction in the variability of ambient temperatures, eating out of home, passive leisure activities, and unsafe cities (Bezerra, Curioni, & Sichieri, 2012; Fox, Feng, & Asal, 2019).

If precisely which factors bear the greatest responsibility for the increasing prevalence of obesity remains unclear (McAllister et al., 2009), these 'universal truths' about behaviours and environmental factors support anti-obesity strategies on a worldwide scale (Nutter et al., 2016). In Spain, a set of measures aimed at reversing the upward trend has been implemented through the 2005 Strategy for Nutrition, Physical Activity and the Prevention of Obesity (NAOS Strategy, 2005). After 15 years of unprecedented implementation of anti-obesity campaigns and protocols of early diagnosis derived from the NAOS Strategy (2005), the obesity prevalence continues to rise, and it is necessary to ask why.

This chapter discusses some of the results of a broader study[2] based on the analysis of anti-obesity policies developed by Spanish health authorities at the national, state, and local levels. Here, we present a critical analysis of the NAOS Strategy (2005), the broad policy framework that has guided all the anti-obesity actions implemented in Spain up to date. In particular, it is argued that focusing on the responsibility individuals and their food and

DOI: 10.4324/9780429344824-41

exercise behaviours bear for ill health – as the NAOS Strategy does – is inadequate to grasp the contextual complexity and structural factors that are involved in weight gain. An example of this complexity has been evidenced by the recent economic crisis and its effects on the daily lives of the most vulnerable people. Spanish epidemiological sources and statistics for this period indicate that obesity rates have increased most quickly among individuals of low socioeconomic status and with a low level of education, particularly women. However, paradoxically, most of the anti-obesity measures adopted have excluded, or minimized, the social determinants of health. This chapter argues that, in the process of translating international guidelines into national action plans, there has been a failure to address the effects of recent socioeconomic changes – job insecurity, reduced wages, social programs cuts – through them. This lack of attention on their impact challenges the adequacy of certain anti-obesity measures. It is suggested that Spanish policymakers should rethink diagnosis and interventions and consider the health effects of their own economic policies in the increase of poverty and social inequality.

Universal causes, local strategies

In February 2005, Spain designed the NAOS Strategy, swiftly responding to the World Health Organization (WHO) mandate to its member states to adhere to the Global Strategy on Diet, Physical Activity and Health (WHO, 2004). Thus, the NAOS follows the general guidelines of the WHO and the European Union (EU), echoing the global diagnosis and concern for its economic impact. Its aim is to overturn so-called 'unhealthy lifestyles' through multifaceted initiatives focused on environmental and policy change, proposing programmes requiring the collaboration of various social actors and interventions in different spheres (school, workplace, healthcare and community).

Although the NAOS Strategy (2005, p. 12) subscribes to the view that "comprehensive knowledge of the causes and of their multiple and complex interrelations is essential to changing public habits and intervening in the causes of obesity", the preventive programs included under this strategy have been developed from the evidence that suggest that obesity results from: (a) the sustained increase in sedentary behaviours and (b) the shift in eating patterns over the past 40 years from a healthy to a less healthy diet. In this same sense, a group of nutrition researchers have reported that 61 percent of the calories currently ingested by Spaniards come from highly processed foods, and 71 percent of the population can be classified as sedentary (FESNAD-SEEDO Consensus, 2011). In the NAOS Strategy (2005, p. 11), it has been highlighted that "obesogenic" factors such as mechanization, industrialization, or urbanization have to be considered responsible for this tendency, and therefore, it is proposed to tackle sedentary lifestyles and poor diets by "promoting a decisive and sustained change towards a healthy diet and regular physical activity" (NAOS Strategy, 2005, p. 19). To that end, diverse programs derived from the NAOS Strategy have been released to reformulate food packaging, ban 'unhealthy' food from schools, reduce portion sizes in restaurants, and to train more health professionals for obesity prevention and treatment. Food reformulation, however, has been left to the goodwill of food and drink corporations, and so far, the government has opted not to tax foods high in sugar or salt.

The kind of actions linked to the NAOS Strategy is wide-ranging. However, most of these actions are focused on promoting a standardized model of diet and physical exercise, indicating what, when, where, and how much to eat or move. Food is reduced to a set of repetitive habits, where it is more important to know the nutritional and caloric composition of food than to find out why people eat, what they eat, and for what purpose.

The NAOS Strategy actions are directed, above all, to children and young people. Schools have been the sector of choice for nutrition and physical activity interventions. For instance, Spanish schools have joined the European 'School Fruit, Vegetable and Milk Scheme' that aims to fund the free distribution of those items to school children from nursery to secondary school age. Also, multiple information and education campaigns have been run, mainly involving the distribution of 'food pyramids', eating guides and nutrition workshops with audio-visual activities and games. In campaigns with slogans like *Come Sano y Muévete* [Eat Healthy and Get Moving], the target groups are usually depicted as mere receptors of the recommendations made by the expert system on what to do during meal, work and leisure times. One example of these messages is the campaign, "10 tips for being more active at work", run by the Health Department in the state if Catalonia. Its aim is to transform people's habits by providing standing or walking time during meetings, taking a stroll instead of having a coffee break, or going to talk to colleagues face-to-face rather than calling them on the phone.

Following the new policy directions resulting from the European Food and Nutrition Action Plan 2015–2020 (WHO-EU, 2014), some programmes have targeted people in lower social socioeconomic strata, but adopting similar approaches, mainly directed at changing behaviour. One example is the POIBA project (2010–2014) devised by the Barcelona Public Health Agency for children aged 11–12, half of whom live in the poorest *barrios* of the city (Ariza et al., 2014). The aims of this programme are to promote physical activity and healthy eating through educational workshops and recreational activities involving teachers, children, and their families. An initial evaluation of the programme's efficacy revealed positive changes in a decrease in the obesity rate over the short term. However, these were greater and longer-lasting among children from better-off areas (Sánchez-Martínez et al., 2016).

While it is true that the NAOS strategy is very similar to the anti-obesity strategies deployed by other countries, what determines its implementation is ultimately the particular context. For instance, in the broader study that informs that chapter, the Spanish, Argentine, and Brazilian strategies were compared. While the three countries designed their strategies following WHO and PAHO recommendations, in practice, significant differences are observed. Unlike Spain and Argentina, for instance, Brazil gives priority to facilitating physical access to food and traditional recipes. The aim is to encourage smaller-scale marketing, taxes on food and inputs, and the institutional purchase of food produced by family farms through public appeals to philanthropic institutions.

Obesity in a context of increasing precarisation

In Spain, since the beginning of the global economic crisis in 2008, living conditions have significantly changed, especially among socially disadvantaged groups. The government responded to the initial effects of the economic recession by focusing its efforts on bank bailouts, liberalizing labour regulations, reducing health spending, and increasing direct and indirect taxes (Navarro, 2015). At the same time, it took regressive actions that affected social rights, restricting family allowances, emancipation benefits, and support for dependents, while also decreasing salaries, freezing pensions, and cutting school-lunch subsidies (Mateos & Penadés, 2013). Austerity measures affected the whole population, but the poor lost more than the rich, making Spain the European country where inequality has grown most in the last decade (Martín, 2019).

Although some macroeconomic indicators such as GDP have improved since 2015 and, according to the Active Population Survey (EPA, 2019), the unemployment rate went down to 13.78 percent in 2019, there are still 3.1 million people out of work. What is more, the quality of employment has worsened, with more temporary contracts and lower salaries preventing many workers from escaping the poverty trap (Fernández, 2017) – 16 percent of working people are in a situation of social exclusion, two percentage points more than in 2018 (FOESSA-Cáritas, 2019). As Llanos Ortiz (2019) shows, the proportion of population at risk of social exclusion grew from 23.3 percent in 2007 to 29.2 percent in 2014, reaching more than 13 million people, many of whom now depend on social assistance to cover their basic necessities. The European authorities have warned Spain that it must improve on fairness and are calling for urgent economic, fiscal, and social policies to reduce the high inequality in income and opportunities.

Although the increase in inequality and social exclusion has been widely confirmed by Spanish surveys and third-sector reports, the effects of the economic crisis on health are still hotly disputed. Some researchers have linked Spain's economic difficulties to an increase in type 2 diabetes, depression, or alcoholism (Gili et al., 2014), and others have established a relationship between the increase in poverty and the rise in obesity (Radwan & Gil, 2014). Research has indicated that the volume of food bought and the quality of meals consumed have decreased during this period, with the incidence of specific nutritional deficiencies rising (Antentas & Vivas, 2014). However, the real socioeconomic and health consequences of precarisation are not well known because, as in other European countries, research on people's access to food has for many years been sporadic and fragmented, based on a variety of definitions and methodologies.

Ethnographic studies have revealed, however, substantial changes in eating itineraries. These include changes in locations for purchase, in the frequency and types of product purchased and brand chosen, with the cheapest sought out in order to reduce spending; fewer meals consumed in restaurants and bars; and changes in the ways meals are prepared, with dishes requiring elaborate preparation avoided and care taken to minimize waste and recycle leftovers for future meals. One of the most important consequences of recession is the decreased ability to regularly and autonomously obtain food among people in financially precarious situations, which has led to terms such as 'shortage', 'eating what you can and what you get', or 'skipping meals' reappearing in their everyday language (Gracia-Arnaiz, 2019).

Most of the preventive actions have failed not only to take into account these possible effects of the crisis but also to adjust to the available epidemiological data (Panetta & López-Valcárcel, 2016), particularly as it relates to social class and gender. According to the 2017 Spanish National Health Survey (ENSE, 2017), the rate of obesity in the adult population reached 17.5 percent, more than 2 percent higher than the figure recorded in 2006.

ENSE (2017) shows that obesity affects all groups, but that it looms larger among people with lower levels of education, especially women, and also among the unemployed, the disabled, and domestic workers. According to this survey, obesity and overweight increase in line with the socioeconomic condition of the head of the family (Group I includes the highest income level and Group VI the lowest). Although obesity affects 9.29 percent in Group I, the rate of obesity and overweight is more than double for Group VI, affecting 22.37 percent of the population. If we look at gender differences, obesity in the case of Group VI women (23.98 percent) is more than three times the 7.26 percent of those in Group I. Moreover, an analysis of the course of obesity between 2006 and 2017 reveals a faster increase among disadvantaged classes. Whereas Group I decreased by −0.99 percent, Groups V and VI saw a 3 percent increase over the same period (ENSE, 2017).

According to the ENSE (2017), the same has occurred with physical activity. Almost half (46.7 percent) of those on the lowest incomes have a sedentary lifestyle, while only

24.3 percent among those earning the most appear under this category. Unemployed people with a low educational level also do less sport.

There are various interpretations as to why the current preventive model has proved ineffectual in reversing the rise in obesity. Some sources attribute the poor results specifically to the economic recession (OECD, 2014). Some studies hold that the prevalence has increased more slowly in recent years (Sánchez-Cruz et al., 2013) or even that it has flattened out among children (Garrido-Miguel et al., 2019), while others insist that Spain is one of the European countries where obesity has grown the most (García-Goñi & Hernández Quevedo, 2012). Some also attribute the limited impact of anti-obesity actions to not having taxed sugar-sweetened beverages and ultra-processed foods or to the lack of better food marketing and labelling regulations (Royo-Bordonaba et al., 2019).

In reality, the texts analysed here contain few references to the cost-effectiveness of community-level interventions that go beyond short-term results and very specific age bands, so it remains hard to fathom whether such measures are having the expected effect. Likewise, few programmes have been directed towards the most vulnerable or focused on gender, which would indicate that addressing social inequalities in health has not been a policy priority to date.

Discussion and conclusion

Spanish public policies have been paradoxical. While the recognition of obesity as a 'costly disease' led to identification of multiple environmental causes and to the proposal of myriad state-developed solutions, in practice, most of the adopted measures have not addressed the broad causes and have instead energetically focused on exhorting people to adopt 'healthier lifestyles'. 'Eating better and moving more' represents the ideological driving force behind health interventions, which has meant prioritizing dietary and exercise activities and deflecting attention away from other relevant questions. In our view, the chief limitations of these actions lie in having reproduced a diagnosis without first having a comprehensive knowledge of the complex factors that shape social practice and without determining how inequalities in overweight and obesity are produced.

Although certain phenomena related to mechanization, industrialization, or urbanization are global in scope, their socioeconomic and political dimensions are local. In Spain, all these factors are present, but it is not well known to what extent they have influenced health and whether this influence has necessarily been negative. According to Varela-Moreiras et al. (2013, p. 5), there is not enough evidence to properly understand the causes of obesity and that there is a tendency to 'believe' rather than to 'find out'. Health experts are still debating whether the increase in body weight is more influenced by a lack of physical activity than diet (Serra-Majem, 2014) or if overweight necessarily entails a higher risk of dying (Flegal, Kit, Orpana, & Graubard, 2013).

In this context, it seems fair to question whether it is true that the Spanish have worsened their diet in recent decades and become more sedentary. Studies provide contradictory evidence. Assuming that their nutritional status has deteriorated due to a weaker adherence to the Mediterranean diet (Blas, Garrido, Unver, & Willaarts, 2019) conflicts with the epidemiological data that today places this society as the healthiest on the planet due, in part, to its eating habits. It is also surprising that, whereas the accepted opinion is that Spaniards are increasingly sedentary (Varela-Moreiras et al., 2013), studies analysing health trends, like the Survey of Sporting Habits in Spain (EHDE, 2015), indicate that sedentarism has fallen by 15 points in the last 20 years (EHDE, 2015). Likewise, according to the EHDE (2015), levels of sporting activity increased by nine points during the period 2010–2015. Given the discrepancies in findings about the nature and consequences of excess body weight, political measures should be applied once the health problem and who it affects have been identified, which means that causality must be examined critically before starting to put specific programmes into practice.

The data on the rising prevalence of obesity cast doubt on the reach of campaigns based on socially uniform messages proposing easy solutions that appeal to the responsibility of homogenous and rational citizens (Lupton, 1995), while at the same time obliging them to learn more. Fatness is an ambiguous concept and experience. From the point of view of body size, some conceive of it as a continuum of natural body diversity which need not be corrected (Casadó-Marín & Gracia-Arnaiz, 2020), arguing that what does require correction are the effects of lipophobia, which by incorporating many negative value judgments involves the discriminatory treatment of fat people (Gracia-Arnaiz, 2013). Not all fat people are unwell, and they do not all eat badly. What is more, not even all those who eat badly, from a nutritional point of view, become fat. Conversely, diagnosis presents fat people as 'big eaters' (Stearns, 2002), laying more emphasis on the food consumed and calories spent than on the economic and social factors conditioning consumption and practice. Food should not be reduced to its nutritional value, however important that is. Food is also culture, and both need to be considered as complex spaces of social relations in which people think and act from their particular and various social positions, resources, and opportunities. There is a lack of references in the literature to lived experiences, to how and why people eat what they do, and how they understand risk, health and bodies in cross-cultural settings. Most campaigns have involved very little participation in their design by citizens in general and less still by those diagnosed as overweight or obese.

The NAOS Strategy was not able to draw on an established understanding of how factors such as employment, wages, housing, foodstuff prices, and food supply influence food consumption and shape Spaniards' way of life, explaining why the obesity prevalence is greater in the lower classes. Although on paper the recognition of social distribution of obesity is mentioned in The Food Safety and Nutrition Law of 2011, and a specific tool for evaluating all the actions was applied using, among other things, gender and social class indicators (Ballesteros et al., 2011), in practice, few programmes have been focused on gender or universal access to healthy foods, especially for the most vulnerable groups.

Given that poverty has a more than slight effect on health (Deaton, 2013), it should be ascertained whether the progressive increase in financial inequality in Spain has influenced obesity rates and if this can be related to social and economic deprivation as in other countries (Bambra, Hillier, Moore, Cairns-Nagi, & Summerbell, 2013). The pressures exerted on people's lives (tax increases, co-payment for health services, salary decreases, etc.) through the current demands of neo-capitalist governments in order to decrease public expenses, raise serious obstacles that prevent individuals from adopting the officially sanctioned dietary recommendations and lifestyles (Riches & Silvasti, 2014).

As we noted previously (Gracia-Arnaiz, 2017; Gracia-Arnaiz, Kraemer and Demonte, 2020), the preventive proposals for combating obesity put forward since the end of the last decade overlap with one of the deepest crises that Spain has experienced since the transition to democracy. Today, we are witnessing yet another crisis, both in terms of health and of economy, leading to a social emergency affecting the most vulnerable. In fact, since the state of emergency was declared in March 2020 in response to the COVID-19 pandemic, requests for social assistance to Caritas have tripled, mostly to cover basic needs, while large cities are registering increases of up to 50 percent in requests for food aid. In Madrid, four out of every five calls to 010 (the citizens' assistance number) refer to requests for food or living allowances. Barcelona has increased its food-aid services by 30 percent, and in one single month, 5,100 lunch-aid cash cards have been distributed among disadvantaged families for students who cannot attend school. We will have to wait to see the social, and health-related, impact that government economic policies, and in particular, the management of aid from the European recovery fund, will have on this group of people. Efforts to get people to live more healthily have been accompanied by a deterioration rather than an improvement in living conditions. This is demonstrated by the fact that, according to data taken from the survey on living standards, plus the active population and third-sector reports, during the last decade, factors that generate inequality and poverty (unemployment, low wages, evictions, declining social aids) have progressively increased.

It is known that, while there may be a certain element of choice in occupation and life-style, poor people lead heavily constrained lives in terms of money, time, emotions, and choices, and some of their choices, even with the poor health consequences they entail, cannot easily be avoided under the circumstances (Deaton, 2013). The daily demands placed on many people do not allow for a healthier and more balanced diet, at least not to the extent that health authorities would like to see because changing diet means changing lifestyles – which, as socio-anthropological works have shown in Spain (Egbe, 2015), can be very difficult, if not impossible, for those living in the most precarious situations. Consequently, an appeal to change food practices or physical activity when these do not depend on the individual – or do so only relatively – makes little sense, and it is of little use for health authorities to recognize that overweight and obesity are closely related to social inequality if, on the other hand, those same authorities endorse economic and social policies that have left so many in a state of poverty.

Notes

1 The research project entitled, 'The precariousness of daily life in Spain: Food (in)security, gender and health' (grant number CSO2016 74941-P, 2016–2019) was funded by the Ministry of Education in Spain. The findings of this project have been presented in Gracia-Arnaiz (2013, 2017, 2019).
2 The research project entitled, 'The precariousness of daily life in Spain: Food (in)security, gender and health' (grant number CSO2016 74941-P, 2016–2019) was funded by the Ministry of Education in Spain. The findings of this project have been presented in Gracia-Arnaiz (2013, 2017, 2019).

References

Antentas, J. M., & Vivas, E. (2014). Impacto de la crisis en el derecho a una alimentación sana y saludable. Informe SESPAS 2014 [Impact of the economic crisis on the right to a healthy diet. SESPAS report 2014]. *Gaceta Sanitaria, 28*(Suppl 1), 58–61. https://doi.org/10.1016/j.gaceta.2014.04.006

Ariza, C., Ortega-Rodriguez, E., Sánchez-Martínez, F., Valmayor, S., Juárez, O., Pasarín, M.I.; Grupo de Investigación del Proyecto POIBA. (2014). La prevención de la obesidad infantil desde una perspectiva comunitaria [Childhood obesity prevention from a community view]. *Atención Primaria, 47*(4), 246–255. https://doi.org/10.1016/j.aprim.2014.11.006

Ballesteros, J. M., Pérez Farinós, N., Quiles i Izquierdo, J., Echeverría Cubillas, P., Castell i Abat, C., Muñoz Bellerín, J., ... Lizalde Gil, E. (2011). *Evaluación y seguimiento de la Estrategia NAOS: Conjunto mínimo de indicadores [Evaluation and monitoring of the NAOS Strategy: Minimum set of indicators]*. Madrid: Ministerio de Sanidad, Política Social e Igualdad.

Bambra, C. L., Hillier, F. C., Moore, H. J., Cairns-Nagi, J-M., & Summerbell, C. D. (2013). Tackling inequalities in obesity: A protocol for a systematic review of the effectiveness of public health interventions at reducing socioeconomic inequalities in obesity among adults. *Systematic Reviews, 2*, 27. https://doi.org/10.1186/2046-4053-2-27

Bezerra, I., Curioni, C., & Sichieri, R. (2012). Association between eating out of home and body weight. *Nutrition Reviews, 70*(2), 65–79. https://doi.org/10.1111/j.1753-4887.2011.00459.x

Blas, A., Garrido, A., Unver, O., & Willaarts, B. (2019). A comparison of the Mediterranean diet and current food consumption patterns in Spain from a nutritional and water perspective. *Science of the Total Environment, 664*, 1020–1029. https://doi.org/10.1016/j.scitotenv.2019.02.111

Bray, G. A., & Tartaglia, L. A. (2000). Medicinal strategies in the treatment of obesity. *Nature, 404*, 672–677. https://doi.org/10.1038/35007544

Brownell, K., & Horgen, K. (2003). *Food fight*. New York: McGraw-Hill Companies.

Casadó-Marín, L., & Gracia-Arnaiz, M. (2020). "I'm fat and proud of it": Body size diversity and fat acceptance activism in Spain. *Fat Studies, 9*(1), 51–70. https://doi.org/10.1080/21604851.2019.1648994

Deaton, A. (2013). What does the empirical evidence tell us about the injustice of health inequalities? In N. Eyal, S. A. Hurst, O. F. Norheim, & D. Wikler (Eds.), *Inequalities in health: Concepts, measures and ethics*. Oxford: Oxford University Press.

Dinsa, G. (2012). Obesity and socioeconomic status in developing countries: A systematic review. *Obesity Reviews, 13*(11): 1067–1079. https://doi.org/10.1111/j.1467-789X.2012.01017.x

Egbe, M. (2015). Food insecurity and poverty in Sub-Sahara African immigrant population in Tarragona Province, Spain. *Journal of Food Security, 3*(5), 115–124.

EHDE. (2015). Encuesta de hábitos deportivos en España 2015 [Survey of sporting habits in Spain]. http://es.calameo.com/read/000075335a18c80405ea7

ENSE. (2017). *Encuesta Nacional de Salud de España 2017 [2017 Spanish National Health Survey]*. https://www.mscbs.gob.es/estadEstudios/estadisticas/encuestaNacional/encuesta2017.html

EPA. (2019). *Encuesta población activa 2019 [2019 Spanish employment survey]*. https://www.ine.es/dyngs/INEbase/es/operacion.htm?c=Estadistica_C&cid=1254736176918&menu=ultiDatos&idp=1254735976595

Fernández, D. (2017). Los salarios en la recuperación Española [Wages in the Spanish recovery]. *Cuadernos de Información Económica, 260*, 1–12.

FESNAD-SEEDO Consensus. (2011). Recomendaciones nutricionales basadas en la evidencia para la prevención y el tratamiento del sobrepeso y la obesidad en adultos [Evidence-based nutritional recommendations for the prevention and treatment of overweight and obesity in adults]. *Revista Española de Obesidad, 10*(Suplemento 1), 1–80. https://doi.org/10.3305/nh.2012.27.3.5678

Flegal, K. M., Kit, B. K., Orpana, H., & Graubard, B. I. (2013). Association of all-cause mortality with overweight and obesity using standard body mass index categories. *JAMA, 309*(1), 71–82. https://doi.org/10.1001/jama.2012.113905

FOESSA-Cáritas. (2019). *VIII Informe sobre exclusión y desarrollo social en España [VIII Report on exclusion and social development in Spain]*. Retrieved from https://caritas-web.s3.amazonaws.com/main-files/uploads/sites/16/2019/05/Informe-FOESSA-2019-completo.pdf

Fox, A., Feng, W., & Asal, V. (2019). What is driving global obesity trends? Globalization or "modernization"? *Globalization and Health, 15*, 32. https://doi.org/10.1186/s12992-019-0457-y

García-Goñi, M., & Hernández -Quevedo, C. (2012). The evolution of obesity in Spain. *Eurohealth, 18*(1), 22–25.

Gard, M., & Wright, J. (2005). *The obesity epidemic: Science, morality and ideology*. London: Routledge.

Garrido-Miguel, M., Cavero-Redondo, I., Álvarez-Bueno, C., Rodríguez-Artalejo, F., Moreno, L. A., Ruiz, J. R., Ahrens, W., & Martínez-Vizcaíno, V (2019). Prevalence and trends of overweight and obesity in European children from 1999 to 2016: A systematic review and meta-analysis. *JAMA Pediatrics, 173*(10), e192430. https://doi.org/10.1001/jamapediatrics.2019.2430

Gili, M., García Campayo, J., & Roca, M. (2014) Crisis económica y salud mental. Informe SESPAS 2014 [Economic crisis and mental health. SESPAS Report 2014]. *Gaceta Sanitaria, 28*(S1), 104–108. https://doi.org/10.1016/j.gaceta.2014.02.005

Gracia-Arnaiz, M. (2013) Thou shalt not get fat: Medical representations and self-images of obesity in a Mediterranean society. *Health, 5*, 1180–1189. https://doi.org/10.4236/health.2013.57159

Gracia-Arnaiz, M. (2017). Taking measures in times of crisis: The political economy of obesity prevention in Spain. *Food Policy, 68*, 65–76. https://doi.org/10.1016/j.foodpol.2017.01.001

Gracia-Arnaiz, M. (2019). Eating outside the home: Food practices as a consequence of economic crisis in Spain. In P. Collinson, I. Young, L. Antal & H. Macbeth (Eds.), *Food and sustainability in the twenty-first century. Cross-disciplinary perspectives* (pp. 185–196). Oxford: Berghahn Books.

Gracia-Arnaiz, M., Bom Kraemer, F. & Demonte, F. (2020) Acting against obesity: a cross-cultural analysis of prevention models in Spain, Argentina and Brazil. *Critical Reviews in Food Science and Nutrition.* https://doi.org/10.1080/10408398.2020.1852169

Lang, T., & Rayner, G. (2007). Overcoming policy cacophony on obesity: An ecological public health framework for policymakers. *Obesity Reviews, 8*(Suppl. 1), 165–181.

Llanos Ortiz, J. C. (2019). *El estado de la pobreza seguimiento del indicador de riesgo de pobreza y exclusión social en España 2008–2018 [The state of poverty monitoring the indicator of risk of poverty and social exclusion in Spain 2008–2018].* Madrid: EAPN España.

Lupton, D. (1995). *The imperative of health. Public health and regulated body.* London: SAGE Publications.

Martín, J. M. (2019). *Nueva desigualdad en España y nuevas políticas para afrontarla [New inequality in Spain and new policies to face it].* Barcelona: Observatorio social de La Caixa.

Mateos, A., & Penadés, A. (2013). España: crisis y recortes [Spain: crisis and cuts]. *Revista de Ciencia Política, 33*(1), 161–183. https://doi.org/.4067/S0718-090X2013000100008

McAllister, E., Dhurandhar, N. V., Keith, S. W., Aronne, L.J., Barger, J., Baskin, M., ... Allison, D. B. (2009). Ten putative contributors to the obesity epidemic. *Critical Reviews in Food Science and Nutrition, 49*(10), 868–913. https://doi.org/10.1080/10408390903372599

NAOS Strategy (2005). *Estrategia para la Nutrición. Actividad Física y Prevención de la Obesidad [Strategy for Nutrition. Physical Activity and Obesity Prevention].* Madrid, ES: Agencia Española de Seguridad Alimentaria.

Navarro, V. (2015). *Ataque a la democracia y al bienestar [Attack on democracy and well-being].* Barcelona: Anagrama.

Ng, M., Fleming, T., Robinson, M., Thomson, B., Graetz, N., Margono, C., ... Gakidou, E. (2014). Global, regional, and national prevalence of overweight and obesity in children and adults during 1980–2013: A systematic analysis for the Global Burden of Disease Study 2013. *The Lancet, 384*(9945), 766–781. https://doi.org/10.1016/S0140-6736(14)60460-8

Nutter, S., Russell-Mayhew, S., Alberga, A. S., Arthur, N., Kassan, A., Lund, D. E., Sesma-Vazquez, M., & Williams, E. (2016). Positioning of weight bias: Moving towards social justice. *Journal of Obesity, ID 3753650.* https://doi.org/10.1155/2016/3753650

OECD. (2014). *Health at a glance: Europe 2014.* Paris: OECD Publishing. doi: 10.1787/health_glance_eur-2014-en

Panetta, J., & López-Valcárcel, B. (2016). El gradiente social de la obesidad en España. ¿Qué sabemos y qué deberíamos saber? [The social gradient of obesity in Spain. What do we know and what should we know?]. *Icade, 99,* 45–68.

Popkin, B. M., & Gordon-Larsen, P. (2004). The nutrition transition: Worldwide obesity dynamics and their determinants. *International Journal of Obesity, 28*(s2–s9). https://doi.org/10.1038/sj.ijo.0802804

Radwan, A., & Gil, J. M. (2014, April 9–11). *On the nexus between economic and obesity crisis in Spain: Parametric and nonparametric analysis of the role of economic factors on obesity prevalence.* 88th Annual Conference, AgroParisTech, Paris, France 170341, Agricultural Economics Society. https://doi.org/10.22004/ag.econ.170341

Riches, G., & Silvasti, T. (Eds.). (2014). *First World hunger revisited. Food charity or the right to food?* (2nd Ed.). London: Palgrave Macmillan.

Royo-Bordonaba, M., Rodríguez-Artalejo, F., Bes-Rastrollo, M., Fernández-Escobar, C., González, C. A., Rivas, F., ... Vioque, J. (2019). Políticas alimentarias para prevenir la obesidad y las principales enfermedades no transmisibles en España: querer es poder [Food policies to prevent obesity and the main non-communicable diseases in Spain: Wanting is power]. *Gaceta Sanitaria, 33*(6), 584–592. https://doi.org/10.1016/j.gaceta.2019.05.009

Sánchez-Cruz, J-J., Jiménez-Moleón, J. J., Fernández-Quesada, F., & Sánchez, M. J. (2013). Prevalence of child and youth obesity in Spain in 2012. *Revista Española de Cardiología, 66*(5), 371–376. https://doi.org/10.1016/j.recesp.2012.10.016

Sánchez-Martinez, F., Capcha, P. T., Cano, G. S., Safont, S. V., Abat, C. C., Cardenal, C. A., & Grupo de Evaluación del Proyecto POIBA (2016). Factors associated with overweight and obesity in school children from 8 to 9 years old. Barcelona, Spain. *Revista Española de Salud Pública, 90:* e1–e11.

Serra-Majem, L. (2014). Childhood obesity: have we bottomed out? Can we bring out the bubbly? *Medicina Clínica, 14*(11), 489–491. https://doi.org/10.1016/j.medcli.2014.02.007

Shelley, J. J. (2012). Addressing the policy cacophony does not require more evidence: an argument for reframing obesity as caloric overconsumption. *BMC Public Health, 12,* 1042.

Stearns, P. N. (2002). *Fat history: Bodies and beauty in the Modern West*. New York: New York University Press.

Swinburn, B. A., Egger, G., & Raza, F. (1999). Dissecting obesogenic environments: The development and application of a framework for identifying and prioritizing environmental interventions for obesity. *Preventive Medicine, 29*(6), 563–570. doi: 10.1006/pmed.1999.0585

Varela-Moreiras, G., Alguacil Merino, L. F., Alonso Aperte, E., Aranceta Bartrina, J., Ávila Torres, J. M., Aznar Laín, S.,... & Garaulet Aza, M. (2013). Obesidad y sedentarismo en el siglo XXI: ¿Qué se puede y se debe hacer? [Obesity and sedentary lifestyle in the 21st century: What can and should be done?]. *Nutrición hospitalaria, 28*, 1–12.

WHO. (2004). *Global strategy on diet, physical activity and health* (DPAS). France: Library Cataloguing-in-Publication Data.

WHO-EU. (2014). *Obesity and inequalities*. Copenhagen: WHO Regional Office for Europe.

35

NEW LANGUAGE, OLD ASSUMPTIONS

The shifting language in British Columbia's physical and health education curricula

LeAnne Petherick and Moss E. Norman

Notwithstanding the bold proclamation of Monaghan and colleagues (2018), we suggest that evidence of an all-out war on obesity is somewhat difficult to find in the Canadian context. Therefore, it was curious to us that the authors point to the 2016 release of the Parliamentary report, *Obesity in Canada: A Whole-of-Society Approach for a Healthier Canada* as evidence of the reinvigorated war on obesity. This report received almost no mainstream media attention (actually *no* media attention that we were able to find), and it is difficult for us to see where the report has been supported either through legislation or budgetary resources. This policy apathy and relative media silence contrasts sharply with the height of the obesity epidemic rhetoric in Canada, where coverage of obesity-related stories was a weekly feature in national news (Holmes, 2009), and federal governments were openly partnering with private industry in launching a full-fledged war on obesity (see Norman, Rail & Jette, 2014, 2016). Indeed, there has been a noticeable, if not precipitous, decline in obesity rhetoric in Canada over the past five or so years. Indeed, it may come as a surprise to readers to learn that the words 'obesity', 'obese', or 'overweight' do not appear in British Colombia's (BC) most recent Physical and Health Education (PHE) curricula, while the word 'weight' only appears twice. This may lead the readers to question why include a chapter on BC's PHE curricula in a book on critical obesity studies? We argue that the lack of explicit language dedicated to obesity is not to suggest that obesity discourse is absent from the BC PHE curricula. It does mean, however, that critical readers have to do a little bit of work to trace the ongoing effects of obesity discourse in the Canadian context generally and in the provincial curricula in BC specifically. We do just this in this chapter, first by briefly overviewing the public health landscape both in the province of British Columbia as well as across Canada and follow this with a more detailed analysis of BC PHE curricula, carefully tracing the shape-shifting ways in which obesity discourse continues to be a force in influencing public health, even in its apparent absence. We conclude the chapter by arguing that if critical obesity studies are to continue to maintain their critical edge and relevance, the field must refrain from broad proclamations and do the nuanced work of tracing the shifting landscapes across which obesity discourse is taken up and materialized across multiple sectors.

DOI: 10.4324/9780429344824-42

Public health, schools, and crises

In this section, we briefly overview the public health landscape both in the province of British Columbia as well as across Canada, paying attention to the ways in which obesity discourse continues to be present, even in its apparent absence. Nowhere is this obesity silence more obvious than in the annual release of the national *Active Healthy Kids Report Card*[1] where, in 2013, the words 'obesity', 'obese', and 'overweight' appeared a total of 27 times, whereas, in the 2018 report card, 'obesity' and 'overweight' are each mentioned once and 'obese' is not mentioned at all. This shift in focus is particularly telling as the *Active Healthy Kids Report Card* was created in 2005 as a social marketing campaign that evaluated – or graded – how Canada was doing in supporting physical activity opportunities for children and youth. In its early days, obesity and overweight were central themes in the report, but over time, this focus has diminished.

In the first decade of the 21st century, there were two strategic initiatives commissioned by British Columbia's Ministry of Health that specifically targeted overweight and obesity: *A Strategy for Combatting Childhood Obesity and Physical Inactivity in BC* (2006) and the *Recommendations for an Obesity Reduction Strategy* (2010). In addition to making health recommendations for the entire province, both of these initiatives make specific proposals for school health education and education more generally, with obesity prevention and management being a primary focus of these recommendations.

These policies would lead one to believe that school physical and health education would be positioned as critical sites in delivering health messages related to obesity (see Wright & Harwood, 2009; Rich, Monaghan, & Bombak, 2019). However, since 2010, there have been no provincial policies specifically related to obesity, with the most recent report – *#MakeB-CHealthyforKids* (2017) – focusing on education related to healthy lifestyles more generally and no mention of obesity whatsoever. Although it is beyond the scope of this chapter to determine why a shift in language has happened, we nonetheless speculate that it is related to the convergence of a number of factors, including: that rates of obesity appear to have plateaued both globally (Gard, 2011; Monaghan et al., 2018) and in Canada (Gard, 2016); the increased awareness that health interventions that target body types may be stigmatizing and detrimental to health (see Puhl & Heurer, 2009; Puhl, Peterson, DePierre, & Joerg, 2013; McVey & Harrison, 2018); and the emergence of a robust critique emerging from critical obesity and fat studies (Ellison, McPhail, & Mitchenson, 2016; McPhail, 2017; Pausé, 2017) that challenge reductionist assumptions about the relationship between body weight, shape, size, and health. Moreover, when it comes to the role of physical activity and exercise – what has been the traditional foundation of physical education – in combatting obesity, there is now considerable evidence to suggest that exercise alone is a relatively ineffective mechanism for weight loss (Malhotra, Noakes, & Phinney, 2015). With the convergence of these factors and others undermining, if not complicating at the very least, the veracity of the obesity crisis, the assemblage of experts (including scientists, health promoters, and educators) who were once 'obesity amplifiers' have now been forced to find a new crisis as their *raison d'etre*.

Michael Gard (2011) anticipated this shift, arguing that, "by 2010 a new phase of the obesity epidemic has been reached, marking the end of a period of consciousness raising or hyperbole...and a transitioning into something else" (p. 4). For Piggin and Bairner (2016), this something else is the crisis of physical inactivity. They suggest that it is not mere coincidence that, as obesity language receded from health policy, the prestigious and highly influential medical journal, *The Lancet*, declared a global pandemic of physical inactivity and called for global action to address this crisis (see Bauman, Brownwell, Lee, Heath, Pratt,

Kohl, & Hallal, 2015). Since then, the World Health Organization has also released a global action plan to address the crisis of physical inactivity (see WHO, 2018). However, what we have found in our analysis of the BC PHE curricula is that there does not appear to be one overarching crisis (i.e., the obesity or physical inactivity crisis) that informs curricular development, rather the target is far broader, encompassing *life* itself. In fact, in its latest iteration, the BC PHE curricula is shifting away from an emphasis on physical activity, exercise, and sport, a trend that has been identified in PHE curricula across the global north, including in the United States (Gard & Pluim, 2014), United Kingdom (Kirk, 2010; Armour & Harris, 2013; Evans, 2014), Australia (Hickey, Kirk, Macdonald, & Penney, 2014), and New Zealand (Fitzpatrick & Tinning, 2014; Fitzpatrick & Burrows, 2017). In the remainder of this chapter, we trace this shift arguing that the explicit focus on physical activity or body shape and size has given way to an emphasis on the self-regulating subject who is produced through continuous everyday micro-practices of measuring, monitoring, and strategizing. However, we also argue that, notwithstanding the apparent obesity retreat, obesity discourse continues to occupy a force, an argument that requires us to take a brief theoretical detour.

Theorizing the shape-shifting discourse of obesity

Using the work of Michel Foucault, health scholars have argued that healthy lifestyle operates as a form of governmentality, where certain lifestyles are incentivized (e.g., healthy eating and active living), as opposed to simply prohibited, and individuals are supposedly empowered to make the 'right' lifestyle choices (Mayes, 2016). Here, healthy lifestyle operates "as a network of disparate ideas, beliefs and practices through which individual choices and bodies are governed" (Mayes, 2016, p. 2). The 2016 BC PHE curricula certainly lend itself to a Foucauldian analysis, where students are incited to engage in practices of monitoring and evaluating their everyday practices and feelings as well as developing strategies for changing particular behaviours as a means of becoming a healthy subject. In this regard, the student appears to be empowered (if not responsibilized) to make the right choice and take control of life itself, quite irrespective of the social and structural conditions of possibility that both enable *and* constrain one to make such choices. However, neither the school nor curricula are sealed discursive spaces, and so it is important to consider the broader context in which they are embedded.

Drawing on Henri Giroux's (2004) notion of public pedagogy, Rich (2011) suggests that health curricula are not isolated from the world, but rather are rendered meaningful within a broader assemblage of relations. Rich (2010) uses the term "obesity assemblage" to describe the manner in which obesity discourse circulates relationally across diverse institutions (e.g., government, commercial, and educational institutions), agents (e.g., policy writers, allied health professions, and educators), and artefacts (e.g., health promotion campaigns, social media representations, digital technologies, and physical health education curricular) and, through circulating, comes to take on a material and affective force. Moreover, the assemblage of obesity also becomes culturally intelligible in relation to broader health discourses, thus merges with, and becomes part of a broader health assemblage that cannot be reduced to concerns, meanings, and practices related to body weight, shape, and size alone. For our analysis, this means that PHE curricula must always be read relationally, recognizing that there is leakage between the curricular, extracurricular, and beyond, "defying what for other subject areas may be more traditional bounded learning, nestled comfortably within the school's" clearly delineated spaces (Macdonald, Johnson, & Leow, 2014, p. 27). This means that even though the 2016 BC PHE curricula does not contain explicit references to obesity, when examined in relation to broader public pedagogies of obesity, we assume that obesity discourse still has a material and affective force in shaping how teachers and students understand and experience the curricula. In other words, PHE teachers and students across British Columbia are always already haunted by the spectre of the unhealthy, obese "Other" who threatens to sabotage the healthy subject and they bring these experiences with them into PHE classes.

Shifting language in British Columbia's physical and health education curricula

In this section, we examine the two most recent Physical Education curricula for British Columbia, specifically looking for shifts that have happened in the decade between 2006 and 2016 curricula. The two documents emerged within very different socio-political contexts, with the 2006 Physical Education (K–7) curricula being conceptualized during the height of obesity epidemic discourse in Canada, whereas the 2016 Physical and Health Education (K–9) curricula comes into being within what we might call the 'post-obesity' epidemic moment (British Columbia Physical Education, 2006; British Columbia Physical and Health Education, 2016). Tellingly, neither document explicitly mentions the terms 'obesity', 'overweight', 'body weight', or 'obesity epidemic'. Notwithstanding this absence, we argue that the effects of the obesity epidemic discourse (see Evans, Rich, Davies, & Allwood, 2008) are still very much present, albeit giving rise to two very different documents.

In order to illustrate these differences, we examine the language used in each with the assumption that language will provide insight into the emphasis of the respective curricula. In order to get at this language, each author closely read both curricula with the intention of identifying reoccurring terms and their related concepts. Once we identified the key terms, we then searched each document for these terms. Table 35.1 overviews the results of this search, revealing two overarching and significant trends in addition to a number of minor trends, that while interesting, are beyond the scope of this chapter.

Table 35.1 British Columbia's physical education curricula

	Physical education curricula	*Physical and health education curriculum*
	2006	*2016*
Physical activity	667	74
Active living	121	20
Movement	733	83
Sport	21	1
Fitness	72	44
Physical literacy	0	28
Health	107	295
Mental	12	56
Well-being	5	81
Emotion	72	57
Fun	25	2
Enjoyment	24	2

The first trend we want to highlight is the de-emphasis on physical activity between 2006 and 2016. Whereas terms related to physical activity including 'sport', 'fitness', 'movement' and 'active living' are mentioned a total of 1,614 times in 2006, these terms (plus, a new, but related term 'physical literacy') are only mentioned 250 times in 2016. This shift represents a nearly 6.5-fold decrease in the language of physical activity over the course of a decade. The second trend is the shift in emphasis to health. In 2016, health and health-related terms (e.g., mental health and well-being) are mentioned 412 times, while they are only mentioned 124 times in 2006, representing a 3.3-fold increase in health and health-related terms between 2006 and 2016. Accompanying this shift to health is the proliferation of strategies related to life where knowledge is linked to an array of practices in the production of healthy lifestyles.

The emphasis on inciting a particular healthy lifestyle is not new. Indeed, both the 2006 and 2016 version of the BC PHE curricula focus on health and well-being; however, the pathway to achieving health is distinctive in the respective documents. Whereas the 2006 curricula centres on fostering health through physical activity, in 2016, the emphasis is far broader and more diffuse and infiltrates almost every aspect of life. In this regard, we argue that, in the 2016 curricula, the healthy active living net, so to speak, is at once cast wider, in that it targets multiple dimensions of life beyond physical activity, at the same time, that the mesh is finer, as it increasingly attends to ever greater details of everyday life. This reflects both an extensification of power relations, where discourses of healthy active living are spread across ever-greater aspects of life, at the same time that there is an intensification of those relations (Gill, 2010), where the healthy student subject learns evermore-minute techniques of self-surveillance and self-management. Here, no aspect of life, no matter how trivial, escapes the imperative of self-surveillance and self-improvement. The 2016 BC PHE curricula invites learners to measure, monitor, and assess an array of 'problems', at the same time that it purports to endow students with the agency, choice, and freedom to work on improving the self in the process of becoming the healthy active living ideal implicitly rendered in the curricula.

In the 2016 curricula, students are responsibilized for crafting a healthy life not just in the here and now, but across the entire life span. As such, the curricula establishes a particular set of power relations whereby students are incited to take up micro practices of the self not solely because of the authoritarian directives of the teacher, but through the internalization of the discursive and affective force of PHE knowledge. For example, across the curricula, students are repeatedly asked to 'describe', 'apply', 'identify', and 'explore' strategies to attain a healthy social, emotional, physical, or environmental outcome. Moreover, in each successive grade, students are asked to devise progressively more sophisticated healthy-living strategies. For instance, Kindergarten and grade 1 students are asked "to identify opportunities to make choices that contribute to health and wellbeing" (British Columbia Physical and Health Education, 2016, pp. 1, 5), and in grade 4, students are expected to "identify and apply strategies for pursuing personal healthy living goals" (p. 19). Expectations in Kindergarten and grade one state students should be able to "identify opportunities to be physically active at school, at home, and in the community", and then expectations in grade 4 require students to "identify and describe opportunities for and potential challenges to participation in preferred types of physical activity at school, at home and in the community" (p. 19). Across these examples, students are called upon to take responsibility for their actions, which gives the impression that students have the freedom to choose healthy strategies of their own making. Notwithstanding the ostensible freedom the curriculum appears to offer students in negotiating their own life circumstances in devising these strategies, we suggest that there are always preferred subjects, leading to preferred healthy strategies, in these documents. Although not explicitly defined, we nonetheless suspect that the spectre of the 'unhealthy' subject is implicitly conjured throughout the curriculum. Here, the curriculum is not an isolated document, but is rendered intelligible in relation to broader discursive and affective public pedagogies. Thus, when students are asked to identify and devise strategies for addressing their worries, it is unlikely that smoking, vaping, or eating energy-dense foods – all practices that could be identified as mechanisms for coping with stress (Shankar & Park, 2016) – would be recognized as 'healthy' strategies. Therefore, the curriculum operates by enabling some strategies while foreclosing others, so what at first glance appears to be a document that enables students to account for their own lived circumstances, ends up being an imperative to make the 'right' choice, where such 'choices' are too often divorced from the social, economic, and cultural conditions that structure one's ability to exercise life choices in the first instance (Gard & Wright, 2005; Gard, 2008; Halse, 2009; Kwauk, 2012).

The shift in the approach to the emotional aspect of health and well-being between the 2006 and 2016 curricula is quite telling. The focus on the emotional dimensions of physical activity, health, and wellness is present in both curricula; with 'emotions' being mentioned a total of 72 times in 2006 and 57 times in 2016. In this regard, both documents situate emotions as a core aspect of holistic health; however, the analysis should not stop there, as there are also significant differences in how emotions are framed. For instance, in 2006, the pleasurable aspects of movement are clearly evident with 49 references to 'fun' and 'enjoyment'. In contrast, 'fun' and 'enjoyment' are only mentioned four times in the 2016, and with a comparably greater emphasis placed on 'managing' and 'regulating' emotions such as depression, anxiety, and stress. Here, the relatively ill-defined dimensions of the emotional benefits of physical activity found in 2006, and in 2016, simultaneously dis-articulated from visceral embodied aspects of movement specifically and re-articulated as broader lifestyle risk factors to be managed and controlled in the production of a healthy subject. For instance, Kindergarten and grade 1 students are asked "to identify and describe feelings and worries" (British Columbia Physical and Health Education, 2016, pp. 1, 5), and then in grade 2, students are asked "to identify feelings and worries, and strategies for dealing with them" (p. 10). In upper grades, students are later asked to "describe and assess strategies for managing problems related to mental-well-being and substance use" (see grades 6–8, pp. 32, 38, 44). Moreover, in the 2016 document, students are invited to monitor, assess, and regulate emotions such as anxiety (mentioned nine times) and depression (mentioned six times) that are considered a threat to healthy student growth and development. Tellingly, anxiety and depression are not explicitly mentioned at all in 2006, although they are certainly implied in some of the language. Although we do not want to discount the importance of attending to student mental health and well-being, we nonetheless want to draw attention to the critical language shifts that are happening in PHE curricula in BC. While skills of strategizing, managing, and planning for better health conditions are valuable, the concentration on the instrumental development and improvement of life overshadows the potential for developing a deeper connection with the body and its visceral and pleasurable responses to physical activity (Pringle, 2010). In doing so, the body and emotion become risks to be managed and regulated as opposed to experienced, a shift that has led Tinning (2014) to suggest that PHE is increasingly 'health work' and not play.

We are not suggesting that situating the body as a site for regulation and self-management suddenly appeared in the PHE curricula in 2016. In fact, there is ample evidence that such technologies of regulation are present in both documents. However, we do argue that, between 2006 and 2016, the pedagogies of self-management have both intensified, providing ever-greater detailed instructions on how to assess, monitor, and control the body, while at the same time, these technologies have increasingly been disconnected from movement specifically and expanded to include all aspects of life (e.g., sleep hygiene, emotional regulation, time management, and so on). Tellingly, there is no mention of obesity in either version of the curricula, but this is not to suggest that the effects of obesity epidemic discourse (Evans et al., 2008) are not present even in their apparent absence. However, to discern these obesity effects requires that we look to those less explicit, shadowy influences that shape curriculum.

Conclusion

Although our analysis in this chapter has focused on the shifting language used in the BC PHE curricula between 2006 and 2016, the point of our argument is not words alone, but the effects these words have in shaping the relationship between students, their bodies, and broader society. In other words, we are using words to get at the power relations embedded in the curricula, where students are incited to perform a particular relationship with the self. We opened this chapter with the recognition that the rhetoric associated with the obesity epidemic is in decline in dominant media and public health policy in Canada. However, we have argued that this does not mean that obesity epidemic discourse does not have a material and affective force, shaping PHE curricula as well as the implementation and experiences of PHE. In their analysis of the histories of school health in the United States, Gard and Pluim (2014) (see also Gard & Vander Schaee, 2011) suggest that one of the lasting consequences of the obesity epidemic crisis is that the fear and concern it generated functioned as a wedge that opened up school curricula to the vested interests of various stakeholders, with public health experts being foremost among them. Within this context, school curriculum was increasingly understood as a site for the promotion and production of students as morally responsible subjects capable of looking after their own health as a pathway to citizenship and healthy nations. Although the circumstances surrounding curricular shifts in the United States differ from the Canadian context, we nonetheless suggest that there are also striking similarities to be found in our analysis of the British Columbia PHE curricula. In particular, it would seem that the crisis generated by the obesity epidemic was at the very least an alibi that created the conditions for the transformation of a PHE curriculum in 2006 that was primarily organized around physical activity, sport, and health to a curriculum that is now dominated by health and, even when movement is discussed, it is the serious work of movement *for* health, as opposed to play and pleasure. This is most apparent in two policy documents – A *Strategy for Combatting Childhood Obesity and Physical Inactivity in BC* (2006) and the *Recommendations for an Obesity Reduction Strategy* (2010). Notwithstanding the explicit focus on obesity in these two documents, the translation of these policies into curriculum did not focus narrowly on body shape, size, and weight. Rather, the focus broadened to form a health assemblage, of which obesity serves an important component, that is at once an intensified and extensified targeting of all aspects of life itself.

Furthermore, when identifying those obesity effects on PHE curricula, it is important to remember that the BC PHE curricula are not stand-alone pedagogical technologies but are always understood in relation to the broader assemblage of obesity that Rich (2010) identifies (see also Monaghan et al., 2019). Here, teaching and learning are more porous, where lessons that pathologize the fat body are learned across multiple socio-cultural sites, as are those that celebrate the thin, lean, and toned body, with these public pedagogies being produced at the nexus of gender, race, ethnicity, social class, and so on (see Rich, 2018). Here, the affective dimension of obesity does not cease to exist simply because it is not explicit in the curriculum but continues to circulate and occupy a force within schools, shaping how PHE curricula are understood, taken up, and experienced for both students and teachers.

Note

1 Re-named to *ParticipACTION Report Card on Physical Activity for Children and Youth* in 2016 (see ParticipACTION, 2018).

References

Active Healthy Kids Report Card. (2013). *Are we driving our kids to unhealthy habits? Report on physical activity for children and youth.* Canada: Active Healthy Kids.

Armour, K., & Harris, J. (2013). Making the case for developing new PE for health pedagogies. *Quest, 65*(2), 201–219. http://doi.org/10.1080/00336297.2013.773531

Bauman, A., Brownell, R., Lee, I.M., Heath, G., Pratt, M., Kohl, H., & Hallal, P. (2015). Correspondence. *The Lancet Obesity Series, 386,* 742–742.

British Columbia Centre for Disease Control. (2010, June 7). *Recommendations for an obesity reduction strategy in BC.* Vancouver.

British Columbia Healthy Living Alliance. (2017). *#MakeBCHealthyforKids.* Vancouver.

British Columbia Legislative Assembly. (2006). *A strategy for combatting childhood obesity and physical inactivity in BC.* Select Standing Committee on Health. Victoria.

British Columbia Physical Education. (2006). *Physical Education K-7. Integrated Resource Package.* British Columbia: Ministry of Education.

British Columbia Physical and Health Education. (2016). *Physical and Health Education. BC's New Curriculum.* British Columbia: Ministry of Education. Retrieved from https://curriculum.gov.bc.ca/curriculum/physical-health-education

Ellison, J., McPhail. D., & Mitchinson, W. (2016). *Obesity in Canada. Critical perspectives.* Toronto, ON: University of Toronto Press.

Evans, J. (2014). Equity and inclusion in physical education PLC. *European Physical Education Review, 20*(3), 219–233. http://doi.org/10.1177/1356336X14524854

Evans, J., Rich, E., Davies, B., & Allwood, R. (2008). *Education, disordered eating and obesity discourses: Fat fabrications.* London: Routledge.

Fitzpatrick, K., & Burrows, L. (2017). Critical health education in Aotearoa New Zealand. *Sport, Education and Society, 22*(5), 552–568. http://doi.org/10.1080/13573322.2015.1131154

Fitzpatrick, K., & Tinning, R. (2014). *Health education. Critical perspectives.* New York: Routledge.

Gard, M. (2008). Producing little decision makers and goal setters in the age of obesity crisis. *Quest, 60*(4), 488–502.

Gard, M. (2011). *The end of the obesity epidemic.* New York: Routledge.

Gard, M. (2016). Hearing noises and noticing silence: Toward a critical engagement with Canadian body weight statistics. In J. Ellison, D. McPhail, & W. Mitchinson (Eds.), *Obesity in Canada. Critical perspectives* (pp. 31–55). Toronto, ON: University of Toronto Press.

Gard, M., & Pluim, C. (2014). *Schools and public health. Past, present and future.* Plymouth: Lexington Books.

Gard, M., & Vander Schaee, C. (2011). The obvious solution. In M. Gard, (Ed.) *The end of the obesity epidemic* (pp. 82–107). New York: Routledge.

Gard, M., & Wright, J. (2005). *The obesity epidemic. Science, morality and ideology.* New York: Routledge.

Gill, R. (2010). Breaking the silence: The hidden injuries of the neoliberal university. In R. Ryan-Flood & G. Gill (Eds.), *Secrecy and silence in the research process: Feminist reflections* (pp. 228–244). New York: Routledge.

Giroux, H. (2004). Public pedagogy and the politics of neoliberalism: Making the political pedagogical. *Policy Futures in Education, 2*(3–4), 494–503. http://doi.org/10.2304/pfie.2004.2.3.5

Halse, C. (2009). *Biopolitics and the obesity epidemic. Governing bodies.* New York: Routledge.

Hickey, C., Kirk, D., Macdonald, D., & Penney, D. (2014). Curriculum reform in 3D: A panel of experts discuss the new HPE curriculum in Australia. *Asia-Pacific Journal of Health, Sport and Physical Education, 5*(2), 181–192. http://doi.org/10.1080/18377122.2014.911057

Holmes, B. (2009). Media coverage of Canada's obesity epidemic: Illustrating the subtleties of surveillance medicine. *Critical Public Health, 19*(2), 223–233. http://doi.org/10.1080/09581590802478048

Kirk, D. (2010). *The history of physical education.* New York: Routledge.

Kwauk, C. T. (2012). Obesity and the healthy living apparatus: Discursive strategies and the struggle for power. *Critical Discourse Studies, 9*(1), 39–57. http://doi.org/10.1080/17405904.2011.632139

Macdonald, D., Johnson, R., & Leow, A. (2014). Health education and health promotion: Beyond cells and bells. In K. Fitzgerald & R. Tinning (Eds.), *Health education. Critical perspectives* (pp. 17–30). New York: Routledge.

Malhotra, A., Noakes, & Phinney, S. (2015). It's time to bust the myth of physical inactivity and obesity: You cannot run a bad diet. *British Journal of Sports Medicine, 49*(15), 967–968. http://doi.org/10.1136/bjsports-2015-094911

Mayes, C. (2016). *The biopolitics of lifestyle. Foucault, ethics and healthy choices.* New York: Routledge.

McPhail, D., (2017). *Canada weighs in: Gender and Race and the making of "obesity", 1945–1970.* Toronto, ON: UT Press.

McVey, L., & Harrison, P. (2018). This girl can('t): A risk of subjectification and self-surveillance in Sport England's behaviour change campaign. *Leisure Studies,* 1–24. http://doi.org/10.1080/01490400.2018.1519472

Monaghan, L., Bombak A., & Rich, E. (2018). Obesity, neoliberalism and epidemic psychology: Critical commentary and alternative approaches to public health. *Critical Public Health, 28*(5), 498–508. http://doi.org/10.1080/09581596.2017.1371278

Monaghan, L., Rich, E., & Bombak, A. (2019). Media, 'fat panic,' and public pedagogy: Mapping contested terrain. *Sociology Compass, 13,* 1–17. http://doi.org/10.1111/soc4.12651

Norman, M., Rail, G., & Jette, A. (2014). Moving subjects, feeling bodies: Emotion and the materialization of fat feminine subjectivities in Village on a Diet. *Fat Studies, 3*(1), 17–31. http://doi.org/10.1080/21604851.2013.778166

Norman, M., Rail, G., & Jette, S. (2016). Screening the un-scene: Deconstructing the (bio)politics of storytelling in a Canadian makeover weight loss series. In J. Ellison, D. McPhail & W. Mitchinson (Eds.), *Obesity in Canada. Critical perspectives.* Toronto, ON: University of Toronto Press.

Parliamentary Report. (2016, March). *Obesity in Canada: A whole-of-society approach for a healthier Canada.* Standing Senate Committee on Social Affairs, Science and Society. Ottawa, ON: Government of Canada. Retrieved from www.senate-senat.ca/social.asp

ParticipACTION. (2018). *The Brain + Body Equation: Canadian kids need active bodies to build their best brains. The ParticpACTION Report Card on Physical Activity for Children and Youth.* Toronto, ON: ParticipACTION. Retrieved from https://www.participaction.com/en-ca/resources/report-card

Pausé, C. (2017). Borderline: The ethics of fat stigma in public health. *The Journal of Law, Medicine & Ethics, 45,* 510–517. http://doi.org/10.1177/1073110517750585

Piggin, J., & Bairner, A. (2016). The global physical inactivity pandemic. An analysis of knowledge production. *Sport, Education and Society, 21*(2), 131–147. http://doi.org/10.1080/13573322.2014.882301

Pringle, R. (2010). Finding pleasure in physical education. A critical examination of the educative value of positive movement effects. *Quest, 62*(2), 119–134. http://doi.org/10.1080/00336297.2010.10483637

Puhl, R., & Heurer, C. (2009). Obesity stigma: A review and update. *Obesity, 17*(5), 941–964. http://doi.org/10.1038/oby.2008.636

Puhl, R., Peterson, J., DePierre, J., & Joerg, L. (2013). Headless, hungry, and unhealthy: A video content analysis of obese persons portrayed in online news. *Journal of Health Communication, 18*(6), 686–702. http://doi.org/10.1080/10810730.2012.743631

Rich, E. (2010). Obesity assemblages and surveillance in schools. *International Journal of Qualitative Studies in Education, 23*(7), 803–821. http://doi.org/10.1080/09518398.2010.529474

Rich, E. (2011). "I see her being obesed." Public pedagogy, reality media and the obesity crisis. *Health, 15*(1) 3–21. http://doi.org/10.1177/1363459309358127

Rich, E. (2018). Gender, health and physical activity in the digital age: Between post-feminism and pedagogical possibilities. *Sport, Education and Society, 23*(8), 736–747. http://doi.org/10.1080/13573322.2018.1497593

Rich, E., Monaghan, L., & Bombak, A. E. (2019). A discourse analysis of school girls' engagement with fat pedagogy and critical health education: Rethinking the childhood obesity scandal. *Sport, Education & Society, 25*(2), 127–142. http://doi.org/10.1080/13573322.2019.1566121

Shankar, N., & Park, C. (2016). Effects of stress on students' physical and mental health and academic success. *International Journal of School and Educational Psychology, 4*(1), 5–9. http://doi.org/10.1080/2 1683603.2016.1130532

Tinning, R. (2014). Getting which message across? The (H)PE teacher as health educator. In K. Fitzpatrick & R. Tinning (Eds.), *Health education. Critical perspectives* (pp. 204–219). New York: Routledge.

World Health Organization. (2018). Global action plan on physical activity (2018–2030). A more active people for a healthier world. Geneva: World Health Organization.

Wright, J., & Harwood, V. (2009). *Biopolitics and the obesity epidemic. Governing bodies.* New York: Routledge.

36

THE ETHICS OF OBESITY POLICY

T. M. Wilkinson

Governments have tried to limit obesity by advising, exhorting, educating, and encouraging their citizens and by taxing and regulating some food and drink while subsidising others. Should governments try to affect their citizens' consumption? This chapter focuses on tax and regulation, and it treats with some scepticism these arguments for them: (1) "costs to others" arguments, such as the cost in health care caused by obesity, (2) paternalistic arguments that people need to be protected from themselves, and (3) social justice arguments that intervening would reduce health inequities.

Since many policies could affect obesity, the term "obesity policy" is potentially very broad. Public transport policy and environmental design could increase the amount of exercise people do. Reducing agricultural price supports or taxing freight transport could increase the price of food and decrease consumption. The effect on obesity might be reasons for these policies, which could be called "stealth interventions" in obesity (Swinburn, 2008). However, the effect would not be the only or main reason for these policies, which are also argued for because of the benefits they might have for reducing congestion, preserving communities, or reducing pollution. For the sake of focus, let us take a narrow definition and have "obesity policy" refer to policies, actual or proposed, that have as a main aim the reduction of obesity. We might roughly classify these policies as:

- Aiming to alter people's beliefs. In this category might fall mandating providing information about calories in food or healthy-tick style labelling requirements. Also, in this category might fall censorship, as with restrictions on the marketing of junk food.
- Aiming to change behaviour by increasing the costs of obesity-promoting behaviour. Into this category might fall taxes on sugar, mandatory restrictions on portion sizes, and planning regulations that make it harder to buy fast food.
- Aiming to change behaviour by decreasing the costs of behaviour that would counteract obesity, such as subsidizing gym memberships or removing sales tax from fruit and vegetables.
- Altering the environment – mandatory reformulation to reduce sugar in food and drink might be one example. Other examples could be reducing plate sizes, making healthy food prominent in shops, and making visible the stairs in public buildings, all of which can be called "nudging," a currently fashionable idea to manipulate the environment

DOI: 10.4324/9780429344824-43

so as to steer people into behaving healthily in an automatic way (Thaler & Sunstein, 2009).

Some obesity policies are not very ethically controversial. For instance, mandatory labelling of ingredients might be ineffective (Downs & Loewenstein, 2011), but it does not really interfere with people's autonomy or harm them. Other policies need more ethical justification. About decreasing costs, the main questions concern how it would be financed and what else the resources could have been used for. For instance, a subsidy for fruit and vegetables could primarily benefit the middle class using revenue that could have gone to worse-off people (Child Poverty Action Group, 2010). As for environmental changes, mandatory reformulation is likely to raise costs for consumers (Wilkinson, 2019b) and nudging is sometimes claimed to manipulate people's minds and constitute a worrying exercise of unaccountable governmental power (Rebonato, 2012; Wilkinson, 2013).

What clearly needs ethical evaluation are government policies to reduce obesity that use the power to regulate and tax, and they are the focus of this chapter. To keep the chapter manageable, I concentrate on evaluating the arguments in favour of these policies rather than the arguments against government interference. The arguments have some merit, but they make assumptions with too little support to justify tax and regulation.

The leading ethical arguments for obesity policy are:

- Fairness: obesity imposes costs, especially in health care and lost production, and it is unfair that people who are not obese should pay them.
- Welfare: obesity is bad for people, in particular, people's health.
- Social justice: obesity follows a social gradient and reducing obesity would reduce health inequities.

All of these arguments presuppose that obesity is bad for people's health. Other chapters in this book have gone thoroughly into whether obesity is bad for health and, if it is, whether it is as bad as is often claimed. Suffice to say that if obesity is not bad for health, then cost-raising policies to reduce obesity would have no serious justification. For the sake of argument then, I mainly proceed as if obesity were bad for health.

Before considering the arguments in more detail, observe that whether a policy is ethically justified depends in part on what it does, and what it does is a factual question with answers that may well vary in time and place. Take the proposal to remove sales tax on fruit and vegetables. This proposal is a hardy perennial in New Zealand, which has a sales tax on almost everything. The proposal assumes that removing the tax would make fruit and vegetables cheaper so people would eat more of them. But if the food retail market were uncompetitive, then retailers could keep the old price and pocket the difference, with the result that no more fruit and vegetables are eaten and tax revenue is lost. By contrast, dropping the tax in a competitive market really might get people to eat more fruit and vegetables because retailers would have to pass on the tax cut or lose their customers. Hence the same policy, in this case removing sales tax, might be justified in one market and not in the other because the effects vary.

The final general point is that the different arguments need not support the same policies in practice. A tax on sugary drinks might be argued for as fair because it offsets the costs to non-drinkers or as promoting welfare by discouraging people from drinking them. But fairness and welfare may support different rates of taxation. For instance, a tax that offsets the costs people impose on others when they consume soft drinks may be much lower than the tax that would most reduce their consumption.

Fairness arguments

A fairness argument can be understood like this. It is unfair to impose costs on other people. More strictly, the idea is that it is unfair for people who could have done otherwise to impose net costs on other people who do not consent, and it is reasonable for the government to prevent such costs being imposed. Thus, people may be legitimately prevented from driving unsafe cars. Drivers may reasonably have to pay a congestion charge. Developers may reasonably be required to provide a number of parking spaces to keep residents' cars from clogging up local streets. Similarly, food and drink and activities that cause obesity may be taxed or discouraged to prevent the non-obese having to pay the costs of health care and lost productivity. (My discussion of fairness arguments skips over many complications, some of which can be found in Cappelen and Norheim, 2005.)

Arguments for obesity policy frequently cite social costs with "scary numbers." For example, Wang, McPherson, Mash, Gortmaker, and Brown (2011) estimate a \$46–48 billion per year increase in medical costs by 2030 in the US from the effect of rising obesity on diabetes, heart disease, stroke, and cancer, and they claim that "the monetary value of lost productivity is several times larger than medical costs" (Wang et al., 2011, p. 817). Leaving aside whether these figures are even approximately correct, notice that the "scary numbers" often lump together costs that fall on the people who are obese, such as an economic valuation of the loss of Quality Adjusted Life Years due to dying early and those that fall on others (Bhattacharya & Sood, 2011). For the purposes of a fairness argument, only costs to others are relevant. A fairness argument must be distinguished from a utilitarian argument that claims that reducing obesity would lead to more overall benefit when aggregated across everyone, including those who would otherwise be more obese.

I do not think that the fairness argument can be entirely ruled out but, for several reasons, one may doubt whether it applies in typical developed countries. The fairness argument claims that obesity imposes costs on the non-obese. When broken down, the argument would have to show (a) that obesity did impose net costs and (b) that those costs did not fall entirely on the obese themselves. Both of these claims have been asserted but not definitively proved.

Obviously, if obesity did not cause ill health, then obesity would not directly cause increased health expenditure. Another, inconsistent, possibility is that obesity is bad enough for people's health that it causes their early death, in which case, the non-obese might get a substantial saving in not paying out pensions (Anomaly, 2012, p. 218). This apparently cynical observation is not supposed to be an argument for encouraging early death; it simply emphasizes that a fairness argument has to show that obesity really does have costs to others (a point missed by Wang et al., 2011, p. 822). It is also possible that obesity has costs, but they are borne by the obese themselves. To the extent that health care is provided privately, those who use health care more could pay more, if only in insurance premiums (Bhattacharya & Sood, 2011). The alleged costs in production caused by absenteeism might well be paid by the absent workers themselves, for instance, in lower wages or foregone promotion (Averett, 2011).

Suppose nonetheless that, in some society, obesity really does impose uncompensated costs on the non-obese. Then, it must be asked whether obese people can fairly be held liable for these costs. Lost production might not be due primarily to absenteeism but to discrimination. Obese people might be kept out of certain jobs or assumed to be incompetent (Cawley, 2011, p. 128). This would be a cost to them but it would also be a social cost because of the inefficient use of workers. But while obesity would be, in some sense, a cause of the discrimination, it would be manifestly unfair to expect the people discriminated against to pay the social costs.

Discrimination aside and other things equal, some tax might make matters more fair by either preventing obesity and thereby its costs or raising revenue to offset the costs. But other things might not be equal. In developed economies, obesity tends to occur on a social gradient – the poorer tend to be more obese than the richer (McLaren, 2011). If, as public health advocates hope, an offsetting tax would be passed on to consumers in higher prices, the tax would be regressive, that is, a transfer from poorer people to richer people, and that would be in one way unfair. Put another way, fairness may not overall justify a tax even if obesity does have costs to the non-obese, which it might well not anyway. For all these reasons, I doubt that the fairness argument for tax and regulation can be made out.

Welfare

The fairness argument for obesity policy is about avoiding the costs some people might impose on others. By contrast, the welfare argument is about the costs the obese might impose on themselves. To make explicit what is often only implicit, here is the common structure of arguments grounded in promoting the welfare of the targets of policy.

1   This policy (sugar tax, fast food regulation, etc.) would reduce obesity.
2   Reducing obesity increases health.

Therefore

3   This policy would make its targets better off (i.e., have more welfare).

This is just the structure of an argument and public health advocates would want to qualify it in various ways. For instance, it is widely acknowledged in public health that some anti-obesity policies could be ineffective (see e.g., Toomath [2016] on the ineffectiveness of encouraging dieting) and that policy needs to be grounded in evidence (Swinburn et al., 2011). It is also acknowledged by many public health advocates that policies risk stigmatizing, with consequent bad effects on the welfare of their targets, although they often claim (quite likely correctly) that taxing and regulating are less stigmatizing than many interventions (Toomath, 2016, chs. 8 & 9). Granted the qualifications, the basic structure of the welfare argument is to be found over and over again in advocacy of obesity policies. However, the argument raises difficult ethical questions. To use the language of political theory, the argument is paternalistic when concluding in favour of tax and regulation, which uses government coercion to alter people's decisions on the grounds that they would otherwise act contrary to their own welfare. Paternalism is controversial in politics and ethics (Dworkin, 2017). One leading objection is that paternalism wrongly infringes upon people's autonomy, that is, is contrary to the principle that people should be free to run their own lives for themselves. Another objection is that paternalism is self-defeating, that when coercion steers people away from doing what they would otherwise prefer it is likely to make them worse off, not better off (Mill, 1982, pp. 142–143 is the classic statement). It is this second objection I focus on because it would be decisive if paternalistic anti-obesity policy really would worsen the lives of the people it is supposed to help.

The rest of this section points out that health is not identical with well-being; that anti-obesity policies tend to reduce choices; that people might quite reasonably act in ways that make them obese; that the claim that anti-obesity policies would improve the welfare of their targets has to give grounds to think that people make mistaken decisions; and that we do not have such grounds for many people. First, though, a word about children. In what follows, I shall leave children aside although, of course, childhood obesity is a major concern of public health advocates. Children are generally considered legitimate targets for paternalism because they do not meet the conditions for being autonomous (Buchanan & Brock, 1989). At least to some extent they can be the object of anti-obesity policy that does not spill over to adults, such as policies banning sugary drinks in schools. Those bald statements leave some problems: what of children who are nearly adults; are they to be treated as non-autonomous? Why think obesity is bad for the overall welfare of children? What of policies that might be good for children but bad for adults, such as an enforced price rise of junk food? Regrettably, space precludes attempting to answer these questions.

Returning to the argument above about how anti-obesity policy would benefit adults, notice the major gap when it moved from "reducing obesity increases health" to "this policy increases welfare." A policy could increase health and yet reduce welfare.

Neither health nor welfare can be defined simply and uncontroversially. Health is often thought of in terms of biological functioning, a view that usually has to be modified in some way given an adequate account of mental health (Powers & Faden, 2006, ch. 2). Welfare is sometimes thought to be a function of having desirable mental states, sometimes the fulfilment of one's desires, and sometimes of having items on a list which includes health but also other goods, such as attachments and self-respect (Parfit, 1984, appendix I; Powers & Faden, 2006). The important point for this discussion is that on no plausible view of either welfare or health are they identical with each other (Wilkinson, 2019b). Thus, it cannot be said that health is just welfare and so whenever health increases, welfare necessarily increases. Nor is health so important in welfare that any loss in health outweighs any gain in other components of welfare. Of course, health is important in welfare, so a gain in welfare often would be a gain in overall welfare. But a gain in someone's health could make them worse off overall.

I should acknowledge that the World Health Organization actually does define health in such a way that it seems identical with welfare (WHO Constitution, Article 1). The WHO says that "Health is a state of complete physical, mental and social well-being and not merely the absence of disease or infirmity." While I think that the WHO definition is obviously wrong, I can rephrase the problem with the welfare argument in its terms – a policy might reduce obesity without increasing health because health is now the whole of welfare, and so any gain in avoiding, say, cardiovascular disease or diabetes might be outweighed by the loss of other parts of "complete physical, mental and social well-being."

Go back to a view of health as not the whole of welfare. That a policy could increase health but reduce welfare is not merely an abstract possibility as we can begin to see if we appreciate these two points. First, obesity comes about in most cases through people's decisions. Second, taxation and regulation will often reduce people's options because, given a limited budget, increasing the money or time price of some goods will reduce the overall quantity of what they can obtain. Let me explain.

To say that obesity occurs as a result of decisions about what to consume and how to exercise is not to say that obesity is solely the result of decisions, only that obesity comes about through some function of consumption and exercise and that consuming and exercising involve actions. They are unlike non-voluntary movements, so unlike the functioning of the kidney, and they do not merely befall people, so unlike being hit by a meteorite (Smith & Jones, 1986, ch. IX). That obesity is the result of decisions is consistent with the decisions being irrational or against the decider's interest or not reflected upon properly.

Tax and regulations generally reduce options. A sugary drink might still be affordable, and so available, even if it costs more; but the overall set of what one can do is reduced if the price of the drink increases (and the budget does not). The point is sometimes obscured in public health arguments. Many scholars do not seem to see the ethical difference between choice-restricting measures, such as taxes, and choice-enhancing ones, such as subsidies (e.g. Hawkes et al., 2015). Public health advocates often use the slogan *Make the healthy choice the easy choice* in a tendentious way by applying it to making unhealthy options harder to take (see e.g. Obesity Action Scotland, 2017). If sugary drinks or junk food were banned, taxed, or compulsorily moved into the next suburb, then water and healthy food would in one sense have become relatively easier to consume. But the method would be by worsening options. The more honest slogan would be "Make the unhealthy choices the hard choices."[1]

If we now combine the points so far, we have this question: how could reducing people's options make them better off when it stops them doing what they would otherwise decide to do? We know that the answer "it makes them thinner and therefore healthier" is inadequate. Even if reducing options would make people healthier, it could still make them worse off in welfare.

At this stage, the debate turns to how people decide to consume or exercise and whether they decide mistakenly or irrationally. We must not assume that decisions that result in obesity must be irrational. We must not, as some public health advocates do, conflate "healthy choices" with "informed choices" (Rajczi, 2008, p. 276). If people dislike exercise or enjoy junk food, or if they lack the time and money to exercise or to shop for and cook with raw ingredients, they may reasonably judge weight gain to be a price worth paying for "unhealthy choices."

If people make rational choices, reducing their options would not make them better off and likely would make some people worse off, even if it made them thinner. What if people do not make rational choices? What if, as many writers assert, their consumption is influenced by marketing, or unconscious cues, or temptation? Since we can be influenced to do the right things as well as the wrong, showing influence alone is not enough. The argument needs to show that the choices would make people worse off. This task can be broken down into two elements:

1   Explain how someone's choices can make them worse off in welfare.
2   Provide the evidence that people's choices in fact do make them worse off in this way.

When it comes to the first element, the usual idea is that people do not choose in a way that gives them what they want in the long term, namely health. For instance, people might be myopic, that is, they give too much weight to the short-term benefits of consuming and not exercising and not enough to the long-term benefits that they themselves think are more important (Conly, 2013). Remove or raise the price of the option that brings short-term benefits but greater long-term costs and people will choose a better option. Leaving aside various complications, I agree that it may be possible to make people better off by restricting their options (Wilkinson, 2019b).

What, then, of the evidence? Some literature claims that the rise in obesity in developed countries can be explained by changes in costs and benefits. Obesogenic food and drink have become cheaper and easier to get, and possibly, the alternatives to exercise have become more desirable (Cutler, Glaeser, & Shapiro, 2003; Offer, 2006). For some writers, people make rational choices and consume more and exercise less (Cutler et al., 2003), whereas, for others, people have become overwhelmed by temptation and act irrationally (Offer, 2006). Establishing whether choices are rational or not is very difficult. Some survey evidence finds that people consume more sugary drinks than they themselves think is best and infers that a tax that reduces their consumption to the level they prefer would make them better off (Allcott, Lockwood, & Taubinsky, 2019). Dieting is sometimes cited as showing that people regret their previous consumption and would have been better off not having consumed that way (Offer, 2006). On the other hand, at least some people would not benefit from having their choices reduced. Not everyone is dieting; only 27 percent said that they were trying seriously to lose weight in a recent US poll (Gallup, 2018).

It seems very likely to me that some adults could benefit from having their choices reduced by obesity policy. They would be the ones who want to be less fat than they would be if left to their own devices. It also seems very likely that some people would not be better off. Not all citizens would benefit from, nor want, paternalistic interventions (Wilson, 2011). Hence choice-reducing obesity policies raise a question of justice in balancing the interests of those who gain and those who lose. The next section considers the idea that, in balancing, one should give extra priority to the interests of the worse off.

Social justice

The field of public health often uses the language of social justice; some writers even claim that social justice, rather than the value of more health, is the ethical foundation of public health (Powers & Faden, 2006). On a commonly held view, it is unjust that people from some social groups, such as those with low incomes, are less healthy than others, such as those with high incomes; and because it is unjust, it is especially important, ethically speaking, to try to reduce these health disparities. Since obesity is bad for health and more common among low-income people, reducing and preventing obesity is a matter of social justice. Consequently, anti-obesity tax and regulation might be required by social justice even if they would be bad for some people (e.g. Swinburn, 2008; Brownell & Frieden, 2009).

Let me make two initial points about this social justice argument. First, social justice might count in favour of many interventions, say in social welfare, the labour and housing markets, and education. On behalf of the case for obesity policy, it strikes me as irrelevant to say such policies would not alone achieve social justice. Why should any one type of policy achieve full justice? But it also strikes me as intellectual confusion to think that if one opposes taxes and regulations that reduce choice, one can be written off as a neoliberal who is against all interference with the free market. One can instead favour many "interferences" without wanting choice-reducing anti-obesity ones. Second, the justifications given for reducing health disparities often make up a grab bag of anything the authors vaguely think might support it (Braveman et al., 2011, is a prime example) even though the considerations appear to recommend conflicting policies. However, one important and coherent element that usually does underlie "social justice" is giving priority to the welfare of the worst off (Braveman et al., 2011). I think giving priority to the worst off is at least defensible and probably correct (Parfit, 1997). Note, because it matters for later, that the priority is to welfare, not health.

The big problem for arguing from social justice to taxing and regulating is to show that it actually would make poorer people better off in welfare. In advance of the evidence (and we are, I think, in advance of the evidence), we could reason either that the policies increase or reduce welfare. Remember from the previous section that taxing and regulating is designed to affect people's decisions and actions and remember the puzzle: how could making some actions harder or more expensive make people better off? It might be said that it is the worst off who are least able to make sensible decisions (Kniess, 2015). Perhaps, for instance, people who are struggling to get by do not have the mental "bandwidth" to be able to think through and act on what they really want to consume and instead take what is quick and cheap, but unhealthy (Mullainathan & Shafir, 2013). On the other hand, it might be perfectly sensible for people without much money or time to consume quick and cheap but unhealthy food. The very fact that they do not have much money or time means that they could be rational to be willing to pay a price in health to consume such food and drink and indeed be more rational than weak-willed middle-class people who give into temptation (Wilkinson, 2019a).

Thus, a story can be told where social justice speaks in favour of or against tax and regulation. What social justice says depends on whether the badly off would be choosing against their interest, that is, would be making themselves worse off if their choices were not shaped by tax and regulation. Are they? I do not think anyone knows (Wilkinson, 2019a). Public health advocates sometimes think that they know, but it turns out that what they have in mind are, say, some studies showing how a tax reduced consumption of sugary drinks. Such studies obviously would not even show that consumers are healthier for the tax let alone whether they are better off. It may be instructive here to revisit some evidence about dieting. Earlier, I quoted a Gallup poll for the US indicating that only a small minority of adults were trying to lose weight. Other polls indicate that the financially worst off are the least likely to be trying (CDC, 2013–2014), which is some grounds for thinking they are the least likely to benefit (as judged by their preferences) from being pushed into losing weight. In my view, the evidence is not good enough to support a social justice argument for reducing the options of badly off people so as to make them thinner than they would otherwise be.

Conclusion

This chapter has focused on policies that aim to reduce obesity by raising the costs of the decisions that cause it. At least when it comes to adults, such policies need ethical justification. The leading attempts to justify them claim that raising costs would be fair, would improve the welfare of their targets, or would be required by social justice, which is just a way of saying that they would improve the welfare of the socioeconomically badly off. I have raised doubt about all of these arguments. The point is not that they are fundamentally flawed. Under some conditions, these arguments could genuinely justify reducing choices. The point is that working through them shows that the arguments rely on certain assumptions, such as that the obese do impose substantial costs on others or that badly off people really would benefit from having fewer options. These assumptions are insufficiently supported to justify anti-obesity tax and regulations.

Acknowledgements

Geoff Kemp, Kathy Smits, Steve Winter.

Note

1 Thanks to Mike King for this suggestion.

References

Allcott, H., Lockwood, B., & Taubinsky, T. (2019). Regressive sin taxes, with an application to the optimal soda tax. *The Quarterly Journal of Economics, 134*(3), 1557–1626. doi: 10.1093/qje/qjz017.
Anomaly, J. (2012). Is obesity a public health problem? *Public Health Ethics, 5*(3), 216–221. doi: 10.1093/phe/phs028

Averett, S. L. (2011). Labor market consequences: Employment, wages, disability, and absenteeism. In J. Cawley (Ed.), *The Oxford handbook of the social science of obesity*. Oxford: Oxford University Press.

Bhattacharya, J., & Sood, N. (2011). Who pays for obesity? *Journal of Economic Perspectives, 25*(1), 139–158. doi: 10.1257/jep.25.1.139

Braveman, P. A., Kumanyika, S., Fielding, J., LaVeist, T., Borrell, L. N., Manderscheid, R., & Troutman, A. (2011). Health disparities and health equity: the issue is justice. *American Journal of Public Health, 101*(S1), S149–S155. doi: 10.2105/AJPH.2010.300062

Brownell, K. D., & Frieden, T. R. (2009). Ounces of prevention—the public policy case for taxes on sugared beverages. *New England Journal of Medicine, 360*(18), 1805–1808. doi: 10.1056/NEJMp0902392

Buchanan, A. E., & Brock, D. W. 1989. *Deciding for others: The ethics of surrogate decision making*. Cambridge: Cambridge University Press.

Cappelen, A. W., & Norheim, O. F. (2005). Responsibility in health care: A liberal egalitarian approach. *Journal of Medical Ethics, 31*(8), 476–80. doi: 10.1136/jme.2004.010421

Cawley, J. 2011. The economics of obesity. In J. Cawley (Ed.), *The Oxford handbook of the social science of obesity*. Oxford: Oxford University Press.

CDC [Center for Disease Control]. National Health and Nutrition Examination Survey 2013–2014. Retrieved from https://wwwn.cdc.gov/Nchs/Nhanes/2013–2014/WHQ_H.htm#WHQ040 (August 19, 2019).

Child Poverty Action Group. (2010). Will removing GST on fresh fruit and vegetables achieve its stated aim? Retrieved from https://www.cpag.org.nz/assets/Tax%20Issues/Backgrounder_GSTExemptions%20on%20Food%20final.pdf (August 19, 2019).

Conly, S. (2013). *Against Autonomy: Justifying coercive paternalism*. Cambridge: Cambridge University Press.

Cutler, D. M., Glaeser, E. L., & Shapiro, J. M. (2003). Why have Americans become more obese? *Journal of Economic Perspectives, 17*(3), 93–118. doi: 10.1257/089533003769204371

Downs, J. S. & Loewenstein, G. (2011). Behavioral economics and obesity. In J. Cawley (Ed.), *The Oxford handbook of the social science of obesity*. (pp. 138–157). Oxford: Oxford University Press.

Dworkin, G. (2017). Paternalism. *Stanford Encyclopedia of Philosophy*. Retrieved from https://plato.stanford.edu/entries/paternalism/ (August 17, 2019).

Gallup. (2018). Personal Weight Situation. Retrieved from https://news.gallup.com/poll/7264/personal-weight-situation.aspx (August 19, 2019).

Hawkes, C., Smith, T. G., Jewell, J., Wardle, J., Hammond, R.A., Friel, S., Thow, A. M., & Kain, J. (2015). Smart food policies for obesity prevention. *The Lancet, 385*(9985), 2410–2421.

Kniess, J. (2015). Obesity, paternalism and fairness. *Journal of Medical Ethics, 41*(11), 889–892. doi: 10.1136/medethics-2014–102537

McLaren, L. (2011). Socioeconomic status and obesity. In J. Cawley (Ed.), *The Oxford handbook of the social science of obesity*. Oxford: Oxford University Press.

Mill, J. S. (1982). *On liberty*. Harmondsworth: Penguin.

Mullainathan, S., & Shafir, E. 2013. *Scarcity: Why having too little means so much*. Basingstoke: Macmillan.

Obesity Action Scotland. (2017). Make the healthy choice the easy choice. Retrieved from https://www.obesityactionscotland.org/campaigns/make-the-healthy-choice-the-easy-choice (August 19, 2019).

Offer, A. (2006). *The challenge of affluence: Self-control and well-being in the United States and Britain since 1950*. New York: Oxford University Press.

Parfit, D. (1984). *Reasons and persons*. Oxford: Oxford University Press.

Parfit, D. (1997). Equality and priority. *Ratio, 10*(3), 202–221. doi: 10.1111/1467–9329.00041

Powers, M., & Faden, R. (2006). *Social justice: The moral foundations of public health and health policy*. New York: Oxford University Press.

Rajczi, A. (2008). A liberal approach to the obesity epidemic. *Public Affairs Quarterly, 22*(3), 269–287.

Rebonato, R. (2012). *Taking liberties: A critical examination of libertarian paternalism*. Basingstoke: Palgrave Macmillan.

Smith, P., & Jones, O. R. (1986). *The philosophy of mind: An introduction*. Cambridge: Cambridge University Press.

Swinburn, B. (2008). Obesity prevention: the role of policies, laws and regulations. *Australia and New Zealand Health Policy, 5*(1), 5–12. doi: 10.1186/1743–8462–5–12

Swinburn, B., Sacks, G., Hall, K., McPherson, K., Finegood, D., Moodie, M., & Gortmaker, S. 2011. The global obesity pandemic: Shaped by global drivers and local environments. *The Lancet, 378*(9793), 804–814. doi: 10.1016/S0140–6736(11)60813-1

Thaler, R., & Sunstein, C. 2009. *Nudge: Improving decisions about health, welfare, and happiness.* New Haven, CT: Yale University Press.

Toomath, R. (2016). *Fat science: Why diets and exercise don't work--and what does.* Auckland: Auckland University Press.

Wang, Y. C., McPherson, K., Marsh, T., Gortmaker, S. L., & Brown, M. (2011). Health and economic burden of the projected obesity trends in the USA and the UK. *The Lancet, 378,* (9793), 815–825. doi: 10.1016/S0140–6736(11)60814-3

Wilkinson, T. M. (2013). Nudging and manipulation. *Political Studies, 61,* 2, 341–355. doi: 10.1111/j.1467–9248.2012.00974.x

Wilkinson, T. M. (2019a). Obesity, equity and choice. *Journal of Medical Ethics, 45*(5), 323–328. doi: 10.1136/medethics-2018–104848

Wilkinson, T. M. (2019b). Obesity policy and welfare. *Public Affairs Quarterly, 33*(2), 115–136.

Wilson, J. (2011). Why it's time to stop worrying about paternalism in health policy. *Public Health Ethics, 4*(3), 269–279. doi: 10.1093/phe/phr028

World Health Organization (n.d.) Constitution. Retrieved from https://www.who.int/about/who-we-are/constitution (August 19, 2019).

PART H

Future directions

To have a section called 'future directions' can be slightly challenging, especially because 'critical obesity studies' are, to be fairly generous, a couple of decades old. There was, of course, the fat movement and academic fat studies which matured many years before the emergence of the 'obesity epidemic.' And as editors of this present volume, which was also created partly by our publishers, we are comfortable with this name but, as a new field, we are somewhat apprehensive about asking authors to describe what the future may hold. But, having read these three chapters which we selected for the final section, there are many challenges and opportunities to build more optimistic view of research and attitudinal changes.

In her chapter, Anna Kirkland reflects on the 'chequered' US history of civil rights activism for fat people. She describes the difficulties for people who want to balance civil rights change, particularly medical services, with an intellectual satisfying position. For example, despite the major intellectual and practical problems in one's thinking, the direction of US research suggests that one's body shape is relatively out of one's control. To quote her from this chapter:

> I'm left in the regrettable position of wishing civil rights protections on the basis of weight existed much more widely, while also doubting their effectiveness and wanting more and better medical care and insurance coverage at the same time as I see the sites where that care is currently provided as among the most unjust and cruel. In the twenty years that I have been researching these issues, I have not found a way out of these binds.

This chapter might be seen as pessimistic by some readers but, at least from the editors' view, these moments of reflection should not be needlessly wasted, and therefore, this moment can be an offer to pursue different course of action including thinking, researching, and activism. This chapter should be particularly useful to any reader who wants to converge one's knowledge of what happened before with what future possibilities.

In slightly more optimistic tone, written by Patricia Cain, Ngaire Donaghue, and Graeme Ditchburn, this chapter explores more hopeful directions, particularly but not only in public health and weight stigma research. Many readers might have serious doubts about many areas of research, whether conducted by psychologists or other professionals. But they are

DOI: 10.4324/9780429344824-44

interested in looking seriously at the assumptions of previous researchers and building new more positive futures, especially, but not only, for fat people. Whether this is a particular area is relevant or not to the reader of this volume, there is a message here for all critical thinkers; the practice of studies is an ongoing and shifting story.

Finally, this volume concludes with a chapter, written by Gyorgy Scrinis, suggesting that the technical terms around 'obesity' as a form of malnutrition should urgently be reassessed. Scrinis's work has been extremely important for thinkers and researchers for some time, and this particular chapter is partly a summary of previously published material. And while this chapter is focused on nutrition research, he is also asking wide-ranging questions about technical terms and its wider circulations throughout society. For example, Scrinis shows how the framing of obesity as a 'complex problem' of malnutrition 'obscures the structures and power relations that create food systems that produce poor-quality, ultra-processed products and unbalanced diets'. It is for this precise reason that he proposes to change the technical terms conceptualizing obesity as a form of 'over-nutrition' to 'ultra-processed malnutrition' when referring to one of the forms that malnutrition can take the focus on nutrition research on body size and BMI and the 'multiple and interconnected biological pathways' of one's life complicates one's understandings of these terms. He also writes convincing about the '... characteristics, limitations and consequences' of obesity research in general and nutritional sciences in particular.

Having read all of the chapters that we received and our final thoughts, there are many intellectual and practical differences between authors who have written for this volume, the spirit of doubt and re-thinking is alive and kicking. We hope that this spirit and pleasure that we had in reading these chapters is alive and kicking for readers; through the gratification of reading and change one's directions of one's thinking.

37

FRAMEWORKS AND IDEOLOGIES FOR FAT NON-DISCRIMINATION RIGHTS

Anna Kirkland

Introduction

Empirical studies have well-documented the existence of anti-fat attitudes and the effects of fat prejudice across domains of social life such as employment and pay, treatment by health-care professionals, media representations, and interpersonal relationships (Puhl, Brownell, & DePierre, 2019; Puhl & Heuer, 2009). The people most likely to exhibit anti-fat attitudes also tend to hold beliefs that being fat is unhealthy and dangerous, that fat people are a burden on society, and that being fat is within one's personal control. Needless to say, it is very difficult to mobilize broad support for civil rights protections from discrimination and harassment on the basis of weight if it is considered an undesirable trait that people could control if they tried hard enough (Oliver & Lee, 2005). Updated survey research in the US suggests that if people think of body weight as strongly genetically determined, they are more likely to recognize that weight discrimination is common, to have sympathy for fat people, and to support non-discrimination policies (Joslyn & Haider-Markel, 2019). It might seem that convincing more people that one's weight is not entirely within one's control is the best way to win rights, reduce health disparities, and push back stigmatization and humiliation. I certainly use this argument all the time.

But as I take stock of where we are with fat rights as a scholar, things are more complicated. Critical obesity studies at its most useful illuminates many other things in addition to helping us better understand the meaning and power of body sizes. It tells us about what kinds of arguments resonate in our law and political systems, thereby helping us to see what forms of power delimit the possible. I will argue that the possibilities for fat rights remain extremely limited because rights overall are extremely limited. Fatness tends to be overwhelmed by health, disease, and disability frames, which are difficult to assimilate into rights discourses at all, and are much more likely to be rerouted to more narrowed forms of medicalization, pity, or moral disapproval. Where large-scale inequalities seem to account for why heavier people suffer more than others, we rarely manage to come up with a social policy that remedies those inequalities on a large scale. Instead, we paste together narrowly constructed medical approaches while ignoring what we wish our non-existent civil rights provisions would have the capacity to point out: stigmatization, harassment, indignity, and deprivation throughout these medicalized solutions. I'm left in the regrettable position of

DOI: 10.4324/9780429344824-45

wishing civil rights protections on the basis of weight existed much more widely, while also doubting their effectiveness and wanting more and better medical care and insurance coverage at the same time as I see the sites where that care is currently provided as among the most unjust and cruel. In the 20 years that I have been researching these issues, I have not found a way out of these binds.

When there are fat rights, what do they look like?

Weight is not a protected category in most non-discrimination laws in the United States, appearing only in the state of Michigan and in a few cities and municipalities such as San Francisco, Santa Cruz, Washington DC (as 'appearance,' not weight specifically). The non-inclusion of weight or attention to fatness as a civil rights problem has not shifted much over the past 20 years, with little movement to increase statutory protections but no removals of existing protections. Rep. Byron Rushing of Massachusetts introduced multiple bills to add height and weight to his state's non-discrimination law between 2007 and the 2017–2018 legislative session, but none passed. (Rep. Rushing lost a primary election in 2018 and no longer serves in the legislature.) On the one hand, exclusion from civil rights laws is stigmatizing, and especially when inclusion is taken up and rejected, it affirms the idea that fat people deserve to be treated badly. On that view, civil rights inclusion would certainly count as progress. On the other hand, civil rights inclusion is much less likely to bring about substantive social change than many people assume.

I have argued that fat rights and the difficulties in justifying and extending them reveal larger limitations in the US civil rights project in general. These limitations are in many ways limited to the state of the law and rights cultures of the contemporary United States, although other countries have not done much better in protecting fat citizens from discrimination. The main way to justify fat rights is to talk in a superficial way about functional capacities and deservingness, stripping away attention to stigmatized traits and elevating the individual. This functional view shares a lineage to the superficial and inaccurate trope of so-called colorblindness in approaching racial difference (Obasogie, 2013). Functional individualism, as I have termed it, can be useful for defending someone in a particular job context where the task at hand is easily measured or assessed and does not turn much on body size (such as typing a certain number of words per minute, talking on the phone at a call center, and so on). But as soon as the employer can describe the job in terms of making a favorable impression in person, seeming 'energetic,' or looking attractive, then the door is open to pull in weight stigmatization as part of the assessment of the employee's functional capacity. If doing so is perfectly legal (and in most jurisdictions everywhere it is), then there is little to stop it, and the counterargument of functional capacity has lost its power. It does little for people whose bodies really are different from the norm and who may require accommodations in public spaces to be secure and comfortable. It gives way entirely to whatever account of functioning the employer wants to impose.

I have praised the San Francisco height and weight ordinance because it extends civil rights recognition while not also requiring that a person describe herself as disabled if she needs a size-based accommodation such as an armless chair to participate fully in public life (Kirkland, 2008a). The San Francisco Human Rights Commission enforces their non-discrimination ordinance in the city by investigating and mediating disputes. However, it seems that weight-based complaints are nearly non-existent. Weight claims are not listed among all the types of complaints the commission handled in any of its annual reports between 2011 and 2016 (the only ones available online), and much of the annual reports focus on the high numbers of housing discrimination complaints such as landlords' refusals to accept Section 8 housing vouchers (Kauff McGuire & Margolis LLP, 2000; San Francisco Human Rights Commission, 2020). Given the dire economic conditions in San Francisco for lower income people looking for housing, it is not surprising that housing claims are about 60–70 percent of all complaints. It may be that there are not very many people whose civil rights problems can be described as only weight-based rather than intersectional with other categories used to classify them, or intertwined with their housing problems in San Francisco these days, that those people have chosen not to make claims for a variety of common reasons, or that weight-based discrimination in the city has declined. An absence of claims does not tell us very much.

Representing intersectional fat identities in legal claims would be difficult even if there were clear protections, as the long history of attempts to articulate race and gender discrimination simultaneously has illustrated (Cortina & Kirkland, 2018). Courts have recognized, for example, that forms of discrimination may happen to only the black women in a workplace, not to the black men or to the white women, and that singularity does not endanger their claims automatically as it has in the past cases. But progress on this well-studied issue has been agonizingly slow, and Dean Spade argues that even a patched-up civil rights regime that can somewhat integrate categories nonetheless cannot represent and respond to white supremacy and other forms of oppression and just ends up providing cover for the status quo (2013). Just a few states have recently enacted civil rights laws protecting, for example, African-American hair styles such as twists, natural curls, and dreadlocks from differential treatment and bans (Padilla, 2019). There has been little room in legal rights discourse to elaborate on ways that anti-fat prejudice trades on and shares in racism, nativism, misogyny, and other forms of hatred and structural inequality. Scholarship in fat studies has come a long way here (Cooper, 2012; Prohaska & Gailey, 2019; Sanders, 2019; Schalk, 2013; Strings, 2019), but law lags far behind, even when connections to clearly covered categories such as race are available for linkage. The mutual reinforcement of fat hatred and misogyny is well-documented (Rinaldi, Rice, Kotow, & Lind, 2020), but all we have in US law is 'sex plus' discrimination, which prohibits employers from applying weight-based rules to one sex, that it does not apply to the other, such as requiring the women to be thin but hiring men of a wider weight range. (The 'plus' factor does not have to be a legally protected trait itself since the underlying gender inequality is the key to the legal claim.) This provision has kept airlines from requiring female flight attendants to be thinner than their male counterparts, for example, so it has had some real-world impact.

The primary option for employment discrimination and public accommodation rights based on weight or body size has been a disability frame. Despite some broadening of US disability rights law since I published *Fat Rights* in 2008, this general picture has not shifted much either. Legal coverage continues to turn on the question of an underlying medical cause for the person's size. After the passage of the ADA Amendments Act, which made it easier to sustain disability claims based on actual or perceived disabilities, the Equal Employment Opportunity Commission pursued cases against employers who fired otherwise-qualified fat workers without regard to whether there was a proven underlying condition (*EEOC v. Resources for Human Development, Inc.*, 2011; US Equal Employment Opportunity Commission, 2012). Washington State's Supreme Court recently declared that obesity is a disability without a finding of an underlying cause (*Taylor v. Burlington Northern Railroad Holdings Inc.*, 2019), holding that their own state law is broader than the federal ADA. Despite the EEOC's pursuit of cases without underlying conditions, federal courts maintain that requirement and plaintiffs often lose because of it (*Richardson v. Chicago Transit Authority*, 2019).

As I've argued, this frame is unsatisfactory because of its significant legal limitations (because one has to argue that an underlying disease or condition caused the person to be fat under the Americans with Disabilities Act), because of the overall lack of usefulness and transformative power of US disability rights laws generally, and because it requires a person to describe herself as limited and disabled when many fat citizens do not think of themselves that way and would prefer to turn the attention to the structures of a fat-hating world (Kirkland, 2006, 2008b). Harassment counts as a civil rights violation if it can be anchored to a protected trait, so if fatness is a disability, then weight-based harassment could count as disability-based harassment (Weber, 2007). But that form of protection would only work if the underlying disability claim itself was valid, and much of the harassment that larger citizens endure occurs outside the workplace: in public spaces and from intimates in private.

When I interviewed fat rights activists to understand how they made arguments about deserving civil rights, I found the same celebration of functional individualism and unease about disability rights (Kirkland, 2008b). People wanted to be treated as individuals with dignity and worried that claiming disability status would only entrench medicalization and stigmatization further. Not even committed fat rights activists could get far beyond the limited moral range of US civil rights law, showing:

> ... how the dominant logics in our antidiscrimination consciousness – reasoning through the narrow list of analogous traits that should be ignored while true merit is measured instead – demarcate and sustain a very narrow range of imaginable injustices. Only harms that come to an otherwise normal, striving person can be fit in easily. That person is just like the other deserving people but for this one little irrelevant thing.
>
> *(Kirkland, 2008b, p. 424)*

Fat not-rights: increased medicalization and expanded health insurance access

While I would not call them rights expansions, there is another major dimension of policy change related to fatness that has been important – its disease classification and medicalization within a recently expanded healthcare delivery and insurance system in the US. Medical professional organizations now endorse the idea that obesity itself is a disease. The American Medical Association voted in 2013 to classify obesity itself as a disease, not simply a risk factor (2013), joining clinical endocrinologists and cardiologists (Pollack, 2013). It remains a controversial idea (and the AMA House of Delegates vote overrode an internal recommendation against it) because it tags so many people with a disease label that is actually a stigmatized and inaccurate proxy (Charrow & Yerramilli, 2018). Paying for obesity treatments in the US health insurance system is easier with an explicit disease classification and, indeed, increased medicalization of obesity has meant expanded coverage. These changes have come primarily through expanded healthcare access under the Affordable Care Act signed by President Obama in 2010, but also through legislative actions across the states. Healthcare has always been a site of misunderstanding and humiliation for fat people but being excluded from the health insurance market because of one's weight, for example, was a common injustice too (and indeed, was the event that prompted US fat activist Marilyn Wann's rise to national prominence). The Affordable Care Act re-shaped the US health insurance market to make gaining healthcare coverage much easier for many Americans. It expanded Medicaid eligibility for lower income people, prohibited insurance companies from refusing coverage based on pre-existing conditions, and created health insurance marketplaces where individuals and small businesses could shop for policies with subsidies for those unable to pay the full cost.

None of these general coverage reforms were aimed at fat people specifically of course, but it helped a lot of people of all sizes who were self-employed (perhaps, as a result of discrimination avoidance, as some of my interview subjects told me), who had been previously shut out of the individual insurance market, or who would have been considered to have a disqualifying pre-existing condition. The ACA also prompted states to offer more homogeneous insurance plans that required coverage for obesity treatments such as bariatric surgery and nutritional counseling and therapy (some states required a diabetes-related diagnosis before access) (Jannah, Hild, Gallagher, & Dietz, 2018; National Conference of State Legislatures, 2019). Medicare also began covering in-person visits with a primary care physician for obesity treatments in 2011 (Centers for Medicare and Medicaid Services, 2011). Charging extra for health insurance because of obesity status is prohibited across the US (National Conference of State Legislatures, 2019). These policy shifts are a double-edged sword from a critical obesity studies perspective because they entrench the notion of fat as pitiable disease but also provide services and protection from medical bankruptcy for some people who may benefit significantly.

Explicit rules and norms regularly restrict patients' access to certain treatments or procedures because of their weight despite these recent reforms. Many surgeons who perform gender confirmation surgeries will not operate on a trans person who is overweight or obese (Martinson, Ramachandran, Lindner, Reisman, & Safer, 2020), although a study at the University of Michigan showed that there was no significant effect of obesity on complication rates for patients who had undergone penile inversion vaginoplasty there (Ives et al., 2019). Similarly, many people are turned away from orthopedic surgeries such as knee replacements because of their weight, but evidence also shows that patients at higher weights still experienced significant functional gains and pain relief after total joint replacements, just as patients of lower weights did (Li et al., 2017). Many surgeons still require significant weight loss before treatment access (meaning that those patients are likely permanently turned away given the difficulty of sustained weight loss), but these shifts in the professional evidence base may mean that fat patients must shop around, perhaps traveling far distances or resorting to out-of-network providers or cash payments to receive care. There are no laws that prevent this gatekeeping. We would need state insurance regulations and national laws to require payment regardless of weight, and individual physicians could still refuse to operate. These examples show the power of professional norms and practices beyond the reach of the formal law.

The disease frame and the employment rights frame clash directly in yet another closely related policy arena – the corporate wellness program. The ACA also allowed employers to expand their wellness programs and to make incentives and punishments a bit stronger, especially for smoking status. I have worried that employer wellness programs would operate to discriminate against anyone who seems less healthy or energetic, but especially older workers, fat workers, workers with chronic illnesses, and disabled workers (Kirkland, 2014a, 2014b). Corporate wellness programs remain common, but it has been difficult to get data about whether they are discriminatory in practice because private firms have no incentive to allow research on this question. We need transparency laws to reveal salary and compensation discrimination as well as wellness incentive or punitive policy impacts on employees, and currently, there are no legal requirements for firms to disclose. The debate about wellness (or the newer term, well-being) programs has continued in terms of return on investment (ROI), with a recent clinical trial suggesting that employees may report more engagement with their health but that clinical markers of health, spending, and absenteeism may not really change (Song & Baicker, 2019). If it is true that the programs mostly reward healthy workers for things they are already doing and if any money is saved, it comes from charging more for employer-based health insurance to unhealthy workers, then these are simply employee relations and discrimination programs, not health promoting programs.

The disease and disability frames are not very empowering, and the non-discrimination employment rights frame is politically unpopular. It is also reductive and difficult to harness to a full-throated intersectional social justice defense of the dignity of fat lives. One solution, popular in well-meaning and health-focused professions like public health, has been to turn the lens away from fat citizens themselves and onto the environments in which they live (Colls & Evans, 2014; Kirkland, 2011; Yancey, Leslie, & Abel, 2006). The turn to the so-called obesogenic environment has been well studied from many angles, and it certainly does not seem to be an easy solution practically, politically, or ethically. The problem with this environmental frame from a critical perspective is that it builds in assumptions about causes of weight gain and the makeup of the social and economic world, but does not acknowledge how these presumptions act to coproduce that same world (Guthman, 2011). Are prosperous, healthy environments a cause or an effect of the bodies and economic statuses of the people living in them? Connecting this impulse with rights protections would mean saying that people have rights to environments in which they can thrive, or at least the ones that do not actively harm them. This argument has great potential for transformative links to issues such as police violence, security from private violence, climate change, or environmental contamination. But transforming environments requires a level of political change and investment that cannot be commanded by rights discourses and which does not currently enjoy any realistic level of support in the US. Indeed, as political scientist Julia Lynch points out, attempts to use health as a way to gain resources for vulnerable people have a poor record in European wealthy industrialized countries, where neoliberal scolding about individual behaviors has been much more popular than evidence-based policies that would transfer wealth (Lynch, 2019). Predictably, all the attention to health inequalities and the social determinants of health in the US and Europe has had little effect on reducing these gaps, and there has been little policy energy directed towards root causes such as systemic and entrenched poverty (Lynch, 2017). Handwringing about fat people not being able to get to a good farmer's market is just one example of how pitiably thin our conceptions of social transformation can become when we face vast and powerful systems of inequality but are distracted by the shiny things of moral disapproval and fat bodies instead.

Conclusion: what will follow the politics of distraction?

In the years since I published research on fat rights and discrimination, I moved on to work on other topics such as vaccine injury claims, wellness discrimination, and civil rights in healthcare settings. I wondered if the anti-fat rhetoric of the turn of the 21st century had really toned down, or if it just seemed like it because I was not following the topic as closely. Headlines used to regularly scream that obesity would cut many lives short and cost enormous amounts, and public health scholars debated whether shaming fat people would help motivate them to get thinner. The scholarly call for shaming has quieted a bit. Daniel Callahan recently called for 'stigmatization lite' against fat people, hoping to pressure them but not to outright promote discrimination (2013, p. 39). The scholarly positions staked out by scholars at the Rudd Center for Food Policy and Obesity (Puhl et al., 2019) – hardly fat activism but also clearly against the harms of what they prefer to call weight bias – have gained considerable traction and, at least among the medical professionals I spoke to over the years, it became clear that simply pushing people to lose weight was not effective and did not make them healthier, especially if it drove them from care or increased marginalization.

But I would argue that it is not so much that experts and the lay public have consciously re-considered their anti-fat prejudice in the United States, but rather that they have been distracted by other issues. In 2015, American life expectancy decreased for the first time since 1993, and all attention turned to so-called 'diseases of despair' such as opioid use and suicide to explain the downturn (Acciai & Firebaugh, 2017; Case & Deaton, 2015). (The decline in 1993 was because of AIDS and an unusually lethal influenza epidemic that year.) US life expectancies continued to drop for the next three years, the longest sustained period of decline since the post-World War I period that included the 1918 flu epidemic (Solly, 2018). The opioid crisis, in particular, has captured our attention (as well it should) and perhaps, writing dramatic headlines about obesity just seems like old news. It has helped us to focus more on patterns of corporate exploitation and economic isolation (and the whiteness of the epidemic also keeps it from being pushed down as simply a racialized problem, best solved with increased criminalization). Gun violence as a public health issue has also moved in to take up some national space for attention at a new level. The roller coaster of the Trump administration, with its barrage of tweets, crises, impeachment, and general dysfunction has also soaked up so much of the national media conversation that it has surely drowned out many other topics, including obesity trends, that we used to pay much more attention to.

When and if more sustained political attention turns back to framing obesity as a social problem, what will have changed in that conversation? Increased medicalization may have come hand in hand with expanded health care access (particularly if a Democrat wins the presidency in 2020), but it is unclear which way this development cuts. Does it promote greater awareness among physicians that pushing for weight loss is untenable and that the relationship of body fat to health is variable, and dignified care for people as they are, is the better option? Or does it simply multiply opportunities for humiliation? Continuing to make Health at Every Size (HAES)-based arguments (Bacon & Aphramor, 2014) is one of the best routes for activism in the conservative field of medicine and health care delivery. Greater attention to overall economic inequality and generating political commitments to change it would also answer Lynch's argument that too much attention to health dispar-ities undercuts those bigger structural responses. (Again, future readers will know if we have voted in the political changes necessary to do that or not.) The rights frames I have presented here will be mostly useful if they come as an effect of a consensus embrace of acceptance, dignity, and thriving for all. Rights language will be useful if it can be mobi-lized for that end, but without it, rights protections are feeble validations of only one type of mythical individual.

References

Acciai, F., & Firebaugh, G. (2017). Why did life expectancy decline in the United States in 2015? A gender-specific analysis. *Social Science & Medicine, 190*, 174–180. doi: 10.1016/j.socscimed.2017.08.004

American Medical Association. (2013). *Recognition of obesity as a disease. Resolution 420, (A-13). American Medical Association House of Delegates.* Chicago, IL: American Medical Association.

Bacon, L., & Aphramor, L. (2014). *Body respect: What conventional health books get wrong, leave out, and just plain fail to understand about weight* (1st Ed.). Dallas, TX: BenBella Books.

Callahan, D. (2013). Obesity: Chasing an elusive epidemic. *Hastings Center Report, 43*(1), 34–40. doi: 10.1002/hast.114

Case, A., & Deaton, A. (2015). Rising morbidity and mortality in midlife among white non-Hispanic Americans in the 21st century. *Proceedings of the National Academy of Sciences, 112*(49), 15078. doi: 10.1073/pnas.1518393112

Centers for Medicare and Medicaid Services. (2011, November 29). *Decision memo for intensive behavioral therapy for obesity (CAG-00423N).*

Charrow, A., & Yerramilli, D. (2018). Obesity as disease: Metaphysical and ethical considerations. *Ethics, Medicine and Public Health, 7,* 74–81. doi: 10.1016/j.jemep.2018.10.005

Colls, R., & Evans, B. (2014). Making space for fat bodies? A critical account of 'the obesogenic environment.' *Progress in Human Geography, 38*(6), 733–753. doi: 10.1177/0309132513500373

Cooper, C. (2012). A queer and trans fat activist timeline: Queering fat activist nationality and cultural imperialism. *Fat Studies, 1*(1), 61–74.

Cortina, L. M., & Kirkland, A. (2018). Looking forward: What lies ahead in employment discrimination research? In *Oxford Library of Psychology. The Oxford handbook of workplace discrimination* (pp. 435–442). New York: Oxford University Press.

EEOC v. Resources for Human Development, Inc., 827 F. Supp. 2d 688 (District Court, E.D. Louisiana 2011).

Guthman, J. (2011). *Weighing in: Obesity, food justice, and the limits of capitalism.* Oakland: University of California Press.

Ives, G. C., Fein, L. A., Finch, L., Sluiter, E. C., Lane, M., Kuzon, W. M., & Salgado, C. J. (2019). Evaluation of BMI as a risk factor for complications following gender-affirming penile inversion vaginoplasty. *Plastic and Reconstructive Surgery – Global Open, 7*(3), e2097. doi: 10.1097/GOX.0000000000002097

Jannah, N., Hild, J., Gallagher, C., & Dietz, W. (2018). Coverage for obesity prevention and treatment services: Analysis of Medicaid and state employee health insurance programs. *Obesity (Silver Spring, Md.), 26*(12), 1834–1840. doi: 10.1002/oby.22307

Joslyn, M. R., & Haider-Markel, D. P. (2019). Perceived causes of obesity, emotions, and attitudes about discrimination Policy. *Social Science & Medicine, 223,* 97–103. doi: 10.1016/j.socscimed.2019.01.019

Kauff McGuire & Margolis LLP. (2000, May 12). Height and weight are now protected categories in San Francisco. Retrieved February 3, 2020, from *News: Employment Discrimination.* https://www.kmm.com/articles-66.html

Kirkland, A. (2006). What's at stake in fatness as a disability? *Disability Studies Quarterly, 26*(1). https://dsq-sds.org/article/view/648/825

Kirkland, A. (2008a). *Fat rights: Dilemmas of difference and personhood.* New York: New York University Press.

Kirkland, A. (2008b). Think of the hippopotamus: Rights consciousness in the fat acceptance movement. *Law & Society Review, 42*(2), 397–432.

Kirkland, A. (2011). The environmental account of obesity: A case for feminist skepticism. *Signs: Journal of Women in Culture and Society, 36*(2), 463–485.

Kirkland, A. (2014a). Critical perspectives on wellness. *Journal of Health Politics, Policy and Law, 39*(5), 971–988. doi: 10.1215/03616878-2813659

Kirkland, A. (2014b). *What is wellness now?* Durham, NC: Duke University Press.

Li, W., Ayers, D. C., Lewis, C. G., Bowen, T. R., Allison, J. J., & Franklin, P. D. (2017). Functional gain and pain relief after total joint replacement according to obesity status. *The Journal of Bone and Joint Surgery. American Volume, 99*(14), 1183–1189. doi: 10.2106/JBJS.16.00960

Lynch, J. (2017). Reframing inequality? The health inequalities turn as a dangerous frame shift. *Journal of Public Health, 39*(4), 653–660. doi: 10.1093/pubmed/fdw140

Lynch, J. (2019, December). *Regimes of inequality: The political economy of health and wealth.* Cambridge: Cambridge University Press. doi: 10.1017/9781139051576

Martinson, T. G., Ramachandran, S., Lindner, R., Reisman, T., & Safer, J. D. (2020). High body mass index is a significant barrier to gender-confirmation surgery for transgender and gender-nonbinary individuals. *Endocrine Practice, 26*(1), 6–15. doi: 10.4158/EP-2019-0345

National Conference of State Legislatures. (2019, January 23). Health reform and health mandates for obesity. Retrieved February 11, 2020, from https://www.ncsl.org/research/health/aca-and-health-mandates-for-obesity.aspx

Obasogie, O. K. (2013). *Blinded by sight: Seeing race through the eyes of the blind.* Stanford, CA: Stanford University Press.

Oliver, J. E., & Lee, T. (2005). Public opinion and the politics of obesity in America. *Journal of Health Politics, Policy and Law, 30*(5), 923–954. doi: 10.1215/03616878-30-5-923

Padilla, M. (2019, December 20). New Jersey is third state to ban discrimination based on hair. *The New York Times*. Retrieved from https://www.nytimes.com/2019/12/20/us/nj-hair-discrimination.html

Pollack, A. (2013, June 18). A.M.A. Recognizes obesity as a disease. *The New York Times*. Retrieved from https://www.nytimes.com/2013/06/19/business/ama-recognizes-obesity-as-a-disease.html

Prohaska, A., & Gailey, J. A. (2019). Theorizing fat oppression: Intersectional approaches and methodological innovations. *Fat Studies, 8*(1), 1–9. doi: 10.1080/21604851.2019.1534469

Puhl, R. M., Brownell, K. D., & DePierre, J. A. (2019). Bias, discrimination, and obesity. In G. A. Bray & C. Bouchard (Eds.), *Handbook of obesity* (pp. 461–470). Boca Raton, FL: CRC Press.

Puhl, R. M., & Heuer, C. A. (2009). The stigma of obesity: A review and update. *Obesity, 17*(5), 941–964. doi: 10.1038/oby.2008.636

Richardson v. Chicago Transit Authority. 926 F. 3d 881 (Court of Appeals, 7th Circuit 2019).

Rinaldi, J., Rice, C., Kotow, C., & Lind, E. (2020). Mapping the circulation of fat hatred. *Fat Studies, 9*(1), 37–50. doi: 10.1080/21604851.2019.1592949

San Francisco Human Rights Commission. (2020). Budget reports, performance data & annual reports. Retrieved February 6, 2020, from https://sf-hrc.org/budget-reports-performance-data-annual-reports

Sanders, R. (2019). The color of fat: Racializing obesity, recuperating whiteness, and reproducing injustice. *Politics, Groups, and Identities, 7*(2), 287–304. doi: 10.1080/21565503.2017.1354039

Schalk, S. (2013). Coming to claim crip: Disidentification with/in disability studies. *Disability Studies Quarterly, 33*(2). doi: 10.18061/dsq.v33i2.3705

Solly, M. (2018, December 3). U.S. life expectancy drops for third year in a row, reflecting rising drug overdoses, suicides. Retrieved February 6, 2020, from *Smithsonian Magazine*: https://www.smithsonianmag.com/smart-news/us-life-expectancy-drops-third-year-row-reflecting-rising-drug-overdose-suicide-rates-180970942/

Song, Z., & Baicker, K. (2019). Effect of a workplace wellness program on employee health and economic outcomes: A randomized clinical trial. *JAMA, 321*(15), 1491–1501. doi: 10.1001/jama.2019.3307

Spade, D. (2013). Intersectional resistance and law reform. *Signs, 38*(4), 1031–1055. doi: 10.1086/669574

Strings, S. (2019). *Fearing the Black Body*. New York: NYU Press. Retrieved from https://nyupress.org/9781479886753/fearing-the-black-body

Taylor v. Burlington Northern Railroad Holdings Inc., 904 F. 3d 846 (9th Circuit 2019).

US Equal Employment Opportunity Commission. (2012, July 24). BAE systems subsidiary to pay $55,000 to settle EEOC Disability Discrimination Suit. Retrieved February 13, 2020, from https://www.eeoc.gov/eeoc/newsroom/release/7-24-12c.cfm

Weber, M. C. (2007). *Disability Harassment*. New York: NYU Press.

Yancey, A. K., Leslie, J., & Abel, E. K. (2006). Obesity at the crossroads: Feminist and public health perspectives. *Signs: Journal of Women in Culture and Society, 31*(2), 425–443. doi: 10.1086/491682

38

CHANGING ATTITUDES

A review and critique of weight stigma intervention research

Patricia Cain, Ngaire Donaghue and Graeme Ditchburn

Introduction

As public discourse has increasingly entrenched a view fatness as a major cause of disease burden in western countries, so too has stigmatization of fat people become an endemic feature of cultural, social, and psychic life (Lupton, 2014). One of the main goals of fat acceptance movements is to remove this stigma, and a considerable body of research in social psychology and related fields has developed around creating and testing the efficacy of interventions designed to reduce weight stigma (see Cain, 2019, for a review). In reviewing the extant body of work around weight stigma reduction, we are less interested in the outcomes or effectiveness of particular approaches; instead, we turn a critical lens on the types of interventions carried out and the materials and the messages presented to participants as part of these interventions. Although weight stigma reduction interventions are clearly motivated by a desire to reduce animosity and improve the lives of fat people, we worry that elements of their design may have the paradoxical effect of perpetuating and legitimizing some aspects of the negative stereotypes of fat people. In this chapter, we will review the typical forms of stigma reduction interventions with a critical eye towards the issues that researchers need to consider in designing interventions that embody the values of critical fat scholarship.

Most weight stigma reduction interventions conducted by psychologists employ experimental designs. These studies typically involve an experimental comparison of some form of positive presentation of fat people/fatness (an 'intervention condition') against a normative (negative) presentation (a 'control' condition). By exposing participants to different interventions, researchers gain insight into the efficacy of different approaches to stigma reduction. Many different kinds of materials have been used to form the 'intervention' conditions, but most of these can be broadly classified as either explanation-focused, empathy-enhancing, or stereotype-challenging (see Cain, 2019, for a fuller review and discussion). Explanation-focused interventions involve presenting participants with material that challenges the assumption that a fat body is a straightforward result of personal choices around eating and exercise, focusing instead on explanations for fatness that emphasize genetic, environmental, and/or socioeconomic factors that impact body weight (e.g., Deidrichs & Barlow, 2011; Lippa & Sanderson, 2012). Empathy-enhancing interventions usually involve either providing participants with first-person accounts from fat people of the negative impact of

DOI: 10.4324/9780429344824-46

stigmatizing experiences (e.g., Teachman, Gapinski, Brownell, Rawlins, & Jeyaram, 2003) or involve creating positive encounters between non-fat participants and fat people (e.g., Koball & Carels, 2015). Stereotype-challenging interventions reframe the ways in which fat people are presented in order to disrupt assumptions about fatness. There are three main elements of many stigma reduction interventions that concern us: (1) the reproduction of fatness as a condition requiring explanation; (2) the nature of the 'control' materials used in experimental weight-stigma reduction research; and (3) the anti-fat tone of the measurement tools used to assess whether an intervention has successfully reduced weight stigma. We discuss each of these in turn below.

Our first concern is that many weight-stigma reduction interventions inadvertently reinforce the status of fatness as a bodily condition that needs to be accounted for. This is particularly an issue in explanation-focused interventions, which provide alternatives to the assumption that fatness is a straightforward result of an individual's eating and exercise, nonetheless reinforcing the view that fatness is an abnormal form of embodiment the cause of which needs to be identified and 'blamed'. Even though assigning individual responsibility for fatness is a key part of the logic of weight stigma, and thus an obvious and potentially important target for change, there is a danger that efforts to absolve individual fat people of 'blame' for their bodies nonetheless reinforce a view of fatness as an unfortunate and undesirable condition. As one of the goals of fat acceptance movements is to challenge the abject status of fat bodies and to instead understand fatness as part of the normal variation in body size, interventions that offer alternative explanations for fatness may unwittingly reinforce prejudice against fat bodies.

Our second concern arises from the nature of the materials used in the 'control' conditions of experimental intervention studies. While the 'intervention' materials are often carefully and creatively designed to disrupt normative ideas and representations of fat people, the 'control' materials against which they are assessed tend to reproduce widely accepted negative beliefs about fat people/fatness (e.g., McClure, Puhl, & Heuer, 2011; Smith, Schmoll, Konik, & Oberlander, 2007). In an experimental design, participants are randomly assigned to one of these conditions; those participants in the 'intervention' condition received positive, stereotype challenging material, but others in the 'control' condition may have negative stereotypes reinforced. Although the material presented in these control conditions is generally no worse than participants would be exposed to in everyday life, the fact that it is presented in a research context, often under the imprimatur of a prestigious institution, may lend an authority to these messages that is contrary to the goals of weight-stigma reduction.

Our final concern involves the methods by which the effectiveness of interventions is assessed. Typically, participants complete one of the widely used anti-fat attitudes scales, for example, the Antifat Attitudes Questionnaire (Crandall, 1994) or the Antifat Attitudes Scale (Morrison & O'Connor, 1999), in which participants are asked to rate the extent of their (dis)agreement with a series of mostly negative and derogatory statements about fat people. It seems to us that presenting participants with statements based in negative, often offensive, stereotypes of fat people in order to measure whether the stigma reduction intervention has led to more positive attitudes towards fat people, is far from ideal. (For fuller discussion of these issues, and the development of a new, fat-positive measure of attitudes towards fat people, see Cain, Donaghue, & Ditchburn, 2021).

In the following section, we explore how the issues we identify above play out in examples of weight-stigma research published since the 1990s. We draw on studies identified in four reviews of weight-stigma research (Alberga et al., 2016; Danielsdottir, O'Brien, &

Ciao, 2010; Lee, Ata, & Brannick, 2014; Puhl & Heuer, 2009) as well as additional research published between 2013 and 2017. In this review, we focus on the most commonly employed strategies in research, using materials that attempt to change beliefs on attributions (causes of fatness), elicit empathy towards fat people, reframe negative fat stereotypes, and manipulate contact with fat people.

Explanation-focused intervention: changing attributions for fatness

Attribution theory suggests that events lead people to seek an explanation or a cause (Weiner, 1986). In doing this, people attribute a reason for an outcome they perceive. In the case of fatness, fat people are typically considered responsible for their weight. As such, interventions based on attribution theory will provide participants with information that suggest different attributions for fatness, explanations that, in particular, challenge the assumptions of personal controllability (e.g., Crandall, 1994; Deidrichs & Barlow, 2011).

If viewing body weight as within the individual's control is associated with negative attitudes towards fat people (Crandall & Resser, 2005), it then follows that shifting such beliefs should result in less negative attitudes. By far, the most common intervention method in stigma-reduction research attempts such a shift. This approach typically provides participants with information that suggest that weight is the result of complex factors, in the expectation that this will reduce person-centred attributions. In this exploratory research, information on individual attribution is often set against another explanation. For example, Lewis, Cash, Jacobi, & Bubb-Lewis (1995) presented information on behavioural control (individual attribution) to one group of participants and information on biogenic control to another group, while Lippa and Sanderson (2012) presented information on behavioural control, genetic attribution, and environmental attribution to three different groups. Although we appreciate the need to demonstrate how material focused on personal behaviours leads to more negative appraisals of fat people, in comparison to factors positioned as outside of personal control, the concern we have with these methods is that they perpetuate stigma by presenting material (to some participants) that maintains the notion of individual responsibility.

As negative attitudes towards fat people have been identified among primary health care providers (Foster et al., 2003; Malterud & Ulriksen, 2011; Setchel, Watson, Jones, Gard, & Briffa, 2014; Teachman & Brownell, 2001; Tomiyama, et al., 2015) including providers specializing in "obesity" (Schwartz, Chambliss, Brownell, Blair, & Billington, 2003), stigma-reduction research is frequently conducted with public health and health professional students. One study with health professional and public health students compared the impact of depicting controllable attributions (diet/exercise) against uncontrollable (genes/environment) attributions (O'Brien, Puhl, Latner, Mir, & Hunter, 2010). Diedrichs and Barlow (2011) used a similar design with undergraduate psychology students, where some students received a lecture on weight bias and the multiple determinants of weight, and others a lecture on the behavioural determinants of weight. These studies by O'Brien et al. (2010) and Diedrichs and Barlow (2011), although framed as research designed to reduce stigma, have nonetheless included normative messages of individual attribution as points for comparison. What is particularly concerning about these studies is that they have taken place in an educational setting. While we appreciate that the use of control and experimental groups are necessary for comparison, our concern is that students may only receive one perspective. The studies by Diedrichs and Barlow (2011) and O'Brien et al. (2010) do not provide details on debriefing protocols or materials, indicating that some students may have received information of a normative nature only.

Some interventions move away from comparing normative and critical attribution and instead present participants with a range of alternate explanations. Participants may be presented materials providing, genetic (Teachman et al., 2003), biomedical (Lewis et al., 1995), psychological (Kahn, Tarrant, Weston, Shah, & Farrow, 2018), and environmental attributions (Lippa & Sanderson, 2012; O'Brien et al., 2010). While omitting the message of individual responsibility, these materials still perpetuate the idea of cause and consequence. Although depicted as outside individual control, messages suggesting genetic or biomedical attribution maintain the notion of fatness as a 'problem', and one that requires explanation. To divert from this narrative, Donaghue (2014) includes an alternative message. Together with messages of individual responsibility and 'obesogenic' environment is a third message detailing how the harm of the 'obesity' epidemic has been overstated. Also, an important feature of this study is that, during the debriefing phase, participants were given all three messages. With this design, debriefing becomes a beneficial extension to the intervention, as the contested nature of claims about fatness/fat people is presented to all participants.

Countering stereotypes of fat people: reframing fatness

Another commonly employed stigma reduction strategy entails manipulating the way fat people are framed. The way that an event or person is 'framed' has implications for how it is/ they are perceived and acted upon (Goffman, 1974). The framing of a social phenomenon has an impact not only on public response but also the solutions considered appropriate (Entman, 1993). Fatness has typically been framed in terms of personal responsibility and negative outcomes for both self and society (Gearhart, Craig, & Steed, 2012; Lawrence, 2004; Saguy & Almeling, 2008). Reframing interventions seek to challenge negative stereotypes and frame fatness and the fat person in a more positive light. Reframing may be achieved through the selection, emphasis, or omission of particular representations (Entman, 1993). Framing differs from attribution focused interventions, in that reframing does not necessarily need to reattribute cause, although it often does.

Reframing interventions are popular with exploratory studies, where the strategy is to compare the impact of competing frames (e.g., Carels et al., 2013). This is achieved in various ways, often with images, although sometimes with text. For example, Frederick, Saguy, Sandhu, and Mann (2016) constructed news articles framing fatness as either (a) unhealthy, controllable, and acceptable to stigmatize or (b) healthy, uncontrollable, and unacceptable to stigmatize. Similarly, Smith et al. (2007) presented participants with a personal advertisement in which a female used either a negative, positive, or an objective descriptor of her large-sized body. Images are used in similar ways, with stereotypical or unflattering photographic images of fat people presented to one group of participants, while non-stereotypical or positive images are presented to another (McClure et al., 2011; Pearl, Puhl, & Brownell, 2012). Once again, information relating to debriefing practices is limited for these studies, so it is unclear if participants engaging with negative frames are later debriefed or presented with the alternate positive or critical content.

Perceptions can also be reframed by presenting critical messages, that is, messages that disrupt negative stereotypes and normative weight-centric ideas of fatness. Health professional and medical students have participated in online education modules that promote size acceptance (Hague & White, 2005) and viewed educational videos on the prevalence and consequence of weight-based prejudice in health care (Poustichi, Saks, Piasecki, Hahn, & Ferrante, 2013; Swift et al., 2013). The material used by Hague and White (2005) focused on a non-diet approach to health and was particularly comprehensive including coverage of controversy around the aetiology of obesity; the physical, psychological, and social effects of weight stigma; risks associated with weight loss efforts; and promoting bias-free behaviour in the classroom. Prior to use, the module was reviewed by experts in nutrition and obesity as well as size acceptance. In contrast to the research presented so far, these studies take a pre-test/post-test design to assess attitude change, so there is no need for a comparison group to be presented negative messages or images. However, the effectiveness of the intervention was assessed using the Antifat Attitudes Test (Lewis et al., 1995) – a scale that presents participants with a list of negative statements about fat people and fatness – meaning that the intervention, despite its many exemplary aspects, did still involve some reproduction of negative social attitudes around fatness.

Research promoting critical frames of fatness has also been conducted with practicing health professionals. Such studies tend to take the form of professional development – often in the form of online modules. Falker and Sledge (2011) conducted a self-learning Bariatric Sensitivity Program with health care professionals. The program sought to "improve knowledge and understanding of obesity" (p. 74) as a means of promoting patient sensitivity and decreasing stigma. The program included information on the multiple causes of obesity, discriminatory actions, and improper/inappropriate responses by health care professionals. The day-long workshop, designed for health promoters, was over a year in the making and included input from an interdisciplinary team. Measures were completed prior to the module, with a follow-up one month after. Another positive feature of this study is that rather than use an anti-fat attitude measure, the study used a purpose-built measure to assess knowledge and sensitivity towards patients.

Last, the manipulation of intergroup contact has also been adopted as a strategy for challenging stereotypes of fat people. Intergroup contact has previously been shown to reduce negative bias with groups defined by race, ethnicity, sexual orientation, physical and mental disability, and age (Pettigrew & Tropp, 2006). Manipulating contact with fat people to improve attitudes seems an unlikely strategy at first glance; given that the majority of many western populations are considered 'overweight' or 'obese' (World Health Organization, 2014), contact with fat people is something that most 'normal' weight people would experience in their everyday lives. However, an important factor in contact theory is that an interaction has particular positive qualities that may not be present in 'naturally occurring' contact. As Allport (1954) advised, for contact to reduce negative bias, interaction should include engagement that fosters positive experiences; perceived equality of status; common goals; cooperation; and social support. Intergroup contact uses fat people as the stimuli materials and limits research participants to those who are themselves not fat.

Weight stigma-reduction research based on contact theory is limited. Koball and Carels (2015) exposed self-reported 'normal' weight participants to one of the three different research conditions: engaging in direct contact with an 'obese' confederate; engaging in imagined contact based on a photograph of an 'obese' confederate; or engaging in vicarious contact through watching a video of 'obese' and 'normal' weight confederates interacting positively. Kushner, Zeiss, Feinglass, and Yelen (2014) had medical students engaged in a communication skills unit with standardized patients (already selected and trained to work with students) who identified as 'overweight' or had a family member who struggled with 'obesity'. Student self-reported weight was not reported or controlled for in this study.

Research in medical settings has also employed a contact research strategy using both real and virtual patients. Persky and Eccleston (2011) created a virtual female patient with standardized patient history and behaviours, except for weight and then had medical students interact with either the normal weight or 'obese' patient through virtual technology.

Roberts et al. (2011) paired medical students with patients undergoing evaluation for bariatric surgery for one year. Patients volunteer to work with students, although it is not made clear if the patients were fully aware of the nature of the study. The research method covered multiple components, including having the student keep a self-reflection journal regarding their beliefs and stereotypes relating to 'obesity'. While the research of Persky and Eccleston (2011) and Roberts et al. (2011) deviates from typical contact research methods, contact is none the less facilitated. However, the patient/practitioner dynamic of this research protocol could be considered to reflect a lack of equality of status, a feature important for contact to be effective as a change strategy (Allport, 1954).

With contact research, it is important to consider the extent to which the subject is 'othered'. In any research assessing the attitudes of one group towards another, the target group is by default set apart as the 'other'. With contact research, this is more evident than other strategies as the intention is deliberate and explicit. The research discussed here has indicated that people have participated voluntarily, although the participants' level of knowledge about the research is neither fully disclosed nor are participant debriefing practices detailed.

Evoking empathy

Evoking empathy is a strategy that has historically resulted in improved attitudes towards other stigmatized groups, such as racial and ethnic minorities, people who are homeless, or people with HIV/AIDS (Batson et al., 1997). To generate empathic responses, participants need to have an emotional reaction towards the target, individual, or group (Batson, Chang, Orr, & Rowland, 2002). Such a response may come from a state of emotional matching or concern, feeling *for* the other person, or it may arise from a cognitive response, imagining how the other person feels or how one would feel in another's situation (Batson & Ahmad, 2009). Materials documenting the experience of being stigmatized may be employed to evoke empathy, although workshops and simulation exercises have also been used (Batson & Ahmad, 2009).

Research designed to evoke empathy has participants engage with a range of materials or experiences. Swift et al. (2013) and Burmeister et al. (2017) have used video content as a stimulus. Swift et al. (2013) used two videos developed by the Rudd Centre for Food Policy and Obesity, *Weight Prejudice: Myths and Facts* and *Weight Bias in Healthcare*, while Burmeister et al. (2017) presented a segment from the HBO documentary *The Weight of the Nation*. Gapinski, Schwartz, and Brownell (2006) also presented videos, this time constructed from media clips that show fat people giving first-person accounts of the difficulties of being overweight and their experience of cruel treatment. Gloor and Puhl (2016) followed a similar approach showing participants a written account of a man's struggle to lose weight despite concerted effort, while Teachman et al. (2003) presented participants the story of a young woman, who was sent to a 'fat camp' and died after being verbally abused and forced to exercise in hot conditions. This use of first-person narratives in research is particularly noteworthy and commendable. Research by Puhl, Himmelstein, Gorin, and Suh (2017) sought advice on stigma reduction protocols from fat people, and one of the recommendations from participants was to increase public understanding of the difficulties fat people face every day.

Unlike the well-considered research discussed above, one study designed to evoke empathy by Cotugna and Mallick (2010) was particularly concerning to us. In this study, 40 dietetics and health promotion students followed a calorie-restricted diet for one week. For women, calories were restricted to 1,200 and for men 1,500. Attitudes towards fat people were measured before and after the intervention. Participants also completed journal entries, reflecting on the restricted diet and answering questions, including "How did you deal with the level of hunger?" and "What was the most difficult level of compliance?"(p. 322). Using calorie restriction and hunger as a research strategy is concerning because of the potential negative impact such protocols may have on participants. Using this type of intervention to evoke empathy also suggests that fat people are only deserving of empathic response because weight loss is difficult, a premise that assumes that fat people are ubiquitously trying to lose weight.

Going forward: stigma reduction without stereotype reproduction?

In reviewing this body of work, it is apparent that there is some interesting and thoughtful research being conducted. However, we believe that there is still some way to go for this research to better reflect the values of critical obesity scholarship. As mentioned, our interest in intervention research is not only on the strategies for change but also on the types of materials that research participants engage with. We are interested in what they read, what are they are shown, what they are asked, and what they do. What does this research look like from the participants' side, and what kinds of assumptions about fat people are being reproduced in the fine detail of its procedures?

Researchers attempting to reduce negative evaluations of fat people need to consider the possibility that their studies' control conditions and attitude assessment measures may inadvertently be cementing the very attitudes they are attempting to shift. Having some research participants engage with material that presents positive representation (intervention condition) and some negative representations (control condition) of fat people allows a comparison of response patterns – however, at what cost? Messages of control and responsibility are already pervasive (LeBesco, 2011; Lupton, 2014), and the body of research to date has established their relationship with negative judgements of fat people. We suggest that it is now time to focus on research designs that either avoid such material or include debriefing practices intended to mitigate their negative effect. Debriefing after the active phase of an experiment is concluded allows researchers to fully explain the weight-stigma reduction purpose of the research (including the role of any negative/stereotypical content about fat people). In this way, participation in the study constitutes a 'teachable moment' for all participants, not just for those in the intervention condition, and lends the authority and legitimacy of the research institution to the cause of stigma reduction.

Similarly, it is important to consider how the measurement tools used to assess the effectiveness of the intervention sit with the overall weight-stigma reduction agenda of the research. As discussed earlier, most anti-fat attitude measures comprise a series of statements about fat people/fatness with which participants are asked to rate their (dis)agreement. These statements overwhelmingly reproduce negative social attitudes and stereotypical beliefs about the psychological characteristics and personal habits of fat people (Cain, Donaghue & Ditchburn, 2021). In order to provide an alternative set of tools for assessing changes in attitudes towards fat people, we have developed an alternative, fat-positive set of measures in the Fat Attitudes Assessment Toolkit (Cain, 2019). Our aim in developing these measures was to provide researchers working within a critical fat studies/fat positive frame with quantitative tools that can be used to assess the efficacy of stigma reduction efforts without inadvertently reproducing the negative attitudes towards fat people that we are working to change.

It is perhaps also now time to reconsider the appropriateness of attribution-focused research. While we do not argue with the link between personal responsibility and negative attribution, we suggest that it may be time to consider whether shifting this belief is a necessary precursor to more positive evaluations. The continued focus on encouraging participants to consider "what makes people fat?" whether perceived as within or outside of individual control maintains the focus on fatness as a 'condition' that needs explaining. We suggest that moving away from this narrative and instead focusing on interventions promoting critical messages presents more avenues for exploration. Messages that disrupt normative notions of fatness are now beginning to permeate public discourse with people communicating concern over the harms of fat shaming and embracing social movements promoting size acceptance (Cain, Donaghue, & Ditchburn, 2017). We suggest that researchers now focus more on how and where emerging critical discourse has the ability to shift negative evaluations and beliefs about fatness and fat people. Rather than comparing normative and critical messages, comparisons of different critical messages such as Health at Every Size and Fat Acceptance may produce more valuable insights and outcomes when it comes to weight stigma reduction.

We acknowledge that not all weight stigma-reduction research has the same objective. While many seek to reduce stigma because of the discrimination and oppression experienced by fat people, there is a body of work focused on what has been labelled the ironic or paradoxical results of stigma (Major, Hunger, Bunyan, & Miller, 2014; Nolan & Eshleman, 2016). Some research focuses on responses to stigma that include exercise avoidance (Vartanian & Novak, 2011), increased calorie consumption (Schvey, Puhl, & Brownell, 2011), binge-eating behaviour (Ashmore, Friedman, Reichmann, & Musante, 2008), and reduced self-control around food (Major et al., 2014). We mention this to highlight the complex research landscape. If weight-stigma research can incorporate what appears to be a weight-centric agenda, then we can see how stigma reduction research has at times incorporated normative messages and reflected stigmatizing material. We suggest that it is now time to turn a more critical lens to the way stigma-reduction research is conducted. Research attempting to reduce weight stigma is not a disembodied practice, the knowledge gained informs stigma-reduction programs and policies, ultimately impacting the lived experience of fat people. That fat people do not enjoy the protective status or the power of a majority group or many minority groups is all the more reason to promote the positive representation of fat people in research.

References

Alberga, A. S., Pickering, B. J., Hayden, K. A., Ball, G. C. B., Edwards, A., Jelinski, S., ...Russell-Mayhew, S. (2016). Weight bias reduction in health professionals: A systematic review. *Clinical Obesity, 6*(3), 175–188. doi:10.1111/cob.12147

Allport, G. (1954). *The nature of prejudice.* Reading, MA: Addison Wesley.

Ashmore, J. A., Friedman, K. E., Reichmann, S. K., & Musante, G. J. (2008). Weight-based stigmatization, psychological distress, & binge eating behavior among obese treatment-seeking adults. *Eating Behaviors, 9*(2), 203–209. doi:10.1016/j.eatbeh.2007.09.006

Batson, C. D., & Ahmad, N. Y. (2009). Using empathy to improve intergroup attitudes and relation. *Social Issues and Policy Review, 3*(1), 141–177. doi:10.1111/j.1751-2409.2009.01013x

Batson, C. D., Chang, J., Orr, R., & Rowland, J. (2002). Empathy, attitudes, and action: Can feeling for a member of a stigmatized group motivate one to help the group? *Personality and Social Psychology Bulletin, 28*(12), 1656–1666. doi:10.1177/04616702237647

Batson, C. D., Polycarpou, M. P., Harmon-Jones, E., Imhoff, H. J., Mitchener, E. C., Bednar, L., L., Klein, T. R., & Highberger, L. (1997). Empathy and attitudes: Can feeling for a member of a stigmatized group improve feelings toward the group? *Journal of Personality and Social Psychology, 72*(1), 105–118. doi:10.1037/0022-3514.72.1.105

Burmeister, J. M., Taylor, M. B., Rosi, J., Kiefner-Burmeister, A., Borushok, J., & Carels, R. A. (2017). Reducing obesity stigma via a brief documentary film: A randomized trial. *Stigma and Health, 2*(1), 43–52. doi:10.1037/sah0000040

Cain, P. (2019). *Quantifying elements of contemporary fat discourse: The development and validation of the Fat Attitudes Assessment Toolkit.* (Doctoral dissertation, Murdoch University, Perth, Australia). Retrieved from https://researchrepository.murdoch.edu.au/id/eprint/52182/

Cain, P., Donaghue, N., & Ditchburn, G. (2021). Quantifying or contributing to antifat attitudes? In C. Pausé & S. R. Taylor (Eds.). *The Routledge International Handbook of Fat Studies*, pp. 26–36. Abingdon: Routledge.

Cain, P., Donaghue, N., & Ditchburn, G. (2017). Concerns, culprits, counsel, and conflict: A thematic analysis of 'obesity' and fat discourse in digital news media. *Fat Studies, 6*(2), 170–188. doi:10.1080/21604851.2017.1244418

Carels, R., Hinman, N. G., Burmeister, J. M., Hoffman D. A., Ashrafioun, L., & Koball, A. M. (2013). Stereotypical images and implicit weight bias in overweight/obese people. *Journal of Eating and Weight Disorders, 18*(4), 441–445. doi:10.1007/s40519-013-00725

Cotugna, N., & Mallick, A. (2010). Following a calorie-restricted diet may help in reducing healthcare students' fat-phobia. *Journal of Community Health, 35*(3), 321–324. doi:10.1007/s10900-010-9226-9

Crandall, C. S. (1994). Prejudice against fat people: Ideology and self-interest. *Journal of Personality and Social Psychology, 66*(5), 882–894. doi:10.1037/0022-3514.66.5.882

Crandall, C. S., & Resser A. H. (2005). Attributions and weight based prejudice. In K. D. Brownell, R. M. Puhl, M. B. Schwartz, & L. Rudd, (Eds.). *Weight bias: Nature consequences and remedies* (pp. 83–96). New York: Guilford Press.

Danielsdottir, S., O'Brien, K. S., & Ciao, A. (2010). Anti-fat prejudice reduction: A review of published studies. *Obesity Facts, 3*(1), 47–58. doi:10.1159/000277067

Diedrichs, P. C., & Barlow, F. K. (2011). How to lose weight bias fast! Evaluating a brief anti-weight bias intervention. *British Journal of Health Psychology, 16*(4), 846–861. doi:10.1111/j.2044-8287.2011.02022.x

Donaghue, N. (2014). The moderating effect of socioeconomic status on relationships between obesity framing and stigmatisation of fat people. *Fat Studies, 3*(1), 6–16. doi:10.1080/21604851.2013.763716

Entman, R. M. (1993). Framing: Toward clarification of a fractured paradigm. *Journal of Communication, 43*(4), 51–58. doi:10.1111/j.1460-2466.1993.tb01304x

Falker, A. J., & Sledge, J. A. (2011). Utilizing a bariatric sensitivity educational module to decrease bariatric stigmatization by healthcare professionals. *Bariatric Nursing and Surgical Patient Care, 6*(2), 73–78. doi:10.1089/bar.2011.9974

Foster, G. D., Wadden, T. A., Makris, A. P., Davidson, D., Sanderson, R. S., Allison, D. B. (2003). Primary care physicians' attitudes about obesity and its treatment. *Obesity Research, 11*(10), 1168–1177. doi:10.1038/oby.2003.161

Frederick, D. A., Saguy, A. C., Sandhu, G., & Mann, T. (2016). Effects of competing news media frames of weight on antifat stigma, beliefs about weight and support for obesity-related public policies. *International Journal of Obesity, 40*(3), 543–549. doi:10.1038/ijo.2015.195

Gapinski, K. D., Schwartz, M. B., & Brownell, K. D. (2006). Can television change anti-fat attitudes and behaviour? *Journal of Applied Biobehavioral Research, 11*(1), 1–28. doi:10.1111/j.1751-9861.2006.tb00017.x

Gearhart, S., Craig, C., & Steed, C. (2012). Network news coverage of obesity in two time periods: An analysis of issues, sources and frames. *Health Communication, 27*(7), 653–662. doi:10.1080/10410236.2011.629406

Gloor, J. L., & Puhl, R. M. (2016). Empathy and perspective-taking: Examination and comparison of strategies to reduce weight stigma. *Stigma and Health, 1*(4), 269–279. doi:10.1037/sah0000030

Goffman, E. (1974). *Frame Analysis.* New York: Free Press.

Hague, A. L., & White, A. A. (2005). Web based intervention for changing attitudes of obesity among current and future teachers. *Journal of Nutrition Education and Behavior, 37*(2), 58–66. doi:10.1016/S1499-4046(06)60017-1

Kahn, S. S., Tarrant, M., Weston, D., Shah, P., & Farrow, C. (2018). Can raising awareness about the psychological causes of obesity reduce obesity stigma? *Health Communication, 33*(5), 585–592. doi:10.1080/10410236.2017.1283566

Koball, A. M., & Carels, R. A. (2015). Intergroup contact and weight bias reduction. *Translational Issues in Psychological Science, 1*(3), 289–306. doi:10.1037/tps0000032

Kushner, R. F., Zeiss, D. M., Feinglass, J. M., & Yelen, M. (2014). An obesity educational intervention for medical students addressing weight bias and communication skills using standardized patients. *Medical Education, 14*(1), 53–61. doi:10.1186/1472-6929-14-53

Lawrence, R. G. (2004). Framing obesity: The evolution of news discourse on a public health issue. *Press and Politics, 9*(3), 56–75. doi:10.1177/1081180X04266581

LeBesco, K. (2011). Neoliberalism, public health, and the moral perils of fatness. *Critical Public Health, 21*(2), 153–164. doi:10.1080/09581596.2010.529422

Lee, M., Ata, R. N., & Brannick, M. T. (2014). Malleability of weight-biased attitudes and beliefs: A meta-analysis of weight bias reduction interventions. *Body Image, 11*(3), 251–259. doi: 10.1016/j.bodyim.2014.03.003

Lewis, R. J., Cash, T. F., Jacobi, L., & Bubb-Lewis, C. (1995). Prejudice toward fat people: The development and validation of the Antifat Attitudes Test. *Obesity Research, 5*(4), 297–307.

Lippa, N. C., & Sanderson, S. C. (2012). Impact of information about obesity genomics on the stigmatization of overweight individuals: An experimental study. *Obesity, 20*(12), 2367–2376. doi:10.1038/oby.2012.144

Lupton, D. (2014). "How do you measure up?" Assumptions about "obesity" and health-related behaviors and beliefs in two Australian "obesity" prevention campaigns. *Fat Studies, 3*(1), 32–44. doi:10.1080/21604851.2013.784050

Major, B., Hunger, J. M., Bunyan, D. P., & Miller, C. T. (2014). The ironic effects of weight stigma. *Journal of Experimental Social Psychology, 51*, 74–80. doi:10.1016/j.jesp.2013.11.009

Malterud, K., & Ulriksen, K. (2011). Obesity, stigma, and responsibility in health care: A synthesis of qualitative studies. *International Journal of Qualitative Study Health and Well-being, 6*(4), 8404–8414. doi:10,3402/qhw.v6i4.8404

McClure, K. J., Puhl, R. M., & Heuer, C. A. (2011). Obesity in the news: Do photographic images of obese persons influence antifat attitudes? *Journal of Health Communication, 16*(4), 359–371. doi:10/1080/10810730.2010.535108

Morrison, T., & O'Connor W.E. (1999). Psychometric properties of a scale measuring negative attitudes toward overweight individuals. *The Journal of Psychology, 139*, 436–445. doi:10.1080/00224549909840

Nolan, L. J., & Eshleman, A. (2016). Paved with good intentions: Paradoxical eating responses to weight stigma. *Appetite, 102*, 15–24. doi:10.1016/j.appet.2016.01.027

O'Brien, K.S., Puhl, R. M., Latner, J. D., Mir, A. S., & Hunter, J. A. (2010). Reducing anti-fat prejudice in preservice health students: A randomized control trial. *Obesity, 18*(11), 2138–2144. doi:10.1038/oby.2010.79

Pearl, R. L., Puhl, R. M., & Brownell, K. D. (2012). Positive media portrayals of Obese persons: Impact on attitudes and image preferences. *Health Psychology, 31*(6), 821–829. doi:10.1037/a0027189

Persky, S., & Eccleston, C. P. (2011). Medical student bias and care recommendations for an obese versus non-obese virtual patient. *International Journal of Obesity, 35*(5), 728–735. doi:10.1038/ijo.2010.173

Pettigrew, T. F., & Tropp, L. R. (2006). A meta-analytic test of intergroup contact theory. *Journal of Personality and Social Psychology, 90*(5), 751–783. doi:10.1073/0022-3514.90.5.751

Poustichi, Y., Saks, N. S., Piasecki, A. K., Hahn, K. A., & Ferrante, J. M. (2013). Brief intervention effective in reducing weight bias in medical students. *Family Medicine, 45*(5), 345–348. doi:1938-3800

Puhl, R. M., & Heuer, C. A. (2009). The stigma of obesity: A review and Update. *Obesity, 17*(5), 941–964. doi:10.1038/oby.2008.636

Puhl, R. M., Himmelstein, M. S., Gorin, A. A., & Suh, Y. J. (2017). Missing the target: Including perspectives of women with overweight and obesity to inform stigma-reduction strategies. *Obesity Science and Practice, 3*(1), 25–35. doi:10.1002/osp.101

Roberts, D. H., Kane, E. M., Jones D. B., Almeida, B. A., Bell, S. K., Weinstein, A. R., & Schwartzstein, R. M. (2011). Teaching medical students about obesity: A pilot program to address an unmet need through longitudinal relationships with bariatric surgery patients. *Surgical Innovation, 18*(2), 176–183. doi:10.1177/1553350611399298

Saguy, A. C., & Almeling, R. (2008). Fat in the fire? Science, the news media, and the "obesity epidemic". *Sociological Forum, 23*(1), 53–83. doi:10.1111/j.1573-7861.2007.00046x

Setchel, J., Watson, B., Jones, L., Gard, M., & Briffa, K. (2014). Physiotherapists demonstrate weight stigma: A cross-sectional survey of Australian Physiotherapists. *Journal of Physiotherapy, 60*(3), 157–162. doi:10.1016/j.jphys.2014.06.020

Schvey, N. A., Puhl, R. M., & Brownell, K. D. (2011). The impact of weight stigma on caloric consumption. *Obesity, 19*(10), 1957–1962. doi:10.1038/oby.2011.204

Schwartz, M. B., Chambliss, H. O., Brownell, K. D., Blair, S. N., & Billington C. (2003). Weight bias among health professionals specializing in obesity. *Obesity Research, 11*(9), 1033–1039. doi:10.1038/oby.2003.142

Smith, C. A., Schmoll, H., Konik, J., & Oberlander, S. (2007). Carrying weight for the world: Influences of weight descriptors on judgements of large-sized women. *Journal of Applied Social Psychology, 37*(5), 989–1006. doi:10.1111/j.1559-1816.2007.00196.x

Swift, J. A., Tischler, V., Markham, S., Gunning, I., Glazebrook, C., Beer, C., & Puhl, R. M. (2013). Are anti-stigma films a useful strategy for reducing weight bias among trainee healthcare professionals? Results of a pilot randomized control trial. *Obesity Facts, 6*(1), 91–102. doi:10.1159/000348714

Teachman, B. A., & Brownell, K. D. (2001). Implicit anti-fat bias among among health professionals: is anyone immune? *International Journal of Obesity, 25*(10), 1525–1531. doi:10.1038/sj.ijo.0801745

Teachman, B. A., Gapinski, K. D., Brownell, K. D., Rawlins, M., & Jeyaram, S. (2003). Demonstrations of implicit anti-fat bias: The impact of providing causal information and evoking empathy. *Health Psychology, 22*(1), 68–78. doi:10.1037/0278-6133.22.1.68

Tomiyama, A. J., Finch, L. E., Incollingo Belsky, A. C., Buss, J., Finley, C., Schwartz, M. B., & Daubenmier, J. (2015). Weigh bias in 2001 versus 2013: Contradictory attitudes among obesity researchers and health professionals. *Obesity, 23*(1), 46–53. doi:10.1002/oby.20910

Vartanian, L. R., & Novak, S. A. (2011). Internalized societal attitudes moderate the impact of weight stigma on avoidance of exercise. *Obesity, 19*(4), 757–762. doi:10.1038/oby.2010.234

Weiner, B. (1986). *An attributional theory of motivation and emotion.* New York: Springer-Verlag.

World Health Organization. (2014). *Obesity and overweight* (Fact sheet No. 311). Retrieved from http://who.int/mediacentre/factsheets/fs311/en

39

A CRITIQUE OF OBESITY AS A CATEGORY OF MALNUTRITION IN ALL ITS FORMS

Gyorgy Scrinis

Introduction[1]

While the term 'malnutrition' has been synonymous with hunger and undernutrition, it is now commonly understood to take many forms and to relate to the health consequences associated with both undernutrition and so-called 'over-nutrition' and obesity. Malnutrition is sometimes classified into these two forms of undernutrition and over-nutrition/obesity, but is also typically differentiated into three types: undernutrition, micronutrient deficiencies (i.e., 'hidden hunger') and over-nutrition/obesity/over-weight (FAO/WHO, 2018; WHO, 2019a).

The emergence of this tripartite classification of malnutrition—beginning in the 1990s—was an attempt to better capture the changing nature and the new realities of dietary and health patterns over recent decades. The identification of a separate category of micronutrient deficiencies was intended to differentiate those people who may have had 'enough' food in terms of dietary energy, but whose diet quality left them deficient in specific micronutrients. The addition of the 'obesity/over-nutrition' category aimed to broaden the concept of malnutrition from a condition of under-consumption to one of excess nutrient/energy intake in order to capture the rapid rise in rates of obesity and NCDs (WHO, 2000). By the late 1990s, the concepts of the double-burden of malnutrition—and eventually the triple-burden of malnutrition—were also introduced to highlight the co-existence of these forms of malnutrition within countries, communities, families and even within individuals.

While the categories and definitions used by different institutions and experts vary, the World Health Organisation (WHO) classifies malnutrition into three forms: undernutrition (wasting, stunting and underweight); micronutrient-related malnutrition (micronutrient deficiencies or excess); and overweight, obesity and diet-related non-communicable diseases (WHO, 2019a). In this WHO classification, the third 'obesity' category drops any reference to 'over-nutrition', and most experts and institutions have now moved away from using the term 'over-nutrition', although, as will be discussed, the spirit of this term remains.

This framing and classification of malnutrition into three distinct forms will be referred to here as the *tripartite classification* of malnutrition and which forms the basis of the *tripartite paradigm* of malnutrition. I will argue that, within this tripartite paradigm, each of these three categories of malnutrition are defined as being nutritionally and biologically precise and specific categories; as distinct and dualistic categories; as internally uniform and singular

DOI: 10.4324/9780429344824-47

categories; and as de-contextualised and de-socialised categories. The framing of malnutrition in these precise and fragmented terms also inevitably promotes and legitimises nutritionally and biologically precise technological solutions and responses and thereby supports the political and commercial interests that benefit from these types of solutions.

Over the past two decades, a number of these characteristics of the tripartite paradigm have been called into question. For example, some nutrient and biomarker-specific approaches have been criticised, including the energy-focused definition of undernutrition (Herforth 2015); the supplementation and fortification strategies to address micronutrient deficiencies; and the focus on body size and BMI. The recognition and analysis of the double-burden or triple-burden of malnutrition has not only highlighted the co-existence these forms of malnutrition but also the multiple and interconnected biological pathways connecting undernutrition and obesity across the life-course, and the common dietary and socio-economic drivers and common health outcomes (Swinburn et al., 2019; Wells et al., 2020). Many experts and institutions acknowledge that poor quality diets can lead to both nutritional deficiencies and obesity, and that a common dietary solution lies in the provision of nutritious and good quality foods and diets (Farrell, Thow, Abimbola, Faruqui, & Negin, 2017; Hawkes, Ruel, Salm, Sinclair, & Branca, 2019; Pradeilles, Baye, & Holdsworth, 2019). Despite these insights, the classification into two or three distinct forms of malnutrition—and the specific categories themselves—continue to be drawn upon as the default framing of malnutrition, even by the experts and institutions that recognise some of the limitations of the conventional framing.

The aim of this chapter is to identify the characteristics, limitations and consequences of the tripartite paradigm of malnutrition, with a focus on the category of obesity. But I will also question the tripartite classification itself and suggest the need for a re-framing and re-classification of malnutrition in all its forms.

The tripartite classification of malnutrition

Malnutrition in all its forms is typically differentiated into two or three high-level categories: either the binary of undernutrition and over-nutrition/obesity; or the tripartite classification of undernutrition, micronutrient deficiencies and obesity. For example, a recent U.N. Food and Agriculture Organisation (FAO) document differentiated malnutrition in this way: 'The multiple burdens of malnutrition consist of undernutrition, micronutrient deficiencies, and overweight and obesity' (FAO, 2018).

Within the tripartite classification, each of the three forms of malnutrition is attributed with their own specific dietary determinants, nutritional status, health consequences and dietary solutions. Non-dietary biological and environmental factors are also acknowledged (e.g., maternal nutrition status, sanitation, infections and exercise), but these tend not to inform or qualify the primary definitions.

Undernutrition is defined as a nutritional state resulting from an inadequate intake of nutrients, particularly in energy (though also protein and micronutrients), and leading to health conditions such as stunting, wasting, under-weight, kwashiorkor, marasmus and micronutrient-deficiency diseases. The nutritional status of having insufficient energy and protein cannot be directly measured in the body (except for some indicators of protein status). Instead, the nutritional status of undernutrition is usually defined in terms of the anthropometric measures of stunting and wasting, and these are often described as forms of undernutrition in themselves.

Micronutrient deficiencies are defined as a nutritional state of the body being deficient in one or more specific micronutrients for normal bodily growth and functioning and that lead to specific micronutrient-deficiency-related diseases and health conditions. In some cases, these micronutrient deficiencies in the body can be directly measured, but, otherwise, the prevalence of micronutrient deficiencies is represented by the number of people estimated to have a deficiency or that have a deficiency-related disease.

Micronutrient deficiencies are framed as a form of undernutrition, and it is recognised that those classified as undernourished may also be micronutrient-deficient (Gupta et al., 2013). However, in the tripartite classification, people categorised as micronutrient-deficient—and as suffering from 'hidden hunger'—are distinguished from the chronically undernourished on the basis that they are receiving adequate energy but lacking in specific micronutrients. Micronutrient malnutrition is thereby framed as a problem with the quality of the diet rather than quantity with diet quality defined in terms of the micronutrient composition of the diet.

The category of obesity, or over-nutrition/obesity, is more ambiguously defined in terms of both *over-nutrition* (a dietary characteristic) and *obesity* (framed as a physiological consequence of over-nutrition). This broad category is intended to capture the phenomena of over-consumption (especially of meat and processed foods), obesity and NCDs. However, it is obesity—or overweight/obesity—that is the primary signifier and measure of this form of malnutrition, and 'over-nutrition' is usually dropped from the title of this category of malnutrition. The nutritional status of over-nutrition/obesity is defined and measured in terms of body size, based on a BMI greater than 25 or 30.

Even though the term 'over-nutrition' is now commonly silenced in the category of over-nutrition/obesity, the idea of 'over' or 'excess' nutrients and energy intake remains a key aspect of the framing of the dietary drivers of this form of malnutrition (Lean, Astrup, & Roberts, 2018; WHO, 2019b). Poor diet quality is also considered a dietary determinant of obesity and of NCD risk, but in this case, diet quality is primarily defined in terms of the excess intake of nutrients-to-limit (i.e., sodium, sugars, saturated and trans-fats and energy). Processed foods are considered to be important dietary sources of these nutrients-to-limit.

The abstracted ontology of malnutrition

What precisely *is* malnutrition, and what do we mean when we say a person is malnourished or is suffering from malnutrition? What is the nature of this bodily condition—the ontology of malnutrition—and where and when in the body is it located or manifested? In categorising malnutrition into three forms, the tripartite paradigm asserts that these categories exist as distinct nutritional and biological conditions within the bodies of the malnourished. I will argue on the contrary that these reified categories are abstractions, reductions and simplifications of what we know to be the more complex and situated dietary, biological and social realities of malnutrition as will be elaborated in the following sections.

Malnutrition is defined by the FAO as an 'abnormal physiological condition caused by inadequate, unbalanced or excessive consumption of macronutrients and/or micronutrients' (FAO, 2019). Malnutrition occurs after the act of consumption, when the body presumably enters into a state of nutritional imbalance (i.e., deficits or excesses of energy, macronutrients and micronutrients), and which is referred to as the *nutritional status* of the body. The nutritional status of being 'undernourished' or 'micronutrient-deficient' defines the body as in a state of energy or micronutrient deficiency, while the status of 'obesity' points to a state of excess of nutrients/energy in the body. There is a claimed precision in these definitions of malnutrition—that specific forms of malnutrition can be precisely diagnosed and addressed. In practice, however, a person's nutritional status can only be directly measured for some micronutrients and proteins. Instead, anthropometric measures are also included as a measure of nutritional status (including stunting, wasting, underweight, overweight and obesity), thereby stretching the definition of nutritional status. Disease incidence is sometimes also used to measure the prevalence of a form of malnutrition such as anaemia as an indicator of iron deficiency.

Yet, anthropometrically defined conditions, such as stunting and obesity, are arguably better understood as possible health consequences of malnutrition rather than as forms of malnutrition or forms of nutritional status. The category of obesity is particularly difficult to reconcile with the notion of nutritional status. This form of malnutrition is no longer directly referred to as over-nutrition—for what does it mean to be over-nourished? However, the category and measure of 'obesity' make no reference to a type of dietary inadequacy. At the same time, many individuals classified as overweight/obese may be 'metabolically healthy' and consume a very good quality diet, so why are all people with a BMI over 25 or 30 classified as malnourished?

Nutritionally and biologically precise and reductive categories

The tripartite classification and definitions of malnutrition are characterised by a nutritionally and biologically precise understanding of malnutrition, one that attributes the presence or absence of precise nutrient factors with precise and unitary health outcomes. Nutri-biologically precise approaches are evident in the claims that specific nutrients (including energy, micronutrients and nutrients-to-limit) lead to nutrient-specific deficiencies/excesses in the body and then to biologically specific diseases, biomarkers and health outcomes; and that these can be remedied with nutrient-specific dietary interventions. The construction of three distinct forms of malnutrition depends upon these claims to nutri-biological precision. This nutri-biologically precise understanding abstracts from, and tends to conceal or downplay, other dietary and non-dietary factors that contribute to shape and mediate each form of malnutrition and their health consequences.

The nutrient-specific definitions of each of the three forms of malnutrition are consistent with, and draw upon, the nutrient-focused and nutritionally reductive paradigm that has been dominant within nutrition science for much of the past century, which I refer to as the ideology or paradigm of 'nutritionism' (Gyorgy Scrinis, 2013). There are a number of characteristics of nutritionism that are evident in the tripartite paradigm: the decontextualisation and abstraction of nutrients outside of any food, dietary or socio-economic context; the tendency towards single-nutrient reductionism that ignores nutrient, food and dietary-level interactions and synergies; the simplification, exaggeration and deterministic understanding of the role of individual nutrients; and the claimed precision in the scientific understanding of the role of individual nutrients in the body.

The tripartite paradigm also adopts a nutritionally and biologically reductive understanding of the body, such as where the presence or absence of specific nutrients or dietary components in the body is assumed to result in specific biological and health outcomes. It may also take the form of what I call *biomarker reductionism*, the reductive focus on and interpretation of single biological and anthropometric measures to assess and classify health conditions, including 'BMI reductionism' (Gyorgy Scrinis, 2013). Nutritional and medical interventions are then often aimed at addressing and modifying these biomarkers rather than addressing their determining factors (Kraemer & van Zutphen, 2019). In these respects and others, the tripartite paradigm of malnutrition shares a number of characteristics with the dominant biomedical paradigm within the medical sciences (Lock & Nguyen, 2018).

The limitations of this reductive framework for understanding malnutrition are increasingly apparent. There is already considerable evidence to suggest that there are multiple and interconnected dietary and non-dietary factors contributing to nutritional deficiencies or imbalances in the body associated with all three forms of malnutrition, and that each, in turn, contribute to multiple and interconnected health consequences. All of these pathways—from dietary patterns, to malnourished bodies, to health outcomes, to dietary and other solutions—are mediated by a range of biological, environmental and social relations and factors, such as infection, inflammation, overall health status, poor sanitation, socio-economic disadvantage and broader social inequities and power imbalances. There is a need for more integrated and contingent dietary, biological, ecological and social frameworks for understanding these forms of malnutrition as they manifest in specific contexts and individuals. However, the reductive, simplified and siloed categories of the tripartite paradigm do not capture, and tend to work against, such a contextualised understanding of malnutrition.

In the case of obesity, while many experts and organisations have moved away from using the term 'over-nutrition', nevertheless, this category of malnutrition is explained in terms of excess intake of energy or nutrients-to-limit. The focus on excess energy intake to explain weight gain/obesity has been criticised by many experts, in part, because it ignores diet quality and other metabolic processes that mediate fat storage, energy metabolism and drivers of appetite and satiety (Lucan & DiNicolantonio, 2015; Thow et al., 2016; Wells, 2013). Diet quality can affect weight and NCD outcomes independent of energy value.

The more nuanced reference to specific nutrients-to-limit intake as a cause of obesity and NCDs does begin to reference some aspects of food and dietary quality, particularly, the nutrients commonly associated with ultra-processed foods. However, even this focus on excess nutrients-to-limit ignores other aspects of food and dietary quality and their association with NCDs and other health outcomes. It also reduces the health impacts of ultra-processed foods to their high content of nutrients-to-limit, rather than the effects of processing, their lack of nutritious ingredients, and their displacement of minimally-processed foods (Scrinis & Monteiro, 2018).

There is also a tendency within the conventional framing to associate ultra-processed food consumption only with obesity and NCDs, but these foods may also contribute to some types of nutrient deficiencies and deficiency-related diseases (Monteiro, Cannon, Lawrence, da Costa Louzada, & Machado, 2019; Pries et al., 2019). The emphasis on over-nutrition and excess intake doesn't account for how individuals categorised as over-weight/obese, or who contract NCDs, may be *lacking* in nutritious, diverse and good quality foods, and are in this sense undernourished, even if—or precisely because—they may be 'over-consuming' poor quality ultra-processed foods (Golden, 2009; Taren & de Pee, 2017; Webb et al., 2018).

Rapidly rising rates of obesity—or a rapid rise in the weight of individuals—are an indicator of inadequate/unbalanced dietary patterns, and some categories of BMI are more strongly correlated with an increased risk of NCDs. However, the reductive interpretation of BMI (i.e. BMI reductionism) as a single indicator of health status ignores great variation amongst those with the same level of BMI. The use of BMI as the marker of this form of malnutrition thereby obscures other dietary and biological pathways and determinants of NCDs. Whether and how obesity impacts on other health outcomes is also dependent on many other social and individual contextual factors (Chiolero, 2018).

Despite the focus on energy balance and nutrients-to-limit, many obesity experts also now frame obesity as a 'complex problem' with multiple and interconnected biological, socioeconomic and environmental drivers and feed-back loops, and requiring multiple, simultaneous and integrated actions to address. In presenting the 'problem' of obesity—and therefore of this category of malnutrition—as enormously complex, also obscures the structures and power relations that create food systems that produce poor quality, ultra-processed products and unbalanced diets, and thereby obscures the policy actions required to address these structures and products (Gálvez, 2018).

Distinct & dualistic categories

Within the tripartite paradigm, each of these three forms of malnutrition—and their specific dietary causes, health consequences and dietary solutions—are defined as being essentially *separate and distinct*, even if some interconnections are recognised. For each form of mal-nutrition, a linear, unidirectional and siloed pathway from dietary factors to health consequences to dietary/medical solutions is posited. Undernutrition is defined as distinct from micronutrient malnutrition and both of these as distinct from obesity. This framing of distinct and largely separate—if not mutually exclusive—categories necessarily follows from the nutrient and biologically specific understanding of the dietary causes of each form of malnutrition.

As already noted, there is much evidence of the multiple and inter-connected dietary determinants of multiple and interconnected health outcomes, and that cut across the dualisms upon which this classification is based. Research into the double/triple burden of malnutrition, in particular, has provided evidence of these criss-crossing and contingent pathways and interconnections between the dietary determinants and health consequences of all forms of malnutrition, including:

- particular dietary factors may contribute to more than one form of malnutrition and health outcome such as the contribution of micronutrient deficiencies to stunting and NCDs;
- individuals may be classified as suffering from more than one form of malnutrition simultaneously such as being both stunted and obese;
- exposure to one form of malnutrition may increase the risk of exposure to another throughout one's life-course, such as the way early undernutrition followed by rapid weight gain predisposes an individual to central adiposity and NCDs later in life (Wells et al., 2019).

Changes in dietary and health patterns in recent decades have increasingly undermined the explanatory power of these dualisms. The rise of ultra-processed food consumption, for example, cuts across simple distinctions between under/over-consumption of nutrients and energy. At the same time, health problems associated with under and over nutrition have also become increasingly blurred as poor diet quality and the inadequate intake of nutritious foods are implicated in all of these health outcomes. The populations and socio-economic groups affected by these forms of malnutrition are also not separate and distinct, and the most disadvantaged groups are more susceptible to all forms of malnutrition.

Internally uniform and singular categories

Within the tripartite paradigm, the three categories of malnutrition are not only characterised as distinct but also as internally homogenous and uniform. People within each category are represented as sharing the same, singular or unitary form of malnutrition or physiological condition, defined in nutrient and biologically specific terms or on the basis of abstracted anthropometric measures, such as BMI. The dietary causes and health consequences for all people within each form of malnutrition are assumed to be essentially the same, as if they are experienced in the same way and can be addressed with much the same dietary or medicalised solutions (Vernon, 2007). Different degrees of severity of each form of malnutrition are acknowledged, such as between acute and chronic malnutrition, or between categories of obesity (e.g., obese and very obese), but these are differences of degree within an otherwise singular form of malnutrition.

However, this framing of internal uniformity doesn't account for the diversity of dietary patterns and health profiles amongst individuals within each category, often underpinned by significantly different socio-economic and life conditions (Carruth & Mendenhall, 2019). At the same time, people classified as having different forms of malnutrition may have more in common with each other than with other individuals within their own category of malnu-trition, such as in terms of the quality of their diets, the types of health challenges they face and other socio-economic stresses.

Within the over-weight/obese category, for example, all individuals with a BMI over 25 or 30 are categorised as having the same, homogenous form of malnutrition, distinguished only by degrees or severity (Green et al., 2016). Yet, this reductive interpretation of BMI can mask the different dietary pathways that can lead to large body size and the very different health consequences that can arise. Some people who reach a BMI of 30 may do so while consuming a diet that is rich in good quality foods, and they may be classified as 'metaboli-cally healthy' (Guo & Garvey, 2016; Roberson et al., 2014). But the dietary patterns, nutri-tional status and risk profile associated with this form of high-BMI is quite different to that which manifests in disadvantaged communities in low and middle-income countries, where obesity and diabetes may co-exist with nutritional deficiencies and extremely inadequate diets (Carruth & Mendenhall, 2019).

Decontextualised and de-socialised categories

Inherent in these nutritionally and biologically reductive, distinct and unitary categories and definitions of malnutrition is an abstracted and decontextualised framework for under-standing malnutrition. These categories and definitions of malnutrition are, by implication, presented as being universally applicable: they are abstracted from particular dietary, health, environmental and social contexts; it is assumed that they will lead to the same biological and health effects regardless of geography or socio-economic differences; and that the nutritional and medicinal solutions can be universally applied.

By contrast, the evidence presented above suggests that the forms that malnutrition takes—their dietary determinants, their health impacts and the effectiveness of interventions—are also shaped by and contingent upon a range of biological, environmental and social determi-nants. While some of the non-dietary factors are acknowledged in malnutrition discourses, they have not been used to qualify the classification and definitions of malnutrition (Haisma, Yousefzadeh, & Boele Van Hensbroek, 2018; MacAuslan, 2009). Social context is important because social determinants—such as socio-economic class, geography and cultural forms—can determine exposure to these dietary, biological and environmental risk factors and de-terminants of malnutrition. These determinants and risk factors tend to cluster in particular social contexts and amongst disadvantaged social and geographical groups. Malnutrition is primarily—in the first instance—a product of broader social inequities and power imbal-ances, which are inscribed in the bodies of the malnourished, and these need to be accounted for to understand the manifestations and responses to malnutrition.

Many anthropologists and sociologists of health and medicine have been examining the deep social shaping of the onset and experience of disease and ill-health in particular contexts—including of hunger, obesity and diabetes—and they have been critical of universalising and decontextualising analyses of these conditions (Adjaye-Gbewonyo & Vaughan, 2019; Tappan, 2017; Yates-Doerr, 2015). This literature not only highlights the multiple social determinants and pathways of disease aetiology but also the multiple ways in which diseases and health conditions are experienced, including the severity of the conditions. What are commonly framed within the biomedical paradigm as singular diseases can in some cases also be understood as taking multiple forms (Carruth & Mendenhall, 2019).

The concept of syndemics, for example, has been developed by medical anthropologists to highlight the synergies between disease epidemics; this includes the clustering and interaction of two or more conditions in a local context via overlapping biological, social and psychological pathways; and an emphasis on the constitutive role of the multiple stresses and the structural violence associated with being poor and socio-economically disadvantaged (Singer, 2009; Mendenhall, 2016). The 2019 Lancet Commission on the *Global Syndemic of Obesity, Undernutrition and Climate Change* drew upon the syndemics concept to highlight the co-existence, the common social and dietary drivers, and the common policy actions required to address undernutrition and obesity (Swinburn et al., 2019). Even though this report placed great emphasis on the social determinants of malnutrition, it nevertheless continued to frame 'undernutrition' and 'obesity' as largely distinct and globally uniform biological conditions that co-exist. While briefly acknowledging some biological overlaps, the report—which was primarily concerned with obesity—didn't explore the deeper synergies between dietary, biological and social factors as they manifest in local contexts and in people's bodies (Mendenhall and Singer, 2019).

The legitimation of technical solutions and political and commercial interests

Approaches to addressing and solving the problem of malnutrition are scientifically and politically contested, with a significant division between approaches that, on the one hand, focus on technical and medicalised responses and solutions, and on the other, those that draw on traditions of social nutrition and that advocate socio-structural responses (GHW, 2011; Harris, 2019; Jaspars, 2019). These two approaches broadly align with 'nutrition-specific' and 'nutrition-sensitive' types of interventions, respectively (Jaspars, 2019).

Many nutrition experts and organisations promote the need for policy responses that address the social, political and commercial determinants of malnutrition, such as the inequities and forms of disadvantage that deny people access to healthy diets. There is also broad support for integrated solutions and 'double-duty actions' to address the multiple forms of malnutrition, such as calls for diverse and nutritious diets, diverse agricultural systems and higher rates of breastfeeding (Constantinides, Blake, Frongillo, Avula, & Thow, 2019; Hawkes et al., 2019).

By contrast, the tripartite framing of malnutrition as a series of discrete nutrient and biologically specific conditions enables governments and industries to claim to be addressing these problems through the design and delivery of nutritionally and biologically specific dietary, pharmaceutical and technological solutions and interventions. These nutrient-specific approaches often take the form of technological fixes and commodified products (Blesh, Hoey, Jones, Friedmann, & Perfecto, 2019). This narrow framing aims to manage populations' nutritional and health status through targeted interventions that address these abstracted nutrient deficiencies and excesses, while enabling these populations to continue consuming inadequate diets. They are thereby a means of adapting malnourished bodies to these dietary and social realities. At the same time, these technological fixes are not intended to address—and instead function to protect and extend—existing socio-economic inequities and power imbalances that produce malnutrition as well as the interests of the governments, corporations and philanthropic organisations that benefit from these types of solutions (Escobar, 2011; Kimura, 2013; Patel, Bezner Kerr, Shumba, & Dakishoni, 2015). This is one of the ideological functions of the tripartite paradigm.

The category of obesity, for example, promotes policies that focus on the reduction of energy and/or nutrients-to-limit, or else to reduce weight/BMI, such as through the regulation of appetite or metabolism. Policies to improve diet quality may be effective if, for example, they are designed to address the production, availability and marketing of ultra-processed foods, or address food environments that promote consumption of these products. However, policies that simply encourage the food industry to reformulate their ultra-processed products by reducing nutrient-to-limit arguably legitimise the continued production, marketing and consumption of these products (Scrinis & Monteiro, 2018).

At the same time, policies that focus on obesity and on reducing BMI may serve to maintain the focus on body size rather than on good dietary and exercise patterns and may promote practices and behaviours that lead to body image problems, eating disorders and fat shaming (Guthman, 2013; Monaghan, Colls, & Evans, 2013). Given the challenges in achieving effective weight loss through means of diet and exercise, solutions focused on surgery and pharmaceuticals are common and are legitimised as a necessary response to this 'epidemic'. Food and pharmaceutical corporations respond to obesity/fat messaging by developing functional foods and pharmaceuticals that claim to address weight-loss and satiety or reduce health risks. The classification of obesity as a disease by leading obesity organisations and experts is also a blessing for pharmaceutical companies, as it promotes the pharmaceutical treatment of obesity, as well as government funding and subsidies for pharmaceutical treatments (Srivastava & Apovian, 2018). By widening the definition of malnutrition to include all those classified as overweight/obese, the market for these products has been correspondingly increased.

Given that this tripartite framing of malnutrition has been used to benefit particular political and commercial interests, the role of specific stakeholders, organisations and corporations in the development and shaping of these scientific frameworks and categories over recent decades—such as the role of philanthropic organisations and aid agencies in promoting a focus on micronutrient deficiencies and of pharmaceutical corporations in medicalising obesity—also warrants further investigation (Kimura, 2013; Oliver, 2006).

Reframing malnutrition

Developing an alternative classification of malnutrition in all its forms requires rethinking the assumptions upon which this classification is based. I have argued that the existing tripartite classification provides neither a plausible nor consistent way of defining and measuring forms of malnutrition. The category of 'obesity' is particularly problematic in this system of classification, and should not be used as the umbrella category or proxy for poor quality diets and NCDs. Increased body size may in part be a consequence of an inadequate and poor-quality diet, and very high levels of body fat may contribute to poor health outcomes such as increased risk of NCDs. But not all people with a high BMI have severely inadequate or unbalanced diets, nor should be considered to be 'malnourished' in this sense. The dietary patterns and state of health of people with a high BMI will vary widely based on other life conditions and contextual factors. Poor quality diets do not necessarily lead to high BMI; and NCDs can be contracted by those with low BMIs.

Beyond acknowledging that malnutrition can take many forms, on what basis can malnutrition be categorised into specific or general forms? Given that multiple forms of inadequate dietary patterns can contribute to the malnourishment of the body, and in turn can lead to multiple types of disease and health outcomes, the premise that there are neat and siloed pathways—from precise dietary inadequacies to precise forms of nutritional status and disease consequences—is outdated.

Forms of malnourishment should be classified in terms of the types of inadequate diets that they are associated with. But there are no obvious alternatives to the classic undernutrition/over-nutrition distinction. While the category of 'undernutrition' clearly references a diet severely lacking in food and nourishment in a *quantitative* sense, it cannot be divorced from diet *quality*. Yet poor diet quality takes many forms. Given that dietary patterns in many countries are increasingly dominated by ultra-processed foods, we could refer to *ultra-processed malnutrition* as one form that malnutrition takes in the contemporary era.

There are multiple diet-related diseases and conditions associated with inadequate diets, and that can be identified based on nutritional biomarkers, anthropometrically defined conditions or disease incidence, such as stunting, diabetes, high-BMI and iron-related anaemia. However, each of these conditions has multiple dietary and non-dietary determinants, and it is therefore difficult to associate them with any one form of malnourishment.

There is also a need to move beyond classifications of malnutrition based on narrow nutritional or biological criteria, particularly given the way these have been exploited by governments, development agencies and corporations to promote narrow, technological and commodified solutions to malnutrition. Categories of malnutrition can instead be defined so that they reveal the structural drivers and forms of power and disadvantage that shape malnourishment. The proposed category of ultra-processed malnutrition, for example, implicates the large corporations that primarily drive the production and consumption of ultra-processed food products, and is in this respect an already socialised category, and not just a technical category of foods.

Notes

1 Some sections of this chapter are part of an article published in 2020. I thank the publisher, Elsevier, for their permissions to reuse material from the article.

References

Adjaye-Gbewonyo, K., & Vaughan, M. (2019). Reframing NCDs? An analysis of current debates. *Global Health Action, 12*(1), 1641043. https://doi.org/10.1080/16549716.2019.1641043

Blesh, J., Hoey, L., Jones, A. D., Friedmann, H., & Perfecto, I. (2019). Development pathways toward "zero hunger". *World Development, 118*, 1–14. https://doi.org/10.1016/j.worlddev.2019.02.004

Carruth, L., & Mendenhall, E. (2019). "Wasting away": Diabetes, food insecurity, and medical insecurity in the Somali Region of Ethiopia. *Social Science & Medicine, 228*, 155–163. https://doi.org/10.1016/j.socscimed.2019.03.026

Chiolero, A. (2018). Why causality, and not prediction, should guide obesity prevention policy. *The Lancet Public Health, 3*(10), e461–e462. https://doi.org/10.1016/S2468-2667(18)30158-0

Constantinides, S., Blake, C., Frongillo, E., Avula, R., & Thow, A.-M. (2019). Double burden of malnutrition: The role of framing in development of political priority in the context of rising diet-related non-communicable diseases in Tamil Nadu, India (P22-005-19). *Current Developments in Nutrition, 3*(Supplement_1), nzz042. https://doi.org/10.1093/cdn/nzz042.P22-005-19

Escobar, A. (2011). *Encountering development: The making and unmaking of the Third World.* Princeton, NJ: Princeton University Press.

FAO. (2018). Strengthening sector policies for better food security and nutrition results. Retrieved: http://www.fao.org/3/a-i7910e.pdf

FAO. (2019). The State of Food Security in the World. Retrieved: http://www.fao.org/state-of-food-security-nutrition

FAO/WHO. (2018). The nutrition challenge: Food system solutions. Retrieved: http://www.fao.org/3/ca2024en/CA2024EN.pdf

Farrell, P., Thow, A. M., Abimbola, S., Faruqui, N., & Negin, J. (2017). How food insecurity could lead to obesity in LMICs: When not enough is too much: a realist review of how food insecurity could lead to obesity in low-and middle-income countries. *Health Promotion International, 33*(5), 812–826. https://doi.org/10.1093/heapro/dax026

Gálvez, A. (2018). *Eating NAFTA: Trade, food policies, and the destruction of Mexico.* Oakland: University of California Press.

GHW. (2011). UNICEF and the 'medicalisation' of malnutrition in children. In Global Health Watch (Ed.), *Global Health Watch 3: An alternative world health report by people's health movement: Health Action International, Medico International and Third World Network.* Zed Books.

Golden, M. H. (2009). Proposed recommended nutrient densities for moderately malnourished children. *Food Nutrition Bulletin, 30*(3 Suppl), S267–342. https://doi.org/10.1177/15648265090303S302

Green, M. A., Strong, M., Razak, F., Subramanian, S. V., Relton, C., & Bissell, P. (2016). Who are the obese? A cluster analysis exploring subgroups of the obese. *Journal of Public Health, 38*(2), 258–264. https://doi.org/10.1093/pubmed/fdv040

Guo, F., & Garvey, W. T. (2016). Cardiometabolic disease risk in metabolically healthy and unhealthy obesity: Stability of metabolic health status in adults. *Obesity, 24*(2), 516–525. https://doi.org/10.1002/oby.21344

Gupta, A., Patnaik, B., Singh, D., Sinha, D., Holla, R., Srivatsan, R.,... Nandi, S. (2013). Are child malnutrition figures for India exaggerated? *Economic and Political Weekly, 48*(34), 73–77.

Guthman, J. (2013). Fatuous measures: The artifactual construction of the obesity epidemic. *Critical Public Health, 23*(3), 263–273. https://doi.org/10.1080/09581596.2013.766670

Haisma, H., Yousefzadeh, S., & Boele Van Hensbroek, P. (2018). Towards a capability approach to child growth: A theoretical framework. *Maternal Child Nutrition, 14*(2), e12534. https://doi.org/10.1111/mcn.12534

Harris, J. (2019). Narratives of nutrition: Alternative explanations for international nutrition practice. *World Nutrition, 10*(4), 99–125.

Hawkes, C., Ruel, M. T., Salm, L., Sinclair, B., & Branca, F. (2019). Double-duty actions: Seizing programme and policy opportunities to address malnutrition in all its forms. *The Lancet.* https://doi.org/10.1016/S0140-6736(19)32506-1

Herforth, A. (2015). Access to adequate nutritious food: new indicators to track progress and inform action. In D. Sahn (Ed.), *The Fight against Hunger and Malnutrition: The role of Food, Agriculture, and Targeted Policies* (pp. 139–164). Oxford: Oxford University Press.

Jaspars, S. (2019). A role for social nutrition in strengthening accountability for mass starvation. World Peace Foundation Occasional Paper No. 20, Fletcher School at Tufts University. Retrieved from https://sites.tufts.edu/wpf/files/2019/09/A-Role-for-Social-Nutrition-Susanne-Jaspers.pdf

Kimura, A. (2013). *Hidden hunger: Gender and the politics of smart foods.* Ithaca, NY: Cornell University Press.

Kraemer, K., & van Zutphen, K. G. (2019). Translational and Implementation Research to Bridge Evidence and Implementation. *Annals of Nutrition and Metabolism, 75*(2), 144–148. https://doi.org/10.1159/000503675

Lean, M. E. J., Astrup, A., & Roberts, S. B. (2018). Making progress on the global crisis of obesity and weight management. *BMJ, 361,* k2538. https://doi.org/10.1136/bmj.k2538

Lock, M., & Nguyen, V.-K. (2018). *An anthropology of biomedicine.* Hoboken NJ: Wiley-Blackwell.

Lucan, S. C., & DiNicolantonio, J. J. (2015). How calorie-focused thinking about obesity and related diseases may mislead and harm public health. An alternative. *Public Health Nutrition, 18*(4), 571–581. https://doi.org/10.1017/S1368980014002559

MacAuslan, I. (2009). Hunger, discourse and the policy process: How do conceptualizations of the problem of 'hunger' affect its measurement and solution? *The European Journal of Development Research, 21*(3), 397–418. https://doi.org/10.1057/ejdr.2009.13

Mendenhall, E. (2016). *Syndemic suffering: Social distress, depression, and diabetes among Mexican immigrant women.* New York: Routledge.

Mendenhall, E., & Singer, M. (2019). The global syndemic of obesity, undernutrition, and climate change. *The Lancet, 393*(10173), 741.

Monaghan, L. F., Colls, R., & Evans, B. (2013). Obesity discourse and fat politics: Research, critique and interventions. *Critical Public Health, 23*(3), 249–262. https://doi.org/10.1080/09581596.2013.814312

Monteiro, C. A., Cannon, G., Lawrence, M., da Costa Louzada, M. L., & Machado, P. P. (2019). *Ultra-processed foods, diet quality and health using the NOVA classification system.* Rome: FAO. Retrieved from: http://www.fao.org/publications/card/en/c/CA5644EN/

Oliver, E. (2006). *Fat politics: The real story behind America's obesity epidemic.* New York: Oxford University Press.

Patel, R., Bezner Kerr, R., Shumba, L., & Dakishoni, L. (2015). Cook, eat, man, woman: Understanding the New Alliance for Food Security and Nutrition, nutritionism and its alternatives from Malawi. *Journal of Peasant Studies, 42*(1), 22–44. https://doi.org/10.1080/03066150.2014.971767

Pradeilles, R., Baye, K., & Holdsworth, M. (2019). Addressing malnutrition in low- and middle-income countries with double-duty actions. *Proceedings of the Nutrition Society, 78*(3), 388–397. https://doi.org/10.1017/S0029665118002616

Pries, A. M., Rehman, A. M., Filteau, S., Sharma, N., Upadhyay, A., & Ferguson, E. L. (2019). Unhealthy snack food and beverage consumption is associated with lower dietary adequacy and length-for-age z-scores among 12–23-month-olds in Kathmandu Valley, Nepal. *The Journal of Nutrition, 149*(10), 1843–1851. https://doi.org/10.1093/jn/nxz140

Roberson, L. L., Aneni, E. C., Maziak, W., Agatston, A., Feldman, T., Rouseff, M., …Sposito, A. (2014). Beyond BMI: The "Metabolically healthy obese" phenotype & its association with clinical/subclinical cardiovascular disease and all-cause mortality—a systematic review. *BMC Public Health, 14*(1), 14. https://doi.org/10.1186/1471-2458-14-14

Scrinis, G. (2013). *Nutritionism: The science and politics of dietary advice.* New York: Columbia University Press.

Scrinis, G., & Monteiro, C. A. (2018). Ultra-processed foods and the limits of product reformulation. *Public Health Nutrition, 21*(1), 247–252. https://doi.org/10.1017/S1368980017001392

Singer, M. (2009). *Introduction to syndemics: A critical systems approach to public and community health.* San Francisco: John Wiley & Sons.

Srivastava, G., & Apovian, C. (2018). Future pharmacotherapy for obesity: New anti-obesity drugs on the horizon. *Current Obesity Reports, 7*(2), 147–161. https://doi.org/10.1007/s13679-018-0300-4

Swinburn, B. A., Kraak, V. I., Allender, S., Atkins, V. J., Baker, P. I., Bogard, J. R., …Dietz, W. H. (2019). The global syndemic of obesity, undernutrition, and climate change: The Lancet Commission report. *The Lancet, 393*(10173), 791–846. https://doi.org/10.1016/S0140-6736(18)32822-8

Tappan, J. (2017). *The riddle of malnutrition: The long arc of biomedical and public health interventions in Uganda.* Athens, GA: Ohio University Press.

Taren, D., & de Pee, S. (2017). The spectrum of malnutrition. In S. de Pee, D. Taren & M. W. Bloem (Eds.), *Nutrition and Health in a Developing World* (pp. 91–117). New York: Springer.

Thow, A. M., Kadiyala, S., Khandelwal, S., Menon, P., Downs, S., & Reddy, K. S. (2016). Toward food policy for the dual burden of malnutrition: An exploratory policy space analysis in India. *Food and Nutrition Bulletin, 37*(3), 261–274. https://doi.org/10.1177/0379572116653863

Vernon, J. (2007). *Hunger: A Modern History.* Cambridge, MA: Harvard University Press.

Webb, P., Stordalen, G. A., Singh, S., Wijesinha-Bettoni, R., Shetty, P., & Lartey, A. (2018). Hunger and malnutrition in the 21st century. *BMJ, 361*, k2238. https://doi.org/10.1136/bmj.k2238

Wells, J. C. (2013). Obesity as malnutrition: The dimensions beyond energy balance. *European Journal of Clinical Nutrition, 67*(5), 507. https://doi.org/10.1038/ejcn.2013.31

Wells, J. C., Briend, A., Boyd, E. M., Berkely, J. A., Hall, A., Isanaka, S., …Dolan, C. (2019). Beyond wasted and stunted—a major shift to fight child undernutrition. *The Lancet Child & Adolescent Health, 3*(11), 831–834. https://doi.org/10.1016/S2352-4642(19)30244-5

Wells, J. C., Sawaya, A. L., Wibaek, R., Mwangome, M., Poullas, M. S., Yajnik, C. S., & Demaio, A. (2020). The double burden of malnutrition: Aetiological pathways and consequences for health. *The Lancet, 395*(10217), 75–88. https://doi.org/10.1016/S0140-6736(19)32472-9

WHO. (2000). Obesity: Preventing and managing the global epidemic. Retrieved from: https://www.who.int/nutrition/publications/obesity/WHO_TRS_894/en/

WHO. (2019a). Malnutrition fact sheet. Retrieved from: www.who.int/en/news-room/fact-sheets/detail/malnutrition

WHO. (2019b). *Obesity and overweight fact sheet.* Geneva: WHO.

Yates-Doerr, E. (2015). *The weight of obesity: Hunger and global health in postwar Guatemala.* Oakland: University of California Press.

INDEX

Note: **Bold** page numbers refer to tables and *Italic* page numbers refer to figures.

For Product Safety Concerns and Information please contact our EU
representative GPSR@taylorandfrancis.com
Taylor & Francis Verlag GmbH, Kaufingerstraße 24, 80331 München, Germany

www.ingramcontent.com/pod-product-compliance
Lightning Source LLC
Chambersburg PA
CBHW081038220326
41598CB00038B/6918